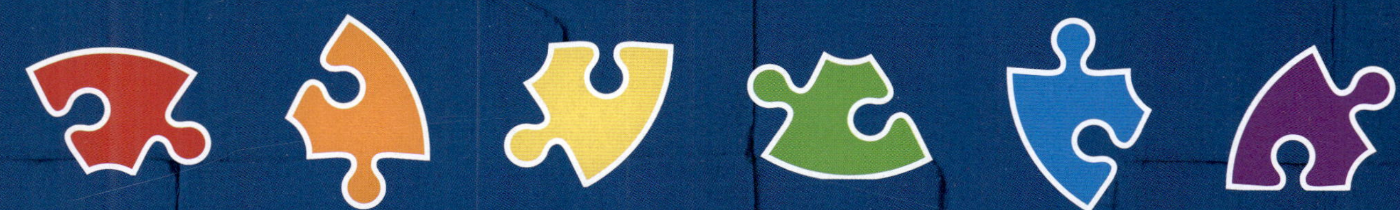

Elsevier's CASE STUDY PRACTICE REVIEW FOR THE NEXT GENERATION NCLEX® (NGN)

Kara Sealock
RN, BN, MEd, EdD, CNCC(C), CCNE
Professor (Teaching)
Faculty of Nursing
University of Calgary
Calgary, Alberta

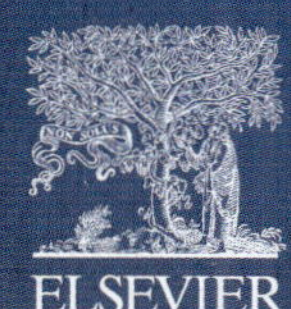

ELSEVIER'S CASE STUDY PRACTICE REVIEW FOR THE NEXT GENERATION NCLEX® (NGN)
ISBN: 978-0-443-12294-1

Executive Editor (Acquisitions, Canada): Roberta A. Spinosa-Millman
Content Development Specialist: Lenore Gray-Spence
Publishing Services Manager: Catherine Jackson
Senior Project Manager: Cindy Thoms
Senior Designer: Amy Buxton

Typeset by GW Tech

Printed in India

Last digit is the print number: 9 8 7 6 5 4 3 2 1

To my daughter Jordyn, my dad, and in memory of my mom. Thank you for your unwavering support, belief in me, and unconditional love.

To nursing students: I am inspired by your dedication, passion, and commitment to our profession. There is always light in moments of darkness, joy in moments of sorrow, and hope in moments of uncertainty. You belong to a profession of strength and resiliency. As an educator, I am inspired by students as you become my teacher, too.

To educators: keep inspiring.

—Kara Sealock

"The mediocre teacher tells. The good teacher explains.
The superior teacher demonstrates. The great teacher inspires."

—William Arthur Ward

Contents

About the Author

Dr. Kara Sealock completed a Bachelor of Nursing in 2000, a Master's of Education in 2012, and a Doctorate of Education, specializing in adult learning, in 2019. Kara has been a nursing educator since 2008 and has worked in various roles, such as a preceptor, in clinical education and theory instruction, focusing on medical–surgical care, critical care, and gerontology. Kara teaches pathophysiology, assessment, pharmacology, and nursing interventions at the University of Calgary. She has considerable years of clinical experience in medical–surgical environments and pharma research experience working with cardiology and endocrinology patients. Most of her career, however, has been positioned in critical care, focusing on nursing care for adult patients in intensive care and coronary care environments. Kara has substantive experience preparing undergraduate nursing students for the NCLEX-RN® and Next Generation NCLEX. She has delivered workshops for students and nursing faculty and facilitated mock examination opportunities, and she assumes an active role in preparing students for success in practice. She co-authored the fifth edition of *Lilley's Pharmacology for Canadian Health Care Practice* and she also serves as an Elsevier Subject Matter Expert for the Next Generation NCLEX® (NGN). Kara has taken on many educational leadership roles locally, provincially, and nationally in nursing education. She recently completed her tenure as vice-chair for the Nursing Education Program Approval Committee at the College of Registered Nurses of Alberta (CRNA). She is the current Chief Editor of the *Canadian Journal of Critical Care Nursing*. Kara's knowledge of adult learning, combined with her clinical and theoretical experience, contributes to an enhanced foundation of understanding, bridging theory and practice for undergraduate nursing education. Kara is a Professor (Teaching) for the Faculty of Nursing at the University of Calgary.

Reviewers

Kim Lauzier, RN, PhD(c)
Department of Nursing
Honours Bachelor of Science — Nursing
Sault College
Sault Ste Marie, Ontario

Kristal Lawson, RN, BN, MN, MScKin, ACCN-ER
School of Health & Community Services
Medicine Hat College
Medicine Hat, Alberta

Laurel MacGray, RN, BSN, MSN
School of Nursing
Thompson Rivers University
Kamloops, British Columbia

Amanda Perkin, RN, BScN, MN
School of Nursing
Saskatchewan Polytechnic
Regina, Saskatchewan

Preface

My Letter to You!

If you are reading this, welcome to the first edition of *Elsevier's Case Study Practice Review for the Next Generation NCLEX® (NGN)!* This textbook is organized to meet your learning needs and provide tips and tricks for success when encountering NGN case studies. I have structured this textbook based on my experience as an educator when teaching undergraduate nursing students pathophysiology, assessment, pharmacology, and nursing interventions. My motivation in preparing this textbook is to help you deepen and strengthen your knowledge when applying the steps necessary for clinical judgement. Preparing for the NCLEX-RN® licensure exam is the last step in your undergraduate nursing chapter and the first step as a registered nurse.

I wish you the best of luck!

Take care,

Kara Sealock

Organization

The content of this book is organized in two main sections. Chapters 1 through 6 introduce NGN concepts to the reader, covering theory and practical approaches to applying current nursing knowledge to solving NGN-style case questions. Two full chapters of NGN-style practice questions follow in Chapters 7 and 8, providing unfolding and stand-alone NGN-style practice case studies organized by body system. Answers with rationales follow in Chapters 9 and 10. Appendix A contains a set of Normal vs. Abnormal vs. Critical Abnormal Condition Tables for use when solving the cases in Chapters 7 and 8. Appendix B (available on Evolve website) provides a list of common laboratory values for use in analyzing case data. Appendix C includes strategies for instructors. Appendix D contains contact information for nursing regulatory bodies in Canada and the United States and Appendix E (available on the Evolve website) provides entry-level competencies and standards.

Practise case studies reflect real-world clinical scenarios that new nursing graduates may encounter in the practice environment. Unfolding and stand-alone case studies are contextually located in medical-surgical units, community settings, emergency departments, labour and delivery, postpartum, internal medicine, mental health, and intensive care units. Many conditions listed in Table 2.7 have corresponding case studies so students can practise applying their knowledge while also identifying gaps in knowledge that require additional study prior to writing the licensure exam.

Unique Features of This Textbook

- Each chapter is intended to build on previously learned information so that students can develop strategies to apply their knowledge when solving nursing problems.
- This textbook incorporates influences of colour psychology and image markers to enhance student engagement and memory retrieval.
- Chapters are designed to address the needs of all learning styles with different *tips and tricks* for transferring knowledge from short-term memory to long-term memory.
- Chapter 2 organizes standard nursing curricula into tangible, easy-to-access information. Several tables are structured for organization, enhanced learning, and memory retention. *Additionally,* a table of medical conditions commonly encountered in nursing practice settings, organized by body systems, can be used to manage various study topics.
- Chapters 3 and 4 break down the clinical judgement model and introduce students to basic elements needed for success.
- Chapter 5 introduces key aspects of unfolding case studies and provides a detailed example of an unfolding case with margin points explaining each part of the case and tips or questions to consider when working through a case.
- Chapter 6 explains the elements of bow-tie and trend cases. A complete case example for each of the two case types is included with important tips and questions to think about in the page margin beside the case example.
- Chapter 7 can be used as a practise exam, for study or additional case-solving practise and features 50 unfolding case studies across medical-surgical, maternal/birth parent health, pediatrics, and mental health topics.
- Chapter 8 contains 50 stand-alone case studies in bow-tie and trend format across medical-surgical, maternal/birth parent health, pediatrics, and mental health topics and can be used for individual case study or as a complete practise exam.
- Chapters 9 and 10 provide complete answers to all cases and include rationales for the correct and incorrect answers so that students can evaluate their answers and identify areas where they need to spend additional time developing their nursing knowledge.
- The student Evolve site contains all 100 cases from the book and an additional 30 case studies for practise in an interactive environment.

All About This Edition

This inaugural edition offers students additional learning opportunities beyond the preparation they received while attending their undergraduate nursing programs. Over the past 13 years, I have developed strategies for making complex concepts regarding pathophysiology, pharmacology, and nursing interventions easier to understand. With the introduction of Next Generation NCLEX®, I altered the delivery of content to incorporate more patterns of presentation so students can recognize even the slightest patient status changes. Using the concept of normal, abnormal, and critical abnormal presentation, students can anticipate and identify the clinical presentation changes during their assessments, ensuring prompt interventions while in practice or choosing the correct answers when practising case studies. Whether students prepare to write their licensure exam or provide care to others, the priority of practice is the delivery of safe and competent care.

Teaching and Learning Features

Putting the Pieces of the Puzzle Together

Each step of the nursing clinical judgement measurement model (NCJMM) is represented throughout the textbook by an individual puzzle piece. Each of the six steps of the NCJMM has a puzzle piece corresponding to the indicated step of the NCJMM. These icons are placed beside the paragraphs discussing that specific step and the rationales throughout the text. Considering the NCJMM as a puzzle in which each piece is essential to complete the full circle wheel will hopefully translate to all steps being considered, even if completing a stand-alone trend case study. The unfolding case studies and the stand-alone bow-tie case studies represent that each narrative is one full-circle moment, requiring each step to be considered to answer the question entirely, while the trend case studies represent a specific moment in time.

Memory Retrieval and Patterns

Additional strategies have been woven throughout the textbook to help users remember the large amount of content needed to be successful on NGN. Each case study represents patterned information that users can identify as part of their knowledge base or an area requiring additional study. For example, the concepts *normal, abnormal,* and *critical abnormal* are used to expect the worst possible acute complication and prepare for the "most normal" or abnormal clinical presentation. Write in your book the patterns of presentation built into each narrative for each condition. These are strategies for memory retrieval. These are three examples of conditions with an existing triad, which help the user remember the requirements for the condition to develop or the most significant clinical manifestations. If any of this information about specific triads is unfamiliar, make note of the areas for growth. Refer back to this table as needed in solving the cases presented in the book.

CONDITION	TRIAD	FACTORS THAT CONTRIBUTE TO DEVELOPMENT OF CONDITIONS OR CLINICAL MANIFESTATIONS
Deep vein thrombosis	Virchow's triad	Venous stasis, hypercoagulability, and endothelial damage
Cardiac tamponade	Beck's triad	Muffled heart sounds, hypotension, and jugular venous distention
Increased intracranial pressure	Cushing's triad	Widened pulse pressure, bradycardia, and irregular respirations

Colour Psychology and Use of Image Markers

The colour schema and image markers were chosen specifically to assist with memory and patterns. There is a direct correlation between attention, colour, and memory. Specific colours increase attention and enhance overall memory (Pi et al., 2021). The colours chosen for the text are vibrant and bright, drawing the reader's attention to the specific image, table, or puzzle piece. There is a colour associated with each step of the NCJMM. Repeated patterns of the same colour ensures there is coding within the brain to associate the colour with the specific step of the NCJMM.

Image markers and visual pictures are meant to break up the written text to both capture the reader's attention and imprint the marker with the intended step of the NCJMM. At the bottom of each page is a legend that repeats consistently throughout the pages. Repeated exposure to the same colour with the same puzzle piece will code within the brain, enhancing working and long-term memory.

Tips for Students

- Use repeating colours to create associations between each step of the NCJMM. When creating study notes, associate these colours with the cognitive level. See the concept map example image in Figure 2.2.
- Add notes to the margins of this textbook when a difficult or easy concept is encountered.
- Underline, highlight, and use this textbook in whatever manner best serves your strength as a learner. If a particular step in the NCJMM is a challenge, note that as well. Recognizing areas for improvement; ensure you address those *before* writing the Next Generation NCLEX-RN® exam.
- Be open to addressing areas of strengths and areas for growth. Nursing is a lifelong learning profession. This is the beginning of being humble enough to know what areas you can improve while also feeling confident in other areas.
- Recognize the type of learner you are as well. I have included tables for linear learners and images for visual learners. You may use a combination of both these learning styles. If so, create notes that reflect how you learn best.
- Be open to recognizing the patterns that are provided in each narrative for each condition and record these in the margins, at the back of the book, or on separate notes.
- Design a study schedule and take the time YOU need to prepare for the Next Generation NCLEX-RN® exam.

Tips for Instructors

- Review Appendix C for additional information.
- Adjust teaching delivery and pedagogical practices needed to reflect the higher cognitive levels required to answer clinical judgement questions.
- Use the case studies as examples in and outside the classroom.
- Become familiar with the patterns of clinical manifestations associated with each condition.

Evolve Website

The Evolve site contains an additional 30 stand-alone and unfolding cases and all 100 practice cases from the textbook for a total of 130 practice NGN-style cases. The clinical judgement stand-alone items provide a clinical scenario and are accompanied by one NGN-style test question in either a bow-tie or trend format. These stand-alone items can measure one or as many as all of the six cognitive skills or steps identified in the NCSBN Clinical Judgement Measurement Model (NCJMM). These cognitive skills include Recognize Cues, Analyze Cues, Prioritize Hypotheses, Generate Solutions, Take Action, and Evaluate Outcomes. Each unfolding case is always accompanied by six NGN test items, each measuring one of the cognitive skills in sequential order.

In Study Mode, filter by Case Type and then Category and click the Begin button to start your study session. Questions have instant feedback and results are not saved so that students can practise as much as they wish. After submitting your answer, the correct answer is displayed. Use the Rationale button for an explanation of why that answer is correct, the Strategy button for the suggested strategy for arriving at an answer, and the Reference button to find further information related to the case topic in an Elsevier textbook.

In Exam Mode, select to filter by Case Type and then Category. Leaving an exam before it is completed suspends it to be resumed at a later time from the History. Completed exams are tallied and archived in the History. Completed exams can be reviewed. The Results Pane displays a completed exam session's results.

In both modes, students can hover their mouse over the NGN Tip button to find additional information about the specific question type, how to approach answering the question, and scoring information.

Next Generation NCLEX®

The National Council for the State Boards of Nursing (NCSBN) is a not-for-profit organization whose members include nursing regulatory bodies. In empowering and supporting nursing regulators in their mandate to protect the public, the NCSBN is involved in the development of nursing licensure examinations, such as the NCLEX-RN®. In Canada, the NCLEX-RN® was introduced in 2015 and is, as of the writing of this text, the recognized licensure exam required for practising RNs in Canada.

The NCLEX-RN® changed, as of 2023, to ensure that its item types adequately measure clinical judgement, critical thinking, and problem-solving skills on a consistent basis. The NCSBN also incorporated into the examination what they call the Clinical Judgement Measurement Model (CJMM), which is a framework that the NCSBN has created to measure a novice nurse's ability to apply clinical judgement in practice. These changes to the examination come as a result of research findings indicating that novice nurses have a much higher than desirable error rate with patients (i.e., errors that cause patient harm) and, upon NCSBN's investigation, that the overwhelming majority of these errors were caused by failures of clinical judgement.

Clinical judgement has been a foundation of nursing education for decades, based on the work of a number of nursing theorists. The theory of clinical judgement that most closely aligns with what NCSBN is basing their CJMM on is the work by Christine A. Tanner. The new version of the NCLEX-RN® is loosely identified as the "Next-Generation NCLEX" or "NGN" and features the following:

- Six key skills in the CJMM: recognizing cues, analyzing cues, prioritizing hypotheses, generating solutions, taking action, and evaluating outcomes.
- Approved item types as of March 2021: multiple response, extended drag and drop, cloze (drop-down), enhanced hot-spot (highlighting), matrix/grid bow tie, and trend. More question types may be added.
- All new item types are accompanied by mini–case studies with comprehensive patient information—some of it relevant to the question, and some of it not.
- Case information may present a single, unchanging moment in time (a "single-episode" case study) or multiple moments in time as a patient's condition changes (an "unfolding" case study).
- Single-episode case studies may be accompanied by one to six questions; unfolding case studies are accompanied by six questions.

For more information (and detail) regarding the NCLEX-RN® and changes coming to the exam, visit the NCSBNs website: www.nclex.com and https://www.ncsbn.org/publications/building-a-method-for-writing-clinical-judgment-items-for-entry-Level-nursing-exams.

For further NCLEX-RN® examination preparation resources, see *Elsevier's Canadian Comprehensive Review for the NCLEX-RN Examination*, Third Edition, ISBN 9780323810333.

Prior to preparing for any nursing licensure examination, nursing students should refer to their provincial or territorial nursing regulatory body to determine which licensure examination is required in order for them to practise in their chosen jurisdiction.

A Note on Terminology

The author of this textbook recognizes and acknowledges the diverse histories of the first peoples of the lands now referred to as Canada. It is recognized that individual communities identify themselves in various ways; within this text, the term *Indigenous* is used to refer to all First Nations, Inuit, and Métis people within Canada, unless there are research findings that are presented uniquely to a population. The author also recognizes that knowledge and language concerning sex, gender, and identity are fluid and continually evolving. The language and terminology presented in this text endeavour to be inclusive of all people and reflect what is, to the best of our knowledge, current at the time of publication.

Elsevier eBooks

More than just words on a screen, Elsevier eBooks on VitalSource come preloaded with interactive learning features that empower students to engage with course content in entirely new ways.

Ideal for use both inside and outside the classroom, Elsevier eBooks on VitalSource give students the ability to access textbook content any time, any place via desktop computer, laptop, tablet, or smartphone.

It includes study aids such as highlighting, e-note taking, and the ability to share notes with other students or with instructors. Even more importantly, it allows students and instructors to do a comprehensive search within the specific text or across several titles. Please check with your Elsevier sales representative for more information.

Acknowledgements

This book would not have been possible without the support of Roberta Spinosa-Millman, Executive Editor at Elsevier, and Lenore Gray-Spence, Content Development Specialist at Elsevier. Thank you, Roberta for being open to creating this book and supporting me from the initial conversations. Lenore, your unwavering support, assistance, and motivation from conception to production have been appreciated. Thank you for allowing my creativity to shine throughout the pages of the textbook and working with my vision of colour, images, and visuals. Thanks are due to Cindy Thoms, Senior Project Manager, and Jerri Hurlbutt, Copy Editor, for keeping me on track and meeting deadlines. Thank you to Catherine Jackson, Publishing Services Manager, and Amy Buxton, Design Direction, for bringing my vision to fruition and ensuring the final production of this book.

Thanks are due to the reviewers who reviewed the content of this book and gave their invaluable comments, expertise, and editing suggestions on the draft manuscript.

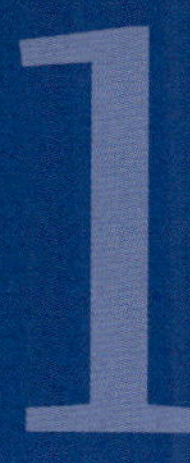

Understanding the New NCLEX-RN® and Next Generation NCLEX®

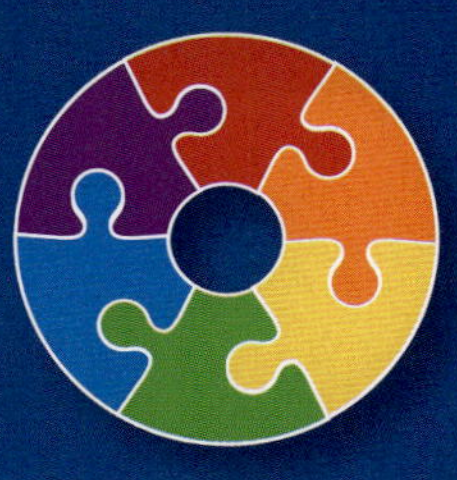

Introduction

Welcome to *Elsevier's Case Study Practice Review for Next Generation NCLEX® (NGN)!* The purpose of this textbook is to help you use knowledge gained in your undergraduate program to engage with questions that test higher-ordered cognitive thinking like the ones you will encounter when writing the Next Generation NCLEX-RN® (NGN®). Each chapter is intended to build on previously learned information so you can develop strategies to apply your knowledge. Chapters include step-by-step advice and show you how to apply clinical judgement to unfolding and stand-alone case studies. The NGN-style questions are meant to elevate your understanding of the complexity of illness and apply this knowledge through real-life case study scenarios. Each case scenario is intended to replicate environments that new nursing graduates may encounter in their first year of practice. This book will provide you with concrete methods of applying your knowledge to NGN-style practice examples and case studies that will increase with complexity throughout the chapters. At the end of the book are unfolding and stand-alone case studies for you to practise with and test your knowledge. Use the rationales provided in Chapter 9 for unfolding case studies and in Chapter 10 for stand-alone case studies to identify gaps in your knowledge and areas where further study is needed so you will be prepared to write the Next Generation NCLEX-RN.

Understanding the New NCLEX-RN

Preparation of undergraduate nursing students for writing the Nursing Council Licensure Exam for registered nurses (NCLEX-RN) is a process that begins on the first day of a baccalaureate nursing program. Educators in nursing programs design undergraduate nursing curricula based on national, provincial, and territorial entry-to-practice or entry-level nursing competencies that ensure graduates are ready to meet the challenges of the dynamic health care system and deliver compassionate, empathic, competent, and safe care to clients on either side of the Canada-United States border. Through collaborative processes between the regulatory bodies, postsecondary institutions, and community stakeholders, nursing educators strive to provide all graduates of nursing programs with the skills and knowledge needed to meet the demands of nursing practice. Taking the NCLEX-RN is the final step for licensure in many Canadian provinces and territories and in all of the United States. Upon completion of your undergraduate nursing program, you are required to successfully pass the NCLEX-RN and become registered to practise in your chosen province, territory, or state.

Currently, the NCLEX-RN, now NGN, is the standard examination that Canadian-educated baccalaureate-prepared nursing students must pass in order to meet provincial and territorial registered nurse requirements, with the exception of Québec and New Brunswick. French- and English-speaking nursing students may choose to write the OIIQ (Ordre des Infirmières et infirmiers du Québec) to become registered to practise in the provinces of Québec or New Brunswick. Successful passing of the OIIQ licensure exam is acknowledged only in these two provinces for practising nursing. All other provinces and territories require the nursing graduate to successfully pass the NCLEX-RN, now NGN, in order to be registered to practise. In the United States, all nursing students who wish to practise as a registered nurse must write the NCLEX-RN. Each US nursing regulatory body has jurisdiction to protect the public and ensure that all regulated members meet standards for nursing care. Appendix B contains contact information for Canadian provincial and territorial and US nursing regulatory bodies.

The National Council of State Boards of Nurses (NCSBN) introduced the Next Generation NCLEX (NGN) on April 1, 2023. Applicants writing the NCLEX-RN will continue to answer NCLEX item types similar to the previous assessment structure of the exam but will also be required to answer NGN case studies in order to assess each test writer's ability to apply clinical judgement to real-life nursing scenarios.

Current NCLEX item types offer a single application of processes that are fundamental to nursing practice, utilizing the nursing process, prioritization, and policies as the foundation for all item types. The addition of NGN case studies provides a multilayered approach that addresses different steps of clinical judgement, taking into account multiple contexts of nursing practice, comparable to what new nursing graduates may encounter when caring for Canadian and American populations. The NCSBN provides up-to-date information for test writers at www.nclex.com.

The NGN was added to the current licensure assessment model to test higher cognitive thinking pertaining to clinical judgement. Testing students' abilities to react to real-world scenarios and apply clinical judgement could not be accomplished in a single-item type question format. While clinical judgement is not a new nursing concept, being tested and graded on this cognitive skill is new for many nursing students, and preparing students for this test is new for many educators as well. NCSBN (2023) describes *clinical judgement* as "the observed outcome of critical thinking and decision-making. It is an iterative process with multiple steps that uses nursing knowledge to observe and assess presenting situations, identify a prioritized client concern and generate the best possible evidence-based solutions in order to deliver safe client care" (p. 4). Embedded within the nursing process is the expectation of critical thinking and application of clinical decision-making. Although similar and often used interchangeably, decision making and enacting clinical judgement are considered different when writing the NGN. Clinical judgement incorporates critical thinking and clinical decision-making. The nursing process remains the foundational core of the NCSBN Clinical Judgement Measurement Model (NCJMM), which means that all of those lectures that you reviewed on the nursing process will still be relevant. This casebook will help take you to the next level, to meet the requirements of clinical judgement for NGN. The NCJMM consists of six cognitive steps: Recognize Cues, Analyze Cues, Prioritize Hypothesis, Generate Solutions, Take Action, and Evaluate Outcomes.

The chapters that follow will show you how to sort through multiple pieces of information and analyze this information in order to establish what is "nice to know," what one "needs to know," and what "must be known" to determine what the clinical problem is for the client. Once you have made a sound decision, based on the evidence provided, you will determine a plan of action for the client, considering orders and nursing priorities; take action; and then evaluate what you have done—just like in practice. This chapter is designed to introduce you to the NGN structure, remind you of the nursing process, and understand how the NCJMM as a tool can be applied to nursing practice.

Clinical Judgement Is an Additional Step Beyond the Nursing Process

The nursing process evolved from Lydia Hall's (1955) introduction of the three-step nursing process, to several iterations published by nursing theorists such as Dorothy Johnson (1959), Ida Lois Orlando (1961/1990), and Helen Petro-Yura and Mary B. Walsh (1973), and finally into the four-step process we as nurses use now: assessment, planning, implementation, and evaluation. The nursing process focuses on assessment, nursing diagnosis (Canada)/analysis (US), planning, implementation, and evaluation. The NCSBN (2023) indicates the nursing process as one of the integrated processes that is fundamental to the practice of nursing and required in the care of clients. *Nursing process* is defined as "a scientific, clinical reasoning approach to client care that includes assessment, analysis, planning, implementation, and evaluation" (NCSBN, 2023). It is important to acknowledge this distinction between the Canadian-taught nursing process and the NCSBN testing requirements. Most NCLEX multiple-choice questions and alternate-format questions include a component of the nursing process. This remains consistent with the Next Generation NCLEX-RN. The nursing process serves as the foundation for the clinical judgement measurement model, which is a systematic, structured way to assess current NCLEX writers' ability to address the complex needs of their clients while providing safe and competent nursing care.

Why Was Clinical Judgement Testing Added?

Every 3 years, the NCSBN conducts a practice analysis of essential skills necessary for safe and competent care. New nursing graduates in Canada (starting after 2015) and the

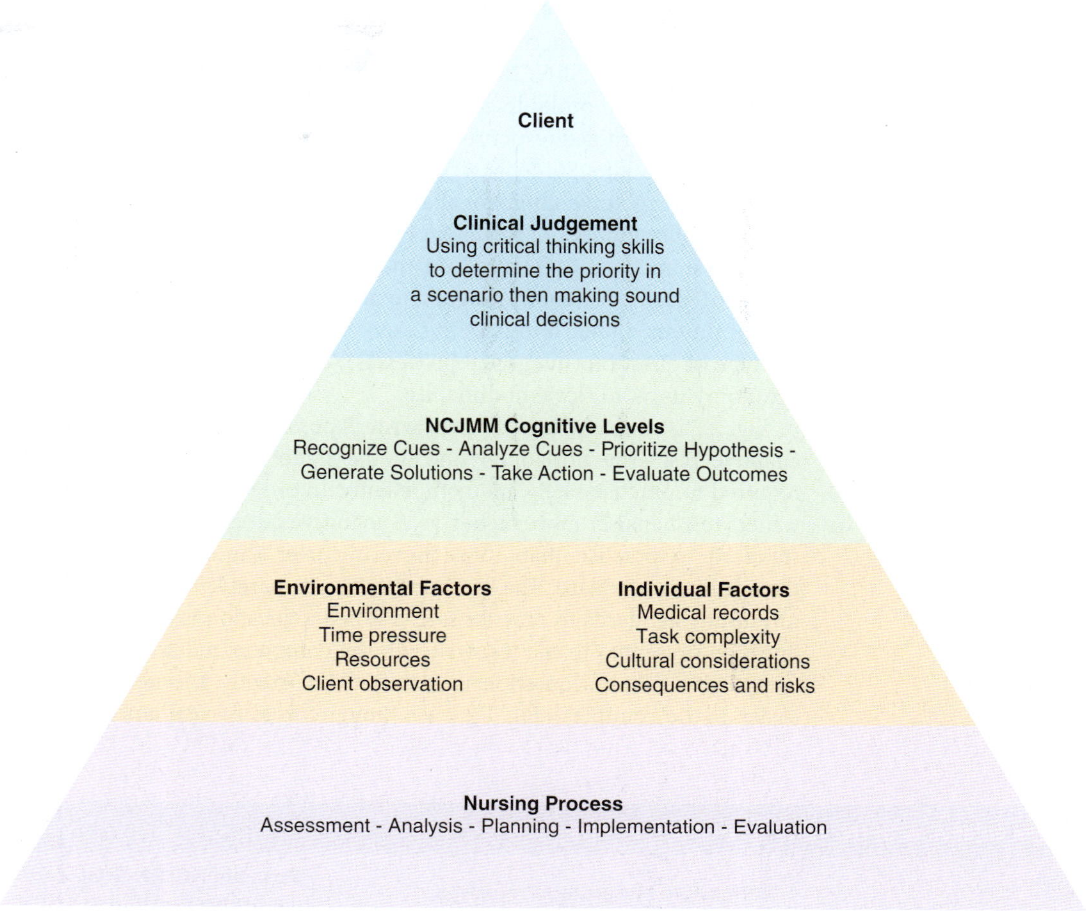

Client

Clinical Judgement
Using critical thinking skills to determine the priority in a scenario then making sound clinical decisions

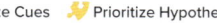

NCJMM Cognitive Levels
Recognize Cues - Analyze Cues - Prioritize Hypothesis - Generate Solutions - Take Action - Evaluate Outcomes

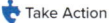

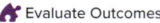

Environmental Factors
Environment
Time pressure
Resources
Client observation

Individual Factors
Medical records
Task complexity
Cultural considerations
Consequences and risks

Nursing Process
Assessment - Analysis - Planning - Implementation - Evaluation

FIG. 1.1 Nursing Clinical Judgement Measurement Model. Adapted from Bloom's Taxonomy concepts and NCSBN (2019). Clinical judgement measurement model and action model. *Next Generation NCLEX News,* Spring, 2019.

United States are randomly selected and provided a survey asking participants activity statements meant to identify the necessary skills and knowledge required in the first year of nursing practice. Year after year, clinical judgement has been shown to be an essential skill embedded within nursing tasks (NCSBN, 2019a). According to the practice analysis conducted in 2017, clinical judgement was woven into 46% of all nursing-related tasks (NCSBN, 2018). Beginning in 2016, the NCSBN began asking all NCLEX writers to voluntarily answer higher-level cognitive questions designed to address the necessary steps required for clinical judgement. The results of this analysis, plus the identification of poor client outcomes and poor nursing clinical decision-making (Nibbelink & Brewer, 2018), initiated steps to develop the nursing clinical judgement measurement model and create higher cognitive-level questions for each writer.

Taking into account several nursing theory models, the NCJMM was developed by the NCSBN. The NCJMM (Fig. 1.1) utilizes the nursing process as a base, then layers on contextual pieces of information that students may encounter, such as environmental and individual factors associated with day-to-day care of the population. Once the context has been set, the NCJMM items are designed to address higher cognitive processing necessary to ensuring that students are competent for practice and that the public is receiving safe and high-quality nursing care.

What Types of Questions to Expect When Writing NCLEX-RN and NGN

Let's Talk About NCLEX-RN

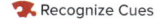

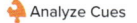

Current item types, as outlined in the NCLEX-RN test plans, offer single-layer application of information. For example, item types on NCLEX-RN are based on one focus area, addressing cognitive levels of Bloom's taxonomy and incorporating integrated processes (nursing process, caring, communication and documentation, teaching/learning, culture and spirituality) (NCSBN, 2019b). Previous NCLEX item types, as described in previous test plans, included multiple-choice, multiple-response, fill-in-the blank calculation, hot spots, exhibits, ordered response, audio, and graphics, which could include charts, tables, graphics, and audio. Students write a minimum number of NCLEX item types, which could include multiple-choice or alternate-format items (Table 1.1) with test questions up to a maximum number of total item types.

These item types are scored on the basis of the *computer adaptive testing* (CAT) structure. Each question is designed to test the student's ability to practise safely. There is a minimum standard to pass the exam successfully. Item types are scored based on the type of question (integrated processes), and each item type is written with Bloom's taxonomy in mind (level of difficulty).

Fig. 1.2 is an example of an item writer's possible attempts when writing a computer adaptive test. The horizontal line in the figure represents the minimum standard required to practise safely and competently. In order to be successful on the exam, test writers must answer more higher-level cognitive questions addressing what is above the standard to practise than those hovering over the standard line or falling below the minimum standard. The first question is comparable to what is required to meet the minimum standards to practise safely. When a question is answered correctly, the next question presented to the test writer in the computerized adaptive testing increases in complexity. When a question is answered incorrectly, the next question presented is easier. In the example in Fig. 1.2, even though this test writer answered several questions

TABLE 1.1 Basic Overview of the Structure of NCLEX-RN

Client Needs	Possible Integrated Processes	Possible NCLEX-Style and Alternate-Format Question Examples

• Safe and Effective Care Environment
  • Management of Care
  • Safety and Infection Control
• Health Promotion and Maintenance
• Psychosocial Integrity
• Physiological Integrity
  • Basic Care and Comfort
  • Pharmacological and Parenteral Therapies
  • Reduction of Risk Potential
  • Physiological Adaptation
	• Caring
	• Clinical judgement
	• Communication and documentation
	• Culture and spirituality
	• Nursing process
	• Teaching/learning
		• Multiple choice
		• Fill in the blanks
		• Hot-spot questions
		• Chart/exhibit questions
		• Drag-and-drop/ordered responses
		• Audio
		• Graphics
		• Multiple response or select all that apply

From National Council of State Boards of Nursing (NCSBN). (2023). *Next Generation NCLEX®: NCLEX-RN® test plan, April 2023.*

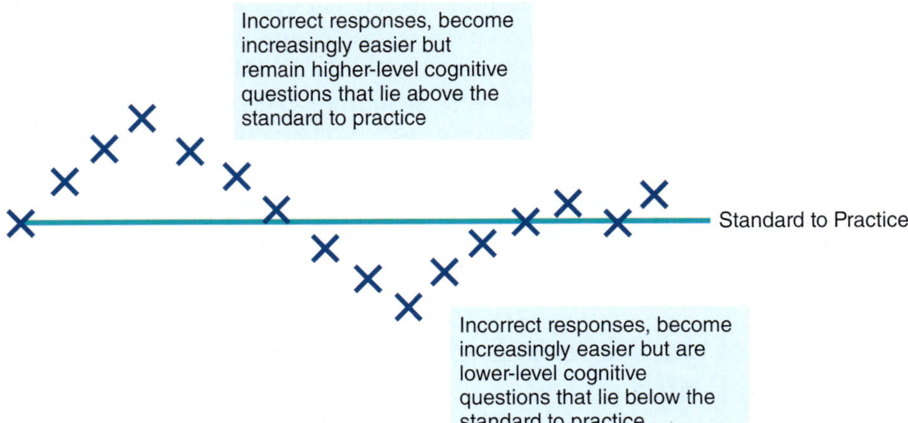

FIG. 1.2 Example of a computerized adaptive test scenario where the complexity of questions offered to a test writer is based on their answer choices. Each correct answer generates a more complex question; each incorrect answer choice generates a less difficult or complex question.

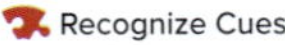

incorrectly at the beginning, the complexity of those questions was higher than the minimum standards to practise. Each test writer will encounter different questions throughout their NCLEX-RN. The program applies a 95% confidence interval rule, whereby it is designed to stop administering questions when the program determines that the test writer has successfully answered more higher–cognitive domain questions positioned above the standard to practise safely. The program can also determine if the test writer has been unsuccessful if a higher number of lower-level cognitive domain questions were answered and fall below the standard to practise.

Each multiple-choice NCLEX question has three components: 1) a singular **topic**; 2) a **stem** (sentence that includes the question which involves the nursing process, delegation of care, or prioritization of care); and 3) four **answers** that consist of three distractors and one correct answer. Alternate-format item types can vary, but they will always include a singular topic and a stem as described above. Answers are written in a unique manner that aligns with the alternate-format item type. Only pertinent information is given in the question; no extraneous, unimportant data are provided to the writer.

The nurse is caring for a postoperative client who required a fasciotomy for compartment syndrome. Which of the following assessment findings would be most important for the nurse to report to the health care provider?

A. Oliguria
B. Temperature: 38.5°C (101.3°F)
C. Heart rate: 89 beats per minute
D. Eupnea

Answer: B

Rationale: The **topic** of this question pertains to fasciotomy as a result of compartment syndrome. *Compartment syndrome* is best described as a complication of a fracture where there is swelling and increased pressure in the compartment at the site of injury. The **stem** of the question is an assessment question based on the nursing process. Each **answer** is a distractor except for the correct answer. The student test writer must recognize what is meant by a fasciotomy. A *fasciotomy* is a surgical intervention where fascia is cut to relieve the pressure and left open for several days to allow soft tissue to decompress. A major complication of this intervention is infection. If the client's condition is progressing to sepsis, a fever would present first prior to renal dysfunction. Oliguria would be a late presentation of monitoring for the potential of sepsis to develop. A heart rate of 89 beats per minute would not be a concern for the nurse. *Eupnea* is defined as normal, regular, and relaxed breathing.

Level of Difficulty: Application

References: Power-Kean et al. (2023), pp. 972–973; Tyerman & Cobbett (2023), pp. 1623–1624.

This structure remains in place for the current NCLEX-RN, where a test writer will be presented multiple-choice or alternate-format questions. The addition of NGN items consisting of three unfolding case studies with the potential of up to seven stand-alone items will allow the NCLEX-RN test model to apply assessment questions based on a multilayered context incorporating both environmental and individual factors. Case studies are based on real-life scenarios. Each NGN **unfolding case study** question will consist of six questions, one for each cognitive step of the NCJMM. Stand-alone case studies can either be a **bow-tie** item, which incorporates all six cognitive steps of the NCJMM into a single question, or a **trend** item, which incorporates one cognitive step of the NCJMM, but the client scenario develops over a span of time.

Let's Talk About Next Generation NCLEX

The first step toward being successful in answering NGN case studies is to learn what is expected of the test writer and breaking down the structure. A brief overview of the NGN, including the six NCJMM cognitive steps, follows. Subsequent chapters will break down each step of the NCJMM, addressing the potential item types that could be asked of writers. Once you understand what is expected of you for the cognitive steps, you can apply this knowledge to either an unfolding case study or a stand-alone item type.

As stated previously, NGN unfolding and stand-alone case studies offer test writers scenarios based on real-life clinical situations where clinical judgement is required to safely and competently care for clients and their families. Scenarios can be situated in community and acute care settings with clients presenting with acute or chronic health issues, from any age across the lifespan. **Unfolding case studies** (Chapter 5, 7, and 9) ask a total of six questions, one from each cognitive step from the NCJMM (see Fig 1.1). Writers may encounter two different types of stand-alone case studies: **bow-tie** and **trend** (Chapter 6, 8, and 10). Bow-tie stand-alone items incorporate all six cognitive steps where test writers must use the information provided in the narrative to identify what the condition may be for the client in the scenario, determine nursing actions required to effectively care for the client, and finally identify specific parameters to monitor for this specific client. Trend stand-alone items ask only one question based on a single cognitive step, but the medical issue occurs over time.

Each case study will have an introductory sentence that includes the client's age and gender, if appropriate, and provides context for the client scenario—that is, emergency department, community care clinic, renal unit, surgical unit, or other locations of practice. If the client is transferred to another unit, a new introductory sentence will accompany the clinical scenario, providing context for the test writer. This alerts the student writer of the change in environment and possible data to re-consider. NGN presents data in a way comparable to how students would encounter client data in the clinical environment. There are 11 potential tabs. During the exam, the test writer can click on the tab, and new information will be presented. In an unfolding case study, there will be a sentence acknowledging new data. New data will not just appear where the test writer could miss new information. The potential 11 tabs for data presentation include the following:

- Nurses' Notes
- History and Physical
- Laboratory Results
- Diagnostic Results
- Flow Sheet
- Progress Notes
- Admission Notes
- Intake and Output
- Medications
- Vital Signs
- Orders

When laboratory data are provided, normal values are also provided, only for NGN case studies. Test writers will not be given normal laboratory values when answering NCLEX-style questions, so be sure you have knowledge of laboratory and acid-based gas values.

As stated earlier, to make sound clinical decisions, nurses use critical thinking to determine the most appropriate and safest action for their clients and families. Case studies utilize the NCJMM to assess the higher cognitive abilities required to make these decisions, through the six cognitive steps:

- Recognize Cues
- Analyze Cues
- Prioritize Hypothesis
- Generate Solutions
- Take Action
- Evaluate Outcomes

Following is a brief overview of the cognitive steps. Chapter 3: What Is Happening With the Client: Recognize Cues, Analyze Cues, and Prioritize Hypothesis, and Chapter 4: What Are Next Steps When Caring for the Client: Generate Solutions, Take Action, and Evaluate Outcomes, will expand further on the NCJMM cognitive steps.

Overview of the NCJMM Six Cognitive Steps

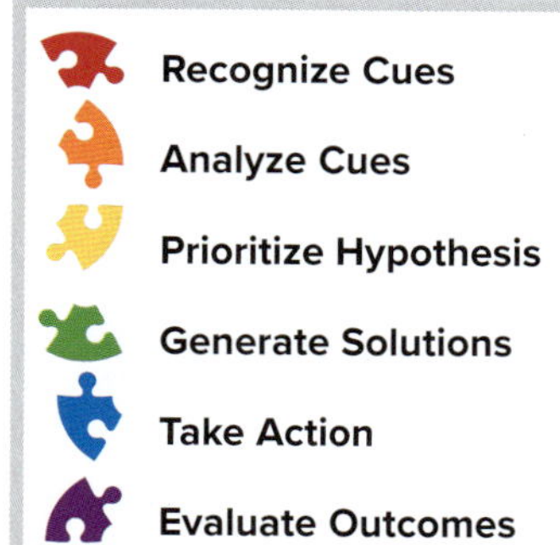

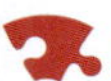

Recognize Cues

When given a client presentation, the nurse determines what would be classified as **normal** assessment data, **abnormal** assessment data, and **critical abnormal** assessment data. Each client condition presents with unique characteristics and patterns of clinical presentation. It is important to remember these patterns in order to determine what data are nice-to-know information as opposed to critically important and valid information. Like a puzzle piece, the nurse then uses each piece of information to put together a larger picture of what could be happening with the client (Box 1.1).

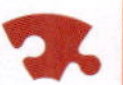

BOX 1.1 NGN Example: Recognize Cues

The nurse is caring for a 76-year-old client in the emergency department.

Nurses' Notes

0800h: The client presents to the emergency department with complaints of chest pain and shortness of breath. The client has returned from an extended 36-hour road trip. The nurse palpates an irregular radial pulse but is unable to determine apical = radial. The client complains of 7 out of 10 pain on a numerical scale, located in the left anterior wall of the chest that increases when taking deep breaths. Skin warm and dry to touch.

When the nurse reads this clinical presentation, key pieces of information to extract include chest pain, shortness of breath, 36-hour road trip, irregular but palpable pulse, and quality of the chest pain (7/10, located left anterior wall of the chest, that increases with deep breaths). Skin warm and dry to touch would be classified as a normal finding.

You will find cognitive step symbols throughout the textbook. Each puzzle piece represents one of the smaller pieces of the NGN larger puzzle. A red puzzle piece represents Recognize Cues; orange indicates Analyze Cues; a yellow puzzle piece represents Prioritize Hypothesis (as in what is the highest potential problem for the client); a green puzzle piece represents Generate Solutions; blue is for Take Action; and purple is for Evaluate Outcomes (as in what are the interventions and outcomes of the interventions).

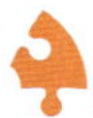

Analyze Cues

This step of the NCJMM takes the data gathered from Recognize Cues and considers *possible conditions* or *complications* that may be associated with the clinical presentation. Understanding the patterns of clinical presentation for conditions is important, as the nurse must bring together multiple pieces of the narrative in order to consider the actual condition. See Box 1.2.

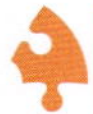

BOX 1.2 NGN Example: Analyze Cues

The nurse is caring for a 76-year-old client in the emergency department.

Nurses' Notes

0800h: The client presents to the emergency department with complaints of chest pain and shortness of breath. The client has returned from an extended 36-hour road trip. The nurse palpates an irregular radial pulse but is unable to determine apical = radial. The client complains of 7 out of 10 pain on a numerical scale, located in the left anterior wall of the chest that increases when taking deep breaths at rest.

Using nursing knowledge, consider what possible conditions or complications the client may be presenting with to the emergency department.

Continued

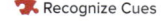

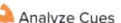

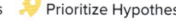

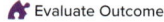

BOX 1.2 NGN Example: Analyze Cues—Continued

Some Possible Conditions That Present With Chest Pain and Shortness of Breath:

- Acute myocardial infarction
- Pleurisy
- Pleuritis
- Pulmonary embolus
- Cardiac tamponade

Environmental Factors:

- Recent return from a 36-hour long road trip

Some Possible Conditions That Present With Irregular Pulse:

- Atrial fibrillation
- Atrial flutter
- Ventricular tachycardia

Are there any data you wish you had in the narrative?

Prioritize Hypothesis

At this stage of the NCJMM, the nurse has reviewed the Recognize Cues data, considered *potential conditions* based on the clinical presentation in the Analyze Cues box, and then come to a conclusion as to what the potential medical issue is for the client or body system that could be most affected (Box 1.3). At the Prioritize Hypothesis cognitive step, the nurse decides what condition the client has the highest potential to develop. The nurse pulls together all pertinent information from the narrative to identify the priority health problem. Although each case study represents a single condition, just as in multiple-choice and alternate-format questions, NGN case studies provide extraneous information that writers will have to sift through and decide if it pertains to the problem given in the scenario.

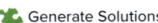

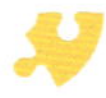

BOX 1.3 NGN Example: Prioritize Hypothesis

The nurse is caring for a 76-year-old client in the emergency department.

Nurses' Notes

0800h: The client presents to the emergency department with complaints of chest pain and shortness of breath. The client has returned from an extended 36-hour road trip. The nurse palpates an irregular radial pulse but is unable to determine apical = radial. The client complains of 7 out of 10 pain on a numerical scale, located in the left anterior wall of the chest that increases when taking deep breaths.

1015h: Client requests assistance to the washroom. Increased shortness of breath with ambulation. Client expectorating blood-tinged sputum and cyanosis noted to lips. Fine inspiratory crackles auscultated posteriorly to bilateral lung fields.

At this stage, the nurse would likely consider the client to be at highest risk for developing a pulmonary embolus. Were you able to determine that this was the problem? The pertinent data to arrive at this condition would include the pleuritic chest pain, shortness of breath, blood-tinged sputum, cyanosis, and fine inspiratory crackles. Taking into account that the client had recently returned from a 36-hour long drive, the likely cause was a deep vein thrombosis that travelled to the lung.

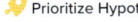

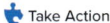

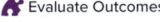

Reference

Power-Kean et al. (2023), p. 692.

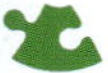

Generate Solutions

This step of the NCJMM considers how the nurse would develop a *care plan* for this client, such as preparation for potential orders or nursing interventions. If a student writer cannot determine the likely condition, anticipating care will be difficult. Clinical judgement is required to identify the potential condition and interventions to treat the client (Box 1.4).

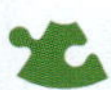

BOX 1.4 NGN Example: Generate Solutions

The nurse is caring for a 76-year-old client in the emergency department.

Nurses' Notes

0800h: The client presents to the emergency department with complaints of chest pain and shortness of breath. The client has returned from an extended 36-hour road trip. The nurse palpates an irregular radial pulse but is unable to determine apical = radial. The client complains of 7 out of 10 pain on a numerical scale, located in the left anterior wall of the chest that increases when taking deep breaths.

1015h: Client requests assistance to the washroom. Increased shortness of breath with ambulation. Client expectorating blood-tinged sputum and cyanosis noted to lips. Fine inspiratory crackles auscultated posteriorly to bilateral lung fields.

When planning care for the client, it is important to consider potential medical interventions as well as nursing interventions. This would include diagnostic tests, blood work, medications, oxygen therapy, client positioning, or other nursing interventions that would improve oxygenation and gas exchange.

Diagnostics:

- Chest radiographic study
- Continuous electrocardiogram (ECG) monitoring
- Arterial blood gas tests (ABGs)
- Venous ultrasound
- Complete blood count (CBC) with white blood cell (WBC) differential
- Spiral (helical) computed tomography (CT) scan
- Ventilation–perfusion (VQ) scan
- Lung scan
- D-dimer level
- Troponin level, B-type natriuretic peptide (BNP) level
- Pulmonary angiography

Potential Nursing Interventions/Orders:

- Supplemental oxygen, intubation may be necessary
- Fibrinolytic agent
- Unfractionated heparin intravenous (IV) infusion
- Low-molecular-weight heparin (e.g., enoxaparin [Lovenox])
- Warfarin (Coumadin) for long-term therapy
- Monitoring of activated partial thromboplastin time (aPTT) and international normalized ratio (INR) levels
- Limited activity
- Opioids for pain relief
- Inferior vena cava filter
- Pulmonary embolectomy in life-threatening situation

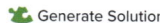

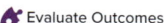

Reference

Tyerman & Cobbett (2023), p. 623.

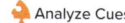

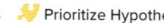

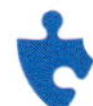

Take Action

When considering this step of the NCJMM, the nurse would decide to take action based on their understanding of the condition. In practice, errors occur for many reasons. Sound clinical decision-making requires knowledge of the condition and being prepared to act in accordance with standards of evidence-informed practice. Knowledge about details to include in a plan of care for a client is similar to knowledge required for the most appropriate and safest actions to take. This would include health care provider orders and specific nursing interventions now, not potential nursing interventions (Box 1.5).

BOX 1.5 NGN Example: Take Action

The nurse is caring for a 76-year-old client in the emergency department.

Nurses' Notes

0800h: The client presents to the emergency department with complaints of chest pain and shortness of breath. The client has returned from an extended 36-hour road trip. The nurse palpates an irregular radial pulse but is unable to determine apical = radial. The client complains of 7 out of 10 pain on a numerical scale, located in the left anterior wall of the chest that increases when taking deep breaths.

1015h: Client requests assistance to the washroom. Increased shortness of breath with ambulation. Client expectorating blood-tinged sputum and cyanosis noted to lips. Fine inspiratory crackles auscultated posteriorly to bilateral lung fields.

When implementing solutions to the identified problem, it is important to apply medical interventions as well as nursing interventions. The same information identified in Generate Solutions, including diagnostic tests, blood work, medications, oxygen therapy, client positioning, or other nursing interventions that would improve oxygenation and gas exchange, would be still applicable for this cognitive step.

Diagnostics:

- Chest radiographic study
- Continuous ECG monitoring
- ABGs
- Venous ultrasound
- CBC count with WBC differential
- Spiral (helical) CT scan
- VQ scan
- Lung scan
- D-dimer level
- Troponin level, BNP level
- Pulmonary angiography

Potential Nursing Interventions/Orders:

- Supplemental oxygen, intubation may be necessary
- Fibrinolytic agent
- Unfractionated heparin IV infusion
- Low-molecular-weight heparin (e.g., enoxaparin [Lovenox])
- Warfarin (Coumadin) for long-term therapy
- Monitoring of aPTT and INR levels
- Limited activity
- Opioids for pain relief
- Inferior vena cava filter
- Pulmonary embolectomy in life-threatening situation

Reference

Tyerman & Cobbett (2023), p. 623.

Evaluate Outcomes

At this cognitive step, the nurse evaluates outcomes of the action that was taken at the previous step. The nurse will determine if the actions improved the client's condition or resulted in no change in client status, or if the client deteriorated as a result of the action. The nurse must account for new assessment information or client statements to determine the client's new status (Box 1.6).

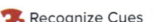

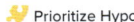

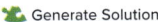

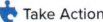

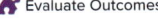

BOX 1.6 NGN Example: Evaluate Outcomes

The nurse is caring for a 76-year-old client in the emergency department.

Nurses' Notes

0800h: The client presents to the emergency department with complaints of chest pain and shortness of breath. The client has returned from an extended 36-hour road trip. The nurse palpates an irregular radial pulse but is unable to determine apical = radial. The client complains of 7 out of 10 pain on a numerical scale, located in the left anterior wall of the chest that increases when taking deep breaths.

1015h: Client requests assistance to the washroom. Increased shortness of breath with ambulation. Client expectorating blood-tinged sputum and cyanosis noted to lips. Fine inspiratory crackles auscultated posteriorly to bilateral lung fields.

1300h: Orders followed and heparin infusion initiated. The client indicates breathing has improved with no complaints of pain but continues to experience shortness of breath with ambulation. Bilateral radial pulse palpable, regular, and strong.

The step of evaluating the outcomes is meant to determine if the client has adequate tissue perfusion and respiratory function, adequate cardiac output, increased level of comfort, and no recurrence of pulmonary embolism. The nurse uses information provided in the scenario to identify if the client's condition has improved, declined, or remain unchanged. In the provided example, the client continues to experience shortness of breath with ambulation (no change), but there are improvements related to no pain with breathing, and radial pulse now regular and strong. Evaluate Outcomes takes into consideration the nurse's knowledge about normal assessment.

Structure of the New NCLEX-RN® With NGN

One of the frequently asked questions from students is how many questions are on the test. Student writers will have 5 hours to complete the exam. The minimum number of test items will be **52** computer adaptive test questions plus 15 unscored test questions (that will be unknown to the student writer but could be used in future examinations) and only 3 unfolding case studies, each with 6 questions. The *minimum number* of total questions a student writer could be asked would be **85** (52 multiple-choice/alternate-format, plus 15 test/unscored questions, plus 18 NGN). If the computer program cannot determine that the student has met the standard to pass the exam successfully, additional questions will be administered. Student writers could write a potential *maximum number* of **150** questions (which includes the initial 85) with a mixture of multiple-choice and alternate-format questions, **three unfolding** case studies, and **up to seven stand-alone** (bow-tie or trend) case studies. Stand-alone items are only provided after the minimum number of questions have been administered, to further assess the student writer's ability to meet the higher cognitive levels required to safely exhibit clinical judgement. To learn more about what to expect on test day and what is meant by "run out of time rule," review the test plan and other information located on www.nclex.com.

Conclusion

Now that you have more information about the NCLEX-RN, NGN case studies, NCJMM, and the six cognitive steps, you are ready to start building your skill set in order to apply knowledge you have learned in your program. Chapter 2 is structured purposefully, to provide accessible ways to prepare for the NGN. Often students need concrete methods when learning material and require opportunities for practice in a safe, nonjudgemental environment (Chapters 7–10). Throughout this book of practice case studies, you will be provided examples of the different item types (questions) you may encounter in relation to an unfolding case study, bow-tie, or trend item. When you understand how to use your knowledge, you will have tangible methods to answer each of the new item types specifically designed for NGN case studies.

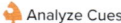

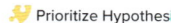

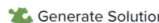

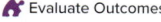

2 Applying Knowledge to Clinical Judgement Scenarios

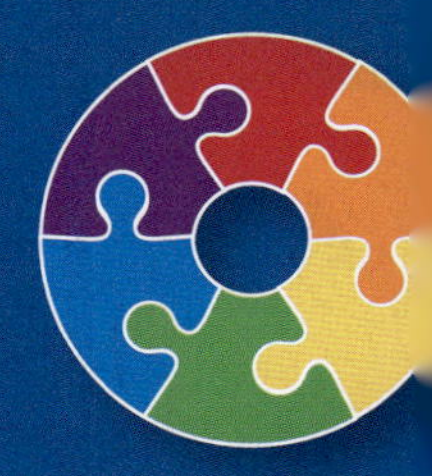

You have learned a lot of information in a very short time during your undergraduate education. It can be challenging to identify methods for keeping all that information organized in a way that helps you remember the information and apply your knowledge when in practice or when writing a standardized test. Next Generation NCLEX (NGN) clinical scenarios present both pertinent and extraneous client data that require knowledge to determine what data are important and require your attention and which data can be discarded. This chapter will focus on how to use the knowledge you have learned throughout your nursing program and apply it to answering NGN questions.

Starting From the Beginning

Reviewing what a **normal** clinical presentation may look like for a client will help you recognize when a client presents with **abnormal** clinical symptoms. With abnormal clinical symptoms, a client's status can deteriorate. When in practice or completing NGN case studies, it is important to anticipate when physiological complications and systemic instability may lead to a **critical abnormal** client presentation. Consider approaching this thinking as steps moving in a progressive nature (Fig. 2.1). Client assessment data will fall within one of the three categories: normal, abnormal, or critical abnormal. Identifying which category the client assessment data fits best will ensure that you can anticipate whether the client's status will improve or further deteriorate.

In order to determine client status, the nurse would include head-to-toe client presentation, incorporating terminology, vital signs, laboratory results, and subjective data or what the client says to the nurse. Each piece of data represents a piece to the puzzle. The nurse must also consider age, environment, previous comorbidities, and culture of the client within the clinical scenario. Understanding the differences in client presentation will help you determine which data to focus on. Through the gathering of evidence, you can determine what is the primary problem of the clinical scenario and what actions you would take, knowing this information. This is how you will proceed with an NGN case study.

Normal assessment data (see Fig. 2.1) include information you would have learned early in your undergraduate nursing program about normal clinical presentation, such as a normal heart rate being 60 to 100 beats per minute and regular with palpation. Abnormal assessment data is any data that deviates from normal: now, that heartbeat is documented as either greater than 100 beats per minute (tachycardia) or less than 60 beats per minute (bradycardia) but still regular with palpation. Critical abnormal assessment data would indicate that the client presentation is compromised and affecting cognition, airway, breathing, or circulation. In the continued example of heart rate, the heart rate is documented at 166 beats per minute, irregular with palpation, and the client is dizzy and has developed shortness of breath. Critical abnormal assessment data often include client status that involves more than one system where the client is at risk for significant complications without treatment.

The following pages contain tables of assessment data, starting with vital signs followed by a systematic head-to-toe breakdown of normal, abnormal, and critical abnormal client presentation. In order to apply clinical judgement, the nurse must think critically about the clinical presentation, including objective and subjective data, prior to making an evidenced-informed decision. Ensuring that all pertinent data are considered is necessary to provide competent and safe care for the public. Only terminology is provided as a reminder of the information you have already learned in your nursing program at this point. Recognizing changes in status is important when reviewing and analyzing data and evaluating those clinical presentations. As you proceed further in this chapter, you will see how to layer this initial yet foundational knowledge in relation to medical conditions. You have learned a great deal of content in the few years of your undergraduate nursing program. By learning to recognize *patterns* in client presentation, from normal, abnormal, to potentially critical abnormal, you will be able to pick up on changes in your client more quickly and recognize changes in the clinical scenario that is standard for all NGN case studies.

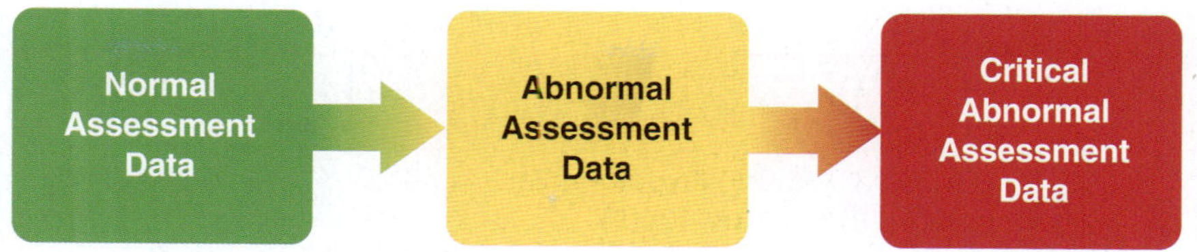

FIG. 2.1 Assessment data will fit into one of these three categories. Recognizing the category will ensure the nurse prepares accordingly for the client's status to improve or deteriorate.

At the beginning of an undergraduate program, you learn normal assessment data. It is imperative to compare client presentations with normal data when in practice. In the beginning, you likely used a memorization strategy to remember the normal rate for heart rate, which is 60 to 100 beats per minute. If the nurse palpates or auscultates a heart rate that is above or below the normal expected, that may be a cause for further investigation. Another example is when the nurse is palpating the pulse, they will need to identify if the pulse is palpable and strong, palpable and weak, or requires the use of a Doppler to identify if a pulse is present. Each abnormal or critical abnormal clinical manifestation represents a corresponding pathophysiological change in the client. Recognizing the progression of client status from normal client presentation to abnormal or critical abnormal clinical manifestations and recognizing complications or changes in overall status keep clients safe. At this point, clients may be provided treatment and return home, or they will be admitted to hospital. A nurse who is able to observe a change in client status and act on critical abnormal clinical assessment indicates preparedness for applying clinical judgement.

Making meaning from the initial client presentation, analyzing what potential complications or conditions each symptom presentation could be related to, and coming to an evidence-informed hypothesis as to the clinical problem is the first half of the NCJMM. The last half of the model involves using the hypothesis of the clinical problem to anticipate nursing or medical interventions, acting on those interventions, and determining the client response to the interventions as it relates back to normal clinical presentation and overall health status of the client.

Each table that follows represents objective data related only to assessment. This information is intended to strengthen your knowledge when applying it to multiple-choice or alternate-format questions and for NGN case studies. Remember, applying your knowledge for clinical judgement is an extension of the nursing process, which many of you have become comfortable with in clinical practice. You may or may not have to consciously think about what to do next with clients and families. Use the tables to refresh your memory. You can also use this information when practising answering multiple-choice, alternate-format, and NGN case study questions.

Assessment Data: Normal, Abnormal, and Critical Abnormal Client Presentation

Nurses use objective assessment data to determine the overall health status of a client. Recognizing the appropriate category for client presentation (normal, abnormal, or critical abnormal) enables the nurse to anticipate changes in status, ensuring safe and competent care. This approach considers the cognitive steps required to meet the Canadian Nurses Association (Almost, 2021) Standards of Practice and Entry-Level Competencies related to delivering competent and safe care. Tables 2.1 through 2.6 divide objective assessment criteria, beginning with vital signs followed by each system presentation, encountered when completing a head-to-toe assessment. Common abbreviations used in such an assessment are as follows:

System	Abbreviation
Neurological	NEURO
Cardiovascular	CV
Respiratory	RESP
Gastrointestinal	GI
Genitourinary	GU
Musculoskeletal	MSK
Endocrine	ENDO

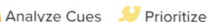

TABLE 2.1 VITAL SIGNS—ADULTS

	Normal Client Presentation	Abnormal Client Presentation	Critical Abnormal Client Presentation
Temperature	36.0–37.9°C (96.8–100.2°F)	≤36.0°C (96.8°F) (hypothermia) 38.0–40°C (100.4–104°F) (hyperthermia)	40.0–41.0°C (104– 105.8°F) (seizures) 41.0–42.0°C (105.8–107.6°F) (requires intervention) ≥42.0°C (≥107.6°F) (without intervention leads to death)
Blood Pressure	≤130–135/80–85 mmHg ≤130/80 mmHg (with diabetes) ≤140/90 (with kidney disease)	≥135/85mmHg (hypertension) ≤95 SBP (hypotension)	≥120 DBP (malignant hypertension or hypertensive crisis)
Heart Rate	60–100 beats per minute	≤60 (bradycardia) ≥100 (tachycardia)	Impacts cardiac output and respirations
Respiratory Rate	12–20 breaths per minute	≥20 breaths per minute	Impacts gas exchange
Pulse Oximetry	95–100%	≤90–92% patient dependent	≤80%

DBP, diastolic blood pressure; *SBP*, systolic blood pressure; ≥, greater than or equal; ≤, less than or equal.

TABLE 2.2 NEUROLOGICAL

	Normal Client Presentation	Abnormal Client Presentation	Critical Abnormal Client Presentation
Level of Consciousness (LOC)	Alert and orientated to person, place, and time (may also include situation)	Confusion, disorientation, lethargy, obtundation, stupor	Light coma, coma, deep coma
Glasgow Coma Scale	15	13–15 (mild) 9–12 (moderate)	3–8 (severe)
Pupils	Equal and reactive to light, shape remains consistent (typically round)	Dilated, unequal in size	Pinpoint, fixed, no reaction, doll's eyes
Motor Power	Strong × 4 extremities, spontaneous and purposeful, withdraws to painful stimuli, equal bilaterally in response	Weak to moderate × 4 extremities or less, dysphagia, may be equal or unequal bilaterally in response	None to weak × 4 extremities or less, paralysis (paraplegia, quadriplegia), decorticate, decerebrate posturing, extensor responses, rigidity, rigor, flaccid with no response to stimuli
Speech	Orientated to person, place, and time, answers questions appropriate	Dysarthria, confusion, inappropriate words, take into consideration tracheostomy, ETT, stroke complications, aphasia (Broca's or Wernicke's)	Incomprehensible to no speech
Gait/Movement	Straight-line ambulation, stable	Incoordination, leaning to one side, history of falls, weakness, imbalance, chorea, tremors, pill rolling, tics, seizures, requiring mobility aids	Unsteady and unsafe, seizures (if airway compromised) even with mobility aids
Pain	Absent	Chronic pain, neuropathy, inability to feel vibration, PQRST assessment (cardiac, pleuritic, bone, muscle, etc.)	Agony, uncontrollable crying, absence (e.g., fourth-degree burns)

TABLE 2.2 NEUROLOGICAL—Continued

	Normal Client Presentation	Abnormal Client Presentation	Critical Abnormal Client Presentation
Numbness and Tingling (paresthesia)	Normal response to reduced blood flow	Agnosia	Inability to feel anything due to spinal cord injury
Mood and Affect	Appropriate for the situation	Restlessness, agitation, anger, depression, euphoria	Harm to self or to others
Thoughts	More positive self-talk compared to negative self-talk, appropriate topics and cognitive processing	Presence or report illusions, hallucinations, delusions, or paranoia	Homicidal or suicidal tendencies
Reflexes	Normal response to stimuli	Delayed	Absent

ETT, Endotracheal tube.

TABLE 2.3 CARDIOVASCULAR

	Normal Client Presentation	Abnormal Client Presentation	Critical Abnormal Client Presentation
Heart Rhythm	Normal sinus rhythm	Sinus bradycardia, sinus tachycardia, first-degree and second-degree heart block, atrial fibrillation, atrial flutter	Third-degree heart block, ventricular tachycardia, ventricular fibrillation, asystole (or any dysrhythmia that compromises cardiac output)
Pulse	Strong, bounding, regular	Weak, thready, irregular,	Absent to palpation and requires Doppler but pulse present; absent even with Doppler assistance
Heart Sounds	S1 and S2	S3, S4, murmurs, bruits, pericardial friction rub	S3, S4, murmurs, bruits, pericardial friction rub with additional CV, RESP, or NEURO clinical manifestations representing hemodynamic instability and impaired gas exchange
Colour (skin)	Pink (conjunctiva, and palms of hands)	Pallor, jaundice, erythema, petechiae, purpura, ecchymosis	Cyanosis, necrotic, purple, petechiae, purpura, ecchymosis (depending on size, location, and progression)
Skin Temperature	Warm and dry	Diaphoresis, flushed	Cool to touch
Jugular Venous Presentation	Absent	Present—must be measured to identify severity	Present and bounding increasing to jaw line
Capillary Refill	<3 seconds	Delayed, sluggish to respond, >3 seconds	Delayed, sluggish to respond, >3 seconds with other accompanying CV decreased perfusion manifestations
Peripheral Edema	Absent	0, +1, +2, +3, +4, dependent or pitting	0, +1, +2, +3, +4, dependent or pitting with other accompanying CV clinical manifestations
Other Systemic Changes	Pink and perfused mucous membranes	Splinter hemorrhages, pale and dry mucous membranes	Splinter hemorrhages, pale and dry mucous membranes with accompanying CV or RESP clinical manifestations associated with infection, and hemodynamic instability

CV, Cardiovascular; *NEURO*, neurological; *RESP*, respiratory; <, less than; >, greater than.

TABLE 2.4 RESPIRATORY

	Normal Client Presentation	Abnormal Client Presentation	Critical Abnormal Client Presentation
Depth	Appropriate lung expansion, easy	Hypoventilation, hyperventilation	Hypoventilation, hyperventilation, tripod position, drooling with other accompanying CV, RESP, or NEURO hemodynamic or impaired gas exchange presentation
Rhythm	Regular and easy	Shallow, Use of accessory muscles	Shallow, use of accessory muscles, tripod position with accompanying CV, RESP, or NEURO hemodynamic or impaired gas exchange presentation
Symmetry	Symmetrical	Asymmetrical	Asymmetrical
Colour	Pink and perfused	Cyanosis	Pallor, grey, cyanosis
Cough	None present	Dry, unable to expectorate sputum, barking cough	Wet with or without sputum
Sputum	Clear to white	Yellow, green, blood-tinged	Hemoptysis (moderate to large amounts of clots in sputum)
Breath Sounds	Absent adventitious breath sounds, bronchial, bronchovesicular, vesicular	Fine crackles, course crackles, pleural friction rub, wheeze, atelectasis (crackles or decreased), tactile fremitus	Course crackles (if impairing gas exchange), atelectasis (absent over area), wheeze if associated with CV, RESP, or NEURO compromise
Breathing Pattern	Regular and easy at rest	Shortness of breath, bradypnea, tachypnea, hyperventilation, hypoventilation, dyspnea, apneic episodes, at rest or with movement/ambulation, pursed-lip breathing	Cheyne-Stokes, apnea, cluster breathing, ataxic breathing, agonal gasps at rest, and unable to move air, signs of increased work of breathing (intercostal, suprasternal, subcostal retractions, nasal flaring, and use of accessory muscles)
Airway Compromise	Absent	Wheeze, stridor; determine if this occurs with inspiratory or expiratory respiratory phase	Wheeze, stridor (determine if this occurs with inspiratory or expiratory respiratory phase), grunting, tripod position, drooling, thoracic retractions
Other Systemic Changes		Clubbing of nail beds	

CV, Cardiovascular; *NEURO*, neurological; *RESP*, respiratory.

TABLE 2.5 RENAL

	Normal Client Presentation	Abnormal Client Presentation	Critical Abnormal Client Presentation
Urine Output Amount	≥30 mL per hour or 0.5–1 mL per kg per hour if given a weight, maintain a neutral fluid balance	Oliguria, hematuria, incontinence, positive 24-hour fluid balance, negative 24-hour fluid balance, polyuria, retention	Anuria, ≤30 mL per hour or ≤0.5–1 mL per kg per hour if given a weight, positive or negative 24-hour fluid balance that leads to CV or RESP compromise
Urine Output Frequency	Output frequency consistent with fluid intake	Increased frequency, urgency, enuresis, fluid and electrolyte imbalance	Diuresis leading to hypovolemia and fluid and electrolyte imbalance that may contribute to CV compromise
Pain	Absent	Costovertebral tenderness, dysuria	

TABLE 2.5 RENAL—Continued

	Normal Client Presentation	Abnormal Client Presentation	Critical Abnormal Client Presentation
Urine Output Colour	Yellow, clear	Concentrated, dark orange, or lacks colour, tissue, hematuria	Concentrated, dark orange, or lacks colour, tissue, hematuria that leads to CV or RESP compromise
Urine Odour	Absent	Present	
Use of Urinary Appliances	None	Catheter, irrigation, dialysis	

CV, Cardiovascular; *RESP*, respiratory.

TABLE 2.6 GASTROINTESTINAL

	Normal Client Presentation	Abnormal Client Presentation	Critical Abnormal Client Presentation
Bowel Sounds	Audible at an appropriate level × 4 quadrants	Hyperactive, hypoactive × 4 quadrants or less than 4 quadrants	Absent
Abdominal Palpation	Soft, non-tender × 4 quadrants	Pain with palpation, distended, hard, round	Pain with palpation, distended, hard, round, rebound tenderness
Weight	Healthy weight with normal BMI and waist-to-hip ratio	Underweight, overweight, obese, morbidly obese, cachexia	Underweight, overweight, obese, morbidly obese that contributes to CV or RESP compromise
Nutritional Intake	Meets caloric needs	Underweight, overweight, obese, morbidly obese, cachexia	Underweight, overweight, obese, morbidly obese that contributes to CV or RESP compromise
Stool Consistency and Frequency	Formed, solid	Loose, frequent, diarrhea, fatty stools, blood in stools	Loose, frequent, diarrhea, fatty stools, blood in stools that contributes to CV or RESP compromise
Nausea and Vomiting	Absent	Frequency, bile, presence of digested or undigested food, medications, colour, blood in emesis, fluid and electrolyte imbalance	Frequency, bile, presence of digested or undigested food, medications, colour, blood in emesis, fluid and electrolyte imbalance that contributes to CV or RESP compromise
Use of Gastrointestinal Appliances	Absent	Ostomies, skin breakdown	

BMI, Body mass index; *CV*, cardiovascular; *RESP*, respiratory.

Normal Considerations for Pediatric Clients

With pediatric clients, understanding normal, abnormal, and critical abnormal assessment data is similar to understanding data for adult clients. Pediatric and older adult clients have a reduced ability for cardiac or respiratory reserve, meaning that these clients have the potential to experience abnormal to critical abnormal clinical manifestations more quickly than adult clients. This requires the nurse to promptly recognize clinical status changes in their client sooner, especially as it relates to airway, breathing, and circulation. Cardiovascular and respiratory compromise can occur without a lot of time afforded to wait for improvement. Normal pediatric vital sign parameters, such as temperature, heart rate, blood pressure, and respiratory rate, based on the age of the client are included here.

Normal Pediatric Vital Sign Parameters

	Normal Temperature Ranges
Method	**Normal Temperature Range**
Rectum	36.6°C to 37.9°C (97.9°F to 100.2°F)
Mouth	35.5°C to 37.5°C (95.9°F to 99.5°F)
Armpit	36.5°C to 37.5°C (97.8°F to 99.5°F)
Ear	35.8°C to 37.9°C (96.4°F to 100.2°F)

Canadian Paediatric Society, Community Paediatrics Committee. Fever and temperature taking. June 2022: https://caringforkids.cps.ca/handouts/health-conditions-and-treatments/fever_and_temperature_taking. With permission.

Normal Vital Signs According to Age

Age	Heart Rate (beats/min)	Blood Pressure (mm Hg)	Respiratory Rate (breaths/min)
Premature	120–170*	55–75/35–45†	40–70‡
0–3 mo	100–160*	65–85/45–55	30–60
3–6 mo	90–120	70–90/50–65	30–45
6–12 mo	80–120	80–100/55–65	25–40
1–3 yr	70–110	90–105/55–70	20–30
3–6 yr	65–110	95–110/60–75	20–25
6–12 yr	60–95	100–120/60–75	14–22
12+ yr	55–85	110–135/65–85	12–18

*In sleep, infant heart rates may drop significantly lower, but if perfusion is maintained, no intervention is required.

†A blood pressure cuff should cover approximately two-thirds of the arm; too small a cuff yields spuriously high pressure readings, and too large a cuff yields spuriously low pressure readings.

‡Many premature infants require mechanical ventilatory support, making their spontaneous respiratory rate less relevant.

From Hartman, M. E., & Cheifetz, I. M. (2020). Pediatric emergencies and resuscitation. In R. M. Kliegman, J. W. St. Geme, N. Blum, et al. (Eds.), *Nelson textbook of pediatrics* (21st ed.). Elsevier.

What Is Missing?

Not all assessment data are included, otherwise this chapter would become the whole book. Other areas for you to consider reviewing prior to writing the NCLEX-RN are the musculoskeletal, integumentary, and reproductive systems. Health patterns that may impact client status and contribute to changes in clinical status include the following: sleep/rest, self-perception/self-concept, roles and relationships with others, coping–stress strategies, health perception, and health management.

Applying Assessment Information to Medical Conditions

Once you are able to recognize and differentiate normal from abnormal or critical abnormal assessment data, you can apply this knowledge to common medical conditions you may encounter in clinical practice. A chart identifying common medical conditions for adult and pediatric clients is included here (Table 2.7). This list is not exhaustive, so feel free to add to it. It is a start for your review.

As previously stated, this list of common medical conditions is comprehensive but not exhaustive. For example, different types of cancers such as tumours (i.e.: breast cancer) are missing. This list is to help you get started with your studying and provide some guidance for your own learning. Students ask me all the time where they should begin, and this list may be a helpful place to start. Please cross-reference conditions that may have appeared in the latest test plan produced by NCSBN (www.nclex.com).

Preparing to Write NCLEX-RN and NGN

The first step in preparing to write the licensure exam is to create a study plan and begin organizing your notes. A study plan consists of an honest appraisal of how much studying is required prior to determining a date to write the NCLEX-RN and NGN. Review and organize all notes from your undergraduate nursing program. If you have made study notes from previous examinations, use that as an initial step. If you do not have previous study notes to review, consider that additional preparation time may be necessary to refresh your knowledge in key areas such as acute medical/surgical topics, pediatrics, maternity, mental health, nursing fundamentals, and community nursing concepts. Once you have determined how much preparation is needed, choose a date

TABLE 2.7 Common Medical Conditions Encountered in Canadian Practice Settings

Neurology	Cardiovascular	Respiratory	Renal	Gastrointestinal	Endocrine
• Increased intracranial pressure (ICP) • Traumatic brain injuries • Concussions • Hematomas (epidural, subdural, and intracerebral • Spinal cord injuries • Neurogenic shock • Autonomic dysreflexia • Transient ischemic attacks (TIAs) • Stroke (ischemic, hemorrhagic) • Cerebral aneurysms • Bacterial meningitis • Encephalitis • Seizures • Dementia • Multiple sclerosis (MS) • Parkinson's disease • Headaches • Guillain Barré • Myasthenia gravis • Amyotrophic lateral sclerosis (ALS) • Huntington's disease • Tumours Pediatrics: • Seizures • Hydrocephalus • Tumours • Epilepsy	• Hypertension • Hypertensive crisis • Hypotension • Hypovolemic shock • Cardiogenic shock • Dysrhythmias (sinus tach, sinus rad, AFib, Aflutter, VTach, VFib, PVCs, heart block, asystole, PEA) • Angina • Atherosclerosis • Acute myocardial infarction (anterior, inferior, lateral locations, NSTEMI, STEMI) • Acute and chronic heart failure • Acute and chronic pericarditis • Pericardial effusions • Cardiac tamponade • Deep vein thrombosis • Abdominal aneurysms • Aortic dissection • Pheochromocytoma • Metabolic syndrome • Endocarditis • Valve stenosis and valve regurgitation • Cardiomyopathy • Peripheral arterial disease Pediatrics: • Pediatric bradycardia • Pediatric hypertension • Congenital heart defects • Kawasaki disease • Rheumatic fever	• Influenza • Pleural effusions • Pneumothorax • Aspiration • Atelectasis • Pulmonary edema • Acute respiratory distress syndrome • Acute lung illness • Chronic obstructive pulmonary disease (COPD) (emphysema, and chronic bronchitis) • Pneumonia • Tuberculosis • Pulmonary embolus • Pulmonary arterial hypertension • Cor pulmonale • COVID-19 • Septic shock • Anaphylaxis shock Pediatrics: • Epiglottitis • Croup • Respiratory syncytial virus (RSV) • Asthma • Pertussis • Foreign body aspiration • Cystic fibrosis	• Kidney stones • Neurogenic bladder • Urinary tract infection • Cystitis • Pyelonephritis • Glomerulonephritis • Nephrotic syndrome • Nephritic syndrome • Acute kidney injury (AKI) • Chronic kidney failure • Rhabdomyolysis • Benign prostate hyperplasia	• Gastritis • Gastroesophageal reflux disease (GERD) • Peptic ulcer disease (PUD) • Upper and lower GI bleed • Bowel obstruction • Hepatitis • Hepatic encephalopathy • Cholelithiasis • Cholecystitis • Cirrhosis • Portal hypertension • Non-alcoholic fatty liver disease (NAFLD) • Non-alcoholic steatohepatitis (NASH) • Ascites • Celiac disease • Celiac crisis • Ulcerative colitis • Crohn's disease • Irritable bowel syndrome • Hepatorenal syndrome • Obesity	• Acute and chronic pancreatitis • Diabetes (type 1, type 2, diabetic ketoacidosis, hyperglycemia, hyperosmolar state) • Hypothyroidism • Myxedema coma • Hyperthyroidism • Grave's disease • Thyroid storm • Cushing's disease • Addison's disease • Addisonian crisis • Syndrome of inappropriate antidiuretic hormone (SIADH) • Diabetes insipidus

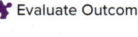

Continued

TABLE 2.7 Common Medical Conditions Encountered in Canadian Practice Settings—Continued

Musculoskeletal	Hematology	Immunity/ Autoimmunity	Mental Health	Pregnancy-Labour/ Delivery-Post-Partum	Integumentary
• Fractures • Compartment syndrome • Avascular necrosis • Osteomyelitis • Osteoporosis • Osteoarthritis • Scoliosis • Muscular dystrophies • Cerebral palsy • Spina bifida	• Disseminated intravascular coagulation (DIC) • Anemia (pernicious and iron deficient anemia) • Polycythemia vera • Leukemias • Myelodysplastic syndrome • Hodgkin's lymphoma • Non-Hodgkin's lymphoma • Lymphadenopathy • Hemochromatosis • Sickle cell syndrome • Sickle cell disease • Sickle cell crisis (vaso-occlusive thrombotic, splenic sequestration, aplastic) Pediatrics: • Hemolytic disease of the newborn	• Human immunodeficiency virus (HIV) • Acquired immune efficiency syndrome (AIDS) • Systemic lupus erythematosus (SLE) • Rheumatoid arthritis • Juvenile idiopathic arthritis • Severe combined immunodeficiency	• Depression • Anxiety • Bipolar disorder • Schizophrenia • Psychosis and psychotic disorder • Delusional disorder • Dissociative identity disorder • Personality disorders • Obsessive–compulsive disorder • Suicidal ideations • Eating disorders • Post-traumatic disorder • Substance use disorder	• Gestational diabetes mellitus • Gestational hypertension • Pre-eclampsia • Eclampsia • Seizures • Hyperemesis gravidarum • Spontaneous abortion (miscarriage) • Placenta previa • Placenta abruption • DIC • Fetal decelerations • Dystocia • Postpartum hemorrhage	• Burns • Varicella • Shingles • Measles • Mumps • Rubella • Pinworms • Hand and foot • Lice • Scabies • Mites • Ringworm • Eczema • Psoriasis • Contact dermatitis • Impetigo • Pressure ulcers

Afib, Atrial fibrillation; *Aflutter*, atrial flutter; *GI*, gastrointestinal; *NSTEMI*, non-ST-elevation myocardial infarction; *PEA*, pulseless electrical activity; *PVCs*, premature ventricular contractions; *STEMI*, ST-elevation myocardial infarction; *Vfib*, ventricular fibrillation; *Vflutter*, ventricular flutter.

and create a study plan. Determine how much time you will need per topic and be realistic with addressing your knowledge level on the topics. There may be nursing areas in which you have higher or lower levels of knowledge. Include in your study plan adequate time to prepare for each topic prior to the date of the exam. Use Table 2.7 to help organize your study notes into common medical conditions and start an assessment of areas in which you may have strengths or gaps in knowledge.

Depending on your individual learning strengths and the areas needing improvement, two possible methods that may help you prepare for doing formative assessments, clinical practice, and writing the NCLEX-RN and NGN are to organize study material in 1) an organized table or 2) concept maps. Students learn best and remember content more effectively when information is presented in a manner congruent with their individual learning preferences (Brown et al., 2014). These two strategies often benefit many different types of learners. When studying for formative assessments or during preparation for NCLEX-RN and NGN, be sure to review the material and create individual study notes. The table and concept map are to be used for study notes, not for initial learning of the content. If any of your professors were to ask you to explain something on your study notes, such as what is a beta blocker, you could easily provide the information. This is also a way to highlight gaps in knowledge. It is important that all students prepare for NCLEX-RN and NGN case studies by learning, reviewing, and applying content and then practising with item examples and NGN-style case studies, such as the ones in this book. If you identify any gaps in knowledge while preparing and practising, make a note, in the margins of this book, on a separate piece of paper or digital file. You can return to this area for further review prior to writing the exam.

The Nursing Process Organized in a Table

If your mind works in a logical, streamlined, organized manner, then a table may be a great way to keep your thoughts and notes presented in linear fashion. This is for study purposes. Anything you put in this table would be a content area you could explain to another nurse or your teacher or provide in client teaching. Table 2.8 shows an example of the nursing process organized as a table with an introductory concept.

When using an introductory concept, such as hypertension, content can be distributed in smaller chunks of information, which can be easier to remember if the table strategy works for student learning. The nursing process applied to NCLEX-RN and NGN uses the acronym AAPIE: **A**ssessment, **A**nalysis, **P**lanning, **I**mplementation, and **E**valuation. Test writers are expected to use assessment information to determine medical conditions and then use this knowledge to think critically and make a judgement that would ensure safe delivery of care for clients. Table 2.8 illustrates how to

TABLE 2.8 Example of Nursing Process Organized as a Table With an Introductory Concept

Condition	Pathophysiology	Clinical Manifestations/ Assessment	Pharmacology/ Labs	Planning/ Implementation	Evaluation
Hypertension	Results from sustained increase in peripheral resistance; increases venous return and more volume back to the heart	Headache, high BP, vision changes, renal insufficiency, vascular occlusions, peripheral edema	• Beta blocker • ACE inhibitor • Diuretics • Adrenergic inhibitors • Vasodilators • Calcium channel blockers Labs: • Electrolytes (sodium, potassium, creatinine, BUN); troponin, BNP	• DASH diet • Weight reduction • Reduce alcohol consumption • Recommend exercise • Stress management	• Reduction in BP • Patient adherence • Improved feeling of health

ACE, Angiotensin-converting enzyme; *BP*, blood pressure; *BNP*, B-type natriuretic peptide; *BUN*, blood urea nitrogen; *DASH*, dietary approaches to stop hypertension.

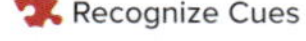 Recognize Cues 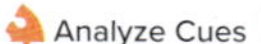 Analyze Cues Prioritize Hypothesis 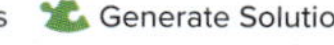 Generate Solutions 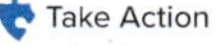 Take Action Evaluate Outcomes

organize content such that it aligns with the nursing process in a condensed manner. Knowledge of key concepts and studying are still required for learning curricular material. For example, students should be able to explain in great detail each of the medications administered to clients experiencing hypertension.

This table can be completed for all conditions. While it may involve extra work, this method of writing down information (particularly using hand-written notes) helps in retaining knowledge. To remain organized, document clinical manifestations in a head-to-toe manner. While in practice, and throughout your undergraduate nursing program, head-to-toe assessment was the standard manner. If you create study notes in the same pattern, the process of assessment, whether during an examination or in real time with a client, will become a habit, as will the cognitive steps necessary for analyzing this data. Be conscientious to **recognize patterns** in how each condition presents and then in specific treatment modalities. For example, Table 2.9 shows a sample table organization of the nursing process that allows comparison of two conditions, pulmonary embolus and pulmonary edema.

Pulmonary embolus and pulmonary edema indicate more concerning abnormal conditions for a client. Identifying and anticipating patterns of clinical presentation can assist the nurse to determine the most appropriate plan of care for the client and act safely and competently. When reviewing Table 2.9, notice how these two pulmonary conditions with differing pathophysiological changes have similar clinical presentation

TABLE 2.9 Sample Table Organization of Nursing Process for Comparison of Two Conditions

Condition	Pathophysiology	Clinical Manifestations/ Assessment	Pharmacology/ Labs	Planning/ Implementation	Evaluation
Pulmonary embolus (PE)	• Blockage of the pulmonary artery by a thrombus, fat, or air embolus, or tumour tissue • Most PEs result from a DVT (Virchow's Triad) or from the right side of the heart, especially as a result of AFib	Abnormal presentation: • **Dyspnea** • Chest pain • **Hemoptysis** • Pleural friction rub • Tachycardia Critical abnormal presentation: • Hypotension • Pallor • Severe dyspnea • Hypoxemia	• Fibrinolytic medications (tPA or alteplase) • Anticoagulation (heparin IV or LMWH) Labs: • PTT, PT, D-dimer, Hgb, platelets	• May require surgical intervention • Plan to take client for a spiral CT • May require oxygen therapy • Pain medication if needed • Promote activity	• Improved gas exchange • Improved respiratory status • Little to no pain with inspiration
Pulmonary edema	• Abnormal, life-threatening accumulation of fluid in the alveoli and interstitial spaces of the lungs • Caused by left ventricular failure secondary to acute myocardial infarction	• Anxiety • Pale to cyanotic • Skin is clammy and cold • Severe **dyspnea** • Orthopnea • Use of accessory muscles • Crackles, wheezes, or rhonchi in the lung fields • **Pink, frothy, blood-tinged sputum** • Tachycardia • Hypertension or hypotension • S3 (volume overload)	• Diuretic as long as blood pressure is within normal Labs: • Electrolytes (sodium, potassium, BNP, creatinine, BUN)	• May require oxygenation • Monitor urine output if given diuretics • Monitor fluid status • Monitor electrolyte imbalances	• Improved gas exchange • Reduction in crackles when auscultated • Less oxygen required • Less shortness of breath • Able to tolerate ambulation and increased mobility

Afib, Atrial fibrillation; *BNP*, B-type natriuretic peptide; *BUN*, blood urea nitrogen; *CT*, computed tomography; *DVT*, deep venous thrombosis; Hgb, hemoglobin; *IV*, intravenous; *LMWH*, low-molecular-weight heparin; *PT*, prothrombin time; *PTT*, partial thromboplastin time; *tPa*, tissue plasminogen activator.

characteristics; however, the diagnostic procedures, laboratory tests, pharmacology, and nursing interventions are uniquely different.

Both conditions can present with dyspnea and hemoptysis or pink, frothy sputum. Note what is different, though, too. A pulmonary embolus occurs as a result of a clot that has travelled to the lung, whereas pulmonary edema is an extension of left ventricular failure due to an acute myocardial infarction. Despite some similar clinical manifestations, the conditions are not the same. By knowing the patterns for each condition and what makes each condition unique when compared to another with similar clinical manifestations, you will be able to recognize the symptoms earlier and choose the correct pharmacological treatment, determine laboratory results to monitor, and identify correct nursing interventions. If you miss details in the narrative, for instance, that an S3 was auscultated during the cardiovascular assessment (if a narrative was provided, such as in an NGN case study), then the potential complication and condition would be pulmonary edema, and not pulmonary embolus. Students make errors when identifying the wrong condition, by not paying close attention to the patterns and proceeding with inappropriate or unsafe nursing actions. Each condition has unique characteristics that will present differently from other conditions.

A Concept Map

Another way to document this type of information is by creating a concept map. The use of a concept map can provide a structured, visual framework of the nursing process, which can help students identify priorities of care (Eisenmann, 2020). Some students find that the aesthetics of a concept map, through colour and organization, are more appealing and make it easier to remember the material. Students can also apply links between concepts and identify relationships between data. For example, when a client arrives at the hospital for assessment and the nurse notices a nitroglycerine patch on their previous medications, and the client is not actively presenting with acute myocardial infarction symptoms, the nurse can identify the relationship between nitroglycerine patches and left ventricular heart failure, likely due to previous coronary artery disease. There are many ways to create a concept map; find one that works for you. Fig. 2.2 shows a sample concept map for reference.

From your concept map, connections can be drawn, if needed, to reinforce relationship patterns. The sample concept map (see Fig. 2.2) uses different colours for each element of the nursing process. When creating concept maps, the use of consistent colours and placement of nursing process categories can facilitate memory recall. Retrieval of learning requires the brain to initially code or place importance on a piece of new material for short-term memory, then consolidate that learning for greater understanding. The repeated and consistent use of colours and spatial placement of the nursing process categories on a page will help provide an association between the material and visual cue. To retrieve that material at another time, the brain must have a retrieval cue (Brown et al., 2014). If material is displayed in a different format each time, the brain has an increasingly difficult time retrieving the information. Consider the structure of a head-to-toe assessment. This basic structure is the foundation for collecting subjective and objective information when caring for clients and their families. If the process of a head-to-toe assessment is repeated several times and in the same manner, the action of collecting the data becomes a habit. For visual learners, if the same colour is always used to represent clinical manifestations (for example), this provides a visual memory cue to remember content for that category of the nursing process.

Additional Strategies for Remembering Content

Once a student learns the **progression of an illness,** it becomes easier to remember data, how to apply the nursing process, and use clinical judgement for NGN case studies. By grouping the progression of similar conditions together, you will see the patterns easier. For example, let's take a look at pericarditis, pericardial effusion, and cardiac tamponade. A client who presents with pericarditis has the potential to develop pericardial effusion and even a cardiac tamponade (Fig. 2.3). Grouping the content together minimizes cognitive overload.

Upon review of content, the cause for a client developing pericarditis could be a viral illness or a condition idiopathic in nature that leads to inflammation of the pericardium.

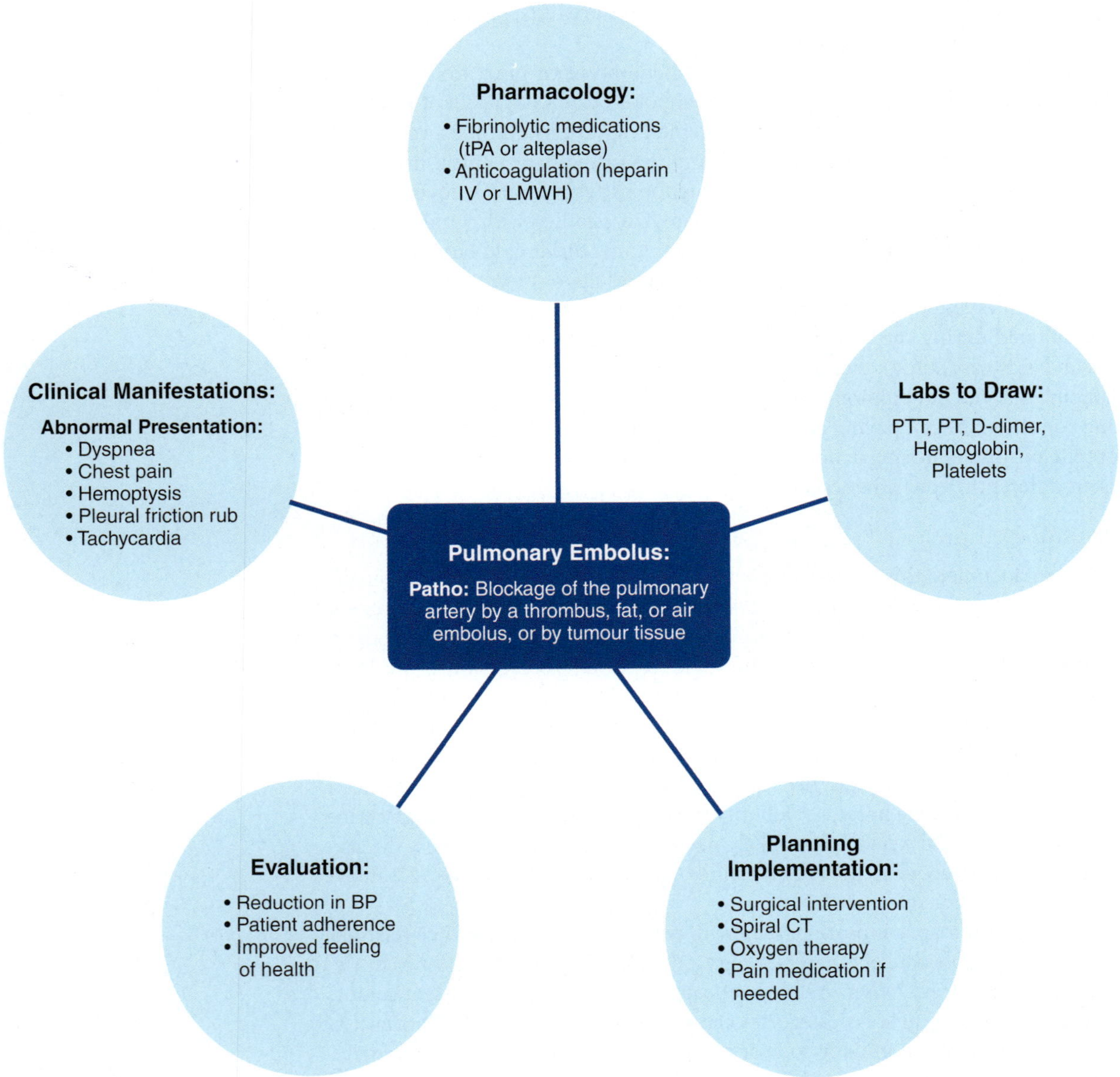

Pharmacology:
- Fibrinolytic medications (tPA or alteplase)
- Anticoagulation (heparin IV or LMWH)

Clinical Manifestations:

Abnormal Presentation:
- Dyspnea
- Chest pain
- Hemoptysis
- Pleural friction rub
- Tachycardia

Labs to Draw:

PTT, PT, D-dimer, Hemoglobin, Platelets

Pulmonary Embolus:

Patho: Blockage of the pulmonary artery by a thrombus, fat, or air embolus, or by tumour tissue

Evaluation:
- Reduction in BP
- Patient adherence
- Improved feeling of health

Planning Implementation:
- Surgical intervention
- Spiral CT
- Oxygen therapy
- Pain medication if needed

FIG. 2.2 Example of a Concept Map. *BP,* Blood pressure; *CT,* computed tomography; *IV*, intravenous; *LMWH,* low-molecular-weight heparin; *PT,* prothrombin time; *PTT,* partial thromboplastin time; *tPa,* tissue plasminogen activator.

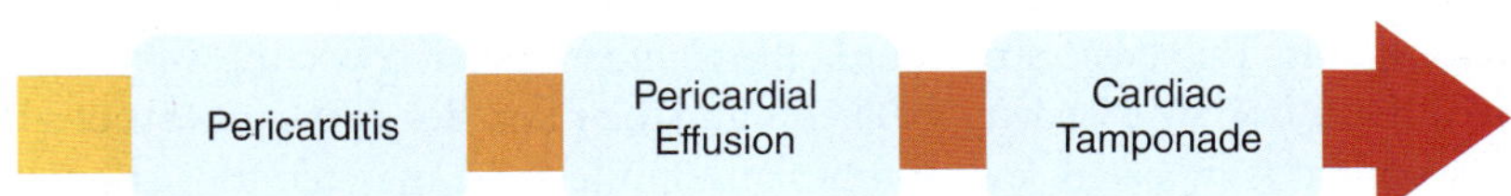

FIG. 2.3 Progression of an Illness Example.

Patterns of illness demonstrate the natural course of progression. Hope for the best possible outcome for clients while preparing for the worst possible outcome in the client situation.

The client who presents with pericarditis may exhibit a pericardial friction rub and complain of left wall chest pain. If the client begins to exhibit respiratory symptoms and impaired gas exchange, an effusion may be developing. Pericardial effusions can occur after a diagnosis of pericarditis leading to minimal hemodynamic compromise, but it is present enough to cause a change in client status. If enough fluid continues to develop in the pericardial sac, the final complication is a cardiac tamponade, resulting in the inability of the heart to have full diastolic stretch, impeding the amount of blood in the left ventricle, and reducing cardiac output and volume of oxygenated blood being delivered systemically. When you are writing down the clinical manifestations, start to recognize the **patterns associated with illness presentation**. Be prepared to identify treatment modalities and nursing interventions related to planning, implementation, and evaluation.

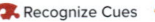

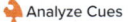

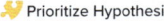

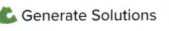

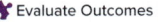

By developing this skill, it will prepare you to address multiple pieces of client data presented in an NGN case study. There may be similar clinical manifestations associated with a respiratory condition, such as dyspnea, which occur in almost all respiratory illnesses. By sifting through the data, you can acknowledge what is a normal clinical presentation as it relates to abnormal presentation, which will help signal a specific condition. From here, you can recognize if the client remains in an abnormal clinical presentation or has progressed to a critical abnormal presentation. These exercises will help you become better prepared when answering multiple-choice and alternate-format questions as well as NGN case studies. There are no shortcuts to answering NGN item types. By learning the content and applying your knowledge, you will have greater success with exhibiting clinical judgement for the NCLEX-RN and, most importantly, with your clients and families in practice.

Acknowledging **patterns in thinking** will help you remember content as well. We have already used the pulmonary embolus and pulmonary edema as an example, but there are other ways to apply patterns of knowledge.

Patterns in thinking help collate information together, which can help create memory cues.

For example, certain conditions have factors that are present either as a cause or as an expression of the condition. These help with remembering large volumes of content. For example, deep vein thrombosis is associated with *Virchow's triad* (intravascular wall damage, status of blood flow, and a hypercoagulable state); *Cushing's triad* (bradycardia, irregular respirations, and a widened pulse pressure) involves clinical manifestations that are present during the development of increased intracranial pressure; complications associated with hypocalcemia can be remembered by the acronym *CATS* (convulsions, arrhythmias, tetany, and stridor). These are just a few memory tricks to help with identifying conditions. Developing strategies to apply when deciding on treatment can also be created to help minimize cognitive overload.

Conclusion

This chapter is meant to remind you how much knowledge you possess while also providing quick references for areas you may have forgotten. By remembering key concepts, such as normal assessment data, and identifying abnormal and critical abnormal assessment data, you can apply this information to medical conditions when in practice or during your preparation to write the licensure examination. Only a small list of common medical conditions, similar to what you may encounter in clinical practice, are provided in this book. Add to the list if any conditions were missed. Learning strategies to assist with memory retention and retrieval is important when writing the licensure exam. An excellent resource for further practice with multiple-choice and alternate-format questions is *Elsevier's Canadian Comprehensive Review for the NCLEX-RN® Examination,* Third Edition.

Chapter 3 breaks down the NCJMM, focusing on recognizing cues, analyzing cues, and prioritizing a hypothesis, and provides strategies for further applying your knowledge. Chapter 4 will follow the same pattern of breaking down the NCJMM but will focus on generating solutions, taking actions, and evaluating outcomes. You will develop skills to use knowledge about assessment data as the data pertain to medical conditions, utilizing the structure of the nursing process as a foundation for applying elevated cognitive thinking for clinical judgement and NGN case studies.

3 What Is Happening With the Client: Recognize Cues, Analyze Cues, Prioritize Hypothesis

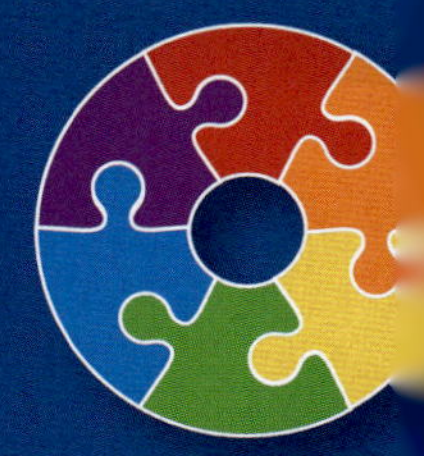

Clinical judgement requires the nurse to first identify a client's health problem correctly before determining the next steps. The first three steps of the NCJMM are intended to test a student's ability to recognize patterns in the client presentation, review those patterns, and then make a hypothesis about the possible condition or the highest risk the client could be experiencing. This chapter breaks down each of these first three steps required for clinical judgement so you will be better prepared to apply your own knowledge to NGN case studies and in clinical practice.

You may be asking, why group these three cognitive steps together? While each step is distinct, they are interconnected, which is why they are presented together in this chapter. As a nurse, you need to cognitively integrate these three steps, and throughout your program, you have developed the skills to do so effectively. Although the NCJMM identifies these items as separate entities, just as the nursing process separates assessment from diagnosis/analysis and diagnosis/analysis from planning, and so on, they are all connected in determining the health problem and the potential treatment necessary to care for the client. As you move through this chapter, with examples provided, ask yourself the following questions:

Recognize Cues	Analyze Cues	Prioritize Hypothesis
• Based on details of the story and clinical presentation of the client, what assessment information would be classified as *normal* or *abnormal?* • Could any assessment data be classified as *critical abnormal*? • What *patterns* of illness or clues (like a puzzle piece or an Easter egg) are present?	• What is the relationship between the *pieces* of information? • What patterns do you see? • What system is most affected? • What pieces of their clinical presentation could help determine the presenting issue or medical condition?	• How does each piece of data *fit together* to identify a specific condition? • What medical condition could the client be at risk for developing? • What possible complications of that medical condition might the client develop?

Recognize Cues

This is where you start to put the pieces of the puzzle together.

When a client seeks out a health care provider for further assessment, they will often provide **objective** and **subjective** data. Over time, the nurse develops observational skills to also assess the client's behaviour, mannerisms and overall safety of the situation. Whether listening, conducting a physical assessment, or observing the client, the nurse needs to recognize that all details are a part of the client's story/clinical presentaiton. Each detail given by the client or that the nurse discovers through assessment, is a puzzle piece the nurse puts together in order to provide safe and competent care for the client and their family. This is where your understanding of conditions and patterns of illness helps in highlighting details in the client's story that deviates from normal clinical assessment and presentation. Use the tables in Chapter 2 to support you while you develop and strengthen this skill. It is the first step toward clinical judgement.

You have been developing this skill since the start of your undergraduate nursing program. Nursing program curricula are designed to scaffold information, layering on more and more pieces of information from the time you entered the program through to graduation. For example, prior to entering a client's room for clinical assessment, you would consider what constitutes normal assessment data, such as a heart rate and characteristics of the pulse and recognize any deviation from normal.

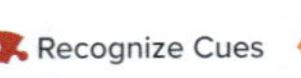
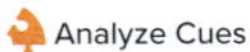
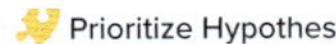
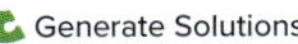
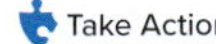
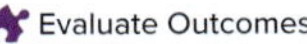

Normal Assessment:

- HR = 60–100 beats per minute
- RR = 12–18 breaths per minute
- Pulse regular with palpation and normal in strength of sensation
- Skin warm and dry to the touch
- No jugular venous distension was noted

All assessments are compared to normal assessment data first when determining baseline status. This is what you will base your heart rate and pulse assessment on when you are with your client.

A client will not typically seek additional medical care from health care providers unless there is a change from their baseline and normal clinical presentation. Now, you may consider that not all emergencies are real emergencies, and you would be correct; however, they are a deviation from the normal client presentation that is enough to concern the client. It is up to the health care provider to determine if the complaint is serious enough for hospital admission or further follow-up care. For example, the client who presents with nausea may be a newly pregnant person who has not eaten enough nutritionally dense food for days and may be becoming dehydrated and nutritionally depleted, leading to compromise for themselves and the fetus. The client may be able to manage their nausea at home.

Developing a skill set to recognize the abnormal presentation from the normal presentation is imperative for doing NGN case studies and clinical practice.

Example 1: Recognize Cues

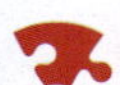

EXAMPLE 1 Recognize Cues

The nurse is caring for a client in the emergency department.

1000h: The client falls with query broken femur bone. They complain of pain and become notably anxious.

- HR = 110
- RR = 20
- Regular pulse with radial palpation but bounding
- Skin warm and dry but flushed
- No jugular venous distension was noted

Consider the client presentation in the brief clinical scenario in Example 1. Identify what could be classified as abnormal assessment data. Write your answers in the space provided. (Answers to each question can be found at the end of the chapter.)

Example 1 Answer

____

____

____

____

Throughout this chapter, the brief clinical scenario in Example 1 will be used as a foundation to explain the "how-to" for the three cognitive steps: Recognize Cues, Analyze Cues, and Prioritize Hypothesis.

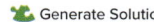

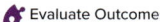

Examples of NCJMM Questions Related to Recognize Cues

To answer these questions correctly, writers must decipher which data from the clinical scenario (classified by the test writer as normal, abnormal, or critical abnormal assessment data) are **most important** and require **prompt attention**. In all questions, writers will be provided more answers to select from for choosing the correct answer than are correct.

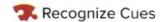

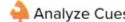

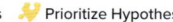

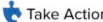

Typical or common ways students may be asked to Recognize Cues in NGN case studies are as follows:

▶ Drag the top 3 clinical client findings that would require **immediate** follow-up to the box on the right.

CLIENT FINDINGS
Heart rate
Respiratory rate
Pulse
Skin
Jugular venous distension

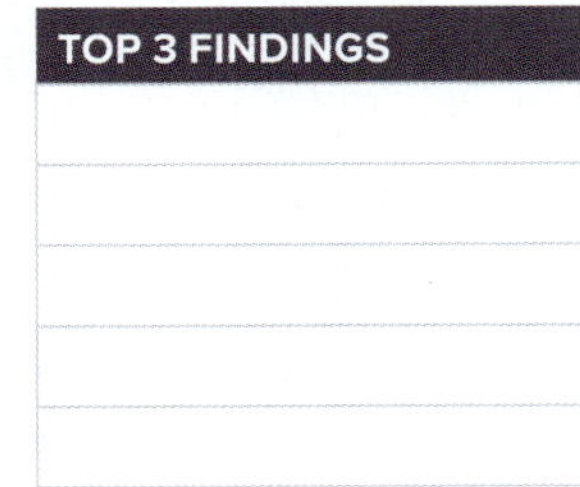

To answer this question, students would identify the top three priority client findings from a list of data that could be found in the client scenario and then drag the data from the left table to the right table. For the purposes of this textbook, the same question will be asked, but instead will use the phrase, "Identify the top 3 clinical client findings that would require follow-up."

▶ Which of the following findings require **immediate** follow-up? **Select all that apply.**

☐ Heart rate
☐ Respiratory rate
☐ Pulse
☐ Skin
☐ Jugular venous distension

▶ Select three client findings that require **immediate** follow-up.

☐ Heart rate
☐ Respiratory rate
☐ Pulse
☐ Skin
☐ Jugular venous distension

The second and third questions require you to have knowledge about what would require you to investigate further. Consider with NGN case studies, extraneous information will be presented. This means you need to identify what catches your attention and provide this immediate follow-up. Immediate means now; it does not mean you can engage in another activity and tend to it later.

▶ Highlight the findings that require **immediate** attention. **Select all that apply.**

> The client falls with query broken femur bone. They complain of pain and become notably anxious.
>
> - HR = 110
> - RR = 20
> - Regular pulse with radial palpation but bounding
> - Skin warm and dry but flushed
> - No jugular venous distension noted

To answer this type of question, test writers highlight the highest priority data directly in the question. It is crucial to be specific and particular about what pieces of data are most important for the care of the client. This clinical scenario is brief, with minimal external and individual factors to consider or other clinical data, such as NEURO, RESP, RENAL, etc. This example only focuses on a small amount of client data pertaining to the cardiovascular system. As you proceed through this textbook, the complexity of the scenarios will increase, just as in real-life practice.

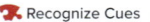

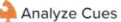

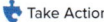

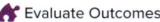

TABLE 3.1 Anticipating Client Compromise Examples

Medical Condition	Potential Complication	Potential Critical Client Deterioration
Traumatic head injury	Increased intracranial pressure	Seizures, airway compromise, strokes, etc.
Hyperthyroidism	Thyroid storm or thyrotoxicosis	Hemodynamic compromise (tachycardia, reduced cardiac output), confusion, delirium, heart failure
Hypothyroidism	Myxedema coma	Confusion, hypotension, paralytic ileus, hypoventilation leading to respiratory distress and requiring intubation

Analyze Cues

Moving to the next cognitive step of the NCJMM, you will use the information ascertained from the initial client clinical presentation to consider complications the client may develop. You are anticipating the presentation of critical abnormal assessment data and will identify any potential conditions that may develop as a result of client compromise. Recall in Chapter 2, the conditions were grouped together using pericarditis, pericardial tamponade, and cardiac tamponade as the example of how to anticipate client deterioration. This process can be done with almost every medical condition. Table 3.1 shows three examples of how to anticipate potential client complications and potential critical client deterioration.

Example 2: Analyze Cues

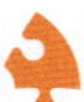

EXAMPLE 2 Analyze Cues

The nurse is caring for a client in the emergency department.

1000h: The client falls with query broken femur bone. They complain of pain and become notably anxious.

- HR = 110
- RR = 20
- Regular pulse with radial palpation but bounding
- Skin warm and dry but flushed
- No jugular venous distension noted

1130h: The client develops shortness of breath, chest pain with inspiration, use of accessory muscles, nasal flaring, and blood-tinged sputum.

- HR = 130
- RR = 28
- Jugular venous distension measured at 7 cm

The above information represents only a few examples. If the information in the table is new for you, review your undergraduate pathophysiology and assessment notes from class. Anticipating a worst-case scenario is a common nursing skill set used to prevent potential complications and harm for your clients. It is at this cognitive step where you will group pieces of assessment data together to identify relationships.

New information has been documented in the above clinical scenario. The client's condition has deteriorated. When considering the client's change in status, would this still be considered abnormal assessment data, or has the client's status progressed to a more critical presentation? What, if any, possible complications do you think could happen with this client? Do you see any relationships between the data? Write your answers in the space provided. (Answers can be found at the end of the chapter.)

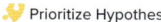

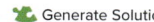

Example 2 Answer

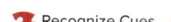

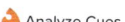

To answer these questions correctly, writers must decipher from data the patterns of illness and progression of the client's status. There has been a change in client presentation, from abnormal to now critical abnormal assessment data. It is imperative to identify the system that is compromised as well as potential complications for the client. There will be **clues** in the clinical scenario based on the assessment data and the story associated with clinical presentation, which will help you identify the most likely medical condition or what the client could be at highest risk to develop. You are collecting the pieces to the puzzle and trying to put them together. In all questions, test writers will be provided multiple answers from which to choose the correct answer.

Common ways students may be asked to Analyze Cues in NGN case studies are as follows:

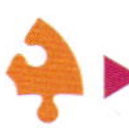

▶ For each client finding, identify if the finding is consistent with the disease process of acute myocardial infarction, pulmonary embolus, or pneumothorax. Each finding may support more than 1 disease process.

CLIENT FINDINGS	ACUTE MYOCARDIAL INFARCTION	PULMONARY EMBOLUS	PNEUMOTHORAX
Shortness of breath	○	○	○
Chest pain with inspiration	○	○	○
Work of breathing	○	○	○
Hemoptysis	○	○	○
Tachycardia	○	○	○
Tachypnea	○	○	○
Jugular venous distension	○	○	○

When answering these types of questions, you must consider if the client data presented in the clinical scenario are related to the clinical manifestations associated with specific medical conditions. The intent is to sift through all the assessment data in order to determine the primary client condition or health problem. To best answer these types of questions, focus on one medical condition at a time. For example, is shortness of breath associated with an acute myocardial infarction? Is chest pain associated with an acute myocardial infarction? Proceed in this way for the acute myocardial infarction column, covering up the pulmonary embolus and pneumothorax columns. Then continue, asking the same questions, by covering up the acute myocardial infarction column and the pneumothorax columns, focusing only on the pulmonary embolus column. Complete this question by covering up the acute myocardial infarction and pulmonary embolus columns and determining if the client findings relate to a pneumothorax. Be thoughtful and specific as to which client findings match which condition.

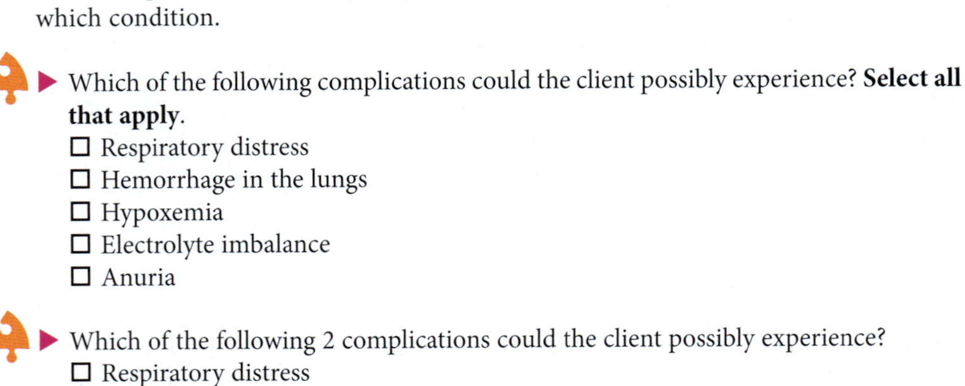

▶ Which of the following complications could the client possibly experience? **Select all that apply**.

- ☐ Respiratory distress
- ☐ Hemorrhage in the lungs
- ☐ Hypoxemia
- ☐ Electrolyte imbalance
- ☐ Anuria

▶ Which of the following 2 complications could the client possibly experience?

- ☐ Respiratory distress
- ☐ Hemorrhage in the lungs
- ☐ Hypoxemia

- ☐ Electrolyte imbalance
- ☐ Anuria

When answering these two types of questions, you will collate together the most pertinent assessment data to anticipate potential complications. Recognizing the patterns as presented by the clinical scenario will help you determine the clinical problem and the complications that would be associated with the condition. Knowledge of patterns of illness progression will help you determine the complications. For example, if a client has increased work of breathing by using their accessory muscles, then a very likely complication would be respiratory distress. This is a critical abnormal assessment piece of data indicating that the client's condition could worsen.

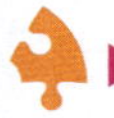

▶ Drag (Identify for the purposes of this textbook) the correct word option from the table to fill in the blank.

The nurse should recognize the client is potentially experiencing _____________ and __________________.

WORD OPTIONS
Respiratory distress
Hemorrhage in the lungs
Hypoxemia
Electrolyte imbalance
Anuria

In fill-in-the-blank questions the writer is asked to use answers from either one column of word options or two columns, where each blank space corresponds to the appropriate column. In the above example, both answers are taken from the list in one column. Answering this type of question pertains to recognizing the potential complications associated with the client presentation.

Prioritize Hypothesis

In order to determine the most probable potential condition the client may be experiencing or what may be the highest risk for the client, you will begin to assemble the puzzle pieces together: Recognize Cues + Analyze Cues = Prioritize Hypothesis. This is where you determine the **highest priority** for the client by addressing the clues presented through the client's subjective and objective data, as well as the additional contextual information presented in the clinical scenario. When determining the highest priority for a condition, consider the **"Easter eggs"** or **specific clues** that are unique and specific to conditions. For example, if the nurse palpates an irregular pulse, the most likely dysrhythmia that contributes to this clinical manifestation would be atrial fibrillation or atrial flutter. If that same nurse palpates an irregular pulse and the client is experiencing confusion or dizziness but is able to speak, the most likely dysrhythmia would be several premature ventricular contractions in a row, contributing to reduced cardiac output. If the client is found unresponsive, then the most likely dysrhythmia would be ventricular tachycardia.

Determining the potential condition occurs in clinical practice often. Putting together the pieces of a clinical situation is what propels the nurse to contact the health care provider, to inform of the change in client status and receive orders. For example, let's say you are caring for a client who has a history of acute myocardial infarction, a percutaneous coronary intervention to their left anterior descending coronary artery, and an ejection fraction of 33%. The client develops shortness of breath with audible coarse crackles (a critical abnormal assessment that is compromising airway). You have learned about left ventricular failure leading to pulmonary edema. This requires you to contact the health care provider. In this scenario, you considered the clinical presentation, prioritized the hypothesis as likely pulmonary edema, and anticipated potential treatment options (this scenario will be continued in Chapter 4).

Example 3: Prioritize Hypothesis

EXAMPLE 3 Prioritize Hypothesis

The nurse is caring for a client in the emergency department.

1000h: The client falls with query broken femur bone. They complain of pain and become notably anxious.

- HR = 110
- RR = 20
- Regular pulse with radial palpation but bounding
- Skin warm and dry but flushed
- No jugular venous distension noted

1130h: The client develops shortness of breath, chest pain with inspiration, use of accessory muscles, nasal flaring, and blood-tinged sputum.

- HR = 130
- RR = 28
- Jugular venous distension measured at 7 cm

Continuing with the current clinical scenario, what do you think is the most likely condition this client is experiencing? Write down your answer here along with any clues you found.

Example 3 Answer

____

____

____

____

Common ways students may be asked to Prioritize Hypothesis in NGN case studies are as follows:

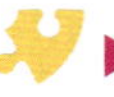

▶ Complete the following sentence by choosing from the list of options.

The client is at **highest risk** of developing ________________.

WORD OPTIONS
Acute myocardial infarction
Pulmonary edema
Pulmonary embolus
Sepsis
Pneumonia
Heart failure

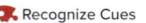

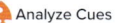

OR

▶ The nurse recognizes that the client is **most** likely experiencing __________.

WORD OPTIONS
An acute myocardial infarction
Pulmonary edema
Pulmonary embolus
Sepsis
Pneumonia
Heart failure

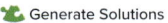

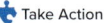

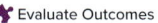

This fill-in-the blank question asks the writer to use knowledge to determine the most probable medical condition based on the abnormal and critical abnormal assessment data. If students are unable to make connections or determine relationships between objective, subjective, and pertinent contextual information and thus choose the incorrect condition, then in any case studies that require the test writer to determine the next steps, all remaining actions chosen will be incorrect. In clinical practice, this is where errors occur, with the potential to cause harm to clients.

▶ The nurse should **first** address the client's ________________.

WORD OPTIONS
Respiratory status
Cardiovascular status
Gastrointestinal status
Pain
Cognitive status
Anxiety

This is another fill-in-the blank type of question that assesses the writer's ability to determine what requires their highest priority or attention. Often, students find these types of questions challenging as there are several priorities and choosing one is difficult. In each question, one body system will be at greatest risk for compromise, causing client decompensation. Start with airway, breathing, and circulation and determine if any of these body systems (respiratory or cardiovascular) is impaired. If none of these three manifestations are associated with the clinical scenario, then determine if cognition or consciousness (neurological) is affected. The two remaining systems are the renal system, which would be closely aligned with cardiovascular status changes, and the gastrointestinal system. If the question pertains to mental health considerations, safety is always the highest priority, whether it is for the client or for others who may be associated with the client.

▶ Identify 2 **priorities** the nurse would address.

- ☐ Respiratory status
- ☐ Cardiovascular status
- ☐ Gastrointestinal status
- ☐ Pain
- ☐ Cognitive Status
- ☐ Anxiety

This type of question allows for a more realistic assessment of competing priorities. Often there is more than one priority that the nurse must attend to with a client.

▶ Select 4 complications the client is at **highest risk** of developing.

- ☐ Pulmonary hypertension
- ☐ Electrolyte imbalance
- ☐ Left-sided heart failure
- ☐ Right-sided heart failure
- ☐ Peripheral edema
- ☐ Syncope

To answer this type of question, the test writer would have to determine what the potential condition may be prior to identifying potential complications of that condition. This type of "complication" question and the type of "complication" question found in Analyze Cues are similar, yet different. In Analyze Cues complication questions, the writer must determine what the client may be at risk for prior to identifying the medical condition. In Prioritize Hypothesis, the writer must already know what the potential condition is without being asked to identify it, and then determine complications as a result of that condition.

How to Successfully Answer Recognize Cues, Analyze Cues, and Prioritize Hypotheses Questions

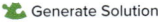

The best strategy for answering these types of questions is:

- Applying sound knowledge of anatomy and physiology
- Determining if the assessment data fall into normal, abnormal, or critical abnormal assessment data
- Understanding basic and advanced pathophysiology to anticipate potential complications prior to acknowledging the medical condition OR identifying complications of the medical condition
- Addressing priority manifestations of airway, breathing, and circulation followed by addressing the body systems according to the clinical scenario
- Recognizing the patterns of words highlighted in the question to know if it is a **Recognize Cues** (requires immediate attention), **Analyze Cues** (patterns of illness and possible conditions and complications to consider), or **Prioritize Hypothesis** (determine priority medical condition or complication of that medical condition)

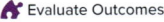

Conclusion

This chapter demonstrates how to group together the three cognitive steps of Recognize Cues, Analyze Cues, and Prioritize Hypothesis in ways that can help you determine a medical condition or complications of that medical condition. By breaking down each cognitive step into more digestible chunks, you can begin to apply your knowledge to the NGN case studies. If you determine you have knowledge gaps, then return back to your notes and strengthen your understanding of anatomy and physiology, pathophysiology, and assessment. Understanding how the body works helps in determining client status. Putting the pieces of the clinical client puzzle together with evidence to support your knowledge allows for safer practice. Fig. 3.1 provides a visualization of the scaffolding of information you may have encountered in your nursing programs. Building on this concept, Chapters 4 to 6 will further expand the step-by-step cognitive processing necessary to apply nursing knowledge to NGN case study questions.

All answers to the questions can be found at the end of the chapter.

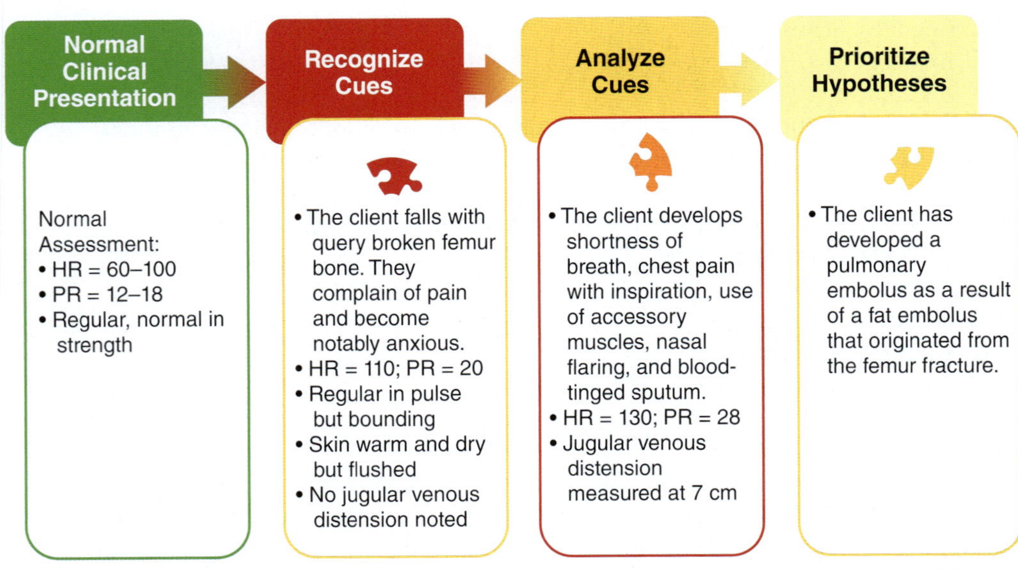

FIG. 3.1 Breaking down Recognize Cues, Analyze Cues, and Prioritize Hypothesis in a simple unfolding clinical scenario.

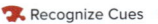

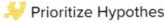

Answers to Typical or Common Questions

Answers to Example 1: Recognize Cues

▶ Drag the top 3 clinical client findings that would require **immediate** follow-up to the box on the right.

TOP 3 FINDINGS
Heart rate
Pulse
Skin

▶ Which of the following findings require **immediate** follow-up? **Select all that apply.**

✔ Heart rate
☐ Respiratory rate
✔ Pulse
✔ Skin
☐ Jugular venous distension

▶ Select 3 client findings that require **immediate** follow-up.

✔ Heart rate
☐ Respiratory rate
✔ Pulse
✔ Skin
☐ Jugular venous distension

▶ Highlight the findings that require **immediate** attention. **Select all that apply.**

> The client falls with query broken femur bone. They complain of pain and become notably anxious.
> - HR = 110
> - RR = 20
> - Regular pulse with radial palpation but bounding
> - Skin warm and dry but flushed
> - No jugular venous distension noted

Answer: The top three client findings are heart rate, pulse, and skin.

Rationale: The heart rate indicates an abnormal rate at 110 beats per minute. This is a deviation from normal, which is 60 to 100 beats per minute. Any rate above 100 is classified as tachycardia, any rate below 60 is classified as bradycardia. The pulse presents as regular (normal assessment data) but is bounding. Although this is a positive abnormal deviation, recognition of a bounding pulse may precede complications (e.g., anxiety attack, fever, pain, etc.) and should be identified as a top finding. Skin is noted to be flushed, indicating a hyperdynamic cardiovascular state. Although this could be a response to the pain, flushed skin could precede complications such as acute myocardial infarction, spinal cord injuries, respiratory conditions. The respiratory rate is 20 breaths per minute; however, this is assessment data to be monitored as it sits at the high end of normal. There is no jugular venous distension acknowledged.

NCJMM Step: Recognize Cues
References: Jarvis et al. (2024), pp. 457–501 (thorax and lungs), pp. 503–547 (heart and neck vessels); Tyerman & Cobbett (2023), pp. 751–772; Power-Kean et al. (2023), pp. 551–578.

Answers to Example 2: Analyze Cues

▶ For each client finding, identify if the finding is consistent with the disease process of acute myocardial infarction, pulmonary embolus, or pneumothorax. Each finding may support more than one disease process.

CLIENT FINDINGS	ACUTE MYOCARDIAL INFARCTION	PULMONARY EMBOLUS	PNEUMOTHORAX
Shortness of breath	✔	✔	✔
Chest pain with inspiration	○	✔	○
Work of breathing	○	✔	✔
Hemoptysis	○	✔	○
Tachycardia	○	✔	✔
Tachypnea	✔	✔	✔
Jugular venous distension	✔	✔	○

Rationale: Acute myocardial infarction (AMI) presents with shortness of breath, tachypnea, and jugular venous distension if there is a right-sided heart problem (inferior myocardial infarction). Chest pain occurs at rest, with exertion, and in the middle of the night. It is not isolated to inspiration only. Although chest pain is a classic hallmark clinical manifestation of an AMI, careful attention to the details is necessary to answer this question correctly. Hemoptysis is not a clinical manifestation associated with AMI. Clients typically present with hypotension, which may result with tachycardia. With the clinical scenario presented, no blood pressure was provided and therefore not needed to answer this question. Given the nature of a brief clinical scenario, all client findings indicative of a pulmonary embolus are included here. Typically, in these questions, not all answers would be correct. This is only an exercise and more opportunities to answer questions like this can be found in subsequent chapters of this textbook. Client findings from the brief scenario that can be found in a pneumothorax are only respiratory manifestations, such as shortness of breath, increased work of breathing, and tachypnea. Tachycardia would accompany difficult breathing. Chest pain with inspiration would not be associated with a pneumothorax, but pleuritic pain may be associated with this condition. The description of chest pain would be pleuritic so involves the wall of the pleura, is sharp and severe, and radiates. Jugular venous distension would not be associated with a pneumothorax, two different locations in the thorax.

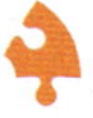

NCJMM Step: Analyze Cues
References: Tyerman & Cobbett (2023), pp. 610–613 (pneumothorax), pp. 622–624 (pulmonary embolus), pp. 796–827 (acute myocardial infarction); Power-Kean et al. (2023), pp. 601–606 (myocardial infarction), p. 624 (pneumothorax), p. 692 (pulmonary embolus).

▶ Which of the following complications could the client possibly experience? **Select all that apply.**

✔ Respiratory distress
☐ Hemorrhage in the lungs
✔ Hypoxemia
☐ Electrolyte imbalance
☐ Anuria

OR

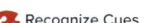

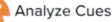

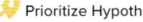

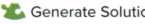

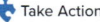

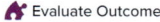

▶ Which of the following 2 complications could the client possibly experience?

- ✔ Respiratory distress
- ☐ Hemorrhage in the lungs
- ✔ Hypoxemia
- ☐ Electrolyte imbalance
- ☐ Anuria

OR

▶ Drag (Identify for the purposes of this textbook) the correct word option from the table to fill in the blank.

The nurse should recognize that the client is potentially experiencing **respiratory distress** and **hypoxemia**.

Rationale: Anticipating respiratory complications would be most pertinent for this client, such as respiratory distress of hypoxemia. There is already increased work of breathing as evidenced by the use of accessory muscles, and the hemoptysis would impede gas exchange, leading to hypoxemia. There may be bleeding in the lungs, but hemorrhaging and a situation where the client continues to bleed represent a critical, extreme situation and would likely occur in the Intensive Care Unit. This client is only in emergency and the clinical presentation does not indicate hemorrhage in the lungs. This is not a cardiac condition; therefore, an electrolyte imbalance would be a rare complication. Finally, anuria would not be associated with a pulmonary embolus at the time of this clinical presentation. Remember, these complications are to identify the medical condition.

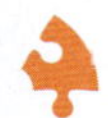

NCJMM Step: Analyze Cues
References: Tyerman & Cobbett (2023), pp. 622–624; Power-Kean et al. (2023), p. 692.

Answers to Example 3: Prioritize Hypothesis

▶ Complete the following sentence by choosing from the list of options.

The client is at **highest risk** of developing **pulmonary embolus**.

OR

▶ The nurse recognizes that the client is **most** likely experiencing **pulmonary embolus**.

Rationale: Based on the critical assessment data in the clinical scenario and contextual information of a femur fracture, the clinical manifestations are a result of a fat embolus travelling from the femur bone. A femur fracture has a high incidence of a fat embolus forming with the outcome of a pulmonary embolus. The clinical manifestations and contextual information do not align with any of the other conditions.

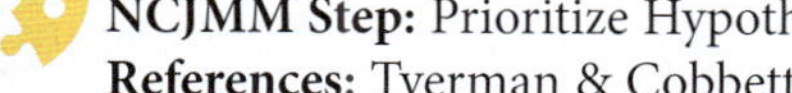

NCJMM Step: Prioritize Hypothesis
References: Tyerman & Cobbett (2023), pp. 622–624; Power-Kean et al. (2023), p. 692.

▶ The nurse should **first** address the client's **respiratory status**.

Rationale: Based on the critical assessment data in the clinical scenario and contextual information of a femur fracture, the clinical manifestations are a result of a fat embolus travelling from the femur bone. A femur fracture has a high incidence of a fat embolus forming with the outcome of a pulmonary embolus. The clinical manifestations and contextual information do not align with other priorities, as only one is requested. The client is presenting with increased work of breathing; therefore, from the critical priority list, airway and breathing (respiratory system) trumps any other options.

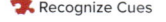

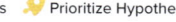

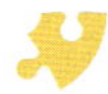
NCJMM Step: Prioritize Hypothesis
References: Tyerman & Cobbett (2023), pp. 622–624; Power-Kean et al. (2023), p. 692.

▶ Identify 2 **priorities** the nurse would address.
- ✔ Respiratory status
- ✔ Cardiovascular status
- ☐ Gastrointestinal status
- ☐ Pain
- ☐ Cognitive status
- ☐ Anxiety

Rationale: Based on the critical assessment data in the clinical scenario and contextual information of a femur fracture, the clinical manifestations are a result of a fat embolus travelling from the femur bone. A femur fracture has a high incidence of a fat embolus forming with the outcome of a pulmonary embolus. The clinical manifestations and contextual information do not align with only two, respiratory and cardiovascular status. The client is presenting with increased work of breathing; therefore, from the critical priority list, airway and breathing (respiratory system) and circulation (cardiovascular) are the immediate priorities. The other priorities are not immediate.

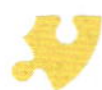
NCJMM Step: Prioritize Hypothesis
References: Tyerman & Cobbett (2023), pp. 622–624; Power-Kean et al. (2023), p. 692.

▶ Select 4 **complications** the client is at highest risk of developing.
- ✔ Pulmonary hypertension
- ☐ Electrolyte imbalance
- ☐ Left-sided heart failure
- ✔ Right-sided heart failure
- ✔ Peripheral edema
- ✔ Syncope

Rationale: Based on the critical assessment data in the clinical scenario and contextual information of a femur fracture, the clinical manifestations are a result of a fat embolus travelling from the femur bone. A femur fracture has a high incidence of a fat embolus forming with the outcome of a pulmonary embolus. Considering that the client is experiencing a pulmonary embolus, complications of this condition affect the right side of the heart, leading to pulmonary hypertension, right-sided heart failure, peripheral edema, and syncope as a result of impaired gas exchange and less cardiac output being pumped into the systemic system. Electrolyte imbalance and left-sided heart failure would not occur.

NCJMM Step: Prioritize Hypothesis
References: Tyerman & Cobbett (2023), pp. 622–624; Power-Kean et al. (2023), p. 692.

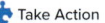

4 Next Steps When Caring for the Client: Generate Solutions, Take Action, Evaluate Outcomes

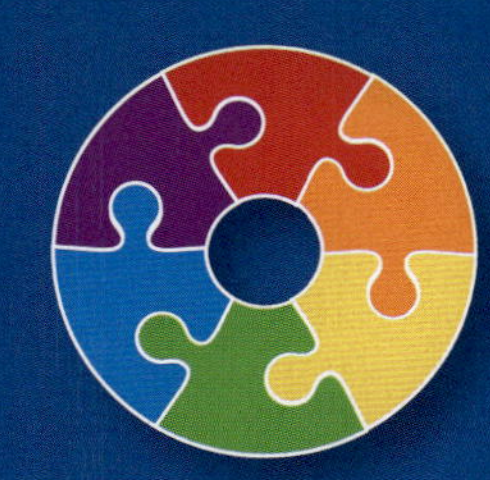

After you have identified the medical problem or the complication the client would be at highest risk of developing based on that identified medical problem, the next steps are planning for care, implementing that plan, and, finally, evaluating the plan to determine the client's overall status. It is important to consider possible nursing interventions, orders, laboratory tests, medications, or even diagnostic procedures associated with the medical problem or complication from the medical problem, then recognize how the interventions and tests affected the client. This chapter will break down each of the final three cognitive steps required for clinical judgement. Knowledge about how to care for clients and then implementing that knowledge is the practice of nurses. It is putting all the pieces of the puzzle together.

In this chapter, the final three cognitive steps are grouped together in the same way as the first three cognitive steps of the NCJMM were grouped in Chapter 3. The final half of the cognitive steps of the NCJMM, Generate Solutions, Take Action, and Evaluate Outcomes, also exist as separate entities and in relationship to one another. As you move through this chapter with the examples provided, ask yourself the following questions:

Generate Solutions	Take Action	Evaluate Outcomes
• What do I need to consider when creating a *plan of care* for this client? • Consider possible nursing or medical interventions such as laboratory tests, diagnostic procedures or tests, any potential orders the health care provider may order for the client's medical condition or complication. • This stage of the NCJMM is the **anticipatory** phase.	• Based on the clinical presentation of the client, what *actions* do I need to implement when addressing the client's highest need? • This stage of the NCJMM is the **doing** phase of the NCJMM.	• Based on the actions, as they relate to the client's medical problem or complication of that medical problem, what is the client's *overall status*; has it improved or declined or is there no change in status? • This stage of the NCJMM is the **reassessment** phase.

Generate Solutions

Once the most probable or likely condition the client is at highest risk of developing, including a complication, you will begin anticipating and planning care for the client. You cannot anticipate or plan care if you cannot determine the correct medical condition. Throughout the case study questions, distractors will often be present that are aligned with an incorrect hypothesis of what is happening with the client. For example, for a client who has been admitted to the hospital for observation after suffering a crushing leg injury, clinical manifestations listed include the client begins to develop edema in the affected limb, loses the pulse distal to the injury, capillary refill becomes greater than 3 seconds, and the affected extremity becomes warm to touch. The nurse may be contemplating whether these clinical manifestations are related to the development of a deep vein thrombosis with all elements of Virchow's triad present (venous stasis, endothelial damage, and hypercoagulability) or compartment syndrome. When planning care for these two possible medical conditions, administration of an anticoagulant in response to a deep vein thrombosis would be warranted but could exacerbate any bleeding if the client actually has developed compartment syndrome. Determining the correct next steps for your client ensures that you are providing safe and competent care.

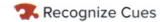

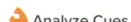

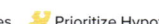

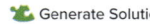

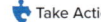

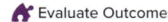

Example 4: Generate Solutions

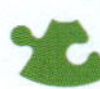

EXAMPLE 4 Generate Solutions

The nurse is caring for a client in the emergency department.

1000h: The client falls with query broken femur bone. They complain of pain and become notably anxious.

- HR = 110
- RR = 20
- Regular pulse with palpation but bounding
- Skin warm and dry but flushed
- No jugular venous distension noted

1130h: The client develops shortness of breath, chest pain with inspiration, use of accessory muscles, nasal flaring, and blood-tinged sputum.

- HR = 130
- RR = 28
- Jugular venous distension measured at 7 cm

Continuing with the current clinical scenario started in Chapter 3, it was determined that the most likely medical condition the client is experiencing is a pulmonary embolus. If you were caring for the client, consider your priorities of care, basing your considerations on the clinical presentation. Priorities in care always start with airway, breathing, and then circulation. In the clinical presentation in Example 4, what do you think are potential nursing interventions; possible medications to be ordered, including oxygen therapy, intravenous fluids, and even supplementations (e.g., multivitamins and thiamine are typically ordered intravenously for clients in alcohol withdrawal); laboratory tests to be ordered; and possible diagnostic tests that would confirm the diagnosis? Use the space below to record your answers.

Example 4 Answer

____

____

____

____

Common ways that students may be asked a Generate Solutions question in NGN case studies are as follows:

▶ For each potential intervention (or could be replaced with potential order), identify whether the intervention is indicated or not indicated for the client.

POTENTIAL NURSING INTERVENTIONS	INDICATED	NOT INDICATED
Prepare the client for a spiral computed tomography scan	○	○
Discuss end-of-life care with the client	○	○
Place the client in low supine position	○	○
Request an order for supplemental oxygen therapy	○	○
Encourage oral fluid intake	○	○
Prepare to initiate a venous access device	○	○

OR

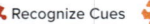

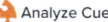

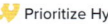

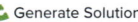

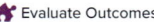

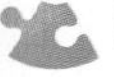 ▶ Drag the top 3 potential nursing interventions (or could be replaced with orders) that the nurse should plan to implement.

POTENTIAL NURSING INTERVENTIONS (OR ORDERS)
Prepare the client for a spiral computed tomography scan
Discuss end-of-life care with the client
Place the client in low supine position
Request an order for supplemental oxygen therapy
Encourage oral fluid intake
Prepare to initiate a venous access device

TOP 3 POTENTIAL NURSING INTERVENTIONS (OR ORDERS)

OR

 ▶ Select the top 3 potential nursing interventions the nurse should plan to implement when caring for the client.

- ☐ Prepare the client for a spiral computed tomography scan
- ☐ Discuss end-of-life care with the client
- ☐ Place the client in low supine position
- ☐ Request an order for supplemental oxygen therapy
- ☐ Encourage oral fluid intake
- ☐ Prepare to initiate a venous access device

OR

 ▶ Which of the following health care orders (or could be replaced with nursing interventions) should the nurse anticipate? **Select all that apply.**

- ☐ Check the client's vital signs every 15 minutes
- ☐ Draw laboratory tests: D-dimer, complete blood count, troponin, brain natriuretic peptide
- ☐ Insert a Foley catheter
- ☐ Initiate oxygen therapy starting at 2 L/min for a pulse oximetry reading of greater than 92%
- ☐ Continuous electrocardiogram monitoring required
- ☐ Initiate unfractionated heparin intravenously
- ☐ Encourage ambulation

In all the Generate Solution questions, knowledge about the expected treatment plan for a client with a pulmonary embolus is important. Improving tissue perfusion, respiratory function, and monitoring adequate cardiac output are primary goals of therapy for a client experiencing a pulmonary embolus. Therefore, anticipating nursing interventions and a potential treatment plan to meet these goals differentiates sound clinical judgement when making decisions during client care.

To successfully answer Generate Solutions *planning of care* questions successfully, knowledge of nursing interventions and the medical treatment plan inclusive of medications, laboratory tests, and diagnostic tests is necessary.

Nursing interventions include addressing critical abnormal assessment data that do not require an order from a health care provider or anticipating the medical plan's orders. For example, positioning a client in the best position associated with the medical condition is important. Be sure to review client positioning, such as Trendelenburg, supine, lateral, semi-Fowlers, high-Fowlers, and even prone position, and when each position would be appropriate for a client's clinical presentation. In the above clinical scenario, the client has identifiable critical abnormal breathing patterns as described by shortness of breath, chest pain with inspiration, use of accessory muscles, and nasal flaring. These manifestations are indicative of impending respiratory distress if treatment is delayed. Although it is recommended that the client be placed in semi-Fowler's position

TABLE 4.1 Pertinent Labs to Monitor

Complete Blood Count (CBC):
- Hemoglobin (Hgb)
- Platelets (Plt)
- Hematocrit (Hct)
- White blood cells (WBC)
- Neutrophils
- Bands

Coagulation:
- International normalized ratio/prothrombin time (INR/PT)
- Partial thromboplastin time (PTT)
- D-dimer

Electrolytes:
- Sodium (Na^+)
- Potassium (K^+)
- Carbon dioxide (CO_2)
- Chloride (Cl^-)
- Magnesium (Mg)
- Phosphorous (Phos)
- Calcium (Ca^+)
- Blood glucose (BG)

Kidney Function:
- Creatine
- Blood urea nitrogen (BUN)
- Glomerular filtration rate (GFR)

Lipids:
- Total cholesterol (TC)
- Triglycerides (TG)
- High-density lipoprotein (HDL)
- Low-density lipoprotein (LDL)

Liver Function Tests:
- Bilirubin (Bili)
- Aspartate aminotransferase (AST)
- Alanine aminotransferase (ALT)
- Alkaline phosphatase (Alk Phos)
- Gamma-glutamyl transpeptidase (GGT)

Specialty Labs:
- Troponin (TNT)
- Brain natriuretic peptide (BNP)
- Creatine kinase (CK)
- Creatine kinase of heart (CK-MB)
- C-reactive protein (CRP)

Pancreatitis:
- Amylase
- Lipase

for comfort, if a client presents with air hunger, then high-Fowler's position with oxygen therapy may be warranted until intubation can occur.

When planning care for clients, it is imperative to include medications, laboratory tests (Table 4.1), and diagnostic tests. The NGN case studies consider holistic care plans; however, the care plans are more closely aligned with a medical plan. If the client has developed clots in their lungs, then anticoagulant therapy would be the chosen medication of choice. It would be important to recognize an abnormal clinical presentation that may warrant subcutaneous injections in contrast to an acute critical abnormal clinical presentation that may warrant an order for fluids to be administered intravenously. It would be up to the student to recognize that a low-molecular-weight heparin is similar in action but not the same medication as unfractionated heparin intravenously. Laboratory tests in general and specific to the medical condition would be helpful when anticipating that laboratory tests may be ordered. For example, a client with a suspected pulmonary embolus would require knowledge about their clotting status, bleeding, arterial blood gases, and, if severe, renal function. The specific test associated with a pulmonary embolus is to include a D-dimer, which may be drawn in the presence of any suspected clot, as in the case of a pulmonary embolus and even a deep vein thrombosis. There are patterns associated with many clinical conditions.

Knowledge of specific diagnostic tests is also helpful for successfully answering these types of questions. It is important to know the difference when common diagnostic tests may be ordered, such as an X-ray, transthoracic ultrasound, echocardiogram, transesophageal echocardiogram, leg/arm Doppler (ultrasound), spiral computed tomography (CT) scan, head/abdominal/chest CT, magnetic resonance imaging (MRI), and positive emission tomography (PET) scan. There are patterns associated with the diagnostic tests that are ordered. For example, a client who presents with clinical manifestations associated with a deep vein thrombosis would likely have leg or arm Dopplers ordered or an ultrasound of the suspected vein that may have developed a clot but is stationary. If the clot becomes embolus (travels) and migrates to the lung, then a spiral CT would be ordered. If there is a suspected clot positioned in either the right or left atrium, a transesophageal echocardiogram is more specific than a transthoracic echocardiogram to visualize the clot.

When laboratory data and diagnostic test information are provided in NGN case studies, the normal results are given in relation to the abnormal test results. You will not have to memorize common laboratory abnormal values for the case studies; however, you are still required to learn the most common laboratory values. Please check the most recent test plan at www.nclex.com to learn which laboratory values you need to know before writing the NCLEX-RN®. Laboratory values are available for review on the Evolve site.

To answer Generate Solutions case study questions successfully, you will need to identify specific knowledge associated with the potential treatment of the clinical presentation of a medical condition. If you are unfamiliar with any of the above tests and patterns of care associated with ordering specific laboratory tests for specific conditions (e.g., troponin is ordered for an acute myocardial infarction), it is recommended that you review this information during your preparation.

Take Action

Now that you have gathered together and carefully considered all the assessment information, determined the most likely or highest-risk medical condition the client may be experiencing, and developed an anticipated plan of care for the client, is it time to put those pieces together and act in accordance with competency, knowledge, and sound clinical judgement to provide safe care for the client. Nursing actions are based on the client's highest need determined in the Prioritize Hypothesis cognitive step and the presenting clinical manifestations.

Prioritizing care begins with addressing issues of airway, breathing, then circulation. Careful consideration of the client's abnormal assessment data and the critical abnormal assessment data will determine the nurse's next steps when making decisions about appropriate actions. For example, if a client is experiencing anxiety, breathing at a rate of 28 breaths per minute, presents with an adequate blood pressure for cardiac output, but does not have any renal output, the airway and taking action to reduce the client's breaths per minute, to minimize symptoms of anxiety, become the priority, not focusing on renal output. Knowledge of anticipating potential nursing interventions and a treatment plan inclusive of potential medications, laboratory tests, and diagnostic tests to be ordered will prepare you to be successful in addressing the highest priority when taking action during the care of a client.

Example 5: Take Action

EXAMPLE 5 Take Action

The nurse is caring for a client in the emergency department.

1000h: The client falls with query broken femur bone. They complain of pain and become notably anxious.

- HR = 110
- RR = 20
- Regular pulse with palpation but bounding
- Skin warm and dry but flushed
- No jugular venous distension noted

1130h: The client develops shortness of breath, chest pain with inspiration, use of accessory muscles, nasal flaring, and blood-tinged sputum.

- HR = 130
- RR = 28
- Jugular venous distension measured at 7 cm

Continuing with the current clinical scenario, what do you think would be the most appropriate actions for a client experiencing a pulmonary embolus? Record your answers here, addressing possible nursing interventions, medications, laboratory tests, and diagnostic tests.

Example 5 Answer

____
____
____
____

Common ways that students may be asked a Take Action question in NGN case studies are as follows:

- For each nursing intervention (or could be replaced with potential order), identify whether the intervention is indicated or not indicated for the client.

NURSING INTERVENTIONS (OR ORDERS)	INDICATED	NOT INDICATED
Prepare the client for a spiral computed tomography scan	○	○
Discuss end-of-life care with the client	○	○
Place the client in low supine position	○	○
Request an order for supplemental oxygen therapy	○	○
Encourage oral fluid intake	○	○
Prepare to initiate a venous access device	○	○

OR

▶ Drag the top 3 nursing interventions (or could be replaced with orders) that the nurse should implement when providing care to the client.

NURSING INTERVENTIONS (OR ORDERS)
Prepare the client for a spiral computed tomography scan
Discuss end-of-life care with the client
Place the client in low supine position
Request an order for supplemental oxygen therapy
Encourage oral fluid intake
Prepare to initiate a venous access device

TOP 3 NURSING INTERVENTIONS (OR ORDERS)

OR

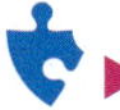

▶ Select 3 priority actions that the nurse should take when caring for the client.

- ☐ Prepare the client for a spiral computed tomography scan
- ☐ Discuss end-of-life care with the client
- ☐ Place the client in low supine position
- ☐ Request an order for supplemental oxygen therapy
- ☐ Encourage oral fluid intake
- ☐ Prepare to initiate a venous access device

OR

▶ Highlight the 3 priority nursing actions that the nurse should take when caring for the client.

- ☐ Prepare the client for a spiral computed tomography scan
- ☐ Discuss end-of-life care with the client
- ☐ Place the client in low supine position
- ☐ Request an order for supplemental oxygen therapy
- ☐ Encourage oral fluid intake
- ☐ Prepare to initiate a venous access device

OR

▶ Which of the following health care orders (or could be replaced with nursing interventions) would the nurse perform? **Select all that apply**.

- ☐ Check the client's vital signs every 15 minutes
- ☐ Draw laboratory tests: D-dimer, complete blood count, troponin, brain natriuretic peptide
- ☐ Insert a Foley catheter
- ☐ Initiate oxygen therapy starting at 2 L/min for a pulse oximetry reading of greater than 92%
- ☐ Continuous electrocardiogram monitoring required
- ☐ Initiate unfractionated heparin intravenously
- ☐ Encourage ambulation

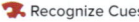

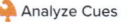

In all the Take Action NGN questions, knowledge about the treatment plan for a client with a pulmonary embolus is necessary in order to answer questions correctly. Improving tissue perfusion and respiratory function and monitoring adequate cardiac output are primary goals of therapy for a client experiencing a pulmonary embolus. Therefore, being certain of nursing interventions and medical treatment plans commonly prescribed when clients are experiencing symptoms associated with a pulmonary embolus is required in order to make sound clinical judgement decisions when providing care to clients. You will get more practice throughout the textbook incorporating the elements of complex case studies to fully understand how these questions are structured. Take Action NGN questions offer the most variability when applying knowledge. This is the time in providing care to clients when preventable nursing errors have a greater chance to occur during client care.

OR

▶ Complete the following sentences by choosing from the lists of options.

The nurse should prepare the client for ________________ (word options 1).

It would be a priority for the nurse to request a prescription for ________________ (word options 2).

WORD OPTIONS 1	WORD OPTIONS 2
Chest X-ray	Amiodarone
Positive emission tomography (PET) scan	Unfractionated heparin
Transthoracic echocardiogram	Apixaban
Spiral computed tomography (CT) scan	Dronedarone
Fluoroscopy	Metoprolol

When answering this type of Take Action question, any of the potential variables necessary for providing care to clients include nursing interventions, medications, laboratory tests, and diagnostic tests provided in drop-down menu options. A strategy to use when answering this specific type of question is to ensure getting the first question correct. This is a new type of scoring for NCLEX-RN, which typically requires the test writer to correctly answer the first fill-in-the-blank item in order to receive full marks for the question if the second fill-in-the-blank item is answered correctly too. Medications may be provided by drug class or by generic names.

Evaluate Outcomes

Finally, you have reached the point where you determine if your actions have had an effect on the client's overall status. This is where you reflect and re-evaluate if the treatment and actions you provided have improved the client's condition, if the client's condition has declined, or if there is no change in the client's status or if the client makes statements demonstrating understanding or no understanding of teaching. Evaluating your actions is a necessary skill to determine the next steps in the care of the client and observe for expected outcomes or determine if the expected outcome was achieved. You are then able to re-evaluate and change the plan of care accordingly in response to the expected outcomes.

Primary ways to identify changes in a client's overall status is to review:

1. The client's assessment data, beginning with their vital signs or clinical presentation
2. Client statements or demonstrations by the client
3. Changes in behaviour

Review Assessment Data

Information will be presented either in a table or through a narrative providing details about a clinical presentation. It will be up to the student to determine if the clinical data have improved, declined, or demonstrated no change as a result of the actions. For example, if oxygen is applied to a client to correct a gas imbalance and the pulse oximetry is less than 90 to 92% originally, an improvement in the client's status would be increased pulse oximetry and improved respiratory function.

When looking at the normal–abnormal–critical abnormal assessment data spectrum (Fig. 4.1), as a nurse you will be required to recognize when the clinical presentation has improved or worsened. Fig. 4.1 represents a visual image of how to conceptualize the progression spectrum. The foundation for all client assessments is the nurse's ability to recognize what would be a clinically normal presentation for the client and how to anticipate and identify improvements or a decline in the client's status.

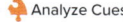

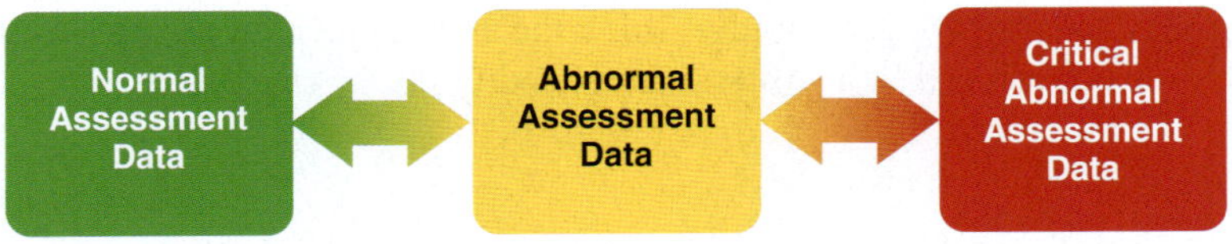

Normal Assessment Data ↔ Abnormal Assessment Data ↔ Critical Abnormal Assessment Data

FIG. 4.1 Normal–abnormal–critical abnormal assessment data spectrum.

For example, at the beginning of an undergraduate nursing program, students learn to identify a "normal" blood pressure. For the purposes of this example, use 120/80 mmHg as the starting value. As more curricular content is learned, students begin to recognize what is meant by abnormal changes in cardiovascular function related to blood pressure, specifically as it relates to higher blood pressure (hypertension) or low blood pressure (hypotension). If a client's status changes, the blood pressure can develop further to an abnormal critical level with particular attention to either critically higher blood pressure, as in the case of a hypertensive crisis, or a critically lower blood pressure, as in the case of shock. When the client's status worsens, the progression will move from left to right and can stop anywhere on the spectrum of normal, abnormal, critical abnormal (Fig. 4.2). When the client's status improves, the progression moves from right to left in the same fashion along the spectrum as in Fig. 4.1. Anticipating these changes will assist new nurses in applying their clinical judgement to provide effective and safe care to clients and families.

It is important to understand that clients can present with abnormal assessment data as well, which can still be considered their baseline. For example, a client may have suffered a previous anterior myocardial infarction, leaving their heart with left ventricular dysfunction and an abnormal ejection fraction of 48%, indicating that client's baseline. This ejection fraction would be considered abnormal but it is also the client's baseline. All new diagnostic data would be based on this client's abnormal baseline. If this client should suffer another acute myocardial infarction, the echocardiogram would report the new ejection fraction, and the health care team would determine if the condition has caused a further decline in the already abnormal ejection fraction or no change in baseline status.

Questions to ask yourself include the following:

- What assessment data tell me the client's status has improved?
- What assessment data tell me that the client's status has declined?
- Is there any change?
- Has the client's status returned to normal assessment data?
- Has the client's status worsened and progressed from either normal assessment data to abnormal assessment data or even critical abnormal assessment data? (Review Chapter 2 to understand improvement and decline in health.)

Analysis of abnormal data is important when anticipating expected medication outcomes. For example, if the client is in pain and the heart rate is elevated, the nurse administers an analgesic and monitors not only for a reduction in pain but also recognizing or anticipating a decrease in the heart rate, indicating that the analgesic relaxed the smooth muscle. The nurse performs a re-evaluation and reassessment of the client to determine if the medication administered altered the client's overall status. For example, consider a cardiac client who presented with anginal pain and was administered nitroglycerine sublingual spray as ordered × 3 for effect, but because of the vasodilatory and afterload effects, the client's blood pressure becomes critically low. This would indicate a decline in the client's

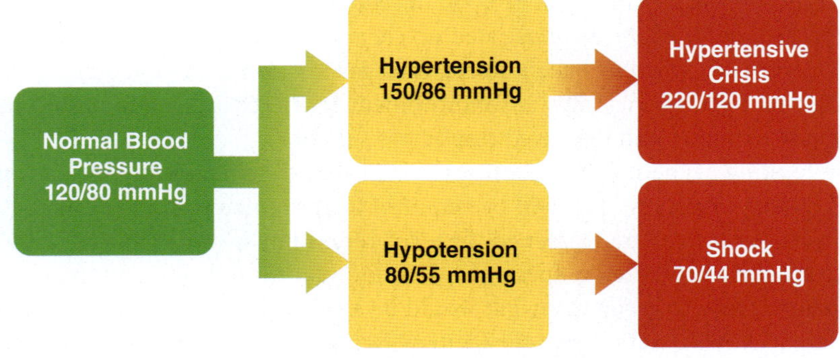

FIG. 4.2 Example of normal–abnormal–critical abnormal assessment data spectrum.

status. Although nitroglycerine was the correct medication to treat the anginal pain, the resulting outcome was hemodynamic instability. Knowledge of the mechanism of action and adverse effects of common medications are helpful when answering these questions.

Client Statements and Demonstrations by the Client

During discharge teaching or client teaching about a medication or condition, the nurse may ask the client to teach back, role-play, or return demonstrate the new information. Client education is intended to maintain and promote health, prevent illness, restore health, and optimize quality of life with impaired functioning (Astle & Duggleby, 2024, p. 330).

Client teaching examples may include teaching back of pre- and postoperative surgical expectations or care, return demonstration of preparation of medications or performing skills (in-and-out self-catheterization), articulation of new information based on statements by the client, and even self-monitoring of data (blood pressure diary or food diary). Effective teaching outcomes are demonstrated by the client having understanding or having no understanding of the intended teaching content or return demonstration.

Changes in Behaviours

Another common way to evaluate expected outcomes is to determine if expected behaviour changes are observed. Changes in behaviours can be a result of medication administration, coping strategies, reduced fear response, or changes in anxiety levels. It is important to determine if the behaviour is a result of the actions or a change in client status. For example, if the client receives quetiapine to assist with sleep but the client is not able to fall asleep, then the medication dose or time of administration was ineffective. Be sure to recognize what the expected behaviour changes may be in relation to the previous actions taken.

Example 6: Evaluate Outcomes

EXAMPLE 6 Evaluate Outcomes

The nurse is caring for a client in the emergency department.

1000h: The client falls with query broken femur bone. They complain of pain and become notably anxious.

- HR = 110
- RR = 20
- Regular pulse with palpation but bounding
- Skin warm and dry but flushed
- No jugular venous distension noted

1130h: The client develops shortness of breath, chest pain with inspiration, use of accessory muscles, nasal flaring, and blood-tinged sputum.

- HR = 130
- RR = 28
- Jugular venous distension measured at 7 cm

1140h: New orders received from the health care provider.

1430h: The client is resting comfortably. Respirations regular and easy at rest. No use of accessory muscles noted. Client denies any pleuritic pain. Client states, "I am not scared I am going to die."

- HR = 87
- RR = 16
- Pulse regular and strong. Skin remains warm and dry to touch. No diaphoresis noted.
- Jugular venous distension measured at 3 cm

Continuing with the current clinical scenario, what do you think would be appropriate responses to the intended nursing actions common for a client experiencing a pulmonary embolus? Write down the expected outcomes of application of oxygen therapy and of appropriate medications commonly administered for a client experiencing a pulmonary embolus. Document appropriate discharge teaching for a client who has recovered from a pulmonary embolus. Record your answers here, addressing possible medications, nursing interventions, and topics for discharge teaching.

Example 6 Answer

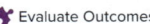

Common ways that students may be asked an Evaluate Outcomes question in NGN case studies are as follows:

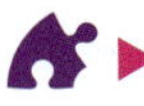

▶ Which of the following findings would indicate that the client's status has improved? **Select all that apply.**

- ☐ Respiratory rate
- ☐ No use of accessory muscles
- ☐ Skin warm and dry
- ☐ Heart rate
- ☐ Jugular venous distension

OR

▶ Highlight the findings that indicate an improvement (or worsening) of the client's status.

> The client is resting comfortably. Respirations regular and easy at rest. No use of accessory muscles noted. Client denies any pleuritic pain. Client states, "I am not scared I am going to die."
> - HR = 87
> - RR = 16
> - Pulse regular and strong. Skin remains warm and dry to touch. No diaphoresis noted.
> - Jugular venous distension measured at 3 cm

OR

▶ For each assessment finding, identify if the finding indicates that the client's condition has improved, has not changed, or has declined.

CLIENT FINDINGS	IMPROVED	NO CHANGE	DECLINED
Respiratory rate 16 breaths per minutes	○	○	○
No use of accessory muscles	○	○	○
Skin warm and dry	○	○	○
Heart rate 87 beats per minute	○	○	○
Jugular venous distension at 3 cm	○	○	○

Note: Each row must have one response option selected.

OR

▶ Drag the top 4 client findings that demonstrate the client's status is improving.

CLIENT FINDINGS
Respiratory rate
No use of accessory muscles
Skin warm and dry to touch
Heart rate
Jugular venous distension

TOP 4 CLIENT FINDINGS

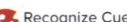

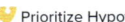

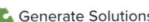

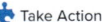

When answering these types of questions, be aware of the knowledge required to evaluate outcomes and determine if the client's status has improved or worsened.

OR

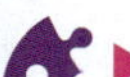 ▶ For each of the statements made by the client during discharge or client teaching, indicate whether the client understands or has no understanding of the information that was provided.

CLIENT STATEMENTS	UNDERSTANDING	NO UNDERSTANDING
"I will stay on blood thinners for 3 months."	○	○
"I am fit and do not need to see my doctor for follow-up."	○	○
"I will need to wear antiembolic stockings when flying."	○	○
"I will need to take more frequent stops when driving."	○	○
"I have to change my diet."	○	○

When answering client statement types of questions, it is important to know what information would be taught during discharge teaching or client teaching. This will include medications post-discharge, any follow-up diagnostic and laboratory tests, diet, exercise restrictions or limitations, mobility, monitoring for adverse effects of clinical manifestations associated with worsening status, and any follow-up care required.

How to Successfully Answer Generate Solutions, Take Action, and Evaluate Outcome Questions

The best preparation for answering these types of questions is:

- Having sound knowledge of plans of care associated with common medical conditions
- Having sound knowledge of common nursing interventions, orders for medications, diagnostic or laboratory tests, and possible client teaching topics covered during client teaching sessions and discharge teaching
- Being able to determine if clinical data would be categorized as normal, abnormal, or critical abnormal assessment data during the reassessment
- Understanding expected outcomes of treatment and medications (mechanism of action and adverse effects)
- Possessing knowledge about expected outcomes associated with client statements demonstrating understanding or no understanding of client teaching
- Being able to recognize the patterns of words highlighted in the question to know if it is a **Generate Solutions** (planning of care), **Take Action** (solutions addressing highest priority that pertains to interventions, orders, medications, or diagnostic or laboratory tests), or **Evaluate Outcomes** (determine if the client status has improved, declined, or not changed, based on the nursing actions) question

Conclusion

This chapter has demonstrated how to group together Generate Solutions, Take Action, and Evaluate Outcomes in ways to determine the plan of care for a client, take nursing actions or carry out orders that address the highest priority for a client, and apply knowledge about expected outcomes associated with appropriate interventions. By breaking down each step of the cognitive processing for these areas of the NCJMM, you can begin to apply your knowledge to the NGN case studies. If you determine that you have gaps, then return back to your notes and strengthen your knowledge in anatomy and physiology, pathophysiology, and assessment. Anticipating a plan and putting that plan into action to improve client outcomes is the basis of nursing practice. You must put the pieces of the puzzle together to determine the problem and then act on that priority to ensure safe client care. See Fig. 4.3 for a continued visualization of the scaffolding of information that you may have encountered

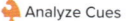

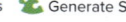

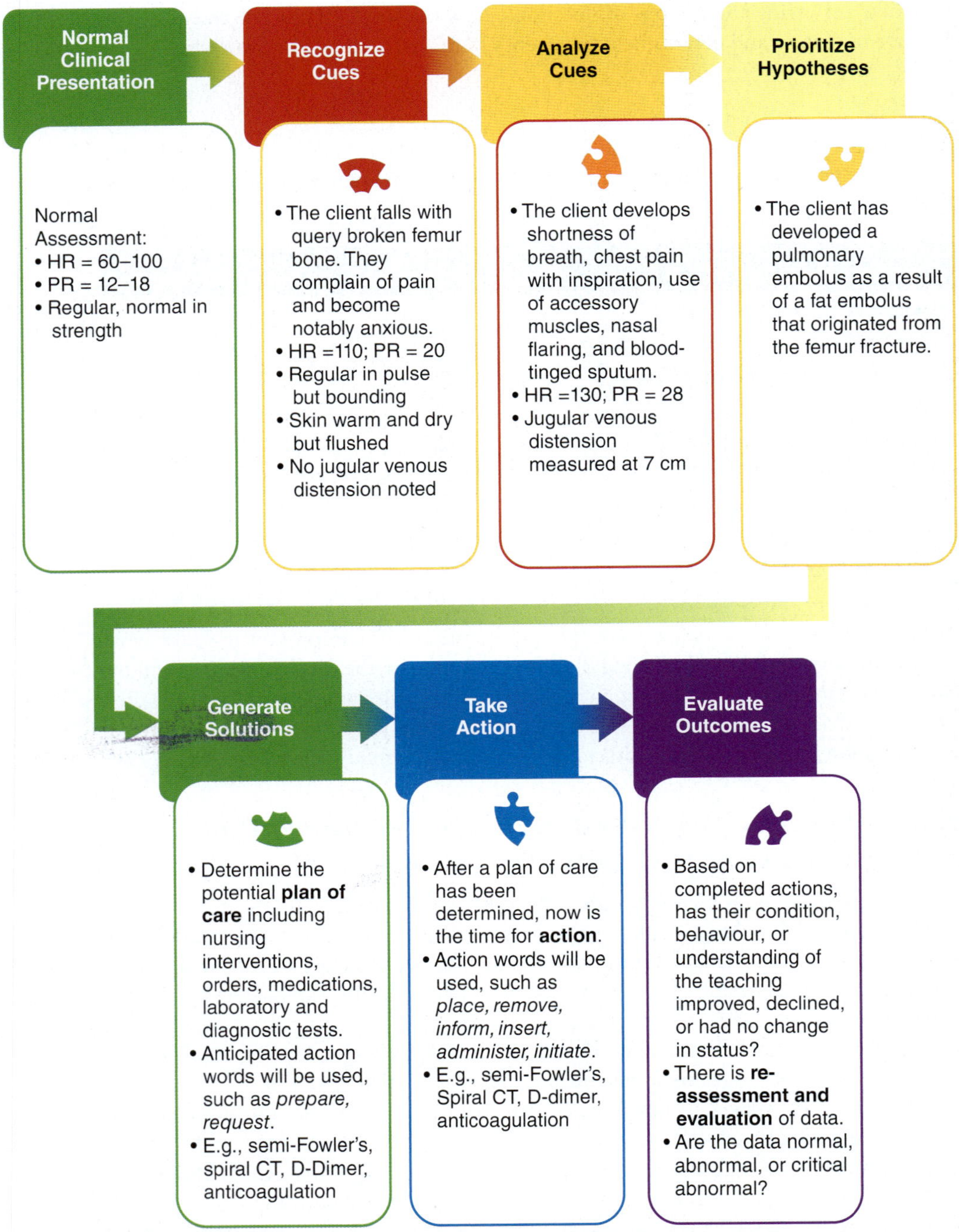

Normal Clinical Presentation

Normal Assessment:
- HR = 60–100
- PR = 12–18
- Regular, normal in strength

Recognize Cues

- The client falls with query broken femur bone. They complain of pain and become notably anxious.
- HR =110; PR = 20
- Regular in pulse but bounding
- Skin warm and dry but flushed
- No jugular venous distension noted

Analyze Cues

- The client develops shortness of breath, chest pain with inspiration, use of accessory muscles, nasal flaring, and blood-tinged sputum.
- HR =130; PR = 28
- Jugular venous distension measured at 7 cm

Prioritize Hypotheses

- The client has developed a pulmonary embolus as a result of a fat embolus that originated from the femur fracture.

Generate Solutions

- Determine the potential **plan of care** including nursing interventions, orders, medications, laboratory and diagnostic tests.
- Anticipated action words will be used, such as *prepare, request*.
- E.g., semi-Fowler's, spiral CT, D-Dimer, anticoagulation

Take Action

- After a plan of care has been determined, now is the time for **action**.
- Action words will be used, such as *place, remove, inform, insert, administer, initiate*.
- E.g., semi-Fowler's, Spiral CT, D-dimer, anticoagulation

Evaluate Outcomes

- Based on completed actions, has their condition, behaviour, or understanding of the teaching improved, declined, or had no change in status?
- There is **re-assessment and evaluation** of data.
- Are the data normal, abnormal, or critical abnormal?

FIG. 4.3 Breaking down Generate Solutions, Take Action, and Evaluate Outcomes in a simple unfolding clinical scenario.

in your nursing program. Fig. 3.1 in Chapter 3 presented clinical data with a focus on the cognitive processing needed to Recognize Cues, Analyze Cues, and Prioritize Hypotheses. Fig. 4.3 proceeds with the same narrative found in Fig. 3.1, but the focus is on the cognitive processing necessary to address Generate Solutions, Take Action, and Evaluate Outcomes. The overall combined example of Fig. 3.1 and Fig. 4.3 represents the application of the cognitive steps in the NCJMM.

All answers to the questions can be found at the end of the chapter.

Answers to Typical or Common Questions

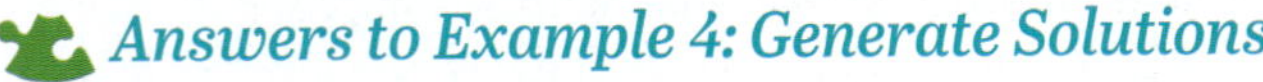

Answers to Example 4: Generate Solutions

▶ For each potential intervention (or could be replaced with potential order), identify whether the intervention is indicated or not indicated for the client.

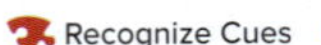 Recognize Cues 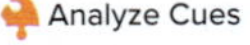 Analyze Cues 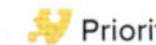 Prioritize Hypothesis 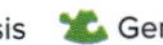 Generate Solutions 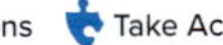 Take Action 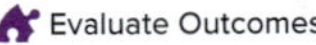 Evaluate Outcomes

POTENTIAL NURSING INTERVENTIONS	INDICATED	NOT INDICATED
Prepare the client for a spiral computed tomography scan	✔	○
Discuss end-of-life care with the client	○	✔
Place the client in low supine position	○	✔
Request an order for supplemental oxygen therapy	✔	○
Encourage oral fluid intake	○	✔
Prepare to initiate a venous access device	✔	○

▶ Drag the top 3 potential nursing interventions (or could be replaced with orders) that the nurse should plan to implement.

TOP 3 POTENTIAL NURSING INTERVENTIONS (OR ORDERS)
Prepare the client for a spiral computed tomography scan
Request an order for supplemental oxygen therapy
Prepare to initiate a venous access device

▶ Select the top 3 potential nursing interventions that the nurse should plan to implement when caring for the client.

✔ Prepare the client for a spiral computed tomography scan
✔ Discuss end-of-life care with the client
☐ Place the client in low supine position
✔ Request an order for supplemental oxygen therapy
☐ Encourage oral fluid intake
✔ Prepare to initiate a venous access device

Rationale: Planning for care requires the nurse to ensure that the client is attending the correct diagnostic test, which in this case would be a spiral CT scan. This is specific for any suspected clots but primarily ordered for clients suspected of developing a pulmonary embolus. The nurse would request supplemental oxygen therapy, even without knowing pulse oximetry data. The client in the above scenario is presenting with respiratory compromise as evidenced by the shortness of breath, chest pain with inspiration, use of accessory muscles, and nasal flaring. This indicates impaired gas exchange with the potential to compromise cardiovascular circulation, leading to further complications. Supplemental oxygen therapy would be required to enhance the overall systemic oxygenation and improve the potential hypoxia and hypoxemia. Given that the client is experiencing respiratory compromise, a venous access device would be inserted in preparation of administering fluids if the client becomes hemodynamically unstable or administering heparin intravenously. The clinical presentation warrants a more aggressive approach to reduce the formation of new clots, because the client is experiencing respiratory compromise. Low-molecular-weight heparin administered subcutaneously or other oral anticoagulant therapy would be ordered and administered in the absence of an acute presentation, as in the case of this client. The client's status does not warrant discussing end-of-life care. Discussing goals of care, which is always important when caring for all clients, is different from discussing end-of-life care. When considering the primary concept of airway, breathing, and circulation interventions, progressing throughout the other systems for appropriate management, focusing on oral fluid intake would not be warranted at this time to ensure proper hydration.

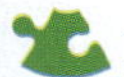
NCJMM Step: Generate Solutions
References: Tyerman & Cobbett (2023), pp. 622–624; Power-Kean et al. (2023), p. 692.

▶ Which of the following health care orders (or could be replaced with nursing interventions) should the nurse anticipate? **Select all that apply**.

- ☐ Check the client's vital signs every 15 minutes
- ✔ Draw laboratory tests: D-dimer, complete blood count, troponin, brain natriuretic peptide
- ☐ Insert a Foley catheter
- ✔ Initiate oxygen therapy starting at 2 L/min for a pulse oximetry reading of greater than 92%
- ✔ Continuous electrocardiogram monitoring required
- ✔ Initiate unfractionated Heparin intravenously
- ☐ Encourage ambulation

Rationale: Common laboratory tests ordered when a client presents with an acute pulmonary embolism are used to determine the degree of bleeding and ability to clot (CBC). The D-dimer test is specific to identifying intravascular clotting, as in the case of a pulmonary embolus, or less is common when querying the development of a deep vein thrombosis. In this case, a troponin would be drawn to assess if there has been any cardiac compromise as a result of lack of oxygen to the myocardium, and a brain natriuretic peptide (BPP) would be drawn to correlate cardiac compromise indicating heart failure, myocardial infarction, or cor pulmonale. Oxygen therapy would be initiated at 2 L and then titrated to the pulse oximetry level. Despite no pulse oximetry level being provided in the narrative, supplemental oxygen therapy would be warranted in this clinical presentation as the client has increased work of breathing and respiratory compromise. Continuous electrocardiogram (ECG) monitoring would be ordered to identify any abnormal ST-segment and T-wave changes associated with lack of oxygen being delivered to the myocardium, in anticipation of a myocardial infarction. Finally, the last order to anticipate would be the appropriate use of an anticoagulant. Unfractionated heparin intravenously would be ordered to prevent any further emboli from forming. It is important for the nurse to recognize in which clinical presentations a fibrinolytic medication (tissue plasminogen activator [tPA] or alteplase-activase) would be necessary to dissolve the clot, or the choice to order other routes of anticoagulant therapy (low-molecular-weight heparin or oral therapy). A Foley catheter would not be necessary to anticipate initiating at this time, as the client's kidney status has not been compromised, based on the narrative. Ambulation should be reserved for when the client is out of the acute active phase of a pulmonary embolus.

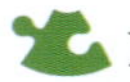
NCJMM Step: Generate Solutions
References: Jarvis et al. (2024), p. 499; Tyerman & Cobbett (2023), pp. 622–624.

Answers to Example 5: Take Action

▶ For each nursing intervention (or could be replaced with potential order), identify whether the intervention is indicated or not indicated for the client.

NURSING INTERVENTIONS	INDICATED	NOT INDICATED
Prepare the client for a spiral computed tomography scan	✔	○
Discuss end-of-life care with the client	○	✔
Place the client in low supine position	○	✔
Request an order for supplemental oxygen therapy	✔	○
Encourage oral fluid intake	○	✔
Prepare to initiate a venous access device	✔	○

▶ Drag the top 3 nursing interventions (or could be replaced with orders) that the nurse should implement when providing care to the client.

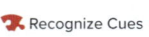

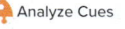

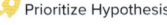

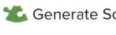

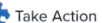

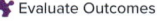

TOP 3 NURSING INTERVENTIONS (OR ORDERS)
Prepare the client for a spiral computed tomography scan
Request an order for supplemental oxygen therapy
Prepare to initiate a venous access device

▶ Select 3 priority actions that the nurse should take when caring for the client.

✔ Prepare the client for a spiral computed tomography scan
☐ Discuss end-of-life care with the client
☐ Place the client in low supine position
✔ Request an order for supplemental oxygen therapy
☐ Encourage oral fluid intake
✔ Prepare to initiate a venous access device

▶ Highlight the 3 priority nursing actions that the nurse should take when caring for the client.

☐ Prepare the client for a spiral computed tomography scan
☐ Discuss end-of-life care with the client
☐ Place the client in low supine position
☐ Request an order for supplemental oxygen therapy
☐ Encourage oral fluid intake
☐ Prepare to initiate a venous access device

Rationale: Initiating action requires the nurse to ensure that the client is getting the correct diagnostic test, which in this case would be a spiral CT scan. This is specific for any suspected clots but primarily ordered for clients suspected of developing a pulmonary embolus. The nurse would request supplemental oxygen therapy even without knowing pulse oximetry data. The client in the above scenario is presenting with respiratory compromise as evidenced by the shortness of breath, chest pain with inspiration, use of accessory muscles, and nasal flaring. This set of symptoms indicates impaired gas exchange with the potential to compromise cardiovascular circulation, leading to further complications. Supplemental oxygen therapy would be required to enhance the overall systemic oxygenation and improve the potential hypoxia and hypoxemia. Given that the client is having respiratory compromise, a venous access device would be inserted in preparation to administer fluids if the client becomes hemodynamically unstable or to administer heparin intravenously. The clinical presentation warrants a more aggressive approach to reduce the formation of new clots as the client is experiencing respiratory compromise. Low-molecular-weight heparin administered subcutaneously or other oral anticoagulant therapy would be ordered and administered in the absence of an acute presentation, such as in the case of this client. The client's status does not warrant discussing end-of-life care with the client. Discussing goals of care, which is always important when caring for all clients, is different from discussing end-of-life care. When considering the primary concept of airway, breathing, and circulation interventions, then progressing throughout the other systems for appropriate management, focusing on oral fluid intake would not be warranted at this time to ensure proper hydration.

NCJMM Step: Take Action
References: Jarvis et al. (2024), p. 499; Tyerman & Cobbett (2023), pp. 622–624; Power-Kean et al. (2023), p. 692.

▶ Which of the following health care orders (or could be replaced with nursing interventions) would the nurse perform? **Select all that apply.**

☐ Check the client's vital signs every 15 minutes
✔ Draw laboratory tests: D-dimer, complete blood count, troponin, brain natriuretic peptide
☐ Insert a Foley catheter
✔ Initiate oxygen therapy starting at 2 L/min for a pulse oximetry reading of greater than 92%

- ✔ Continuous electrocardiogram monitoring required
- ✔ Initiate unfractionated heparin intravenously
- ☐ Encourage ambulation

Rationale: Common laboratory tests ordered when a client presents with an acute pulmonary embolism are used to determine the degree of bleeding and ability to clot (CBC). A D-dimer test is specific to identifying intravascular clotting, as in the case of a pulmonary embolus, or is less common when querying the development of a deep vein thrombosis. A troponin would be drawn to assess if there has been any cardiac compromise as a result of lack of oxygen to the myocardium, and a brain natriuretic peptic would be drawn to correlate cardiac compromise indicating heart failure, myocardial infarction, or cor pulmonale. Oxygen therapy would be initiated at 2 L and then titrated to the pulse oximetry level. Despite no pulse oximetry level being provided in the narrative, supplemental oxygen therapy would be warranted in this clinical presentation as the client has increased work of breathing and respiratory compromise. Continuous electrocardiogram (ECG) monitoring would be ordered to identify any abnormal ST-segment and T-wave changes associated with lack of oxygen being delivered to the myocardium, in anticipation of a myocardial infarction. Finally, the last order to anticipate would be the appropriate use of an anticoagulant. Unfractionated heparin intravenously would be ordered to prevent the further emboli from forming. It is important for the nurse to recognize in which clinical presentations a fibrinolytic medication (tissue plasminogen activator [tPA] or alteplase-activase) would be necessary to dissolve the clot, or the choice to order other routes of anticoagulant therapy (low-molecular-weight heparin or oral therapy). A Foley catheter would not be necessary to anticipate initiating at this time as the client's kidney status has not been compromised, based on the narrative. Ambulation should be reserved for when the client is out of the acute active phase of a pulmonary embolus.

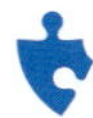
NCJMM Step: Take Action
References: Jarvis et al. (2024), p. 499; Tyerman & Cobbett (2023), pp. 622–624.

▶ Complete the following sentences by choosing from the lists of options.

The nurse should prepare the client for a **spiral computed tomography (CT) scan.** It would be a priority for the nurse to request a prescription for **unfractionated heparin**.

Rationale: This question asks the student to identify the correct diagnostic test as well as the appropriate medication to be ordered. Knowledge of the diagnostic tests associated with particular conditions is important when anticipating therapy and initializing therapy. A chest X-ray may be ordered at a later time, but not during the acute presentation of a pulmonary embolus. A PET scan is ordered to identify glucose metabolism in malignant tumours, and fluoroscopy is used as a tool to assist with other procedures, allowing the radiologist to view the body organs and observe their motion. A transthoracic echocardiogram (TTE) should not be confused with a transesophageal echocardiogram (TEE) as they are used in different cardiac situations. Both a TTE and TEE are diagnostic tests used to evaluate the heart wall motion, detect valvular disease, evaluate the heart during a stress test, and identify and quantify pericardial fluid. The difference between the two is that a TTE is less invasive than a TEE, where a scope is inserted into the client's mouth to obtain better visualization of the posterior portion of the heart and thoracic vessels.

During the practice of nursing, there is the possibility of performing an error by incorrectly choosing the wrong medication, causing harm to the client. Students who encounter this type of question must be familiar with drug classes and common medications. Amiodarone is an antidysrhythmic medication typically ordered for unstable rhythms. Apixaban is a factor Xa inhibitor and platelet aggregator, typically ordered to prevent the formation of thrombus. Dronedarone is another antidysrhythmic ordered for clients who have atrial fibrillation. Metoprolol is a beta blocker typically ordered for clients with mild to moderate hypertension, angina, or acute myocardial infarction.

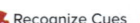

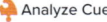

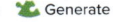

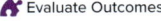

NCJMM Step: Take Action
References: McDonald (2024), pp. 867–871; Tyerman & Cobbett (2023), p. 768.

Answers to Example 6: Evaluate Outcomes

- Which of the following findings would indicate that the client's status has improved? **Select all that apply.**
  - ✔ Respiratory rate
  - ✔ No use of accessory muscles
  - ☐ Skin warm and dry
  - ✔ Heart rate
  - ✔ Jugular venous distension

- Highlight the findings that indicate an improvement (or worsening) of the client's status.

> The client is resting comfortably. Respirations regular and easy at rest. No use of accessory muscles noted. Client denies any pleuritic pain. Client states, "I am not scared I am going to die."
> - HR = 87
> - RR = 16
> - Pulse regular and strong. Skin remains warm and dry to touch. No diaphoresis noted.
> - Jugular venous distension measured at 3 cm

- For each assessment finding, identify if the finding indicates that the client's condition has improved, has not changed, or has declined.

CLIENT FINDINGS	IMPROVED	NO CHANGE	DECLINED
Respiratory rate 16 breaths per minutes	✔	○	○
No use of accessory muscles	✔	○	○
Skin warm and dry	○	✔	○
Heart rate 87 beats per minute	✔	○	○
Jugular venous distension at 3 cm	✔	○	○

- Drag the top 4 client findings that demonstrate the client's status is improving.

TOP 4 CLIENT FINDINGS
Respiratory rate
No use of accessory muscles
Heart rate
Jugular venous distension

Rationale: When answering Evaluate Outcomes questions, recognizing improvements, decline in status, or no change is important during a reassessment. If the orders were carried out that addressed the highest priority, then the client's overall respiratory status would improve, as evidenced by the respiratory rate decreasing from 28 breaths per minute to 16 breaths per minute. The fact that the client is no longer using accessory muscles indicates that there has been an improvement in respiratory function and a reduction in the work of breathing, moving toward a more normal respiratory function. The heart rate has reduced from 130 beats per minute to 87 beats per minute, indicating that the heart is not pumping as hard to try and compensate for the lack of oxygen in the client's systemic system. Finally, the jugular venous distension has decreased from 7 cm to 3 cm, indicating an improvement in overall right ventricular function and less pulmonary artery resistance. There was no change in the client's overall assessment of their skin, which remains warm and dry to touch, indicating well perfused.

NCJMM Step: Evaluate Outcomes
References: Tyerman & Cobbett (2023), pp. 622–624; Power-Kean et al. (2023), p. 692.

▶ For each of the statements made by the client during discharge/client teaching, indicate whether the client understands or has no understanding of the information that was provided.

CLIENT STATEMENTS	UNDERSTANDING	NO UNDERSTANDING
"I will stay on blood thinners for 3 months."	✔	○
"I am fit and do not need to see my doctor for follow-up."	○	✔
"I will need to wear antiembolic stockings when flying."	✔	○
"I will need to make more frequent stops when driving."	✔	○
"I have to change my diet."	○	✔

Rationale: Upon discharge, the client will continue anticoagulant therapy for at least 3 to 6 months. Clients who continuously develop thrombi may require indefinite anticoagulant treatment. There will be a follow-up appointment to review disease progression after an acute episode affecting the heart and lungs. There may be long-term consequences as a result of the acute episode, and the client will need to be monitored and followed closely. It is recommended that clients who develop deep vein thrombosis in their extremities and previously had a pulmonary embolus wear antiembolic stockings while travelling to reduce the incidence of further clot development. Making frequent stops while driving is also recommended to reduce the incidence of clot formation in the lower extremities. Diet is not associated with a pulmonary embolus.

NCJMM Step: Evaluate Outcomes
Reference: Tyerman & Cobbett (2023), p. 624.

5 Understanding Unfolding Case Studies

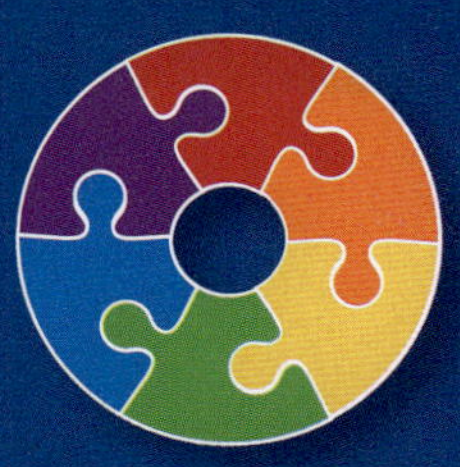

Introduction

Two primary ways that clinical judgement will be assessed for Next Generation NCLEX® (NGN) will be through multisystem **unfolding** or **stand-alone** case studies. Each student who writes the licensure exam will encounter three unfolding case studies, each consisting of six questions (one question for each cognitive step of the nursing clinical judgement measurement model). If, after answering the minimum number of standard NCLEX multiple-choice and/or alternate-format questions plus the three unfolding case studies, the student has not demonstrated enough knowledge to successfully pass the exam, up to seven stand-alone case studies may be asked along with standard multiple-choice and/or alternate-format questions until the program can determine if the student has met the standards for a pass or fail.

After studying Chapters 3 and 4, you are ready to assemble ALL the pieces of each cognitive step and apply this knowledge to unfolding case studies. Previous chapters presented a breakdown of a single-system clinical scenario to demonstrate the basic application of each cognitive step, complete with the most common types of questions to be asked for each cognitive step. Now that you are familiar with the cognitive steps, this chapter will focus on a case study that unfolds with higher complexity. Chapter 6 will address two types of stand-alone case studies: bow-tie and trend.

The **unfolding** case study incorporates all six cognitive steps into one clinical scenario. Utilizing information presented in Chapter 2, this chapter will demonstrate how to further recognize patterns within the clinical scenario and apply this knowledge to each of the six questions. Once you have a grasp on the structure of the unfolding case study, the stand-alone case studies will be presented in the next chapter.

Basic Elements of Any Case Study

The Next Generation NCLEX (NGN) case studies are designed to ensure that each student can demonstrate safe and appropriate clinical judgement when presented with a comparable clinical situation commonly encountered in practice. All case studies have similar basic elements that are needed to present the clinical story in a familiar way consistent with the presentation of medical information. A useful analogy for a case study is to think of it like a recipe; let's use a bread recipe, for example. Each type of bread recipe (whole wheat, oat, sourdough, brioche, raisin, etc.) has different ingredients, but some essential ones are necessary to make bread. The five essential ingredients of most bread recipes are flour (or gluten-free substitute), eggs, yeast, sugar, and oil. Like a recipe, essential ingredients (or elements) can be found within every case study. These essential pieces provide further data so you can answer the questions correctly. The three essential elements of all case studies are:

1. The introductory statement
2. The clinical data
3. The clinical scenario

Pay close attention to the details in these essential elements.

Introductory Statement

Each case study begins with an initial **introductory statement** providing context to the narrative. Information found in the introductory statement may include age, health care location, and gender (if important to the main issue of the narrative). Here are some examples of introductory statements:

The nurse is caring for a 65-year-old female client in the emergency department.

OR

The nurse on a cardiac unit is caring for an 85-year-old male client.

OR

The nurse is caring for a 32-year-old non-binary client on the postpartum unit.

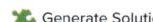

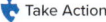

Clinical Data

One main element of all case studies is the presentation of **data,** which familiarize the test writer with the details of the clinical scenario. The clinical data are presented through tabs commonly found in a client's medical chart. When writing the licensure examination, test writers can choose a tab and move through the data as presented throughout the case study. This information is not "taken away" but remains present and can be accessed as the test writer progresses through the question(s). There are 11 possible tabs (Table 5.1): Nurses' Notes, History and Physical, Laboratory Results, Diagnostic Results, Flow Sheet, Intake and Output, Progress Notes, Admission Notes, Medications, Vital Signs, and Orders.

Presentation of NGN Case Studies

All case studies are presented in a similar format. Client information will be presented on the left side of the computer screen or page during practice questions, and the appropriate cognitive step question is located on the right side of the computer screen or page. The writer will always see the full case as presented with the ability to flip between tabs if writing on a computer. No information is hidden from the writer.

During an unfolding case study, as the case unfolds and new information is provided, the writer will be notified in a sentence before the next question to review the new data, which may or may not be pertinent to the cognitive step being tested. Only the question will change on the right side. Test writers are able to access the tabs as presented to gather information and answer the question(s) as needed.

TABLE 5.1 Possible Clinical Data Tabs Used to Represent a Client's Medical Chart

Possible Clinical Data Tabs	Rationale
Nurses' Notes	Narrative data are comparable to the admission notes. This information may include a narrative detail of the initial presentation, vital signs, and head-to-toe system assessment details. This is the most common way for information to be presented in case study formats.
History and Physical	Information is presented in a chart format identifying head-to-toe assessment information and psychosocial information.
Laboratory Results	Client data are presented along with normal values.
Diagnostic Results	Client data are presented along with expected normal results.
Flow Sheet	The information presented in this tab demonstrates data over time and may include fluids, vital signs, blood glucose results, pain scores, weight, height, nutritional intake, etc.
Intake and Output	This tab is specific to fluids only and may include oral intake, intravenous fluid administration volumes, blood and blood product volume administration, nutritional volumes, renal output, chest tube or any surgical drain output, abdominal secretion amounts, blood loss, insensible losses, etc.
Progress Notes	Data are presented as introductory clinical scenario information or as changes over time, as in a community setting. This could include data pertaining to client presentation over time, such as in the case of newborns and infants, outpatient pregnancy clinics, or with home care clients.
Admission Notes	These are clinical data to situate the writer within the client presentation. This is typically presented in a narrative format, including the initial story of what brought the client to the specific clinical context.
Medications	Client data at the time of admission or transfer to another unit may include current medications or, if appropriate, new medication orders, which will alert the writer that new information has been presented.
Vital Signs	This tab may include singular vital sign data or client data presented over a specific time period to demonstrate possible changes. Vital signs include temperature, pulse, respiratory rate, blood pressure, and pulse oximetry reading.
Orders	New orders received can be written in the designated tab.

The intent of each of the presenting case studies is to ensure that students are able to process, analyze, and determine pertinent information when possible extraneous details are also shared in the client chart. NCLEX multiple-choice or alternate-format questions only present pertinent information in the question, whereas Next Generation NCLEX case studies can present additional or extraneous information that will not assist the student in making appropriate decisions regarding client care. This is where your knowledge helps you answer these questions successfully and, when compared to clinical situations, provide safe and competent client care.

Clinical Scenario

Each case study presents the test writer with a clinical scenario comparable to client narratives that students may encounter in practice. By this point, many of you have been in the clinical practice environment and may have received a report from the previous nurse about the clients you will be assuming care of during your shift. The clinical scenario in the NGN case studies is similar to a nurses' report complete with SBAR elements (**S**ituation, **B**ackground, **A**ssessment, and **R**ecommendation). As you know, the client's medical chart is a communication tool necessary to keep all health care providers up to date on the latest clinical data. The clinical scenario is the centre of any client's story or the reason for them to seek additional care. The details of the clinical scenario often consist of patterns of information that, when recognized by the student, demonstrate their knowledge and, ultimately, make safe decisions for client care.

A key important fact to remember is NGN case studies are meant to test student knowledge at higher cognitive levels by presenting multiple pieces of data on one *medical/clinical* scenario that may or may not lead to client deterioration. There may be multiple pieces of information to sift through to determine the singular health problem, but there is one *connected problem* in each case study. Remember the Chapter 2 discussion of knowing how conditions progress through the example of pericarditis, pericardial effusion, and cardiac tamponade? The clinical manifestations of this scenario are connected and require the student to recognize the main problem, identify solutions, and determine if the client's status is improving or getting worse. The student would account for multiple physiological system presentations to decipher the main issue. This is where knowledge again is needed to recognize patterns of care to identify the primary medical concern. There is a difference in client presentation between pericarditis and a cardiac tamponade with more than just cardiovascular clinical manifestations.

NGN case studies *do not* test theoretical knowledge. Each case study is associated with a clinical problem, not theory. For example, students may encounter a clinical scenario associated with addictions, such as alcohol withdrawal, but would not encounter a case study with the core topic of Prochaska and DiClemente's (1984) Transtheoretical Model (TTM), otherwise known as Stages of Change. Clinical judgement is not associated with application of a theory into clinical practice scenarios. Theory has its place in undergraduate nursing programs; however, students are not tested on theory in the clinical judgement problems found on the Next Generation NCLEX (NGN).

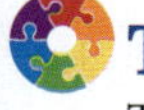

The Unfolding Case Study

The unfolding case study presents one clinical/medical scenario addressing all six cognitive steps of the clinical judgement measurement model. This is where you will apply concepts learned in Chapters 3 and 4 with the knowledge base you developed from your undergraduate program to identify the medical problem and make appropriate decisions about how to care for the client, and then recognize if the client is improving or deteriorating in status. You are going to be putting together all the pieces of the puzzle. Unfolding Case Study Example 1.0 will walk you through an unfolding case study.

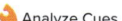

The introductory sentence indicates the condition is **pediatric** in nature and **serious** enough to be requiring care in the **emergency department**.

Always start with **airway, breathing**, and **circulation**. What do you notice is an immediate concern for this client?

Determine the system that is **most affecte**d with this client. Is it NEURO, CV, RESP, GI, GU, MSK, and/or ENDO?

Then differentiate normal, abnormal, and critical abnormal assessment data as documented in the chart.

RECOGNIZE CUES

Consider clinical data that have the potential to develop or are already at a critical level for the client. Ask yourself: Are there any concerns with the airway, breathing, and circulation, followed by NEURO, CV, RESP, GI, GU, MSK, ENDO systems? Look for patterns and determine which manifestations are **normal, abnormal,** or **critical abnormal** based on the narrative and then in the questions.

ANALYZE CUES

When considering client presentation, it is best to consider the **potential complications** the client could develop and the patterns of presentation.

Unfolding Case Study Example 1.0

The nurse is caring for a 16-year-old female client in the emergency department (ED).

Nurses' Notes

- **1030h:**
  The client was found on the floor at school by two students who witnessed the client's body stiffen, followed by jerking movements. 911 was called. Emergency medical services (EMS) found the client in the same position, with irregular breaths, cool and clammy skin to touch, with diaphoresis noted. No further movement noted. Client remained unresponsive with a GCS 9. Initial ED vital signs: T: 37.7°C (99.8°F); BP: 121/78; P: 110; RR: 28; with pulse oximetry of 90% on room air. Upon arrival at the ED, the client was difficult to rouse, unable to follow commands, but withdraws from painful stimuli and groans with movement. Pupils equal in size and react sluggish to light and measured at 2 mm. Skin remains cool to touch. Bilateral radial pulses regular and strong × 2 with palpation. S1, S2 auscultated with no adventitious heart sounds noted. Apical = radial. Bilateral dorsalis pedis pulses regular and strong × 2. Capillary refill less than 3 seconds. No peripheral edema was noted. No jugular venous distension. Chest auscultated posteriorly for fine inspiratory crackles noted to bilateral bases. Lips noted to be cyanotic. Respirations noted to be irregular and shallow. No cough noted. Client's pants were soiled with urine. Hyperactive bowel sounds auscultated × 4 quadrants. Abdomen is soft to touch. A peripheral venous access device was inserted into the left antecubital fossa. No known comorbidities.

▶ Select 4 client findings that require immediate follow-up.

- ☐ Pupillary response
- ☐ Level of consciousness
- ☐ Bowel sounds
- ☐ Skin temperature
- ☐ Lung sounds
- ☐ Incontinence
- ☐ Cyanosis

▶ Which of the following complications could the client develop? **Select all that apply.**

- ☐ Bleeding on the brain
- ☐ Respiratory distress
- ☐ Peripheral edema
- ☐ Bacteria in the urine
- ☐ Skin breakdown
- ☐ Sepsis
- ☐ Dysrhythmia

Nurses' Notes | Laboratory Results

1210h: Client found with stiffening × 4 limb extremities, followed by jerking motions. Eyes remained open but no eye movement noted and unable to determine pupil reactivity. Stiffening and jerking movements lasted × 25 seconds. Client extremely fatigued, moaned only to questions, observed moving all four extremities independently but not to command. Vital signs: T: 37.9°C (100.2°F); BP: 130/88; P: 122; RR: 16; with pulse oximetry of 91% on room air. Client's breathing noted to be shallow and irregular breaths with occasional coughing and snoring noted. Health care provider notified.

Nurses' Notes | **Laboratory Results**

1050h:			
Hemoglobin 140–180 g/L 14–18 g/dL (male) 120–160 g/L 12–16 g/dL (female)	152 g/L (15.2 g/dL)	**Sodium** 136–145 mmol/L	151 mmol/L
Platelets 150–400 × 10^9/L (150 000–400 000/mm^3)	250 × 10^9/L (250 000/mm^3)	**Potassium** 3.5–5.1 mmol/L	4.4 mmol/L
White blood cells 3.5–12.0 × 10^9/L (3 500–12 000/mm^3)	8.8 × 10^9/L (8 800/mm^3)	**Creatinine** 53–106 mcmol/L (male) 44–97 mcmol/L (female)	76 mcmol/L
Neutrophils 3.0–5.8 × 10^9/L (3 000–5 800/mm^3)	4.5 × 10^9/L (4 500/mm^3)	**Blood urea nitrogen (BUN)** 2.9–8.2 mmol/L	0.65 mmol/L
Arterial blood gas pH: 7.35-7.45 CO_2: 35-45 mmHg HCO_3: 22-26 mEq/L PaO_2: 80-110 mmHg	**ABG results:** pH: 7.48 CO_2: 58 mmHg HCO_3: 22 mEq/L PaO_2: 81 mmHg	**Blood glucose (random)** 3.9–6.1 mmol/L (70–110 mg/dL)	2.6 mmol/L

When more clinical data information is provided, focus on what system is being presented (NEURO, CV, RESP, GI, or GU), then make note of what has changed from the previous information. Remember, you are looking for patterns.

The nurse has reviewed the Nurses' Notes entries at 1030h, 1210h, and the new Laboratory Results drawn at 1050h.

New clinical data is always reported to the writer. It is up to the writer to determine the importance of this information.

▶ Complete the following sentence by choosing from the lists of options.

The client is at **highest risk** of developing _________________ (word options 1) as evidenced by the client's _______________ (word options 2) and ______________ (word options 2).

WORD OPTIONS 1	WORD OPTIONS 2
Increased intracranial pressure	Sodium levels
Renal failure	Arterial blood gas results
Hypoxemia	Glucose levels
Seizure	Cyanosis
Ventricular tachycardia	Potassium levels

PRIORITIZE HYPOTHESIS

This is where you put all the pieces of the assessment clinical data together to determine the medical issue. Recognizing the patterns of clinical presentation will help you determine **which condition the client is likely experiencing**.

GENERATE SOLUTIONS

Once you have determined the correct medical issue, this cognitive skill assesses your ability to create an appropriate **plan of care.** If you determined the incorrect medical issue, distractors will lead you to create the wrong plan. Use your knowledge to anticipate nursing interventions or orders from the health care provider and plan accordingly.

▶ For each potential nursing intervention, identify whether the intervention is indicated or not indicated for this client.

POTENTIAL NURSING INTERVENTIONS	INDICATED	NOT INDICATED
Prepare to administer intravenous dextrose	○	○
Place the LIFEPAK monitor outside the client's room	○	○
Ensure safety by placing bed in lowest position, suction is working, and bedrails are padded	○	○
Request an order for supplemental oxygen therapy	○	○
Prepare phenytoin for administration	○	○
Prepare the client for a chest X-ray	○	○
Encourage oral fluids for rehydration	○	○
Prepare to administer sodium bicarbonate	○	○

TAKE ACTION

When considering priority orders to implement or nursing interventions, consider client safety and if the **critical nature of the medical issue would be resolved.** Ensure that the actions meet the expectations of appropriate client care.

▶ Highlight below the 3 priority health care orders the nurse should perform immediately.

Orders

1218h:

- 0.9% sodium chloride (normal saline) at 125 mL/hr per IV
- Dextrose 50% half amp, IV STAT
- Insert an oral pharyngeal airway
- Insert in-dwelling urinary catheter
- Maintain pulse oximetry levels greater than 92%, initiate oxygen therapy at 2 L/min per nasal prongs
- Place client in Trendelenburg position
- Phenytoin, start with loading dose of 15 mg/kg IV then 100 mg IV q8hr
- Insert an additional venous access device

The nurse performed the interventions as ordered by the health care provider.

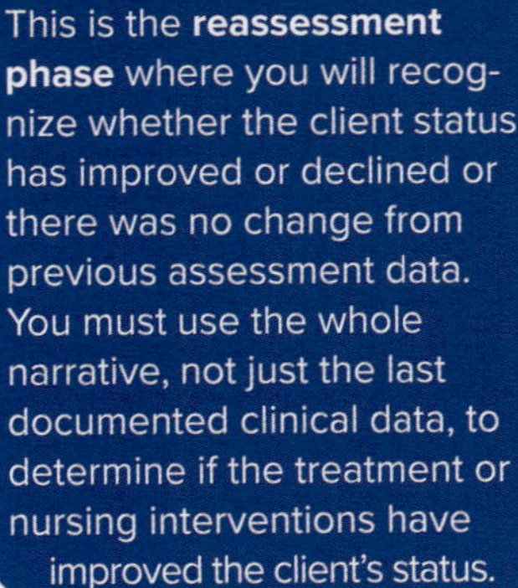

EVALUATE OUTCOMES
This is the **reassessment phase** where you will recognize whether the client status has improved or declined or there was no change from previous assessment data. You must use the whole narrative, not just the last documented clinical data, to determine if the treatment or nursing interventions have improved the client's status.

▶ For each assessment finding, identify if the finding indicates that the client's condition has improved, not changed, or has declined.

CLIENT ASSESSMENT FINDINGS	IMPROVED	NO CHANGE	DECLINED
RR 18 regular and easy at rest	○	○	○
HR 77	○	○	○
Cyanotic lips	○	○	○
Pulse oximetry 88%	○	○	○
Unable to remember anything that happened after arriving at school	○	○	○
Obeys commands	○	○	○

Summary of the Unfolding Case Study

In the above unfolding scenario, you have been provided with a guided process to answer the questions. These *tips and tricks* consist of specific **language** that you can use when you are answering the question types pertaining to each cognitive step. It is important to use this knowledge about interpreting the questions so you can translate this skill to stand-alone items, which will be covered in Chapter 6. The answers to the case study are provided at the end of this chapter for your reference.

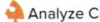

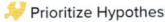

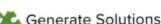

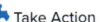

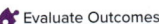

Answers to Unfolding Case Study Example 1.0

Answer to Recognize Cues

- ☐ Pupillary response
- ✔ Level of consciousness
- ☐ Bowel sounds
- ✔ Skin temperature
- ✔ Lung sounds
- ☐ Incontinence
- ✔ Cyanosis

Rationale: The three most important client findings pertain to level of consciousness (neuro), skin temperature (CV–circulation), and cyanosis (CV–circulation leading to respiratory compromise). The client is difficult to rouse and unable to follow commands. It is important to rule out potential neurological complications (head injury, seizure disorder, hematoma, increased intracranial pressure, etc.) associated with these clinical manifestations. The skin temperature remains cool to touch and has been consistent since the client was found by EMS. This may contribute to a lack of circulation issues, leading the client to have sluggish blood flow. Finally, the cyanosis around the lips is an immediate concern indicating that the low circulation levels may be contributing to respiratory distress, especially since the client is taking fast, shallow breaths (as evidenced by the vital signs). The lung sounds indicate fine inspiratory crackles, which could develop into aspiration pneumonia or, worse, septic shock. The pupils, albeit sluggish, are still equal in size and shape and remain equally reactive. This indicates normal nerve function. The bowel sounds are hyperactive but present in all four quadrants. The incontinence is an addition to the client's narrative but does not need to be immediately followed up on at the moment.

NCJMM Step: Recognize Cues
References: Tyerman & Cobbett (2023), pp. 1516–1522; Eli Lily Canada (2019).

Answer to Analyze Cues

- ✔ Bleeding on the brain
- ✔ Respiratory distress
- ☐ Peripheral edema
- ☐ Bacteria in the urine
- ☐ Skin breakdown
- ✔ Sepsis
- ☐ Dysrhythmia

Rationale: The client was lying on the floor. It would be too soon to rule out any potential head injuries that may have occurred, despite the lack of blood. It would be prudent to monitor neurological status for any increased intracranial pressure, monitoring for high blood pressure, changes in pupillary response, and additional changes to levels of consciousness. The client does present with fine inspiratory crackles to the bases. Again, since the client was found unconscious and unresponsive on the floor, there is no way to determine if the client aspirated. Monitoring the temperature and changes in respiratory status would be appropriate as changes could indicate a progression of client status to the critical complication of sepsis. The client is 16 years old and presents as healthy despite the unresponsiveness. The client would not be at risk for peripheral edema, which is associated with cardiac dysfunction. There is nothing in the initial narrative to indicate the client would be at risk for introduction of bacteria into the urethra, warranting the need to monitor for a urinary tract infection. There were no open areas identified indicating the need to monitor for skin breakdown. The client presents with regular heart rate and palpable pulses. There are no clinical manifestations to indicate the client may develop a dysrhythmia.

CLIENT PRESENTATION	POTENTIAL COMPLICATION	POTENTIAL CRITICAL CONDITION
Client found on the floor, unknown if injury to the head	Bleeding on the brain	Increased intracranial pressure, subdural or intracerebral hematoma
Fine crackles to bilateral lung bases, cyanosis	Aspiration pneumonia, impaired gas exchange	Sepsis, respiratory distress

If you consider how to use the clinical manifestations associated with the narrative, consider potential complications and critical conditions the client may encounter by **recognizing patterns**. With any injury to the head the client has the potential to develop bleeding on the brain, which could lead to increased intracranial pressure. The pattern to recognize would be Cushing's triad—irregular breathing pattern, bradycardia, and widened pulse pressure.

NCJMM Step: Analyze Cues
Reference: Tyerman & Cobbett (2023), pp. 1516–1522.

Answer to Prioritize Hypothesis

The client is at **highest risk** of developing **seizure** as evidenced by the client's **sodium levels** and **glucose levels**.

Rationale: The initial presentation and subsequent observed clinical data of limb stiffening followed by jerking motions and extreme fatigue point to the client developing a seizure, likely a tonic-clonic seizure. The body stiffens (tonic phase) for 10 to 20 seconds and the extremities jerk (clonic phase), possibly for another 30 to 40 seconds. Main clinical manifestations postseizure include cyanosis, excessive salivation, tongue or cheek biting, and incontinence. The primary system of concern is the neurological system. The seizure activity is a result of likely dehydration and low blood sugar. When sodium levels are greater-than-normal levels of lower-than-normal levels, the client has a propensity for seizure activity. The glucose levels are classified as severe low as per Diabetes Canada (2023). Classic symptom presentation of Cushing's triad is missing from the client narrative data; therefore, at this time, you can remove increased intracranial pressure from the list. The client's creatinine and BUN levels are within normal so you can rule out renal failure. Although the client may have aspirated, the client is not experiencing hypoxemia, based on the PaO_2 levels in the arterial blood gas (ABG) result. The client's potassium levels remain within normal, and no other contributing factor is present with this client for development of ventricular tachycardia.

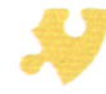
NCJMM Step: Prioritize Hypothesis
References: Tyerman & Cobbett (2023), pp. 1516–1522; McDonald (2024), pp. 241–244 (glucose), pp. 427–430 (sodium).

Answer to Generate Solutions

POTENTIAL NURSING INTERVENTIONS	INDICATED	NOT INDICATED
Prepare to administer intravenous dextrose	✔	○
Place the LIFEPAK monitor outside the client's room	○	✔
Ensure safety by placing bed in lowest position, suction is working, and bedrails are padded	✔	○
Request an order for supplemental oxygen therapy	✔	○
Prepare phenytoin for administration	✔	○
Prepare the client for a chest X-ray	○	✔
Encourage oral fluids for rehydration	○	✔
Prepare to administer sodium bicarbonate	○	✔

Rationale: Interventions would be related to airway, breathing, and circulation first, then address safety, followed by prevention for any other seizures to occur. Ensuring client safety is a priority when seizure activity occurs. The bed should be in the lowest position to prevent injury. The nurse must also ensure that suction is on and working correctly in the event the client has emesis and ensure the bedrails are up × 4 and padded with either padding or blankets. Supplemental oxygen therapy may be necessary, especially if the client becomes hemodynamically unstable and requires airway support. Administration of medication to prevent and control the development of other seizures is important. Other medications include phenobarbital, benzodiazepines, midazolam, or lorazepam. The client presents with severe hypoglycemia (less than 2.8 mmol/L), which places the client at risk for a seizure. Administration of dextrose intravenously will increase the client's blood sugar more quickly than other routes of administration. Distractors are present in the event the wrong potential condition was chosen. A LIFEPAK monitor would be necessary if the client was experiencing ventricular tachycardia and require support during a cardiac arrest. A chest X-ray would be warranted if the client was experiencing respiratory distress or hypoxemia. Oral fluids would be inappropriate and a safety hazard given the client's lethargy. Finally, sodium bicarbonate could be administered in the event of an acidotic state. Based on the ABG in the laboratory results, the client is experiencing uncompensated respiratory alkalosis, plus the sodium levels are already elevated. Administering sodium bicarbonate would further increase sodium levels, potentiating other seizures.

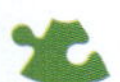

NCJMM Step: Generate Solutions
References: Power-Kean et al. (2023), pp. 118–119; Tyerman & Cobbett (2023), pp. 1516–1522.

Answer to Take Action

- ☐ 0.9% sodium chloride (normal saline) at 125 mL/hr per IV
- ☐ Dextrose 50% half amp, IV STAT
- ☐ Insert an oral pharyngeal airway
- ☐ Insert in-dwelling urinary catheter
- ☐ Maintain pulse oximetry levels greater than 92%, initiate oxygen therapy at 2 L/min per nasal prongs
- ☐ Place client in Trendelenburg position
- ☐ Phenytoin, start with loading dose of 15 mg/kg IV then 100 mg IV q8h
- ☐ Insert an additional venous access device

Rationale: The priority is to prevent further seizures from happening, so the cause must be addressed, which is either the low blood sugar or high sodium levels. The client's blood sugar is significantly low as per the laboratory draw and will require treatment to raise the glucose level. A half amp of dextrose 50% (D_{50}) would be most appropriate at this time given the additional seizure activity. A full amp of D_{50} is 25 mg and a half amp would be 12.5 mg. This has the potential to raise the blood sugar by 8 mmol/L, giving much needed sugar to cells. It would be important to initiate medication for seizure control. The most common medication for a tonic-clonic seizure would be phenytoin, carbamazepine, phenobarbital, and divalproex. There is a loading dose with phenytoin followed by consistent administration to maintain an appropriate serum level to prevent further seizure activity. An additional venous access device would be imperative as most medication is incompatible with phenytoin. The order of 0.9% sodium chloride should be verified prior to initiating therapy, as this will continue to raise the sodium levels. Possibly a 0.45% normal saline or D_5W would be a better solution to choose for this client. There is no indication that the client is having airway issues; therefore, an oral pharyngeal airway would be unnecessary. An in-dwelling urinary catheter may be an appropriate order for this client; however, it is not an immediate action. The client has already been incontinent prior to coming to the hospital with little hydration. Initiating oxygen therapy would be important, as would continuing to monitor respiratory status. The client should not be placed in Trendelenburg position but in a side-lying position, also called a *lateral position*, to prevent aspiration of stomach contents.

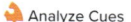

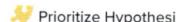

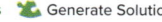

NCJMM Step: Take Action
Reference: Tyerman & Cobbett (2023), pp. 1516–1522.

Answer to Evaluate Outcomes

CLIENT ASSESSMENT FINDING	IMPROVED	NO CHANGE	DECLINED
RR 18 regular and easy at rest	✔	○	○
HR 77	✔	○	○
Cyanotic lips	○	✔	○
Pulse oximetry 88%	○	○	✔
Unable to remember anything that happened after arriving at school	○	○	✔
Obeys commands	✔	○	○

Rationale: In the postictal phase the client may experience muscle soreness and fatigue and may require additional sleep. The client may not have any memory of the seizure or events during the postictal phase either. This client has improved respiratory effort as the breaths are now easy and regular at rest. The heart rate has returned to a more rest-and-digest phase rather than staying in a sympathetic fight-or-flight state. The client's lips remain cyanotic due to the impaired gas exchange, as evidenced by the drop in pulse oximetry levels. Oxygen can be applied as ordered. The lack of memory is normal. The nurse needs to reorientate the client and provide reassurance of their safety. The client's ability to obey commands indicates that their neurological status has improved overall, with clear messaging being interpreted by the brain followed by the action.

NCJMM Step: Evaluate Outcomes
Reference: Tyerman & Cobbett (2023), pp. 1516–1522.

6 Understanding Stand-Alone Case Studies

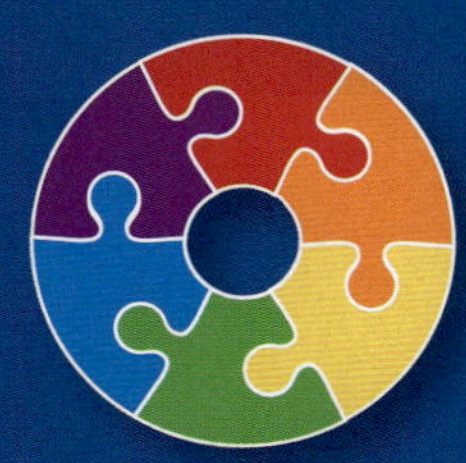

Introduction

Chapter 5 presented a more complicated multisystem presentation of an unfolding case study than the basic single-system case study found in Chapters 3 and 4. Once you have the foundational pieces to understand how to move through the cognitive steps of a complex unfolding clinical presentation, applying this knowledge to stand-alone case studies like the bow-tie and trend formats will become easier. When writing NCLEX-RN®, if more questions are needed, beyond the minimum number of multiple choice and/or alternate format questions plus the three unfolding case studies, test writers may encounter up to seven additional **stand-alone** case studies. You may never encounter a stand-alone question; however, it is best to be prepared to answer all types of questions used to assess your ability to apply clinical judgement to clinical scenarios.

Basic Elements of the Stand-Alone Case Studies

Stand-alone case studies will be presented in either the bow-tie or trend structure. The **bow-tie** stand-alone case study incorporates all six cognitive steps for clinical judgement. By recognizing patterns of presentation in the clinical scenario (Recognize Cues + Analyze Cues), the student will determine the potential condition that the client is experiencing (Prioritize Hypothesis), two appropriate actions to take (Generate Solutions + Take Action), then two appropriate parameters to monitor for the client (Evaluate Outcomes).

In contrast, a **trend** stand-alone case study will ask one question associated with one cognitive step. As in previous chapter examples, common types of questions aligned with each cognitive step is presented, enabling you to become familiar with each type of question type through repeated exposure and practice and learn how to apply your knowledge to answer each question successfully. The trend stand-alone case study presents a clinical scenario that develops over time and may or may not state a diagnosis in the introductory statement. Test writers will be assessed by a single question representing any one of the cognitive steps (Recognize Cues *or* Analyze Cues *or* Prioritize Hypothesis *or* Take Action *or* Generate Solutions *or* Evaluate Outcomes).

This book contains practice case studies and exposure to various questions associated with each cognitive step used to assess clinical judgement. Make notations of the phrasing patterns in the questions explained in Chapters 3 and 4 when working through the practice case studies to help you identify the cognitive step being addressed in the single question. You will find practice stand-alone case studies in Chapter 8.

Like the unfolding case study, both the bow-tie and trend case studies continue to include an introductory statement, clinical data, and the clinical scenario. There are small differences in the presentation of this information when comparing unfolding to stand-alone case studies.

Introductory Statement

The introductory statements for trend stand-alone case studies differ from those in unfolding and bow-tie case studies, which present the client, age (if applicable), and health care environment. In addition to the basic information provided to the exam writer, the introductory sentence of a trend stand-alone case study may also present a stated diagnosis or additional relevant clinical assessment data. For example:

The nurse is caring for a 5-year-old in the Critical Care Unit who is intubated following an anaphylaxis reaction to a bee sting.

Clinical Data

For bow-tie and trend stand-alone case studies, the same tabs are used to present clinical data as in Chapter 5 for unfolding case studies. See Table 5.1 to review the 11 possible tabs used to present clinical data for the case study for a review. Client data can be presented using the various tabs in a manner necessary to determine the correct answer.

Clinical Scenario

Bow-tie clinical scenarios contain all the information necessary to identify the possible condition, which in turn will determine which actions to take and parameters to monitor for the client. The clinical scenario includes enough information to inform exam writers. Trend case clinical scenarios present information that occurs *over* time. This could include a change in client presentation, changes in vital signs, or input and output values. In either clinical scenario, use information presented in Chapter 2 to assist with identifying patterns in the data and clues within the narrative.

This chapter will break down the bow-tie and trend case studies further.

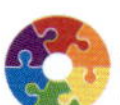

Bow-Tie Stand-Alone Case Study

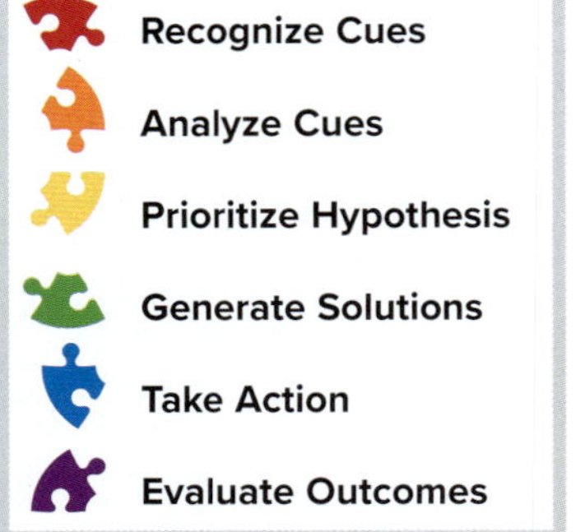

Bow-tie stand-alone case studies incorporate all six cognitive steps into one question. Students will be asked to synthesize recognized patterns of assessment data, further analyze these clues independently from the clinical narrative to determine the correct medical condition, then determine two nursing actions to take and two parameters to monitor (see the bow-tie table shown below).

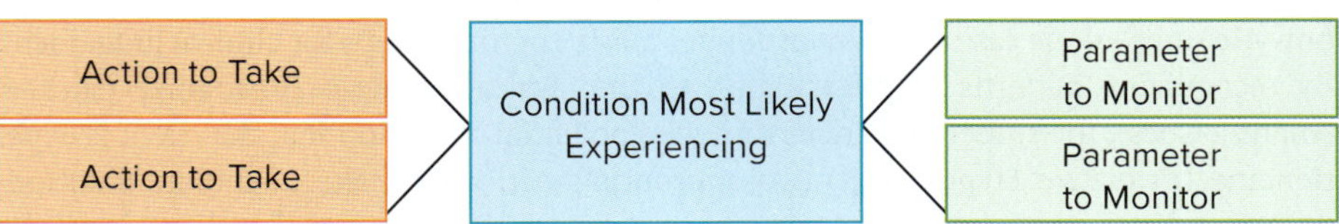

The bow-tie stand-alone case study incorporates the application of the six cognitive steps of the NCJMM in a single question that has three main elements: determining the presenting condition the client is most likely experiencing, actions to take related to that condition, and, finally, parameters to monitor for ensuring safe care.

What can confuse students about this question is determining the correct medical condition. Ensure you have prepared well and studied your pathophysiology notes to have a good understanding of the clinical manifestations associated with medical conditions. Recognizing those patterns of clinical presentation will be helpful in answering these questions correctly. Then it is a matter of choosing the correct actions to take and parameters to monitor that are associated with the correct medical condition the client is experiencing in the clinical scenario. Distractors will be present, which will align with an incorrect hypothesis of the medical condition. If you choose the incorrect medical condition, then there is a higher chance of choosing the incorrect actions to take or parameters to monitor. Focus on identifying the correct medical condition, then apply your knowledge to the remainder of the question.

Let's practise! Notice that the same consistent elements of case study presentation are presented in both the bow-tie and trend case studies.

Stand-Alone Case Study Example 1.0—Bow-Tie

The nurse is caring for a 62-year-old client on the internal medicine unit.

Which system is most affected? Differentiate between what is normal, abnormal, and critical abnormal assessment data.

Nurses' Notes	History and Physical
1012h: Client presented to the emergency department (ED) accompanied by their partner. Primary complaints of extreme fatigue, palpitations, and shortness of breath precipitated the need for further assessment. Temp: 37.3°C (99.1°F); BP: 99/60; HR: 117; RR: 28; pulse oximetry of 86% on room air.	

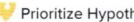

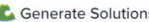

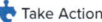

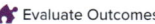

Nurses' Notes | **History and Physical**

1012h:

Body System/History	**Findings**
Neurological	Alert and orientated to person, place, and time. Cooperative, obeys commands. Motor power strong × 4. Gait steady. Denies headache, double vision, dizziness. Denies any pain.
Cardiovascular	Skin warm and dry to touch. Capillary refill less than 3 seconds. No jugular venous distension noted. Bilateral radial pulses palpable but irregular. Client complaints of feeling fast heart rate in chest at rest then it disappears. Denies any chest pain but feels a "fluttering" in the left upper chest wall. Bilateral dorsalis pedis pulses strong. Posterior tibial pulses × 2 weak but palpable. +1 non-pitting peripheral edema noted on bilateral lower extremities.
Pulmonary	Shortness of breath with minimal exertion. Coarse crackles noted to left lower lobe with fine crackles noted to right lower lobe. No cyanosis noted. No use of accessory muscles noted. Nonproductive cough noted. Client taking short, shallow breaths and states, "I feel like I am running a marathon."
Renal	Urinal at the bedside with concentrated small amount of foul-smelling urine.
Psychosocial	Married, CEO of a company in an urban centre with over 500 employees.
Past Medical History	Type 2 diabetes diagnosed 3 years ago, controlled with oral hypoglycemic agents; coronary artery disease with acute myocardial infarction 10 years ago with percutaneous coronary intervention to distal right coronary artery and coronary artery bypass graft × 2 vessels—left anterior descending coronary artery and circumflex. Client developed acute renal failure post-bypass.

What clinical patterns of presentation do you see leading up to identifying the most likely condition this client is experiencing?

The nurse is reviewing the collected client data to assist with preparing the client's plan of care.

▶ Complete the diagram from the choices below to specify what condition the client is most likely experiencing, 2 actions the nurse should take to address the condition, and 2 parameters the nurse should monitor to assess the client's progress.

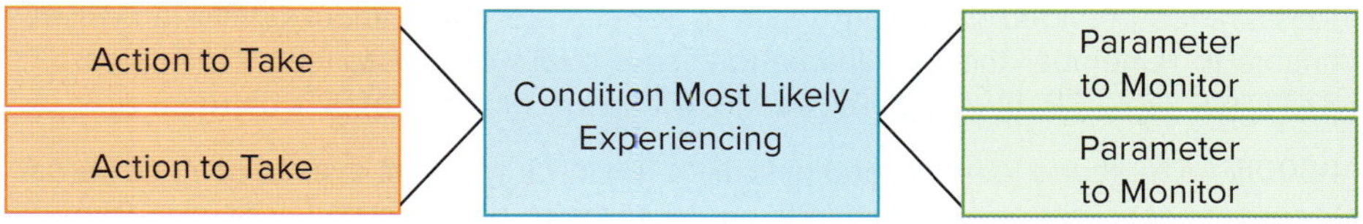

Action to Take	Condition Most Likely Experiencing	Parameter to Monitor
Action to Take		Parameter to Monitor

What are you going to monitor in this client, taking into consideration the condition and plan of care and actions?

Action to Take	Potential Condition	Parameters to Monitor
Request a D-dimer be added	Pulmonary embolus	Urine output
Request an order to administer furosemide	Pneumonia	Temperature
Request an order to administer 0.9% sodium chloride at 175 mL/hr	Cardiomyopathy	Corrected calcium
Prepare for intubation	Chronic pericarditis	Weight loss
Initiate oxygen therapy at 2 L/min per nasal prongs		Continuous electrocardiogram (ECG)

What is the most appropriate plan of care and actions for this client, based on your determination of the most likely condition?

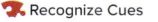

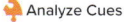

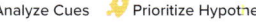

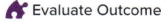

Answer to this bow-tie stand-alone question can be found at the end of this chapter.

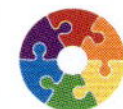

Trend Stand-Alone Case Study

Trend stand-alone case studies have similar elements to the clinical narrative, such as the introductory statement (which may or may not include a stated diagnosis), a narrative of the clinical scenario, plus the use of tabs commonly found in a client's medical chart. What is unique about these stand-alone case studies is that the narrative is presented as details of the clinical scenario unfold over time, thereby indicating that the condition is often deteriorating in some way. The test writer is often tasked with identifying the problem to determine next nursing interventions or actions or to evaluate the client's overall condition. Any one of the 13 possible question item types can be asked as only a single question is asked. The appropriate question style will still reflect the cognitive step being assessed. You will continue to use the same strategies from the previous case study examples to apply your knowledge to these unique questions.

Stand-Alone Case Study Example 2.0—Trend

The nurse is caring for a 23-year-old male client in the emergency department (ED).

Nurses' Notes

2015h: Client presented to the ED via emergency medical services (EMS) after being found at the bottom of a stairwell. Client was found at the scene by a Good Samaritan, unconsciousness lying on right side of body. EMS was notified and spinal collar applied as a precaution. Vital signs: T: 37.2°C (99.0°F); BP: 122/70; P: 88; RR: 20; with pulse oximetry of 92% on room air. Client opens eyes to speech, obeys commands, but presents confused, with intermittent difficulty understanding words the client is speaking. Motor power strong × 4 extremities. Client requires reorientation several times as he cannot remember reason for admission. Agitation noted with memory loss and client requires ++ reassurance. Client able to speak his own name but cannot remember the date or year. GCS 12. Right pupil dilated to approximately 4 mm and no reaction to light. Left pupil noted to be 3 mm in size with sluggish reaction. Pupils both present as round. Client complaining of a headache rated 7 out of 10 on a numerical pain scale. Denies halos around lights or diplopia. Capillary refill less than 3 seconds. Radial pulses × 2 noted to be normal and regular. Bilateral dorsalis pedis pulses normal × 2 with posterior tibial pulses weaker × 2. Skin warm and dry to touch. Respirations regular and easy at rest. Lung fields clear on auscultation. Urinal at bedside.

0116h: Client became agitated when the nurse tried to take blood pressure, waving arms yelling, "No, you can't do this to me. I have rights. You can't keep me here." Client noted to be taking deep, but rapid breaths when trying to communicate. Additional reassurance provided in a calm voice to reorientate client about admission. Client unable to remember the fall. Unable to assess pupils due to agitation. Vital signs: T: 37.7°C (99.86°F); BP: 144/66; P: 97; RR: 26; with pulse oximetry of 97% on room air.

0300h: Client found lethargic and difficult to rouse. Only opens eyes to pain, no verbal response, does not obey commands but localizes to painful stimuli with extension of bilateral upper extremities. Vital signs: T: 38.6°C (101.5°F); BP: 156/54; P: 57; RR: 26; with pulse oximetry of 90% on room air. Right pupil fixed and dilated, left pupil 1 mm and remains sluggish to light. No change in shape of pupils. Irregular respirations with short, fast breaths followed by long expiratory phase. Health care provider notified immediately.

▶ Complete the following sentence by choosing from the lists of options.

The client is at highest risk of developing __________ (word options).

WORD OPTIONS
Epidural hematoma
Increased intracranial pressure
Concussion
Guillain-Barré syndrome
Meningitis
Arteriovenous malformation

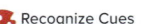

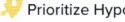

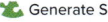

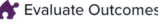

The answer to this trend question can be found at the end of this chapter.

Remember, any of the 13 different types of questions that pertain to each cognitive step could be asked of the test writer when assessing for clinical judgement. As you move through this textbook, you will gain more practise at recognizing the patterns of how each question is structured to identify if it is a Recognize Cues, Analyze Cues, Prioritize Hypothesis, Generate Solutions, Take Action, or Evaluate Outcomes question. The table below outlines things to consider when reading the clinical narrative scenario and key phrases that can help you recognize and identify the cognitive step being tested in a trend case question.

Cognitive Step	What to Consider in the Clinical Narrative Scenario	Key Phrases in Questions to Help Identify the Cognitive Step
Recognize Cues	Based on the story of the client, what assessment information would be classified as *normal* or *abnormal*, or is there anything *critical abnormal*? What patterns of illness or clues (like a puzzle piece or an Easter egg) are present?	"Immediate attention" "Immediate follow-up"
Analyze Cues	What is the relationship between the *patterns* of information (what system is most affected, what pieces of their clinical presentation could help determine the medical condition)?	"Potential complications" "Potential disease process"
Prioritize Hypothesis	How does each piece of data *fit together* to identify a specific condition or what the client could be at risk of developing or complications of that medical condition? This is where you are starting to put together the pieces of the puzzle.	"Highest risk of developing" "Complications or conditions the client is at risk for"
Generate Solutions	What do I need to consider when creating a *plan of care* for this client? Consider possible nursing or medical interventions, such as laboratory tests, diagnostic procedures or tests, or any potential orders the health care provider may place for the client's medical condition or complication. This stage of the NCJMM is the **anticipatory** phase.	"Potential nursing intervention" "Potential nursing action" "Potential health care provider orders that would be indicated or not indicated"
Take Action	Based on the client clinical presentation, what *actions* do I need to implement when addressing the client's highest need? This stage of the NCJMM is the **doing** phase of the NCJMM.	"Intervention, action, or orders that are a priority"
Evaluate Outcomes	Based on the actions, as they relate to the client's medical problem or complication of that medical problem, what is the client's *overall status*; has it improved, declined, or not changed? This stage of the NCJMM is the **reassessment** phase.	"Assessment findings that indicate improved, not changed, or declined" or any of these changes in status alone

Scoring of NGN Case Study Questions

NGN case study questions are scored differently than traditional NCLEX-RN style multiple-choice and alternate-format questions. For some NGN questions, students may receive partial credit for their answers, and they are not penalized for an incorrect response. What this means is that students may respond to a question, and despite an incorrect response, they could receive partial credit for their correct responses. If there are three correct responses but the student only answers two correctly and one incorrectly, the student could be scored as two out of three. One prime example would be **Select all that apply** (SATA). In traditional NCLEX-RN SATA questions, a student must correctly identify all the responses to receive full credit for this question. If a SATA question is asked within an NGN case study, students will receive partial credit if there are more correct responses than incorrect responses. A bow-tie stand-alone case study would be scored out of five, as there are only five possible correct responses. There are other NGN clinical judgement questions where students can be penalized for incorrect responses. Some questions are scored by the incorrect responses being subtracted from the correct responses. For example, if a student identifies one correct response and one incorrect response, the student will receive a zero for that question. Each question is designed to assess the test writer's ability to apply clinical judgement to commonly encountered clinical situations. For example, in a question about a code situation you cannot correctly choose choose chest compressions for a response while also choosing to administer oral fluids. This extreme example illustrates the need to prepare for this exam. Further information can be obtained from www.nclex.com if you are curious about the scoring of NGN items.

When taking the test, answer each question to your highest ability. Knowledge of the NGN case study structure, curricular content, and patterns in care; understanding the cognitive processing skills associated with answering clinical judgement questions; and exposure to the variability of NGN questions are all more important than the scoring of these items. This section is only for information purposes to inform you that NGN questions are scored differently than traditional NCLEX-RN questions.

Conclusion

Chapter 5 presented you with a step-by-step guide to answering unfolding case studies, and Chapter 6 has explained bow-tie and trend stand-alone case studies. Exposure to the different types of questions and clinical scenarios will provide you with practise and help you identify gaps in knowledge, thereby giving you time to further prepare to write the NGN. Each clinical narrative in this book is written specifically to demonstrate question patterns. Head-to-toe clinical data will include normal, abnormal, and critical-abnormal client data. Practising this pattern will help you identify what is present or missing when you write the NGN. Use your knowledge, take notes on questions you got wrong, and use the resources provided to increase your ability for success! You have come this far in your undergraduate nursing program, with only one more step to becoming a registered nurse. Now, let's practise!

Answer to Stand-Alone Case Study Example 1.0—Bow-Tie

Action to Take	Condition Most Likely Experiencing	Parameters to Monitor
Request an order to administer furosemide	Cardiomyopathy	Urine output
Action to Take		**Parameters to Monitor**
Initiate oxygen therapy at 2 L/min per nasal prongs		Continuous electrocardiogram (ECG)

Rationale:

Potential Conditions: The client is experiencing symptoms associated with cardiomyopathy. Although crackles are auscultated, along with palpitations, irregular pulses, and shortness of breath, atrial fibrillation is not associated with pulmonary embolus. The client presents afebrile, which eliminates pneumonia. The vital signs indicate a lower blood pressure associated with reduced cardiac output. At this time, the client is not hemodynamically unstable. Peripheral edema could be an indicator for chronic pericarditis; however, clinical presentation of chronic pericarditis includes weight loss, edema, jugular venous distension, arial fibrillation, exercise intolerance, dyspnea on exertion, fatigue, and anorexia.

Actions to Take: The primary focus for this client should be airway, breathing, and circulation, which would be accomplished by administering a loop diuretic (furosemide) and applying oxygen therapy for a low pulse oximetry reading of 86% on room air. A D-dimer would be appropriate if the client was experiencing symptoms of a deep vein thrombosis or pulmonary embolus. The appropriate blood test for this client would be a brain natriuretic peptic (BNP) level. The client presents in volume overload as indicated by the coarse crackles and higher respiratory rate + short shallow breaths; therefore, administering IV fluids would only put the client in further distress. The client is not in respiratory failure requiring intubation.

Parameters to Monitor: Urine output would need to be monitored as well as dysrhythmias, which can be observed via continuous ECG monitoring. When in heart failure, furosemide would assist with pulmonary edema, reduce peripheral edema, and improve oxygenation. Monitoring urine output would assist in identifying a fluid shift for the client. The blood pressure is not low enough that administration of a diuretic would make the client's blood pressure plummet. It is always a consideration. Clients with cardiomyopathy are prone to dysrhythmias, particularly atrial fibrillation, tachycardia, or bradycardia. The client does not have pneumonia, owing to the absence of a fever; therefore, monitoring the temperature would not be appropriate. Corrected calcium would be unnecessary in this circumstance, and finally, weight would be associated with chronic pericarditis, not with cardiomyopathy. Monitoring for weight gain would be appropriate if the client develops long-term heart failure as a result of the cardiomyopathy. There is no indication in the narrative that the client has reached a chronic state. In the acute phase, monitoring weight would demonstrate no benefit to evaluate if the actions were appropriate or if the condition warrants this observation. The primary goal would be to reduce the volume overload then provide education upon discharge.

NCJMM Step: Recognize Cues, Analyze Cues, Prioritize Hypothesis, Generate Solutions, Take Action, Evaluate Outcomes
References: Power-Kean et al. (2023), pp. 608–609; Tyerman & Cobbett (2023), pp. 891–895.

Answer to Stand-Alone Case Study Example 2.0—Trend

The client is at highest risk of developing **increased intracranial pressure**.

Rationale: The client presents with a fall and likely head injury and is developing an acute deterioration of increasing intracranial pressure. The spinal collar is only a precaution; however, given the client presentation at 0016h, the client can move all extremities without further injury. It is important to recognize the progression of the client's neurological status. Initially, the client presents with a Glasgow Coma Scale (GCS) of 12, but as the unfolding case study progresses, the GCS decreases to 5. There are pupillary changes throughout the unfolding case study as well, indicating increasing pressure within the brain. The vital signs indicate widening pulse pressure, bradycardia, and irregular breathing, which are all indicative of Cushing's triad. The client presented with clinical manifestations associated with a moderate concussion and acute subdural hematoma that progressed to increasing intracranial pressure requiring immediate interventions.

NCJMM Step: Prioritize Hypothesis
References: Power-Kean et al. (2023), pp. 367–368, 383–387; Tyerman & Cobbett (2023), pp. 1453–1485.

7 Let's Practise Unfolding Case Studies

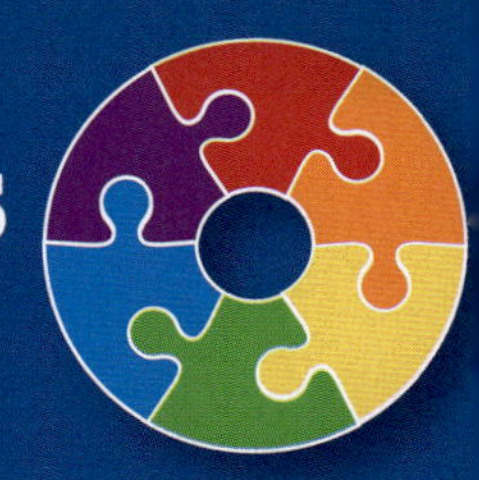

The following unfolding case studies will cover content from medical-surgical topics, maternity/postpartum, pediatrics, and mental health. As you practise these case studies and review the answers, it is good to not only address your strengths and gaps in knowledge but also identify strengths and areas for improving when considering the process behind each cognitive step. Remember, each question in an unfolding case study will assess the writer's ability to address concerns associated with recognizing cues, analyzing those cues, developing a hypothesis, generating a solution or plan of care, taking action, and evaluating client outcomes. Complete each question of the case study before confirming answers. Make notes about your strengths and areas for improvement, then plan to work on these gaps.

Note that in the test environment, the scenario data will be available by clicking on the tabs in order to review the full unfolding scenario information. Within the restrictions of a textbook, you may need to refer back to an earlier part of the question within the case to re-read the earlier client information and data. The answer key to these cases is in Chapter 9.

Medical-Surgical Unfolding Cases

Medical-Surgical 1.0

The nurse on the cardiology unit is caring for a 68-year-old male client.

History and Physical	Nurses' Notes	Vital Signs

1400h:

Body System	**Findings**
Neurological	Alert and oriented to person, place, time, and situation. Cooperative, obeys commands, moves all four extremities independently, gait steady.
Cardiovascular	Client was a direct admit to the unit with a "fast heartbeat" so strong that the client reports it felt like his heart was going to beat out of his chest.
Pulmonary	Complaints of shortness of breath at rest that worsen with any physical activity. Reports lack of energy most of the day.
Renal	Client denies any issue with voiding. Urinal at bedside and client encouraged to use.
Psychosocial	No previous cardiac history. Past medical history includes previous COVID-19 infection 7 months ago, prediabetes, body mass index (BMI) 37.

History and Physical	**Nurses' Notes**	Vital Signs

1420h: Client was directly admitted to the unit for further follow-up. Client denies a headache or any pain. Pupils equal and reactive to light at 3 mm. Motor power strong × 4. S1 and S2 noted, no S3 or S4 auscultated. Client denies chest pain but can feel his heart beating fast, even at rest when he is not doing anything physically active. Client noted to be well perfused, with mucous membranes pink in colour, and client well hydrated. Apical = radial pulses × 2, noted to be irregular but strong. Lungs clear with auscultation, no adventitious breath sounds noted.

▶ Highlight the findings below that would require follow-up.

History and Physical	Nurses' Notes	Vital Signs

1400h:

Body System	**Findings**
Neurological	Alert and oriented to person, place, and time. Cooperative, obeys commands, moves all four extremities independently, gait steady.
Cardiovascular	Client was a direct admit to the unit with a "fast heartbeat" so strong that client reported it felt like his heart was going to beat out of his chest.
Pulmonary	Complaints of shortness of breath at rest that worsen with any physical activity. Reports lack of energy most of the day.
Renal	Client denies issue with voiding. Urinal at bedside and client encouraged to use.
Psychosocial	No previous cardiac history. Past medical history includes previous COVID-19 infection 7 months ago, prediabetes, BMI 37.

History and Physical	**Nurses' Notes**	Vital Signs

1420h: Client was directly admitted to the unit for further follow-up. Client denies headache or any pain. Pupils equal and reactive to light at 3 mm. Motor power strong × 4. S1 and S2 noted, no S3 or S4 auscultated. Client denies chest pain but can feel his heart beating fast, even at rest when he is not doing anything physically active. Client noted to be well perfused, with mucous membranes pink, and client well hydrated. Apical = radial pulses × 2, noted to be irregular but strong. Lungs clear with auscultation, no adventitious breath sounds noted.

History and Physical	Nurses' Notes	**Vital Signs**

	1415h:
T	36.9°C (98.4°F)
P	155
RR	26
BP	132/77
Pulse oximetry reading	97% on room air

The nurse on the coronary care unit is caring for a 68-year-old male client.

History and Physical	**Nurses' Notes**	Vital Signs

1450h: Electrocardiogram (ECG) shows atrial fibrillation. Client is transferred to the coronary care unit for a cardioversion.

History and Physical	Nurses' Notes	**Vital Signs**

	1415h:	**1500h:**
T	36.9°C (98.4°F)	36.9°C (98.4°F)
P	155	176
RR	26	30
BP	132/77	128/72
Pulse oximetry reading	97% on room air	92% on room air

History and Physical	Nurses' Notes	**Vital Signs**

	1415h:
T	36.9°C (98.4°F)
P	155
RR	26
BP	132/77
Pulse oximetry reading	97% on room air

The nurse has reviewed the History and Physical at 1400h, the Vital Signs at 1415h, and Nurses' Notes at 1420h.

▶ Which of the following issues is the client at risk of developing? **Select all that apply.**

- ☐ Venous thrombosis
- ☐ Pulmonary embolism
- ☐ Stroke
- ☐ Peripheral arterial disease
- ☐ Atherosclerosis
- ☐ Cardiac tamponade
- ☐ Pleural effusion

▶ Complete the following sentence by choosing from the list of options.

The nurse should **first** address the client's _______________.

WORD OPTIONS
Heart sounds
Urine output
Respiratory status
Previous COVID-19 infection
Heart rhythm
Gait

The nurse has reviewed the Nurses' Notes from 1450h and Vital Signs at 1500h.

▶ For each potential nursing intervention, identify whether the potential intervention is **indicated** or **not indicated** for the client.

POTENTIAL NURSING INTERVENTIONS	INDICATED	NOT INDICATED
Place the client in the tripod position	○	○
Prepare to apply oxygen	○	○
Prepare to administer metoprolol	○	○
Consult spiritual care	○	○
Provide reassurance to the client	○	○
Insert venous access device	○	○

Note: Each row must have one response option selected.

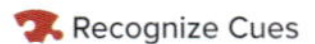 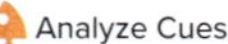 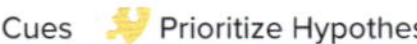 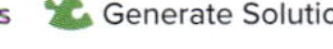 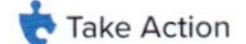 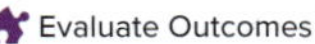

▶ The health care provider has placed an order for the client to have a cardioversion. Select 2 actions the nurse should take.

- ☐ Assist with a transesophageal echocardiogram
- ☐ Administer anticoagulation
- ☐ Consult respiratory therapy to monitor airway
- ☐ Keep suction outside of the room in case it is needed
- ☐ Place the client in the recovery position for the cardioversion
- ☐ Draw up paralytic to administer

▶ The client is to be discharged home after the cardioversion. For each of the statements made by the client, select whether the statement indicates an **understanding** or **no understanding** of the discharge teaching provided.

CLIENT STATEMENTS	UNDER-STANDING	NO UNDER-STANDING
"I have taken *Ginkgo biloba* before, so there is no issue taking it now, right?"	○	○
"I will call 9-1-1 if I experience sudden numbness or inability to speak."	○	○
"I have a big project that needs to be dealt with today. I can return back to work."	○	○
"I am to rest if my heart feels like it is racing and monitor if it slows down by feeling my pulse."	○	○
"My partner can drive me home today."	○	○

Note: Each row must have one response option selected.

Medical-Surgical 2.0

The nurse on the urology unit is caring for a 73-year-old male client.

History and Physical | Nurses' Notes | Vital Signs

0720h:

Body System	**Findings**
Neurological	Alert and oriented to person, place, time, and situation. Cooperative, obeys commands, moves all four extremities independently, gait steady. Denies a headache or dizziness.
Cardiovascular	Client presents with S1 and S2, no adventitious heart sounds, apical pulses = radial pulse, which is regular and strong. Denies chest pain.
Pulmonary	Lung sounds clear with auscultation. No shortness of breath noted.
Renal	Client education about transurethral resection of the prostate (TURP) provided. Client reports difficulty with voiding for several years, with multiple urinary tract infections as a result of benign prostate hyperplasia.

The nurse has reviewed the Nurses' Notes at 0800h, 1200h, and 1700h, including Vital Signs at 0720h and 1700h.

▶ Identify 4 assessment findings that require **immediate** follow-up.

- ☐ Lung sounds
- ☐ Heart sounds
- ☐ Nausea
- ☐ Chest pain
- ☐ Vital signs
- ☐ ECG findings
- ☐ Urine drainage

▶ For each client finding, identify if the finding is consistent with the disease process of angina, endocarditis, or cardiac tamponade. Each finding may support more than one disease process.

History and Physical	Nurses' Notes	Vital Signs
Psychosocial	Retired high school science teacher, married × 50 years, with four adult children and eight grandchildren. Previous coronary artery disease (CAD), angina, takes nitroglycerin for pain. Angiogram 3 years ago without any intervention taken.	

History and Physical	**Nurses' Notes**	Vital Signs

0800h: Client transferred to the operating room for TURP. Client in good spirits. Peripheral venous access device noted in right forearm.

1200h: Client returned to the unit post-recovery. Presents as lethargic but rouses easily. Alert and oriented to person, place, time, and situation. Pupils equal and reactive to light at 2 mm. Obeys commands and assisted with transfer from stretcher to bed. S1 and S2, bilateral radial pulses strong with palpation. Bilateral dorsalis pedis pulses strong with palpation. Skin warm and dry to touch. Apical = radial. Diminished air entry to bilateral bases. No adventitious lung sounds noted. Respirations regular and easy at rest. Client presents with three-way Foley catheter with continuous bladder irrigation, drainage device attached. Urine noted to be pink in colour with small clots noted in bag.

1700h: Called to bedside. Client complaining of 8/10 chest pain on a numerical rating scale, reports feeling like an elephant is sitting on his chest. He presents with diaphoresis, nausea but no emesis. Kidney basin placed on the bedside table. Notable tachypnea. 12-lead ECG shows sinus tachycardia with ST elevation in anterior leads.

History and Physical	Nurses' Notes	**Vital Signs**
	0720h:	**1700h:**
T	37.7°C (99.9°F)	37.5°C (99.5°F)
P	103	122
RR	16	26
BP	125/78	82/60
Pulse oximetry reading	99% on room air	85% on room air; oxygen applied at 2 L/min with new reading at 92%

CLIENT FINDINGS	ANGINA	INFECTIVE ENDOCARDITIS	CARDIAC TAMPONADE
Hypotension	○	○	○
Chest pain	○	○	○
ST elevation	○	○	○
Nausea	○	○	○
Tachypnea	○	○	○
Afebrile	○	○	○

▶ Complete the following sentence by choosing from the list of options.

The client is at **highest** risk of developing _____________ (word options 1) as evidenced by the client's _____________ (word options 2).

WORD OPTIONS 1	WORD OPTIONS 2
Acute myocardial infarction	Neurological assessment
Dysrhythmias	Respiratory assessment
Pneumonia	Cardiovascular assessment
Hypoxemia	Neurological assessment
Respiratory failure	Renal assessment

The nurse on the urology unit is caring for a 73-year-old male client.

History and Physical	Nurses' Notes	Vital Signs	**Laboratory Results**

Laboratory Test and Reference Range	**1720h:**
Troponin I <0.35 mcg/L (<0.35 ng/mL)	0.50 mcg/L (0.5 ng/mL)

The nurse has reviewed the Laboratory Results from 1720h.

▶ For each potential order by the health care provider, identify whether the order is **indicated** or not **indicated** for the care of this client.

POTENTIAL ORDERS	INDICATED	NOT INDICATED
Initiate low-molecular-weight heparin (LMWH)	○	○
Apply oxygen 0–5 L/min per nasal prongs to maintain pulse oximetry greater than 9%	○	○
Initiate a nitroglycerine infusion	○	○
Prepare client for an angiogram immediately	○	○

POTENTIAL ORDERS	INDICATED	NOT INDICATED
Discontinue the continuous bladder irritation	○	○
Transfer client to Coronary Care Unit	○	○
Administer dimenhydrinate	○	○

Note: Each row must have one response option selected.

The nurse on the coronary care unit is caring for a 73-year-old male client.

History and Physical	**Nurses' Notes**	Vital Signs	Laboratory Results

1815h: The client is transferred to the Coronary Care Unit. Chest pain persists without any change when given nitroglycerin spray sublingual. The angiography team is notified. The client is prepared for an angiogram. Several large bags of solution are transferred with the client to maintain continuous bladder irrigation (CBI).

The nurse has reviewed the Nurses' Note at 1815h.

▶ Which of the following nursing interventions would be indicated for this client? **Select all that apply**.

- ☐ Discontinue unfractionated heparin IV prior to going to the angiogram catheter suite
- ☐ Contact the client's spouse to join us at the angiogram suite
- ☐ Initiate nitroglycerine IV to achieve pain-free status for the client
- ☐ Apply oxygen at 2 L/min to achieve pulse oximetry above 92%
- ☐ Provide sips of water
- ☐ Mark dorsalis pedis and post-tibialis pulses on right and left feet and ankles

The nurse on a general medical unit is caring for a 44-year-old male client.

History and Physical	**Nurses' Notes**	Vital Signs	Laboratory Results

2200h: The client returns from the angiogram, lethargic. The procedure was completed through a femoral approach and the sheath removed at 2020h. A percutaneous coronary intervention (PCI) was required. Client teaching was provided by the nurse. CBI remains as treatment with urine output noted to be more frank in colour, but no clots noted. CBI reduced in rate.

The nurse has reviewed the Nurse's Notes at 2200h.

▶ For each of the statements made by the client, identify whether the statement indicates an **understanding** or **no understanding** of the discharge teaching provided.

CLIENT STATEMENTS	UNDER-STANDING	NO UNDER-STANDING
"I am going to have to follow the DASH diet now."	○	○
"My wife and I are going to need to speak with a counsellor about our intimate life."	○	○
"I need to drive myself to the foodbank where I volunteer. My next shift is in a couple of days."	○	○
"I cannot wait to sit up in a couple of hours."	○	○
"I can participate in exercise programs."	○	○

Note: Each row must have one response option selected.

Medical-Surgical 3.0

The nurse is caring for an 88-year-old male in the emergency department (ED).

Nurses' Notes | History and Physical | Medications

2220h: Client was brought to the ED by emergency medical services after being discovered on the floor of his apartment. Residential staff reported the client recently experienced a gastrointestinal virus and was isolated to their apartment to prevent spread to other residents. Staff were monitoring the status of the client several times per day to ensure safety and client physical needs were met. The client lives alone, independent with care and active with social activities in the residence. Presenting vital signs: T: 37.3°C (99.1°F); BP: 90/50; P: 102; RR: 16; with pulse oximetry of 92% on room air. #20 venous access device initiated in the left forearm with a 500-mL bolus of 0.9% sodium chloride administered × 1 time.

Nurses' Notes | **History and Physical** | Medications

2220h:

Body System	Findings
Neurological	Alert and oriented to person, place, and time. Pupils equal and reactive to light at 2 mm. Client presents as pleasant and cooperative and obeys all commands. Motor power moderate × 2 bilateral upper extremities, and weak × 2 bilateral lower extremities. Client presents with 2 out of 10 headache on numerical rating scale. Complains of dizziness when head of the bed is raised. A 3-cm bruise noted on left temple. Client indicates he was lying on his left side when the staff found him. Complains of fatigue.
Cardiovascular	Skin warm and dry to touch on bilateral upper extremities with bilateral lower extremities noted to be cool to touch. Capillary refill less than 3 seconds. Bilateral radial pulses moderately palpable but regular. Bilateral dorsalis pedis pulses weak. +3 bilateral peripheral edema noted to ankles. S1, S2 noted, but no S3 or S4 auscultated. No jugular venous distension noted. Mucous membranes dry and pale in colour. Tenting noted on back of the hand.
Pulmonary	Denies shortness of breath. Lung sounds auscultated for fine crackles to bilateral bases with fine crackles. Respirations remain regular and easy at rest, but client presents with mild shortness of breath with change in position.
Gastrointestinal	Nausea remains with bile emesis. Client states he has been unable to ingest solid food × 2 days. Reports limited oral fluid intake due to emesis several times per day. Client also reports diarrhea with last bowel movement in the evening. Hyperactive bowel sounds auscultated × 4 quadrants. Client encouraged to drink fluids. Ice water at the bedside.

▶ Identify 3 assessment findings that require **immediate** follow-up.

- ☐ Pupillary response
- ☐ Oliguria
- ☐ Headache
- ☐ Lung sounds
- ☐ Diarrhea
- ☐ Vertigo
- ☐ Pulses

▶ For each client finding, identify if the finding is consistent with the disease process of an acute subdural hematoma, dehydration, or pulmonary edema. Each finding may support more than one disease process.

CLIENT FINDINGS	ACUTE SUBDURAL HEMATOMA	DEHYDRATION	PULMONARY EDEMA
Headache	○	○	○
Drowsiness	○	○	○
Fine crackles	○	○	○
S1, S2, no S3 or S4	○	○	○
Shortness of breath	○	○	○
Oliguria	○	○	○

▶ Complete the following sentence by choosing from the list of options.

The client is at **highest** risk of developing ____________.

WORD OPTIONS
Hemorrhagic stroke
Acute myocardial infarction
Dysrhythmias
Acute kidney injury
Hip fracture

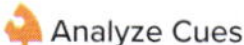 Recognize Cues 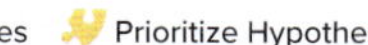 Analyze Cues 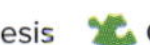 Prioritize Hypothesis 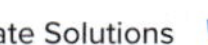 Generate Solutions 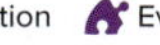 Take Action Evaluate Outcomes

Nurses' Notes	**History and Physical**	Medications
Renal	Client denies voiding for several hours with no reported urgency. Client encouraged to void. Urinal placed at the bedside.	
Psychosocial	Widowed, retired police officer, with two children who live out of province. Past medical history: CAD with PCI to LAD for 80% in 2013, last known ejection fraction 43%. Type 2 diabetes mellitus diagnosed 5 years ago controlled with oral hypoglycemic agents, and benign prostate hyperplasia.	

Nurses' Notes	History and Physical	**Medications**
Furosemide (loop diuretic) 20 mg PO once a day		
Metoprolol (beta blocker) 50 mg PO twice a day		
Ramipril (angiotensin-converting enzyme [ACE] inhibitor) 2.5 mg PO once a day		
Lipitor (HMG-CoA reductase inhibitor) 40 mg PO once a day		
Metformin (biguanide) 500 mg PO twice a day		
Repaglinide (meglitinide) 2 mg PO to be taken with each meal		

The nurse on the internal medicine unit is caring for the 88-year-old male client.

Nurses' Notes	History and Physical	Medications	Laboratory Results
0130h: The client is transferred to the internal medicine unit. **0142h:** The client arrived on the internal medicine unit. Vital signs: T: 37.5°C (99.5°F); BP: 86/48; P: 112; RR: 18; with pulse oximetry of 86% on room air. Required minimal assistance when transferring from stretcher to the bed with stable and equal gait. Client continues to present with dizziness when changing position but states it settles when not moving. Client denies a headache, chest pain, or difficulty breathing. Client reported 8 out of 10 abdominal pain based on a numerical rating scale. Client indicates improved nausea and no more diarrhea × 2 hours but states he has not been able to void since arrival at the hospital. Health care provider notified of status.			

Nurses' Notes	History and Physical	Medications	**Laboratory Results**
2245h: Hemoglobin 140–180 g/L (14–18 g/dL) (male) 120–160 g/L (12–16 g/dL) (female)	198 g/L (19.8 g/dL)	Sodium 136–145 mmol/L	148 mmol/L
Platelets 150–400 × 10^9/L (150 000– 400 000/mm^3)	260 × 10^9/L (260 000/ mm^3)	Potassium 3.5–5.1 mmol/L	5.6 mmol/L

The nurse has reviewed the Nurses' Notes from 2220h, 0130h, and 0142h as well as the Laboratory Results from 2245h.

▶ For each potential nursing intervention, identify whether the intervention is **indicated** or **not indicated** for the client.

POTENTIAL NURSING INTERVENTIONS	INDICATED	NOT INDICATED
Place the crash cart outside of the room in the event of a code blue	○	○
Request an order to administer intravenous (IV) fluids	○	○
Perform a bladder scan	○	○
Prepare the client for chest X-ray	○	○
Administer cardiac medications previously ordered prior to hospital admission	○	○
Request a regular diet tray be delivered to the unit	○	○
Place bed in the lowest position with the brakes on	○	○

Note: Each row must have one response option selected.

Nurses' Notes	History and Physical	Medications	Laboratory Results
White blood cells 3.5–12.0 × 10^9/L (3 500–12 000/ mm^3)	8.1 × 10^9/L (8 100/ mm^3)	Creatinine 53–106 mcmol/L (male) 44–97 mcmol/L (female)	368 mcmol/L
Neutrophils 3.0–5.8 × 10^9/L (3 000–5 800/mm^3)	4.4 × 10^9/L (4 400/ mm^3)	Blood urea nitrogen (BUN) 2.9–8.2 mmol/L	10.7 mmol/L

▶ Which of the following orders should the nurse consider a priority? **Select all that apply.**

☐ Initiate 0.45% sodium chloride at 100 mL/hr
☐ Perform an in-and-out catheter × 1 then monitor urine output
☐ Administer a narcotic analgesic as needed
☐ Draw laboratory tests: type and cross-match, arterial blood gas (ABG)
☐ Apply oxygen starting at 2 L/min per nasal prongs to maintain pulse oximetry greater than 92%.

The nurse on the internal medicine unit is caring for the 88-year-old male client.

Nurses' Notes

0630h: The client was found confused, no oxygen per nasal prongs on, and searching for the door to the washroom, trying to push the IV pole through the door in the hallway. Client redirected and assisted to the toilet and voided concentrated, foul-smelling urine. Identified correctly person, place, and time but slow in response. Pupillary response sluggish with right pupil documented at 2 mm in size and left pupil 4 mm in size. Client denies a headache, chest pain, or difficulty breathing. Indicates relief after voiding. Client repositioned back to the bed and oxygen reapplied at 2 L/min. Vital signs: T: 38.0°C (100.4°F); BP: 92/57; P: 122; RR: 20; with pulse oximetry of 92% on 2 L/min per nasal prongs.

0215h: In and out catheter performed for 600 mL of concentrated, cloudy urine. Client repositioned in bed.

The nurse has reviewed the Nurses' Notes at 0215h and 0630h.

▶ Highlight the findings below that indicate a worsening of the client's status.

Nurses' Notes

0630h: The client was found confused, no oxygen per nasal prongs on, and searching for the door to the washroom, trying to push the IV pole through the door in the hallway. Client redirected and assisted to the toilet and voided concentrated, foul-smelling urine. Identified correctly person, place, and time but slow in response. Pupillary response sluggish with right pupil documented at 2 mm in size and left pupil 4 mm in size. Client denies a headache, chest pain, or difficulty breathing. Indicates relief after voiding. Client repositioned back to the bed and oxygen reapplied at 2 L/min. Vital signs: T: 38.0°C (100.4°F); BP: 92/57; P: 122; RR: 20; with pulse oximetry of 92% on 2 L/min per nasal prongs.

Medical-Surgical 4.0

The nurse is caring for a 72-year-old female on an internal medicine unit.

Nurses' Notes

1100h: Client was admitted to the unit from the emergency department. The client had not been in contact with family for 3 days. Family notified the police, who entered the client's home on a wellness check. Client was found by emergency medical services (EMS) laying on her right side, in a pool of emesis with two empty bottles of wine on the table. The client was found unconscious, unresponsive to sternal rub but noted to have spontaneously irregular breathing. Vital signs: T: 38.2°C (100.8°F); BP: 129/77; P: 60; RR: 22; with pulse oximetry of 93% on room air. Client rouses with stimulation, opens eyes to voice, obeys commands, but easily falls back to sleep. Glasgow Coma Scale (GCS) 10. Client is unable to articulate place and time and remains in bed with side rails × 4. Client noted to be unsteady during transfer from stretcher to bed and when standing at the side of the bed. Pupils equal in size and react sluggishly to light at 2 mm, sclera noted to be yellow in colour. Fine crackles auscultated to bilateral posterior bases. No cough noted. Client taking long, irregular breaths coupled with snorting when at rest. Capillary refill noted to be less than 3 seconds with fingertips pale in colour. Skin warm and dry to touch. Bilateral radial pulses strong and regular with palpation. Bilateral dorsalis pedis weak with palpation and posterior tibial pulses require Doppler. Unable to determine chest pain. Abdomen distended and hard with hypoactive bowel sounds auscultated × 4 quadrants. Client petite in frame with pelvic bones noticeable, spine observable, and on the frailty scale, client scored moderately frail. Client has not voided upon arrival to the unit. Client presents disheveled, unhygienic with dirt noted under nails, and clothes had not been recently washed. Client presented with strong body odour. Full bed bath provided. Palm size red area noted on right hip and toonie-sized redness noted on right shoulder. No open areas noted on client's body. Petechiae and purpura documented on client's lower extremities. A peripheral venous access device was initiated in the left antecubital and saline locked.

▶ Which of the following findings require **immediate** follow-up? **Select all that apply.**

- ☐ Confusion
- ☐ Unsteady gait
- ☐ Irregular breathing with snorting
- ☐ Pale fingertips
- ☐ Frailty
- ☐ Malnourished
- ☐ Yellow-coloured sclera
- ☐ Fever
- ☐ Lung sounds
- ☐ Pupillary response
- ☐ Hypoactive bowel sounds
- ☐ Use of Doppler for bilateral posterior tibial pulses

▶ For each client finding below, click to specify if the finding is consistent with the disease process of cirrhosis, subdural hematoma, and pneumonia. Each finding may support more than one disease process.

CLIENT FINDINGS	CIRRHOSIS	SUBDURAL HEMATOMA	PNEUMONIA
Confusion	○	○	○
Irregular breathing	○	○	○
Fever	○	○	○
Yellow-coloured sclera	○	○	○
Fine inspiratory crackles	○	○	○

▶ Complete the following sentence by choosing from the list of options.

The client is at **highest** risk of developing _______________.

WORD OPTIONS
Thrombocytopenia
Dysrhythmias
Respiratory failure
Heart failure
Renal failure

The nurse is caring for a 72-year-old female on an internal medicine unit.

Nurses' Notes | Laboratory Results

1227h: Client found unresponsive by nurse. The client presents as cool to touch × 4 extremities. Unable to palpate bilateral radial pulses, bilateral carotid pulses are weak and thready. The breathing pattern was noted to be agonal. Unable to obtain pulse oximetry. Vital signs: T: 38.8°C (101.8°F); BP: 70/48.

The nurse has reviewed the Nurses' Notes from 1100h and 1227h as well as the Laboratory Results drawn at 0936h and is planning care for the client.

▶ For each potential nursing intervention, identify whether the intervention is **indicated** or **not indicated** for the care of this client.

Nurses' Notes	**Laboratory Results**		
0936h:			
Hemoglobin 140–180 g/L (14–18 g/dL) (male) 120–160 g/L (12–16 g/dL) (female)	162 g/L (16.2 g/dL)	Sodium 136–145 mmol/L	133 mmol/L
Platelets 150–400 $\times$ 10^9/L (150 000–400 000/mm^3)	43 $\times$ 10^9/L (43 000/mm^3)	Potassium 3.5–5.1 mmol/L	5.7 mmol/L
White blood cells 3.5–12.0 $\times$ 10^9/L (3 500–12 000/mm^3)	16.0 $\times$ 10^9/L (16 000/mm^3)	Creatinine 53–106 mcmol/L (male) 44–97 mcmol/L (female)	200 mcmol/L
Neutrophils 3.0–5.8 $\times$ 10^9/L (3 000–5 800/mm^3)	9.2 $\times$ 10^9/L (9 200/mm^3)	D-dimer <3.0 nmol/L)	5.9 nmol/L

POTENTIAL NURSING INTERVENTIONS	INDICATED	NOT INDICATED
Prepare the client for a chest X-ray and spiral computed topography (CT)	○	○
Check pupillary response	○	○
Call a code blue	○	○
Contact the client's family	○	○
Request an order to administer an intravenous fluid bolus	○	○
Review the client's allergies	○	○

Note: Each row must have one response option selected.

▶ Select 2 nursing actions the nurse would take.

- ☐ Place the client in Trendelenburg position
- ☐ Request an order to administer sodium polystyrene sulfonate (Kayexalate) or sodium zirconium cyclosilicate powder (Lokelma)
- ☐ Perform chest compressions
- ☐ Connect the client to an external pacemaker
- ☐ Prepare for rapid defibrillation
- ☐ Manage temperature regulation

The nurse is caring for a 72-year-old female on an internal medicine unit.

Nurses' Notes	Laboratory Results
1255h: The client was connected to a ventilator for supportive care until the family could arrive to say goodbye. Palliative care will be provided to ensure comfort care has been initiated for the client. The family has been contacted about the client's status.	

The nurse has reviewed the Nurses' Notes at 1255h.

▶ Identify the top 4 client findings to indicate the client is nearing death.

CLIENT OUTCOMES
Weakening pulse
Skin warm to touch
Palliative sedation is required more frequently
Incontinent
Gag reflex intact
"Guppy breathing"

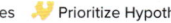

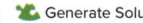

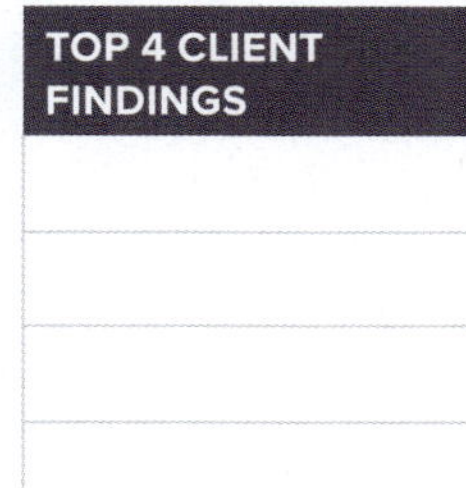

TOP 4 CLIENT FINDINGS

Medical-Surgical 5.0

The nurse is caring for a 63-year-old female client on the oncology unit.

Nurses' Notes

1100h: Client presented to the emergency department complaining of new-onset hemoptysis with complaints of being lightheaded and unstable with walking. Client has been experiencing a nonproductive, dry cough that started approximately 2 months ago with new-onset voice hoarseness that started 2 weeks ago. She had been previously healthy. Her past medical history includes a previous breast cancer diagnosis 1 year prior to this event with bilateral mastectomy with right-sided axillary node removal. She was accompanied by her partner of 35 years.

Vital signs: T: 37.7°C (99.9°F); BP: 102/54; P: 92; RR: 26; with pulse oximetry of 92% on room air. Client presents as pleasant, cooperative, alert and oriented to person, place, time, and situation. Gait steady now, denies any dizziness. S1 and S2 heart sounds, apical heart rate regular and equals radial pulse. Upon lung auscultation, posteriorly there was reduced air entry noted right lower lobe only but clear air entry noted throughout left lobe. No other adventitious lung sounds noted. Client complains of 4 out of 10 pain, based on a numerical rating scale, during inspiration and mild shortness of breath with ambulation. Sputum noted to be blood-tinged. Client voiding clear amber urine. Bowel sounds auscultated × 4 quadrants with abdomen soft and round during palpation.

▶ Which of the following findings require **immediate** follow-up? **Select all that apply**.

- ☐ Sputum
- ☐ Hoarseness
- ☐ Vital signs
- ☐ Bilateral mastectomy 1 year ago
- ☐ Gait
- ☐ Heart sounds
- ☐ Atelectasis
- ☐ Pain

▶ For each client finding below, identify if the finding is consistent with the disease process of pneumonia, pulmonary embolus, or lung cancer. Each finding may support more than 1 disease process.

CLIENT FINDINGS	PNEUMONIA	PULMONARY EMBOLUS	LUNG CANCER
Hemoptysis	○	○	○
Atelectasis	○	○	○
Pleural pain	○	○	○
Voice hoarseness	○	○	○
Shortness of breath	○	○	○
Afebrile	○	○	○

The nurse is caring for a 63-year-old female client on the oncology unit.

Nurses' Notes | Laboratory Results | Diagnostic Results

1245h: Full assessment completed by attending

1500h: Client sent for CT chest

1730h: The health care provider informs the client of the new possible diagnosis of finding a malignant mass

Nurses' Notes | **Laboratory Results** | Diagnostic Results

1330h:

Hemoglobin 140–180 g/L (14–18 g/dL) (male) 120–160 g/L (12–16 g/dL) (female)	79 g/L (7.9 g/dL)	Sodium 136–145 mmol/L	142 mmol/L
Platelets 150–400 × 10^9/L (150 000–400 000/mm^3)	162 × 10^9/L (162 000/mm^3)	Potassium 3.5–5.1 mmol/L	3.5 mmol/L
White blood cells 3.5–12.0 × 10^9/L (3 500–12 000/mm^3)	7.2 × 10^9/L (7 200/mm^3)	Creatinine 53–106 mcmol/L (male)	
44–97 mcmol/L (female)	65 mcmol/L		

The nurse reviews the Nurses' Notes at 1100h, 1245h, 1500h, and 1730h, Laboratory Results at 1330h, and Diagnostic Results at 1500h 1500h, and 1730h, Laboratory Results at 1330h, and Diagnostic Results at 1500h.

▶ Complete the following sentence by choosing from the list of options.

The client is at **highest** risk of developing _______________ (word options 1) and _______________ (word options 1) as evidenced by the ___________________ (word options 2).

WORD OPTION 1	WORD OPTION 2
Anemia	Vital signs
Dysrhythmias	Respiratory assessment
Anorexia	Cardiovascular assessment
Hypoxemia	Neurological assessment
Renal failure	Renal assessment

▶ Select 3 possible nursing interventions when creating a plan of care for this client.

- ☐ Contact client's partner with new diagnosis
- ☐ Encourage exercise and a healthy lifestyle
- ☐ Collaborate with client about end-of-life care
- ☐ Request an order to consult for dietitian
- ☐ Be authentically available to the client and family
- ☐ Assess client needs for counselling and additional resources

Nurses' Notes	**Laboratory Results**	Diagnostic Results	
Neutrophils 3.0–5.8 × 10^9/L (3 000–5 800/ mm^3)	4.8 × 10^9/L (4 800/ mm^3)	Blood urea nitrogen (BUN) 2.9–8.2 mmol/L	5.0 mmol/L

Nurses' Notes	Laboratory Results	**Diagnostic Results**

1500h:
CT scan of chest WITHOUT intravenous contrast, using low-dose lung cancer screening protocol
Comparison: None
Findings: Lines/Tubes: None
Lungs and Airways: 3-cm mediastinal mass located posterior side of the heart by the right atrium and base of esophagus compressing the inferior area of the right lung
Impression: Possible lung mass with malignancy. Requires further investigation by interventional radiology

The nurse is caring for a 63-year-old female client on the oncology unit.

Nurses' Notes	Laboratory Results	Diagnostic Results

2100h: Client preparing for sleep. No voice complaints. Client to remain NPO from midnight in the event of further testing.
1 Day Later:
0325h: The client woke several times with panic attacks. Client expressed difficulty sleeping due to anxiety. Vital signs: T: 37.3°C (99.1°F); BP: 122/76; P: 110; RR: 26; with pulse oximetry of 86% on room air. Oxygen applied at 2 L/min per nasal prongs and pulse oximetry increased to 91%. Client reports increased pleuritic pain at 8 out of 10. Reduced air entry noted to right lobe with atelectasis increased from RLL to RML. Client continues to expectorate clots with sputum. Health care provider notified. Plan is to send client for lung biopsy in a.m. Client provided reassurance and settled with presence.
0730h: Orders received by health care provider for lung biopsy. Vital signs: T: 37.3°C (99.1°F); BP: 132/87; P: 112; RR: 28; pulse oximetry of 94% on 2 L/min per nasal prongs. Client assisted onto the stretcher.

Nurses' Notes	Laboratory Results	Diagnostic Results	**Orders**

0730h:
- Ensure patency of #18 g peripheral venous access device
- Obtain sputum sample
- Initiate 0.9% sodium chloride (normal saline) 100 mL/hr
- Administer lorazepam 0.5 mg SL prior to the procedure
- Consult physiotherapy
- Consult social work
- Regular diet

The nurse has reviewed the Orders written at 0730h.

▶ Highlight the orders that the nurse should consider a priority.

Orders

0730h:
- Ensure patency of #18 g peripheral venous access device
- Obtain sputum sample
- Initiate 0.9% sodium chloride (normal saline) 100 mL/hr
- Administer lorazepam 0.5 mg SL prior to the procedure
- Consult physiotherapy
- Consult social work
- Regular diet

▶ Upon return to the unit from the lung biopsy, identify which of the following findings would indicate the client's condition has improved, has not changed, or has declined.

ASSESSMENT FINDINGS	IMPROVED	NO CHANGE	DECLINED
Lethargy with sternal rub	○	○	○
RR 12	○	○	○
0.9% sodium chloride 200 mL/hr	○	○	○
BP 116/68	○	○	○
Hemoptysis	○	○	○

Note: Each row must have one response option selected.

Medical-Surgical 6.0

The nurse on a general medical unit is caring for a 44-year-old male client.

Nurses' Notes

1100h: Client was seen in the emergency department complaining of constant cramping abdominal pain that has not relented over 2 days, located in the left lower quadrant, accompanied with nausea, emesis, and chills. Vital signs: T: 39.5°C (103.1°F); BP: 143/85; P: 115; RR: 22; with pulse oximetry of 96% on room air. Client presents as pleasant, cooperative, alert and oriented to person, place, and time. Gait steady, denies any dizziness. Found in the fetal position. S1 and S2 heart sounds auscultated only, apical heart rate regular and equals radial pulse. Bilateral radial pulses strong. Mucous membranes pink. Client noted to be diaphoretic. Denies any chest pain. Clear air entry noted bilateral lower lobes. Client complains of 7 out of 10 abdominal pain, based on a numerical rating scale, located left lower quadrant of abdomen. Abdomen rounded, client guards with minimal abdominal palpation. Bowel sounds active and auscultated in four quadrants. Client reports no bowel movement for 4 days, which is not his typical routine as he has regular movements. Client reports passing flatus. Denies any dysuria, frequency, or urgency with voiding but maintaining oral fluid intake has been difficult due to abdominal pain. Client denies a change in eating habits; main diet consists of take-out fast food due to difficult and stressful occupation. BMI 36. Peripheral venous access device (VAD) placed in left forearm.

▶ Which of the following would require **immediate** follow-up? **Select all that apply**.

- ☐ Temperature
- ☐ Blood pressure
- ☐ Pulse oximetry
- ☐ Heart sounds
- ☐ Mucous membranes
- ☐ Abdominal pain
- ☐ Diaphoresis
- ☐ Constipation
- ☐ Body mass index (BMI)

▶ Complete the following sentence by choosing from the list of options.

The nurse should recognize that the client is potentially experiencing a(an) ____________________ (word options 1) based on the ____________________ (word options 2).

WORD OPTIONS 1	WORD OPTIONS 2
Angina	Neurological assessment
Bowel obstruction	Respiratory assessment
Dehydration	Cardiovascular assessment
Dysrhythmia	Neurological assessment
Infection	Renal assessment
Hematemesis	Gastrointestinal assessment

▶ Complete the following sentence by choosing from the list of options.

The client is at **highest** risk of developing ________________.

WORD OPTIONS
Gastroesophageal reflux disease
Appendicitis
Peptic ulcer disease
Ulcerative colitis
Diverticulitis
Gastroenteritis

The nurse on a general medical unit is caring for a 44-year-old male client.

Nurses' Notes

1350h: Called to the client washroom by emergency button pulled by the client. Client found on the floor by the toilet, pale in colour, with frank red blood noted in the basin of the toilet. Client attempted to have a bowel movement but started bleeding and called for help. Client assisted back to the bed. Vital signs: T: 39.9°C (103.8°F); BP: 91/57; P: 140; RR: 26; with pulse oximetry of 84% on room air. Bilateral radial pulses weak and thready. Skin cool to touch. Health care provider notified.

Nurses' Notes | **Laboratory Results**

1145h:

Hemoglobin 140–180 g/L (14–18 g/dL) (male) 120–160 g/L (12–16 g/dL) (female)	90 g/L (9 g/dL)	Sodium 136–145 mmol/L	146 mmol/L
Platelets 150–400 × 10^9/L (150 0000–400 000/mm^3)	140 × 10^9/L (140 000/mm^3)	Potassium 3.5–5.1 mmol/L	5.0 mmol/L
White blood cells 3.5–12.0 × 10^9/L (3 500–12 000/mm^3)	15 × 10^9/L (15 000/mm^3)	Creatinine 53–106 mcmol/L (male) 44–97 mcmol/L (female)	55 mcmol/L
Neutrophils 3.0–5.8 × 10^9/L (3 000–5 800/mm^3)	8 × 10^9/L (8 000/mm^3)	Blood urea nitrogen (BUN) 2.9–8.2 mmol/L	5.0 mmol/L

The nurse has reviewed the Nurses' Notes from 1350h and the Laboratory Results from 1145h.

▶ For each potential nursing intervention, identify whether the intervention would be **indicated** or **not indicated** for this client.

POTENTIAL NURSING INTERVENTIONS	INDICATED	NOT INDICATED
Place client in Trendelenburg position	○	○
Prepare to apply non-rebreather mask to client	○	○
Request an order for stat antibiotic therapy	○	○
Request an order to administer an intravenous fluid bolus	○	○
Offer the client oral fluids	○	○

Note: Each row must have one response option selected.

The nurse on a general medical unit is caring for a 44-year-old male client.

Orders

1405h:
- Cefazolin 2 g, IV, every 8 hours
- 0.9% sodium chloride (normal saline) 500 ml IV bolus once
- Consult general surgery
- Consult dietician
- Draw laboratory tests: CBC, urinalysis
- Insert an additional peripheral venous access device
- Oxygen nasal prongs 0-5 L to maintain pulse oximetry greater than 90%

The nurse has reviewed the Orders from 1405h.

▶ Identify 4 orders that the nurse should consider a **priority**.

- ☐ Cefazolin 2 g, IV, q8h
- ☐ 0.9% sodium chloride (normal saline) 500 mL IV bolus once
- ☐ Consult general surgery
- ☐ Consult dietitian
- ☐ Draw laboratory tests: complete blood count (CBC), urinalysis
- ☐ Insert an additional peripheral venous access device
- ☐ Oxygen at 0–5 L per nasal prongs to maintain pulse oximetry greater than 92%

▶ For each assessment finding, identify if the finding indicates that the client's condition has improved, not changed, or declined.

ASSESSMENT FINDINGS	IMPROVED	NOT CHANGED	DECLINED
Hemoglobin 69 g/L (6.9 g/dL)	○	○	○
P 102	○	○	○
One-person assistance for mobility	○	○	○
Skin warm and dry to touch	○	○	○
BP 98/60	○	○	○
T 38.0°C (99.9°F)	○	○	○

Note: Each row must have one response option selected.

Medical-Surgical 7.0

The nurse is caring for the 40-year-old female client on a general surgical unit.

Nurses' Notes

1100h: Client arrived on the unit post–gastric bypass surgery through the Roux-en-Y gastric bypass procedure. Previous comorbidities include coronary artery disease, type 2 diabetes mellitus controlled with metformin and repaglinide, hypertension but controlled with ramipril, and dyslipidemia controlled by rosuvastatin. Client presented with a BMI of 39. Vital signs: T: 37.4°C (99.3°F); BP: 98/68; P: 90; RR: 16; with pulse oximetry of 92% on 4 L/min of oxygen. Client presents as pleasant, cooperative, lethargic postanaesthetic but rouses easily and oriented to person, place, and time. Client denies any pain or discomfort. Pupils equal and reactive to light at 3 mm. Denies a headache or dizziness. Client presents with S1 and S2 heart sounds, no adventitious heart sounds noted. Apical equals radial pulse. Bilateral radial pulses strong with bilateral dorsalis pedis pulses noted to be weak. Lower extremities' skin cool to touch. Capillary refill less than 3 seconds. Fine inspiratory crackles noted to bilateral lung bases with upper airway wheezing noted. No shortness of breath or distress noted. Client reports feeling thirsty but reminded of NPO. In-dwelling Foley catheter draining clear amber urine. Approximately 400 mL emptied from drainage device. Bowel sounds auscultated × right and left upper quadrants only with absent bowel sounds noted to right lower quadrant and left lower quadrant. Client is not passing any flatus. Abdomen rounded and soft with palpation. Client arrived with intermittent pneumatic compression device going. Peripheral venous access device noted in left antecubital.

▶ Highlight the assessment findings that would require follow-up.

Nurses' Notes

1100h: Client arrived on the unit post–gastric bypass surgery through the Roux-en-Y gastric bypass procedure. Previous comorbidities include coronary artery disease, type 2 diabetes mellitus controlled with metformin and repaglinide, hypertension but controlled with ramipril, and dyslipidemia controlled by rosuvastatin. Client presented with a BMI of 39. Vital signs: T: 37.4°C (99.3°F); BP: 98/68; P: 90; RR: 16; with pulse oximetry of 92% on 4 L/min of oxygen. Client presents as pleasant, cooperative, lethargic postanaesthetic but rouses easily and oriented to person, place, and time. Client denies any pain or discomfort. Pupils equal and reactive to light at 3 mm. Denies a headache or dizziness. Client presents with S1 and S2 heart sounds, no adventitious heart sounds noted. Apical equals radial pulse. Bilateral radial pulses strong with bilateral dorsalis pedis pulses noted to be weak. Lower extremities' skin cool to touch. Capillary refill less than 3 seconds. Fine inspiratory crackles noted to bilateral lung bases with upper airway wheezing noted. No shortness of breath or distress noted. Client reports feeling thirsty. In-dwelling Foley catheter draining clear amber urine. Approximately 400 mL emptied from drainage device. Bowel sounds auscultated × right and left upper quadrants only with absent bowel sounds noted to right lower quadrant and left lower quadrant. Client is not passing any flatus. Abdomen rounded and soft with palpation. Client arrived with intermittent pneumatic compression device going. Peripheral venous access device noted in left antecubital.

▶ Which of the following early complications is the client at risk of developing? **Select all that apply.**

☐ Dehydration
☐ Bowel obstruction
☐ Respiratory failure
☐ Electrolyte imbalances
☐ Venous thromboembolism
☐ Bleeding
☐ Anastomotic leak
☐ Pulmonary embolism
☐ Malabsorption
☐ Dumping syndrome

The nurse is caring for the 40-year-old female client on a general surgical unit.

Nurses' Notes | Laboratory Results

1410h: Client is more awake, less lethargic, maintaining a conversation. Bowel sounds auscultated and hypoactive × 4 quadrants. Client is offered 15 mL of water to start then increased by 15-mL increments every 10 to 15 min. Client denies nausea, abdominal pain. Client progressing well.
0400h: Client complaining of 5/10 abdominal pain on a numerical rating scale, difficulty catching her breath, and left shoulder pain. Head of bed raised to 40-degree angle and client complains of dizziness. Vital signs: T: 38.4°C (101.1°F); BP: 87/52; P: 135; RR: 26; with pulse oximetry of 90% on room air.

Nurses' Notes | **Laboratory Results**

0430h:

Hemoglobin 140–180 g/L (14–18 g/dL) (male) 120–160 g/L (12–16 g/dL) (female)	155 g/L (15.5 g/dL)	Sodium 136–145 mmol/L	140 mmol/L
Platelets 150–400 × 10^9/L (15 0000–400 000/ mm^3)	280 × 10^9/L (280 000/ mm^3)	Potassium 3.5–5.1 mmol/L	5.0 mmol/L
White blood cells 3.5–12.0 × 10^9/L (3 500–12 000/mm^3)	12.3 × 10^9/L (12300/mm^3)	Creatinine	
53–106 mcmol/L (male) 44–97 mcmol/L (female)	90 mcmol/L		
Neutrophils 3.0–5.8 × 10^9/L	5.9 × 10^9/L (5 900/mm^3)	Blood urea nitrogen (BUN) 2.9–8.2 mmol/L	5.2 mmol/L
		Troponin I <0.35 mcg/L	0.30

The nurse has reviewed the Nurses' Notes at 1410h and 0400h and Laboratory Results at 0430h.

▶ Complete the following sentence by choosing from the list of options.

The client is at **highest** risk of developing _______________.

WORD OPTIONS
Acute myocardial infarction
Hemorrhage
Dumping syndrome
Respiratory distress
Anastomotic leak
Abdominal compartment syndrome

▶ For each potential nursing intervention, identify whether the intervention is **indicated** or **not indicated** for the care of this client.

POTENTIAL NURSING INTERVENTIONS	INDICATED	NOT INDICATED
Place the client in Trendelenburg position	○	○
Prepare the client for endoscopy	○	○
Request an order to insert an additional venous access device	○	○
Offer oral fluids	○	○
Increase oxygen delivery	○	○

Note: Each row must have one response option selected.

▶ The health care provider has written the orders. Select 3 actions the nurse should take.

- ☐ Insert an in-dwelling urethral Foley catheter
- ☐ Initiate cefazolin 2 g IV q8h starting now
- ☐ Consult dietitian
- ☐ Administer 0.9 % sodium chloride (normal saline) 500 mL bolus × 1
- ☐ Apply oxygen 0–5 L per nasal prongs to maintain pulse oximetry greater than 90%
- ☐ Consult physiotherapy
- ☐ Administer an opiate

The nurse has instituted the orders as directed. For each assessment finding, identify if the finding indicates that the client's condition has improved, not changed, or worsened.

ASSESSMENT FINDINGS	IMPROVED	NO CHANGE	WORSENED
BP 101/60	○	○	○
Fine inspiratory crackles bilateral lung bases	○	○	○
Client reports nausea with smell of food	○	○	○
Afebrile	○	○	○

Note: Each row must have one response option selected.

Medical-Surgical 8.0

The nurse is caring for a 36-year-old male client in the emergency department (ED).

Nurses' Notes

2153h: Client presented to the emergency department complaining of generalized weakness from a gastrointestinal illness with blood noted in stool. Client reports having increasing numbers of bowel movements (~12 today) over the past 2 weeks. Client queries if it is food poisoning that is continuing the feelings of urgency to have a bowel movement and generalized unwell feeling. Vital signs: T: 38.3°C (100.9°F); BP: 102/54; P: 130; RR: 16; with pulse oximetry of 92% on room air. Client presents as lethargic but as oriented to person, place, time, and situation. Client reports dizziness with ambulation, requiring him to secure his body against the wall or needing to sit down. The lack of energy has increased over the past 2 weeks. Client obeys all commands with moderate motor power × 4 extremities. No assistance required with ambulation at the moment. Client complains of a dull headache, rated 2 out of 10 on a numerical pain scale, located at the front of his head. Client denies double vision, pupils equal and reactive to light at 3 mm in size. Client presents with regular bounding rhythm, palpated bilateral radial pulses, apical = radial. Bilateral dorsalis pedis pulses weak × 2. S1, S2 present. No adventitious heart sounds auscultated. Skin cool and clammy to touch. Capillary refill sluggish and greater than 3 seconds. Conjunctiva pale, palms noted to be pale. Mucous membranes are dry. Anteriorly and posteriorly lung sounds auscultated for clear air entry throughout all lung fields. Respirations are regular and easy at rest. Client noted to be taking shallow breaths. Abdomen flat with hyperactive bowel sounds auscultated × 4 quadrants. Client complains of ++ cramping at the time of bowel movements and has noted streaks of blood in solid stool mixed with foamy pus. Client denies the need to void. Bladder scanner reveals 250 mL of urine in the bladder. A urinal was placed at the bedside. A peripheral venous device was inserted into the right forearm and infusing 0.9% normal saline at 125 mL/hr. Lab to draw a CBC and electrolytes.

▶ Identify the top 3 client findings that require **immediate** follow-up.

- ☐ Mucous membranes
- ☐ Urine output
- ☐ Lung sounds
- ☐ Vital signs
- ☐ Cardiac rhythm
- ☐ Motor power
- ☐ Headache
- ☐ Bowel movements

▶ For each client finding, identify if the finding is consistent with the disease process of gastroenteritis, inflammatory bowel disease, or celiac disease. Each finding may support more than one disease process.

CLIENT FINDINGS	GASTROENTERITIS	INFLAMMATORY BOWEL DISEASE	CELIAC DISEASE
Febrile	○	○	○
Constipation	○	○	○
Dry mucous membranes	○	○	○
Weight loss	○	○	○
Frequent bowel movements	○	○	○
Abdominal cramping	○	○	○
Nausea	○	○	○

▶ Complete the following sentence by choosing from the list of options.

The client is at **highest** risk of developing ______________.

WORD CHOICES
Gastritis
Gluten intolerance
Peptic ulcer disease
Ulcerative colitis
Gastroesophageal reflux disease
Crohn's disease

The nurse is caring for a 36-year-old male client in the emergency department (ED).

Nurses' Notes

0017h: Client calls the nurse to the room with complaint of "feeling something wet" on the sheets. Client was concerned they were incontinent. Upon assessment, nurse finds the bed soaked with bright, frank red blood. Client presents as grey, lethargic, and confused, trying to ambulate without assistance. Vital signs: T: 38.6°C (101.5°F); BP: 80/44; P: 145; RR: 28; with pulse oximetry of 81% on room air.
0020h: Primary health care provider notified about client status. Awaiting orders.

Nurses' Notes | **Laboratory Results**

2330h:

Hemoglobin 140–180 g/L (14–18 g/dL) (male) 120–160 g/L (12–16 g/dL) (female)	82 g/L (8.2 g/dL)	Sodium 136–145 mmol/L	142 mmol/L
Platelets 150–400 × 10^9/L (150 000–400 000/mm^3)	122 × 10^9/L (122 000/ mm^3)	Potassium 3.5–5.1 mmol/L	4.7mmol/L
White blood cells 3.5–12.0 × 10^9/L (3 500–12 000/ mm^3)	15.0 × 10^9/L (15 000/mm^3)	Creatinine 53–106 mcmol/L (male) 44–97 mcmol/L (female)	75 mcmol/L
Neutrophils 3.0–5.8 × 10^9/L (3 000–5 800/ mm^3)	8.2 × 10^9/L (8 200/mm^3)		
Type and screen	AB positive		

The nurse has reviewed the Nurses' Notes at 2153h, 0017h, and 0020h and Laboratory Results drawn at 2330h.

▶ For each potential interventions, identify whether the order is **indicated** or **not indicated** during the **immediacy** for the care of this client.

POTENTIAL NURSING INTERVENTIONS	INDICATED	NOT INDICATED
Request an order to initiate oxygen therapy	○	○
Prepare to insert an in-dwelling urinary catheter	○	○
Encourage oral fluid intake	○	○
Request an order to insert a second peripheral venous access device	○	○
Draw laboratory tests: CBC, electrolytes, type and screen/cross-match	○	○
Inform the client they will be receiving AB negative blood product ASAP	○	○
Prepare to initiate a 500-mL intravenous bolus of 0.9% normal saline × 1 then reassess blood pressure	○	○
Prepare to call a code blue	○	○
Prepare to administer Remicade within the next 30 minutes	○	○
Consult general surgery for possible colostomy	○	○

Note: Each row must have one response option selected.

The nurse is caring for a 36-year-old male on the general surgical unit.

Nurses' Notes

0050h: General surgery arrived for consult, and client taken to the operating room.
0400h: Client admitted to the surgical unit post-laparotomy followed by LLQ colostomy intervention. The client arrived at the unit with a nasogastric tube at a low suction level, lactated Ringer's infusing at 100 mL/hr through the peripheral venous access device inserted in the ED. Vital signs: T: 38.2°C (100.8°F); BP: 102/74; P: 101; RR: 14; with pulse oximetry of 96% on 3 L/min per nasal prongs.

The nurse has reviewed the Nurses' Notes at 0050h and 0400h.

▶ Complete the following sentence by choosing from the list of options.

▶ Identify which of the following nursing actions the nurse should take: _______________ and _______________.

NURSING ACTION OPTIONS
Request an order for laxatives
Monitor stoma viability
Inform the client the colostomy is permanent
Replace stoma and nasogastric tube output with an isotonic IV solution
Administer a regular diet

The nurse is caring for the client in the immediate postoperative period.

▶ For each assessment finding, identify if the finding indicates that the client's condition has improved, not changed, or has declined.

CLIENT FINDINGS	IMPROVED	NO CHANGE	DECLINED
Pulse oximetry reading 98% on room air	○	○	○
Stoma dark red with moderate amount of bleeding noted	○	○	○
Conjunctiva pale and perfused	○	○	○
Dorsalis pedis pulses palpable	○	○	○
Bowel sounds hypoactive × 4 quadrants 12 hours after the procedure	○	○	○

Note: Each row must have one response option selected.

Medical-Surgical 9.0

The nurse in the emergency department (ED) is caring for a 23-year-old male client.

Nurses' Notes

1100h: Client presented to the ED with complaints of urgency, frequency, dysuria, left-sided flank pain rated 8 out of 10 on numerical rating scale, and costovertebral tenderness. Client has vomited × 3 this a.m. with emesis consisting of yellow bile. Client was previously camping with friends × 2 days and needed to return due to the pain. Vital signs: T: 39.0°C (102.2°F); BP: 135/82; P: 122; RR: 22; with pulse oximetry of 99% on room air. Upon general assessment, client noted to have "tenting," dry mucous membranes as documented by the conjunctiva. Client reports camping was hot and he did not consume appropriate hydration during the camping trip. He is alert and appropriate, oriented to person, place, and time. Cooperative and follows commands. S1, S2, no extra heart sounds noted. Skin is cool with diaphoresis noted. Denies any chest pain. Capillary refill noted to be less than 3 seconds. Lung sounds clear. Moderate to severe left-sided flank pain that increased this morning prompted visit to the ED. Client reports not being able to get warm and feeling chilled for the last 12 hours. He cannot remember the last time he voided. Client denies any previous pertinent medical history.

The nurse has reviewed the Nurses' Notes at 1100h.

▶ Highlight the findings that require **immediate** follow-up.

Nurses' Notes

1100h: Client presented to the ED with complaints of urgency, frequency, dysuria, left-sided flank pain rated 8 out of 10 on pain rating scale, and costovertebral tenderness. Client has vomited × 3 this a.m. with emesis consisting of yellow bile. Client was previously camping with friends × 2 days and needed to return due to the pain. Vital signs: T: 39.0°C (102.2°F); BP: 135/82; P: 122; RR: 22; with pulse oximetry of 99% on room air. Upon general assessment, client noted to have "tenting," dry mucous membranes as documented by the conjunctiva. Client reports camping was hot and he did not consume appropriate hydration during the camping trip. He is alert and appropriate, oriented to person, place, and time. Cooperative and follows commands. S1, S2, no extra heart sounds noted. Skin is cool with diaphoresis noted. Denies any chest pain. Capillary refill noted to be less than 3 seconds. Lung sounds clear. Moderate to severe left-sided flank pain that increased this morning prompted visit to the ED. Client reports not being able to get warm and feeling chilled for the last 12 hours. He cannot remember the last time he voided. Client denies any previous pertinent medical history.

▶ Which of the following complications is the client at risk of experiencing? **Select all that apply.**
- ☐ Urinary tract infection
- ☐ Gastrointestinal viral illness
- ☐ Fluid imbalance
- ☐ Dysrhythmias
- ☐ Acute kidney failure
- ☐ Lower back injury

The nurse in the emergency department (ED) is caring for a 23-year-old male client.

Nurses' Notes	**Laboratory Results**	Diagnostic Results

1120h: (Collected in the Emergency Department)

Urinalysis:		**Client Result:**	
Colour	Yellow	Colour	Dark amber
Appearance	Clear	Appearance	Cloudy
Specific gravity	1.005–1.030	Specific gravity	1.25
Ketones	Negative	Ketones	Positive
Protein	Negative	Protein	Negative
Leukocytes	Negative	Leukocytes	Positive
Nitrates	Negative	Nitrates	Positive
Red blood cells	0–3	Red blood cells	7 (moderate)

Nurses' Notes	Laboratory Results	**Diagnostic Results**

1145h: Ultrasound whole abdomen with focus on kidney
Kidney: Right kidney size: 10.5 cm × 3.8 cm
Left kidney size: 11.7 cm × 4.2 cm
Collection systems: Dilated in left kidney
Stones: 3–5, approximate size measured at 2–3 mm, stones noted in both kidneys and one in the left ureter
Bladder: Normal contour, no stones observed

The nurse has reviewed the Laboratory Results at 1120h and the Diagnostic Results at 1145h.

▶ Complete the following sentence by choosing from the list of options.

The client is at **highest** risk of developing _______________.

WORD OPTIONS
Bladder cancer
Urinary retention
Interstitial cystitis
Renal stricture
Pyelonephritis
Glomerulonephritis

▶ For each potential order, identify whether the potential order is **indicated** or **not indicated** for the client.

POTENTIAL ORDERS	INDICATED	NOT INDICATED
Administration of pain medication	○	○
Initiate lactated Ringer's at 200 mL/hr	○	○
Draw CBC, electrolytes, PTT, INR, blood cultures	○	○
Consult Urology	○	○
Administer ibuprofen	○	○
Initiate broad-spectrum antibiotics	○	○

The nurse in the emergency department (ED) is caring for a 23-year-old male client.

Nurses' Notes	Laboratory Results	Diagnostic Results

1215h: Urinal at the bedside. Client attempting to void. Indicates pain improved to 4 out of 10.
1800h: Client to be admitted and transferred to a renal unit for further observation and treatment.

The nurse has reviewed the Nurses' Notes at 1215h and 1800h.

▶ Select 3 actions the nurse should take now that the client has been transferred to the renal unit.
- ☐ Prepare client for lithotripsy
- ☐ Insert a Foley catheter
- ☐ Monitor blood glucose
- ☐ Initiate 0.9% sodium chloride at 200 mL/hr
- ☐ Monitor urine output

The nurse on a renal unit is caring for a 23-year-old male client.

Nurses' Notes | Laboratory Results | Diagnostic Results

2 days later on a renal unit:
1500h: Client's condition resolved, and he is able to be discharged home on oral antibiotics. Client teaching provided prior to discharge from the unit.

▶ For each of the statements made by the client, identify whether the statement indicates an **understanding** or **no understanding** of the discharge teaching provided.

CLIENT STATEMENTS	UNDER-STANDING	NO UNDER-STANDING
"Drinking more hydrating fluids such as water would have helped prevent the stones from forming."	○	○
"I am healed now and do not have to monitor urine output."	○	○
"Until the stones completely pass, I should remain on bed rest."	○	○
"I have more information about which foods contributed to the stone developing along with lower fluid intake."	○	○
"I can adequately control the pain with acetaminophen."	○	○

Medical-Surgical 10.0

The nurse is caring for a 92-year-old male client on a urology unit.

Nurses' Notes

1100h: Client was seen in the emergency department complaining of lower abdominal discomfort rated 4 out of 10 on a numerical rating scale, found to be incontinent of urine in the hallway of the long-term care facility. He was trying to find the bathroom in his room and became disoriented. Client presents with a past medical history of coronary artery disease with PCI to LAD in 1995, benign prostate hyperplasia, chronic obstructive pulmonary disease (COPD), and left hip fracture due to frequent falls. Client accompanied by adult child. Vital signs: T: 38.3°C (100.9°F); BP: 143/86; P: 86; RR: 18; with pulse oximetry of 92% on room air. Client presents as pleasant, cooperative, alert and oriented to person, place, and time. No confusion noted while on Urology but he was placed in a room close to the nurses' station. Gait steady, denies any dizziness, but requires one-person assist for support only. S1 and S2 auscultated with S3, apical heart rate regular and equals radial pulse. Crackles auscultated in bilateral lower lung fields increasing to right middle lobe. Respirations regular and easy at rest. Client encouraged to use urinal at bedside when he is able to void. Client reports the urge to void but cannot, has to get up several times in the night to void, and he is exhausted. There is some discomfort when he starts to void but diminishes with stream. Bowel sounds auscultated × 4 quadrants with abdomen soft and round during palpation.

▶ Highlight the findings below that would require **immediate** follow-up.

Nurses' Notes

1100h: Client was seen in the emergency department complaining of lower abdominal discomfort rated 4 out of 10 on a numerical rating scale, found to be incontinent of urine in the hallway of the long-term care facility. He was trying to find the bathroom in his room and became disoriented. Client presents with a past medical history of coronary artery disease with PCI to LAD in 1995, benign prostate hyperplasia, chronic obstructive pulmonary disease (COPD), and left hip fracture due to frequent falls. Client accompanied by adult child. Vital signs: T: 38.3°C (100.9°F); BP: 143/86; P: 86; RR: 18; with pulse oximetry of 92% on room air. Client presents as pleasant, cooperative, alert and oriented to person, place, and time. No confusion noted while on Urology but he was placed in a room close to the nurses' station. Gait steady, denies any dizziness, but requires one-person assist for support only. S1 and S2 auscultated with S3, apical heart rate regular and equals radial pulse. Crackles auscultated in bilateral lower lung fields increasing to right middle lobe. Respirations regular and easy at rest. Client encouraged to use urinal at bedside when he is able to void. Client reports the urge to void but cannot, has to get up several times in the night to void, and he is exhausted. There is some discomfort when he starts to void but diminishes with stream. Bowel sounds auscultated × 4 quadrants with abdomen soft and round during palpation.

▶ Which of the following complications is the client at risk of experiencing? **Select all that apply**.

☐ Dehydration
☐ Leukopenia
☐ Incontinence
☐ Glomerulonephritis
☐ Distended bladder
☐ Hypertension
☐ Peripheral edema
☐ Syndrome of inappropriate antidiuretic hormone (SIADH)

▶ Complete the following sentence by choosing from the list of options.

The client is at **highest** risk of developing ______________ and ______________________.

WORD OPTIONS
Urosepsis
Dysrhythmias
Anorexia
Acute myocardial infarction
Renal failure

The nurse is caring for a 92-year-old male client on a urology unit.

Nurses' Notes | Laboratory Results

1215h: Client complains of lower abdominal discomfort that has become lower abdominal pain rated 8/10 on the numerical rating scale. Client presents with diaphoresis, pallor, and agitation.
1220h: Orders received from health care provider.

Nurses' Notes | **Laboratory Results**

1130h:

Hemoglobin 140–180 g/L (14–18 g/dL) (male) 120–160 g/L (12–16 g/dL) (female)	155 g/L (15.5 g/dL)	Sodium 136–145 mmol/L	136 mmol/L
Platelets 150–400 × 10^9/L (150 000–400 000/mm^3)	279 × 10^9/L (279 000/mm^3)	Potassium 3.5–5.1 mmol/L	5.8 mmol/L
White blood cells 3.5–12.0 × 10^9/L (3 500–12 000/mm^3)	7.0 × 10^9/L (7 000/mm^3)	Creatinine 53–106 mcmol/L (male) 44–97 mcmol/L (female)	98 mcmol/L
Neutrophils 3.0–5.8 × 10^9/L (3 000–5 800/mm^3)	4.0 × 10^9/L (4 000/mm^3)	Blood urea nitrogen (BUN) 2.9–8.2 mmol/L	7.2 mmol/L

The nurse reviewed the Nurse' Notes at 1215h and Laboratory Results at 1130h.

▶ For each potential nursing intervention, identify whether the intervention is **indicated** or **not indicated** for the care of this client.

POTENTIAL NURSING INTERVENTIONS	INDICATED	NOT INDICATED
Complete a bladder scan	○	○
Offer oral fluids to increase fluid intake	○	○
Request an order to insert a Foley catheter	○	○
Suggest client consume bananas	○	○
Request an order to insert a venous access device	○	○
Speak in a calm, reassuring voice to the client	○	○

Note: Each row must have one response option selected.

▶ Select 3 actions the nurse should take when inserting an in-dwelling catheter.

- ☐ Place the client in high Fowler's position
- ☐ Provide water at the bedside to assist with insertion
- ☐ Ensure client education about not "tugging" on the catheter
- ☐ Maintain sterile technique
- ☐ Educate the client about maintaining perineal care at least twice per day
- ☐ Place the drainage system on the raised bed rail

▶ For each assessment finding, identify if the finding indicates that the client's condition has **improved**, **not changed**, or **worsened**.

ASSESSMENT FINDINGS	IMPROVED	NO CHANGE	WORSENED
T: 37.7°C (99.9°F)	○	○	○
2 out of 10 pain on numerical rating scale	○	○	○
Found wandering, unable to locate room	○	○	○
S1, S2, and S3	○	○	○
Pulse oximetry 92% on room air	○	○	○
Urine output: 750 mL	○	○	○
BP: 92/65	○	○	○

Note: Each row must have one response option selected.

Medical-Surgical 11.0

The nurse is caring for a 78-year-old client on the orthopedic unit.

History and Physical	Nurses' Notes	Vital Signs

1020h:

Body System	**Findings**
Neurological	Alert and oriented to person, place, time, and situation. Cooperative, obeys commands. Denies headache.
Cardiovascular	Skin warm and dry to touch. Capillary refill less than 3 seconds. Bilateral radial pulses strong. Bilateral dorsalis pedis pulses strong. Peripheral edema absent on all extremities.
Pulmonary	Denies shortness of breath. Lung sounds clear with auscultation.
Musculoskeletal	Right leg externally rotated, supported by pillows with 8/10 on the numerical rating scale with minimal touch.
Psychosocial	Married, retired corporate executive for 10 years. Type 2 diabetes diagnosed 3 years ago controlled with oral hypoglycemic agents, coronary artery disease with acute myocardial infarction 10 years ago with PCI to RCA and distal LAD.

The nurse has collected data from the client upon return from the operating room.

▶ Which of the following assessment findings require **immediate** follow-up? **Select all that apply**.

- ☐ Pupillary response
- ☐ Alertness
- ☐ Respirations
- ☐ Lung sounds
- ☐ Pulses
- ☐ Pulse oximetry
- ☐ Skin temperature

▶ For each client finding below, identify if the finding is consistent with the disease process of stroke, hematoma, or venous thrombosis. Each finding may support more than one disease process.

History and Physical	**Nurses' Notes**	Vital Signs

1020h: Client admitted to the orthopedic unit after suffering a ground fall in his home due to spilled water on the floor. Partner unable to help client stand and emergency medical services were notified of the incident. Orthopedic surgery consulted.
1115h: Client to be prepped for surgery to repair a right hip fracture. Left antecubital venous access device inserted.
1600h: Client returned from the operating room after insertion of a femoral head prosthesis. Client lethargic but rouses. Alert and oriented to person, place, time, and situation. Denies pain at present, states right leg feels "heavy." Client moving all four extremities independently. Pupils equal and sluggish but reactive to light at 2 mm. S1, S2, heart sounds regular. Lungs auscultated for diminished air entry to bilateral bases. Right leg hip dressing, dry and intact with mild shadowing noted on the gauze. Right leg warm to touch, right dorsalis pedis pulse weaker as compared to left leg, which has a strong dorsalis pedis pulse. Capillary refill more sluggish on right toes as compared to left toes. Urinal at the bedside. No bruit auscultated at the surgical femoral site. Client NPO.

History and Physical	Nurses' Notes	**Vital Signs**

	1020h:	**1600h:**
T	37.3°C (99.1°F)	37.7°C (99.9°F)
P	102	82
RR	22	12
BP	128/74	101/60
Pulse oximetry reading	97% on room air	94% on 2 L/min per nasal prongs

CLIENT FINDINGS	STROKE	HEMATOMA	VENOUS THROMBOSIS
Weak dorsalis pedis pulses	○	○	○
Level of consciousness	○	○	○
Sluggish pupil response	○	○	○
Skin temperature	○	○	○
Bruit at the surgical site	○	○	○
Moving extremities equally	○	○	○

The nurse is caring for a 78-year-old client on the orthopedic unit.

History and Physical	**Nurses' Notes**	Vital Signs

0030h: Called to the client's room with complaints of extreme right leg tenderness. Right lower leg and right foot edematous, pale in colour, and sharp shooting pain with dorsiflexion of right foot. Dorsalis pedis pulse required Doppler to locate a regular but weak pulse. Skin is red and warm to touch. Popliteal pulse remains palpable on right leg. Left leg, lower leg, and foot remain unchanged in size. Dorsalis pedis pulse remains weak but found with palpation.

History and Physical	Nurses' Notes	**Vital Signs**

	1020h:	**1600h:**	**0030h:**
T	37.3°C (99.1°F)	37.7°C (99.9°F)	37.3°C (99.1°F)
P	102	82	92
RR	22	12	18
BP	128/74	101/60	114/76
Pulse oximetry reading	97% on room air	94% on 2 L/min per nasal prongs	99% on room air

The nurse reviewed the Nurses' Notes at 0030h and the Vital Signs taken at 0030h.

▶ Complete the following sentence by choosing from the list of options.

The client is at **highest** risk of developing ____________.

WORD OPTIONS
Venous thromboembolism
Rejection of the femoral head prothesis
Gangrene
Osteomyelitis
Peripheral arterial disease

▶ Select 2 potential nursing interventions for this client.

- ☐ Elevate the right leg while in bed
- ☐ Use a pillow between the legs
- ☐ Apply a warm blanket to the affected area
- ☐ Notify health care provider
- ☐ Contact client's partner with status

▶ Complete the following sentence by choosing from the list of options.

It would be a priority for the nurse to request a prescription for ___________________.

WORD OPTIONS
Rivaroxaban PO
Unfractionated heparin IV
Low-molecular-weight heparin SC
Clopidogrel PO

▶ Complete the following sentence by choosing from the list of options.

The nurse should prepare the client for the procedure ___________________ to confirm diagnosis.

WORD OPTIONS
Spiral CT
Coronary angiogram
Chest X-ray
Doppler ultrasonography

The nurse is caring for a 78-year-old client on the orthopedic unit.

History and Physical | **Nurses' Notes** | Vital Signs

Day 2 Postoperative:
0800h: Client reports ambulating the hallways several times a day with the use of a walker and increased mobility each day. Right lower leg remains slightly edematous, foot similar in size to the left foot. Dorsalis pedis pulses strong and palpable on the left foot, weak but palpable on the right foot. Capillary refill less than 3 seconds on bilateral toes. Right leg remains cooler to touch as compared to the left. Bilateral lower extremity colour noted to be pink.

The nurse has reviewed the Nurses' Notes from Postoperative Day 2 at 0800h.

▶ Highlight the findings below that indicate an improvement in the client's status.

Nurses' Notes

Day 2 Postoperative:
0800h: Client reports ambulating the hallways several times a day with the use of a walker and increased mobility each day. Right lower leg remains slightly edematous, foot similar in size to the left foot. Dorsalis pedis pulses strong and palpable on the left foot, weak but palpable on the right foot. Capillary refill less than 3 seconds on bilateral toes. Right leg remains cooler to touch as compared to the left. Bilateral lower extremity colour noted to be pink.

Medical-Surgical 12.0

The nurse is caring for a 30-year-old female client in the outpatient sexual health clinic.

Progress Notes

April 20: Client presents to the clinic to request sexually transmitted infection (STI) testing. She reports flulike symptoms: fatigue, fever, muscle aches, headaches, dysuria, and purulent urethral discharge after having condomless intercourse with a male partner. Client is requesting STI panel be completed.

▶ Highlight the assessment findings that would require follow-up.

Progress Notes

April 20: Client presents to the clinic to request sexually transmitted infection (STI) testing. She reports flulike symptoms: fatigue, fever, muscle aches, headaches, dysuria, and purulent urethral discharge after having condomless intercourse with a male partner. Client is requesting STI panel be completed. Full panel including chlamydia, gonorrhea, HIV, herpes, genital warts completed with specimens taken for testing.

▶ Which of the following complications is the client at risk of experiencing? **Select all that apply.**

- ☐ Chlamydia
- ☐ Genital herpes simplex type 2
- ☐ Syphilis
- ☐ Human immunodeficiency virus (HIV)
- ☐ Gonorrhea
- ☐ Pregnancy

The nurse is caring for a 30-year-old female client in the outpatient sexual health clinic.

Progress Notes | Laboratory Results

April 22: Client notified that results are available and to make an appointment at the clinic to review them in person.
April 23: Client informed of STI results and HIV status.

Progress Notes | **Laboratory Results**

April 20: Final Report Results	Status
Test for chlamydia	**** negative
Test for gonorrhea	**** positive
Test for herpes simplex type 1	**** positive
Test for herpes simplex type 2	**** negative
Test for genital warts	**** negative
Test for human immunodeficiency virus	**** positive
Human chorionic gonadotropin	**** negative

Urinalysis:		Client Result:	
Colour	Yellow	Colour	Yellow
Appearance	Clear	Appearance	1.25
Specific gravity	1.005–1.030	Specific gravity	Negative
Ketones	Negative	Ketones	Negative
Protein	Negative	Protein	Negative
Leukocytes	Negative	Leukocytes	Negative
Nitrates	Negative	Nitrates	2 (nil)
Red blood cells	0–3	Red blood cells	Clear

The nurse has reviewed the Laboratory Results from April 20.

▶ Complete the following sentence by choosing from the list of options.

The client is at **highest** risk of developing ______________ and ______________.

WORD OPTIONS
Chlamydia
Gonorrhea
Syphilis
Herpes simplex type 1
Herpes simplex type 2
Human immunodeficiency virus
Urinary tract infection

▶ Select 3 interventions the nurse would make **immediately**.

- ☐ Assess for client suicide risk
- ☐ Report both gonorrhea and HIV to public health
- ☐ Contact client's partners
- ☐ Rebook client for follow-up appointment
- ☐ Reassure client about new antiretroviral medications to lower viral loads
- ☐ Leave client alone to process information

▶ Which of the following health care provider orders should the nurse perform right away? **Select all that apply.**

- ☐ Initiate antiretroviral medication regime at the time of diagnosis
- ☐ Consult spiritual care
- ☐ Initiate cefixime and azithromycin
- ☐ Inform client of abstinence from all sexual activity until gonorrhea infection is cleared

▶ For each of the statements made by the client, identify whether the statement indicates an **understanding** or **no understanding** of the discharge teaching provided.

CLIENT STATEMENTS	UNDER-STANDING	NO UNDER-STANDING
"I can still be intimate with a partner; I will need to use condoms and know my viral load."	○	○
"I do not have to disclose my HIV status to any new partner."	○	○
"I will be taking this ARV therapy for the rest of my life."	○	○
"I can do this on my own."	○	○
"I will contact all partners to recommend getting tested."	○	○

Medical-Surgical 13.0

The nurse in the emergency department (ED) is caring for a 27-year-old male client.

Nurses' Notes

1530h: Client presents to the ED with shortness of breath, chills, and left chest wall discomfort. He had a skin biopsy for a suspicious mole in a dermatologist's office earlier in the day and noticed increasing redness from the biopsy site. Vital signs: T: 39.2°C (102.6°F); BP: 90/60; P: 115; RR: 24; with pulse oximetry of 89% on room air. Client is cooperative, alert and oriented to person, place, and time. Obeys commands. Moving all four extremities independent. Presents as pale, ashen in colour, skin cool to touch. S1, S2, no S3 or S4 heart sounds auscultated. Bilateral radial pulses regular and strong, bilateral dorsalis pedis pulses noted to be weak and thready. Capillary refill less than 3 seconds. Mild cyanosis noted on fingertips. No edema noted. Lungs clear with auscultation, reduced air entry noted to bilateral bases. Client noted to have short, shallow respirations. Abdomen soft and round to touch. Bowel sounds auscultated × 4 quadrants to be hypoactive. Anorexia. Client reports not voiding for several hours. Typically, a healthy male, who exercises 3–5 × per week, eats healthy and planning on competing in a power-lifting competition.

▶ Select the 4 client findings that require **immediate** follow-up.

- ☐ Vital signs
- ☐ Skin biopsy site
- ☐ Shortness of breath
- ☐ Radial pulses
- ☐ Bowel sounds
- ☐ Urine output
- ☐ Skin cool to touch

▶ Fill in each blank in the following sentence using the word options below.

The nurse should recognize that the client is potentially experiencing a(an) _______________ (word options 1) as indicated by ____________________ (word options 2) and ____________________(word options 2).

WORD OPTIONS 1	WORD OPTIONS 2
Sympathetic nervous system response	Low urine output
Volume overload	Orientation
Hypothermia	Lung sounds
Parasympathetic nervous system response	Skin temperature
Urinary tract infection	S3

The nurse in the emergency department (ED) is caring for a 27-year-old male client.

Nurses' Notes | Laboratory Results

1726h: Called to bedside as client is complaining of excruciating pain rated 9 out of 10 on a numerical pain scale, on the left chest wall. Left chest wall noted to be increasing in redness, radiating around to the client's back and down toward the left hip. T: 39.9°C (103.8°F); BP: 85/62; P: 135; RR: 28; with pulse oximetry of 70% on room air. Client presents with confusion, unable to remember why he is in the hospital. He is noted to be grey in colour with cyanosis around the lips and increasing cyanosis on the fingertips. Lung auscultated for reduced air entry to left lower lobe and right lower lobe extending to right mid-lobe with inspiratory crackles noted to bilateral upper lobes. Health care provider contacted for immediate orders.

Nurses' Notes | **Laboratory Results**

1600h: (As Taken in the Emergency Department)

Test	Result	Test	Result
Hemoglobin 140–180 g/L (14–18 g/dL) (male) 120–160 g/L (12–16 g/dL) (female)	174 g/L (17.4 g/dL)	Sodium 136–145 mmol/L	144 mmol/L
Platelets 150–400 × 10^9/L (150 000–400 000/mm^3)	220 × 10^9/L (220 000/mm^3)	Potassium 3.5–5.1 mmol/L	5.5 mmol/L
White blood cells 3.5–12.0 × 10^9/L (3 500–12 000/mm^3)	16 × 10^9/L (16 000/mm^3)	Creatinine 53–106 mcmol/L (male) 44–97 mcmol/L (female)	120 mcmol/L
Neutrophils 3.0–5.8 × 10^9/L (3,000–5 800/mm^3)	7.8 × 10^9/L (7 800/mm^3)	Blood urea nitrogen (BUN) 2.9–8.2 mmol/L	12 mmol/L

The nurse has reviewed the Nurses' Notes at 1726h and the Laboratory Results at 1600h.

▶ Complete the following sentence by choosing from the list of options.

The client is at **highest** risk of developing _______________.

WORD OPTIONS
Pneumonia
Shock
Cardiac tamponade
Cellulitis
Venous thrombosis

The nurse has reviewed the Nurses' Notes from 1726h and is planning care for the client.

▶ For each potential nursing interventions, identify whether the intervention is **indicated** or **not indicated** for the care of this client.

POTENTIAL NURSING INTERVENTIONS	INDICATED	NOT INDICATED
Plan for intubation	○	○
Reposition client in Trendelenburg position	○	○
Apply nasal prongs for oxygen administration	○	○
Draw an arterial blood gas	○	○
Obtain blood cultures	○	○
Prepare client for a chest X-ray	○	○
Request a nutritional consult for parenteral nutrition	○	○

▶ Which of the following health care orders should the nurse perform? **Select all that apply.**

☐ Administer opiates for pain
☐ Initiate broad-spectrum antibiotics
☐ Insert intraosseous access to administer fluids
☐ Initiate 500 mL 0.9% sodium chloride IV bolus then 150 mL/hr continuous
☐ Insert a Foley catheter
☐ Contact general surgery for consult

The nurse in the Intensive Care Unit (ICU) is caring for a 27-year-old male client.

Nurses' Notes | Laboratory Results

Intensive Care Unit:
1845h: Client intubated in the ED and transferred to the ICU for additional monitoring and ventilatory support. General surgery met client in the ICU and an operating room (OR) suite was to be prepped for immediately for abdominal surgery. T: 39.9°C (103.8°F); BP: 88/67; P: 122; RR: 23 on pressure control level of 26, pressure support at 14 cm H_2O, PEEP 8, and FiO_2 at 90%. Client's pulse oximetry noted to be 92%.
2030h: Client returned from the OR intubated and on inotropic support to maintain blood pressure. Resettled into the bed. T: 39.9°C (103.8°F); BP: 91/66; P: 92; RR: 18 on assist control ventilation at a rate of 16. Tidal volume 6 mL/kg, pressure support at 14 cm H_2O, PEEP 8, and FiO_2 at 90%. Client's pulse oximetry noted to be 90%. Bilateral wrist restraints applied. Pupils equal and sluggish to react to light at 2 mm. Client noted to have large left chest wall wound measuring from left nipple to umbilicus. The client's diagnosis is necrotizing fasciitis.

The nurse has reviewed the Intensive Care Unit transfer Nurses' Notes at 1845h and 2030h.

▶ Select 3 assessment data that would indicate the client's status has improved.

- ☐ The client cannot wiggle toes on command
- ☐ BP 100/75; P 78
- ☐ Diaphoresis
- ☐ Capillary refill greater than 3 seconds with no cyanosis noted
- ☐ Urine output documented at 50 mL/hr
- ☐ Right pupil 3 mm and left pupil 2 mm in size

Medical-Surgical 14.0

The nurse is caring for a 25-year-old transgender female client in the emergency department (ED).

Nurses' Notes | History and Physical | Vital Signs

0120h: Client presents to the ED with a primary complaint of chills and generalized feeling of being unwell × 2 days. Client indicates they are experiencing homelessness and have been staying in a shelter.

Nurses' Notes | **History and Physical** | Vital Signs

0130h:

Body System	**Findings**
Neurological	Alert and oriented to person, place, time, and situation. Cooperative, pleasant, with motor power strong × 4. Obeys commands. Speaks in an orderly manner, no deficits in speech, mood, or affect.
Cardiovascular	Skin warm and dry to touch. Capillary refill less than 3 seconds. Bilateral radial pulses palpable and regular. Bilateral dorsalis pedis pulses strong. Peripheral edema absent on all extremities. Mucous membranes dry. Tongue and lips noted to be dry and cracked.
Pulmonary	Denies shortness of breath. Lung sounds clear with auscultation anteriorly and posteriorly. Dry, nonproductive cough noted.
Gastrointestinal	Client presents as underweight, obtaining nutrition from the shelter eating 1–2 meals per day.

The nurse has reviewed the Nurses' Notes at 0120h, the History and Physical at 0130h, and the Vital Signs at 0125h.

▶ Which of the following assessment findings require **immediate** follow-up? **Select all that apply.**

- ☐ Lung sounds
- ☐ Heart rate, respirations, and pulse oximetry
- ☐ Blood pressure and temperature
- ☐ Motor power
- ☐ Pulses
- ☐ Mucous membranes
- ☐ Weight
- ☐ Cough
- ☐ Wounds

▶ Identify each word choice from below to fill in each blank in the following sentence.

The nurse should recognize that the client is potentially experiencing ________________ (word options 1) and ________________ (word options 2).

WORD OPTIONS 1	WORD OPTIONS 2
Anemia	Infection
Dysrhythmias	Pneumonia
Dehydration	Pulmonary embolus
Hypoxemia	Stroke
Impaired cognition	Obesity

Nurses' Notes	**History and Physical**	Vital Signs
Integumentary	Loonie-sized wounds × 1 noted bilateral antecubital fossa areas. Skin presents as excoriated, with yellow–green drainage noted. Skin around the wound noted to be white in colour, nonblanching erythema.	
Psychosocial	Client has been homeless × 3 years at the end of a romantic relationship. Client finds obtaining work difficult and has been left to panhandle or at times engage in sex work. Client reports using intravenous drugs.	

Nurses' Notes	History and Physical	Vital Signs
	0125h:	
T	38.6°C (101.5°F)	
P	106	
RR	16	
BP	92/64	
Pulse oximetry reading	98% on room air	

▶ Complete the following sentence by choosing from the list of options.

The client is at **highest** risk of developing ______________.

WORD OPTIONS
Sepsis
Gangrene
Meningitis
Melanoma
Impetigo

The nurse is caring for a 25-year-old transgender female client in the emergency department (ED).

Nurses' Notes	History and Physical	Vital Signs
0330h: The client rings for assistance by the nurse after noticing increased warmth radiating up from left antecubital fossa to upper bicep. There is increased erythema, tenderness at the side, and presence of +2 edema that extends from bilateral antecubital fossa location to shoulder on the right arm on the forearm side located anterior and posterior. Client presents flushed yet requesting a warm blanket. Client denies shortness of breath but noted to be taking shallow breaths. Health care provider notified of change in status as the client has not been seen by a physician yet.		

Nurses' Notes	History and Physical	**Vital Signs**
	0125h:	**0332h:**
T	38.6°C (101.5°F)	38.9°C (102.0°F)
P	106	115
RR	16	20
BP	92/64	88/60
Pulse oximetry reading	98% on room air	92% on room air

The nurse has reviewed the Nurses' Notes at 0330h and the Vital Signs taken at 0332h.

▶ For each potential nursing intervention, identify whether the intervention is **indicated** or **not indicated** for the care of this client.

POTENTIAL NURSING INTERVENTIONS	INDICATED	NOT INDICATED
Request an order to initiate intravenous fluids	○	○
Prepare to draw blood cultures	○	○
Administer an antipyretic then obtain a covering order from the health care provider when they assess the client	○	○
Prepare to apply oxygen per nasal prongs	○	○
Request to insert a peripheral venous access device	○	○
Place the client in semi-Fowler's position	○	○

Note: Each row must have one response option selected.

▶ Select 5 orders the nurse should perform right away.

- ☐ Administer cefazolin 1 g IV q8h
- ☐ Initiate oxygen therapy at 2 L to 6 L to maintain pulse oximetry greater than 92%. Notify health care provider if respiratory status changes
- ☐ Elevate and apply heat to the wound beds
- ☐ Draw borders of erythema and inform health care provider if borders increase in size

- ☐ Insert an in-dwelling Foley catheter if urine output drops below 30 mL/hr
- ☐ Insert a peripheral venous access device in the left forearm
- ☐ Initiate 0.9% normal saline (sodium chloride at 125 mL/hr)
- ☐ Laboratory draws: complete blood count, electrolytes, and blood cultures (culture and sensitivity)
- ☐ Consult social work
- ☐ Consult addiction services

The nurse performed the interventions as ordered by the physician for the client.

▶ For each assessment finding, identify if the finding indicates that the client's condition has improved, has not changed, or has declined.

ASSESSMENT FINDINGS	IMPROVED	NO CHANGE	DECLINED
Erythema less than original borders on right forearm	○	○	○
BP 125/73	○	○	○
Urine output 700 mL documented at 0730h	○	○	○
RR 20	○	○	○
Erythema extending beyond the shoulder border and now documented at the collarbone	○	○	○

Note: Each row must have one response option selected.

Medical-Surgical 15.0

The nurse is caring for a 74-year-old client on the internal medicine unit.

Progress Notes | Nurses' Notes

Admission note: Client was admitted to the unit to receive medical assistance in dying (MAiD) care. The client was informed 3 months ago that no further treatment options were available for their end-stage chronic obstructive pulmonary disease (COPD) and immediately began the paperwork and necessary process to become eligible for MAiD. According to the client and their family, the client's quality of life has significantly declined over the past 6 months and the client expressed difficulty breathing even with minimal exertion and is currently at 7 L/min of continuous home oxygen therapy. The client was unable to visit friends, engage in social activities outside of the home, and had limited contact with family due to increased susceptibility to infection during the COVID-19 pandemic. The client spoke with family about end-of-life care and prepared their three children and seven adult grandchildren for their plan to proceed with MAiD.

▶ Highlight the findings below that would require follow-up.

Progress Notes | **Nurses' Notes**

0730h: Intended MAiD appointment is scheduled for tomorrow, for end-stage idiopathic pulmonary arterial hypertension. Client did not want to complete MAiD at home. Family to be arriving later in the day. Vital signs: T: 37.7°C (99.9°F); BP: 102/54; P: 105; RR: 26; with pulse oximetry of 92% on 6 L/min of oxygen via high-flow nasal prongs. Client presents as pleasant, cooperative, alert and oriented to person, place, and time. Gait steady, becomes ++ dizzy with sitting at the edge of the bed, requires two-person stand-by assist for ambulation and minimal changes to position (i.e., bed to chair). S1 and S2 heart sounds documented with no other adventitious heart sounds noted. Jugular venous distension noted at 7 cm. Apical heart rate regular, strong, and noted to be equal in rate to radial pulse. +1 peripheral edema noted to bilateral lower extremities. Client denies any pain with extremities. Reduced air entry noted throughout all lung fields. Client complains of ++ shortness of breath even with extended periods of talking. Client noted to have nonproductive wet cough. Client is voiding small amounts of clear amber urine. Client has reduced fluid and food intake over the past few days, states they are not feeling up to it. Hypoactive bowel sounds auscultated × 4 quadrants with abdomen firm and distended during palpation.

Progress Notes | **Nurses' Notes**

0730h: Intended MAiD appointment is scheduled for tomorrow, for end-stage idiopathic pulmonary arterial hypertension. Client did not want to complete MAiD at home. Family to be arriving later in the day. Vital signs: T: 37.7°C (99.9°F); BP: 102/54; P: 105; RR: 26; with pulse oximetry of 92% on 6 L/min of oxygen via high-flow nasal prongs. Client presents as pleasant, cooperative, alert and oriented to person, place, and time. Gait steady, becomes ++ dizzy with sitting at the edge of the bed, requires two-person stand-by assist for ambulation and minimal changes to position (i.e., bed to chair). S1 and S2 heart sounds documented with no other adventitious heart sounds noted. Jugular venous distension noted at 7 cm. Apical heart rate regular, strong, and noted to be equal in rate to radial pulse. +1 peripheral edema noted to bilateral lower extremities. Client denies any pain with extremities. Reduced air entry noted throughout all lung fields. Client complains of ++ shortness of breath even with extended periods of talking. Client noted to have nonproductive wet cough. Client is voiding small amounts of clear amber urine. Client has reduced fluid and food intake over the past few days, states they are not feeling up to it. Hypoactive bowel sounds auscultated × 4 quadrants with abdomen firm and distended during palpation.

▶ Which of the following complications is the client at risk of experiencing? **Select all that apply.**

- ☐ Cor pulmonale
- ☐ Bowel obstruction
- ☐ Deep vein thrombosis
- ☐ Pulmonary edema
- ☐ Atrial fibrillation

The nurse is caring for a 74-year-old client on the internal medicine unit.

Progress Notes | **Nurses' Notes**

1224h: Client used call bell for assistance. Client found in semi-Fowler's position, ++ shortness of breath noted, diaphoretic, and clutching chest. Client noted to be taking short, shallow breaths. Fine inspiratory crackles noted throughout all lung fields when auscultated posteriorly. Client nodded when asked if they were having chest pain. Pulses remain palpable and regular. Abdomen remains firm and distended with hypoactive bowel sounds × 4 quadrants. Vital signs: T: 37.9°C (100.2°F); BP: 95/57; P: 128; RR: 30; with pulse oximetry of 84% on 6 L/min of oxygen via high-flow nasal prongs. Health care provider notified.

The nurse has reviewed the Nurses' Notes from 1224h.

▶ Complete the following sentence by choosing from the list of options.

The client is at **highest** risk of developing ____________ (word options 1) as evidenced by ______________ (word options 2).

WORD OPTIONS 1	WORD OPTIONS 2
Acute myocardial infarction	Temperature
Dysrhythmias	Respiratory assessment
Pulmonary embolus	Cardiovascular assessment
Pneumonia	Neurological assessment
Hepatic dysfunction	Gastrointestinal assessment

▶ For each potential nursing intervention, identify whether the intervention would be **indicated** or **not indicated** for the care of this client.

POTENTIAL NURSING INTERVENTIONS	INDICATED	NOT INDICATED
Prepare to administer nitroglycerin sublingual	○	○
Initiate a peripheral venous access device	○	○
Prepare the client for an electrocardiogram (ECG) to be performed	○	○
Prepare to contact the family	○	○
Reposition the client	○	○
Call a code blue	○	○

Note: Each row must have one response option selected.

▶ Select 3 health care orders that the nurse should perform right away.

- ☐ Initiate oxygen therapy via a non-rebreather mask 0–10 L/min in order to achieve a pulse oximetry of greater than 92%
- ☐ Recommend a regular diet
- ☐ Initiate bowel protocol
- ☐ 12-lead electrocardiogram (ECG)
- ☐ Draw laboratory tests: troponin, complete blood count, electrolytes

▶ Which of the following findings would indicate the client's status has improved? **Select all that apply.**

- ☐ Pulse oximetry recorded at 93% on 5 L/min of oxygen therapy via a non-rebreather mask
- ☐ Respiratory rate 32
- ☐ Client reports chest pain at 2 out of 10 on a numerical rating scale
- ☐ Client denies need to void
- ☐ Client reports feeling less dizzy with changes in position
- ☐ Client noted to be taking short, shallow respirations

Medical-Surgical 16.0

The nurse is caring for a 36-year-old client on an internal medicine unit.

Progress Notes

2254h: Client presented to the emergency department with increased redness, edema, and the feeling of heat on a left anterior/lateral lower leg wound that occurred during a hike. The client had fallen on the muddy path and suffered the cut on what might have been a tree branch on the ground. Vital signs: T: 38.7°C (101.7°F); BP: 120/65; P: 87; RR: 24; with pulse oximetry of 92% on room air. Client presents to the unit alert and oriented to person, place, and time. Pupils equal in size and shape measured at 2 mm and react briskly to light. Gait steady, with movement noted independent and strong × 4. Client denies any numbness, tingling, or dizziness with ambulation. S1 and S2 heart sounds noted with no adventitious heart sounds auscultated. Apical heart rate regular and equals radial pulse. Client denies any chest pain. Respirations regular and easy at rest. No adventitious lung sounds auscultated upon posterior lung field assessment. Client denies a cough. Abdomen soft with bowel sounds auscultated × 4 quadrants. Able to void independently. Client states urine is clear and amber-coloured. Left lower leg wound was dressed with saline-soaked gauze, abdomen pad, and wrapped with gauze Kling wrap, secured with paper tape. Client states wound pain is 3 out of 10 on a numerical rating scale, but manageable. Peripheral venous access device inserted right antecubital fossa and saline locked. Client noted to have an allergy wristband indicating an allergy to penicillin. Client prescribed ciprofloxacin to be administered through a venous access device. Initial antibiotic was provided to client in the emergency department at 2200, prior to arriving to the unit.

0030h: The unit was notified that the client had received cloxacillin in error in the emergency department. Health care provider notified.

▶ Which of the following findings require **immediate** follow-up? **Select all that apply.**

- ☐ Left lower leg wound
- ☐ Heart sounds
- ☐ Lung sounds
- ☐ Pupillary response
- ☐ Gait
- ☐ Medication error

▶ Identify the correct word options from below to complete the following sentence.

The nurse should recognize that the client is potentially developing _______________ (word options 1) as a result of _______________ (word options 2).

WORD OPTIONS 1	WORD OPTIONS 2
Anemia	Gastrointestinal assessment
Dysrhythmias	Respiratory assessment
Anorexia	Cardiovascular assessment
Anaphylaxis	Neurological assessment
Renal failure	Renal assessment
Deep vein thrombosis	Medication error

▶ Complete the following sentence by choosing from the list of options.

The client is at **highest** risk of developing ______________.

WORD OPTIONS
Cellulitis
Respiratory failure
Pulmonary embolus
Pneumonia
Acute kidney injury
Stroke

The nurse is caring for a 36-year-old client on an internal medicine unit.

Progress Notes

0042h: Client found sitting at the edge of the bed in tripod position gasping for air. Audible wheeze and stridor noted. Client's colour pale with cyanosis noted around the lips and fingertips. Vital signs: T: 39.2°C (102.6°F); BP: 87/48; P:132; RR: 28; with pulse oximetry of 82% on room air. Code blue activated.

The nurse has reviewed the Progress Notes 0042h and is planning care for the client.

▶ For each potential nursing intervention, identify whether the intervention is **indicated** or **not indicated** for the care of this client.

POTENTIAL NURSING INTERVENTIONS	INDICATED	NOT INDICATED
Prepare to take the client for a spiral computed tomography (CT)	○	○
Bring oxygen supplies to the room	○	○
Call a code blue	○	○
Offer oral fluids for hydration	○	○
Ensure suction is patent and ready	○	○
Prepare to draw blood cultures	○	○

Note: Each row must have one response option selected.

▶ Select 3 orders the nurse should perform right away.

- ☐ Initiate oxygen therapy with high-flow nasal prongs 0–8 L/min to maintain pulse oximetry greater than 92%
- ☐ Ambulate client as tolerated
- ☐ Give regular diet
- ☐ 0.9% normal saline (sodium chloride) 500 mL IV × 1 bolus then 150 mL/hr
- ☐ Administer bronchodilator
- ☐ Laboratory draws: complete blood count, electrolytes, lipid levels

▶ For each assessment finding, identify if the finding indicates that the client's condition has **improved**, **not changed**, or **worsened**.

CLIENT FINDINGS	IMPROVED	NOT CHANGED	DECLINED
Respirations, 28	○	○	○
Temperature, 37.9°C	○	○	○
Short, shallow breaths	○	○	○
Colour, pink	○	○	○
No stridor noted	○	○	○
Pulse oximetry 92%	○	○	○

Note: Each row must have one response option selected.

Medical-Surgical 17.0

The nurse is caring for a 28-year-old male client in the emergency department (ED).

Progress Notes

0215h: The client arrived at the ED via emergency medical services (EMS) after being involved in a motor vehicle accident in which the client hit the steering wheel from the impact, despite wearing their seatbelt. Vital signs: T: 37.7°C (99.9°F); BP: 135/64; P: 128; RR: 28; with pulse oximetry of 92% on 4 L/min of continuous oxygen per nasal prongs. Client is alert and oriented to person, place, and time. Pupils equal and briskly reactive to light. Motor power strong × 4 with client able to move all four extremities independently. Client denies hitting head on the steering wheel, indicating their chest received the full force. Client denies any numbness or tingling. S1 and S2 heart sounds; apical heart rate regular and equals radial pulse. Bilateral radial pulses palpable, bilateral dorsalis pedis pulses palpable. Lower extremities cool to touch. Capillary refill less than 3 seconds. Client presents with shortness of breath and indicates pain at 3 out of 10 on a numerical rating scale, pleuritic plain with inspiration. Client is noted to be taking short, shallow breaths. Absent air entry is noted in posterior left lower lung, with quiet air entry noted in left upper lung region. Inspiratory crackles noted right lung posteriorly. No open areas noted on the client's thorax. Large anterior lateral bruise noted at the apex of the heart. No cough noted. Abdomen is soft and rounded with active bowel sounds auscultated × 4 quadrants. Client denies need to void. Peripheral venous access device previously inserted by EMS located right antecubital fossa.
0242h: Portable chest X-ray completed.

▶ Select the top 3 client findings that would require follow-up.

- ☐ Orientation
- ☐ Motor power
- ☐ Pupillary response
- ☐ Pulses
- ☐ Pleuritic pain
- ☐ Lung sounds
- ☐ Breathing pattern
- ☐ Bowel sounds
- ☐ Urine output

▶ Identify the potential complications the client is at risk of experiencing. **Select all that apply.**

- ☐ Rib fractures
- ☐ Pulmonary embolus
- ☐ Deep vein thrombosis
- ☐ Pneumothorax
- ☐ Clavicle fracture
- ☐ Cardiac tamponade
- ☐ Bowel obstruction

The nurse is caring for a 28-year-old male client in the emergency department (ED).

Progress Notes

0248h: Health care provider notified of change in status.
0252h: Client presents as confused, unable to follow simple commands. Client noted to be indrawing at the rib cage, nasal flaring, cyanosis of the lips and fingertips and was found in the tripod position over the bedside table. Tracheal deviation noted to be drifting toward the right. Vital signs: T: 38.3°C (100.9°F); BP: 82/56; P: 142; RR: 36; with pulse oximetry of 76% on 6 L/min per nasal prongs.

The nurse has reviewed the Progress Notes at 0242h, 0248h, and 0252h.

▶ Complete the following sentence by choosing from the list of options.

The client is at **highest** risk of developing ____________.

WORD OPTIONS
Pulmonary edema
Pleurisy
Pneumothorax
Pneumonia
Pleural effusion

▶ For each potential nursing intervention, identify whether the intervention is **indicated** or **not indicated** for the care of this client.

POTENTIAL NURSING INTERVENTIONS	INDICATED	NOT INDICATED
Arrange a disposable water-seal chest drainage system with suction ready	○	○
Prepare to administer intravenous fluids	○	○
Reposition client to Fowler's position	○	○
Prepare to insert a nasogastric tube	○	○
Gather in-dwelling Foley catheter supplies	○	○
Laboratory draw: type and cross-match	○	○
Prepare to apply high-flow oxygen with a non-rebreather mask	○	○

Note: Each row much have one response option selected.

The nurse is caring for a 28-year-old male client in the emergency department (ED).

Progress Notes

0300h: The health care provider inserted a rigid chest tube into the fifth intercostal space, and a multichamber chest drainage system was attached to the tube; 130 mL of frank blood collected in the collection chamber. Client on 6 L/min non-rebreather mask of continuous oxygen with pulse oximetry increasing to 89%. Chest expansion symmetrical with air entry noted in left lung. Vital signs: T: 38.3°C (100.9°F); BP: 80/58; P: 140; RR: 28; with pulse oximetry of 89% on 6 L/min continuous oxygen on a non-rebreather mask.

The nurse has reviewed the Progress Notes from 0300h.

▶ Highlight the 4 orders that the nurse should perform right away.

- ☐ Initiate 0.9% normal saline (sodium chloride) 500 mL bolus then 125 mL/hr
- ☐ Chest X-ray
- ☐ Attach chest tube to high suction
- ☐ Oxygen 0–10 L per non-rebreather to achieve pulse oximetry greater than 92%
- ☐ Laboratory draws: complete blood count (CBC), electrolytes, arterial blood gas (ABG)
- ☐ Initiate regular diet or diet as tolerated
- ☐ Monitor input and output

The nurse performed the interventions as ordered by the health care provider.

▶ For each assessment finding, identify if the finding indicates that the client's condition has **improved**, **not changed**, or has **declined**.

ASSESSMENT FINDINGS	IMPROVED	NO CHANGE	DECLINED
BP 101/70	○	○	○
Pulse 102	○	○	○
Respiratory rate 20	○	○	○
4 out of 10 pain at insertion site	○	○	○
Continuous bubbling in the water seal in the multichamber chest drainage system	○	○	○
Chest tube drainage 130 mL for shift	○	○	○

Note: Each row much have one response option selected.

Medical-Surgical 18.0

The nurse is caring for a 54-year-old client on an oncology surgical unit.

Progress Notes

0620h: Client was admitted to the unit post–bowel resection due to a malignant mass that ended with a colostomy. The client's gut is to be rested while the surgical area heals, so the client has been ordered to have a peripherally inserted central catheter placed for the purpose of receiving total parenteral nutrition. Client is aware of the procedure and understands the complications and risks. Vital signs: T: 37.7°C (99.9°F); BP: 102/54; P: 92; RR: 26; with pulse oximetry of 92% on room air. Client presents as pleasant, cooperative, alert and oriented to person, place, and time. Pupils equal and briskly reactive to light at 2 mm. Presents with S1 and S2; no adventitious heart sounds auscultated. Gait steady, denies any dizziness. Assisted with transfer from bed to stretcher to go to interventional radiology for the procedure. S1 and S2 heart sounds. Apical heart rate regular and equals radial pulse. Bilateral radial pulses remain strong, regular, and palpable. Bilateral dorsalis pedis pulses and posterior tibial pulses noted to be weak but palpable. Capillary refill less than 3 seconds. Skin warm and dry to touch. Fine inspiratory crackles located bilateral lower lobes when lungs auscultated posteriorly. Client instructed to perform deep-breathing and coughing exercises. Respirations regular and easy at rest. Abdominal dressing dry and intact. Colostomy stoma pink in colour, no bleeding noted, no blanching, no grey areas noted. No drainage noted in the bag. Client able to void in the washroom but requires stand-by assist for ambulation. A peripheral venous access device was inserted prior to the abdominal surgery and has been infusing Ringer's lactate at 100 mL/hr.

0814h: Client returned from interventional radiology, grey in colour, skin cool to touch. Client rouses easily, complaining of pleuritic pain with inspiration, expectorating blood. Client says they cannot catch their breath. Client noted to be indrawing at neck and with nasal flaring. Coarse crackles auscultated throughout all lung fields posteriorly. Vital signs: T: 38.1°C (100.6°F); BP: 86/64; P: 135; RR: 28; with pulse oximetry of 87% of on 4 L/min of continuous oxygen per nasal prongs.

▶ Identify the top 4 assessment findings that require **immediate** follow-up.

- ☐ Skin colour characteristics
- ☐ Pleuritic pain
- ☐ Cognitive status
- ☐ Hemoptysis
- ☐ Temperature
- ☐ Blood pressure
- ☐ Respiratory retractions
- ☐ Lung sounds

▶ For which of the following complications is the client at risk? **Select all that apply.**

- ☐ Sepsis
- ☐ Asymmetrical breathing
- ☐ Reduced gastric motility
- ☐ Migration of the central line into the carotid
- ☐ Perforation of the vein
- ☐ Dehydration

▶ Complete the following sentence.

The client is at **highest** risk of developing ____________ (word options 1) based on the assessment data of ________________ (word options 2).

WORD OPTIONS 1	WORD OPTIONS 2
Line sepsis	Vital signs
Pneumothorax	Respiratory assessment
Pneumonia	Cardiovascular assessment
Air embolus	Neurological assessment
Pleural effusion	Renal assessment

The nurse is caring for a 54-year-old client on an oncology surgical unit.

Progress Notes

0825h: D-dimer drawn.

Progress Notes | **Laboratory Results**

0530h:

Test	Result	Test	Result
Hemoglobin 140–180 g/L (14–16 g/dL) (male) 120–160 g/L (12–16 g/dL) (female)	124 g/L (12.4 g/dL)	Sodium 136–145 mmol/L	145 mmol/L
Platelets 150–400 × 10^9/L (150 000–400 000/mm^3)	275 × 10^9/L (275 000/ mm^3)	Potassium 3.5–5.1 mmol/L	3.3mmol/L
White blood cells 3.5–12.0 × 10^9/L (3 500–12 000/ mm^3)	8.0 × 10^9/L (8 000/ mm^3)	Creatinine 53–106 mcmol/L (male) 44–97 mcmol/L (female)	65 mcmol/L
Neutrophils 3.0–5.8 × 10^9/L (3 000-5 800/mm^3)	4.3 × 10^9/L (4 300/ mm^3)	Blood urea nitrogen (BUN) 2.9–8.2 mmol/L	3.0 mmol/L

0825h:

	Result
D-dimer	
Negative	Positive

The nurse reviewed the Progress Notes at 0620h and 0814h and Laboratory Results at 0530h and 0825h.

▶ For each potential nursing intervention, identify whether the intervention is **indicated** or **not indicated** for the care of this client.

POTENTIAL NURSING INTERVENTIONS	INDICATED	NOT INDICATED
Ensure all catheter connections are clamped	○	○
Place the client in Trendelenburg position and turn on left side	○	○
Provide supplemental oxygen	○	○
Contact health care provider	○	○
Prepare to administer narcotics for the pain	○	○

Note: Each row must have one response option selected.

The nurse has received orders from the physician.

▶ Highlight below the orders the nurse should perform right away. **Select all that apply.**

Orders

- Piperacillin/Tazocin 2.25 g IV q8h
- Initiate anticoagulant therapy (IV heparin)
- Prepare the client for a spiral computed tomography (CT)
- Laboratory draws: PTT/INR, ABG
- Consult physiotherapy
- Oxygen therapy to maintain pulse oximetry greater than 92%

The nurse has performed the interventions as ordered by the physician for the client.

▶ For each assessment finding, identify whether the finding indicates that the client's condition has improved, has not changed, or has declined.

ASSESSMENT FINDINGS	IMPROVED	NO CHANGE	DECLINED
Pulse oximetry 94% on 3 L/min of oxygen via non-rebreather mask	○	○	○
RR 22	○	○	○
Client able to sit in semi-Fowler's position without chest pain	○	○	○
BP 103/65	○	○	○
T 37.8°C (100.0°F)	○	○	○
Client has feeling of being unable to catch their breath	○	○	○

Note: Each row must have one response option selected.

Medical-Surgical 19.0

The nurse is caring for a 22-year-old client on a general medical unit.

Progress Notes

0730h: Client presents to the unit with failure to thrive. Previous comorbidities include cerebral palsy with bilateral contractures noted on wrists, elbows, and hips and a percutaneous endoscopic gastrostomy (PEG) tube in situ for nutrition. Vital signs: T: 38.4°C (101.1°F); BP: 91/67; P:76; RR: 14; with pulse oximetry of 92% on room air. On assessment, client presents as nonverbal but opens eyes to voice and tracks with eyes. Client is unable to follow commands but moves all extremities independently in the bed. Client moans with repositioning but does not express grimacing, guarding, tachycardia, or diaphoresis. Pupils are equal in size, measuring at 3 mm and briskly reactive to light. Skin is cool to touch with dry mucous membranes, coating noted on tongue, and dry lips noted. Bilateral radial pulses are strong with palpation and regular. Apical = radial pulse. Client takes short, shallow breaths with fine inspiratory crackles noted bilateral lower lungs with minimal cough reflex. Secretions pool at the back of the client's throat, requiring suction. Client positioned in semi-Fowler's position as they slide down the bed when the head of the bed is positioned too high. Foley catheter in situ because client is incontinent of urine. Dark, concentrated urine noted in the Foley bag with 800 mL documented from 8-hour night shift. Client presents as cachectic with low body weight. Redness noted on bilateral shoulder blades, Loonie-sized open area noted on coccyx with yellow slough, purulent drainage, and pink borders, and redness noted on bilateral heels as client rubs heels on the bed for self-soothing. Client to receive tube feeds as per dietitian's caloric requirements for basal metabolic rate through PEG tube, and all pill form medications to be crushed and administered as per institution policy. Skin around tube site has mild excoriation but is dry and intact. No open areas noted around PEG site. Bowel sounds hypoactive × 4 quadrants.

▶ Highlight the findings below that would require follow-up.

Progress Notes

0730h: Client presents to the unit with failure to thrive. Previous comorbidities include cerebral palsy with bilateral contractures noted on wrists, elbows, and hips and a percutaneous endoscopic gastrostomy (PEG) tube in situ for nutrition. Vital signs: T: 38.4°C (101.1°F); BP: 91/67; P:76; RR: 14; with pulse oximetry of 92% on room air. On assessment, client presents as nonverbal but opens eyes to voice and tracks with eyes. Client is unable to follow commands but moves all extremities independently in the bed. Client moans with repositioning but does not express grimacing, guarding, tachycardia, or diaphoresis. Pupils are equal in size, measuring at 3 mm and briskly reactive to light. Skin is cool to touch with dry mucous membranes, coating noted on tongue, and dry lips noted. Bilateral radial pulses are strong with palpation and regular. Apical = radial pulse. Client takes short, shallow breaths with fine inspiratory crackles noted bilateral lower lungs with minimal cough reflex. Secretions pool at the back of the client's throat, requiring suction. Client positioned in semi-Fowler's position as they slide down the bed when the head of the bed is positioned too high. Foley catheter in situ because client is incontinent of urine. Dark, concentrated urine noted in the Foley bag with 800 mL documented from 8-hour night shift. Client presents as cachectic with low body weight. Redness noted on bilateral shoulder blades, Loonie-sized open area noted on coccyx with yellow slough, purulent drainage, and pink borders, and redness noted on bilateral heels as client rubs heels on the bed for self-soothing. Client to receive tube feeds as per dietitian's caloric requirements for basal metabolic rate through PEG tube, and all pill form medications to be crushed and administered as per institution policy. Skin around tube site has mild excoriation but is dry and intact. No open areas noted around PEG site. Bowel sounds hypoactive × 4 quadrants.

▶ Which of the following complications is the client at risk of developing? **Select all that apply**.
- ☐ Deep vein thrombosis
- ☐ Pneumothorax
- ☐ Pleural effusion
- ☐ Pneumonia
- ☐ Pressure injury
- ☐ Bowel obstruction

▶ Complete the sentence by choosing from the list of options.

The nurse should **first** address the client's _______________.

WORD OPTIONS
Vital signs
Skin integrity
Pulse
Urine output
Nutrition
Lung sounds

The nurse is caring for a 22-year-old client on a general medical unit.

Progress Notes

1026h: Dietitian consulted for dietary needs and to determine caloric metrics.
1317h: Client found incontinent of stool with tube feed leaking from PEG tube. Tube feed tubing noted to be caught in the rail of the bed, allowing for increased moisture in the bed. Client had wiggled in the bed, causing increased friction of the pressure injury. Coccyx wound noted to be bleeding during cleaning with slough no longer present and skin erosion of the epidermis noted. Vital signs taken after the client was cleaned: T: 38.8°C (101.8°F); BP: 89/55; P:98; RR: 18; with pulse oximetry of 92% on room air. Full assessment completed. Lungs auscultated posteriorly for scattered fine crackles noted throughout that clear with cough. Repositioning the client triggered a cough and the client's lung sounds auscultated pre- and post-movement. Client diaphoretic from previous assessment, bilateral radial pulses remain strong and regular upon palpation. Abdomen flat with hypoactive bowel sounds × 4 quadrants. Foley draining clear amber urine and bag drained for 537 mL.

The nurse has reviewed the Progress Notes from 1026h and 1317h and is planning care for the client.

▶ Select 2 potential nursing interventions that the nurse should implement when planning care for this client.
- ☐ Place the client in Trendelenburg position
- ☐ Reposition the client to stay off reddened areas
- ☐ Prepare to administer oral fluids
- ☐ Contact the family for update of status
- ☐ Provide reassurance to the client

▶ For each nursing intervention, identify whether the intervention is **indicated** or **not indicated** for the care of this client.

NURSING INTERVENTIONS	INDICATED	NOT INDICATED
Administer laxatives	○	○
Implement the Braden scale	○	○
Place client in an adult incontinence product and secure sides	○	○
Irrigate the wound	○	○
Use friction-reducing sheets	○	○
Hold the tube feeds to reduce risk of tube becoming loose again	○	○
Incorporate a turning schedule	○	○

Note: Each row must have one response option selected.

The nurse performed the interventions for the client.

▶ For each assessment finding, identify whether the finding indicates that the client's condition has improved, not changed, or declined.

ASSESSMENT FINDINGS	IMPROVED	NO CHANGE	DECLINED
Wound identified as stage 1 on Braden scale	○	○	○
Bleeding of wound with fecal incontinence	○	○	○
Caloric and protein needs identified by a dietitian	○	○	○
T 37.6°C	○	○	○
Client wiggles in bed	○	○	○
Client tolerating sitting in chair with foam supports	○	○	○

Note: Each row must have one response option selected.

Medical-Surgical 20.0

The nurse is caring for a 25-year-old client on the orthopedic unit.

Progress Notes

1100h: Client was brought to the emergency department via emergency medical services (EMS). The client was a passenger in a car that was struck from behind and pushed into another vehicle while waiting at a traffic light. The force of the accident caused the client to become pinned under the dashboard, requiring extrication. The client's airway remained patent throughout, and the client was found unconscious prior to extrication but remained alert and appropriate while en route to the hospital. Primary injury presents as an open fracture of the left tibia and ankle dislocation on the same leg. Left lower leg splinted. Vital signs: T: 37.7°C (99.9°F); BP: 143/62; P: 110; RR: 18; with pulse oximetry of 99% on room air. Client presents as pleasant, cooperative, alert and oriented to person, place, and time. Client able to assist with moving from stretcher to bed and has mild dizziness with movement. Client indicates the back of their neck is tender because they remember their head extending forward and then backward from the impact. Pupils equal in size at 3 mm and briskly reactive to light. Client denies hitting head on the dashboard and no bruising is noted. Motor power strong × 3, with client able to wiggle toes; +4 edema noted left leg. Client states they have 7 out of 10 pain on a numerical pain scale. S1 and S2 heart sounds, apical heart rate regular and equals radial pulse. Bilateral radial pulses noted to be strong and bounding. Upper extremity skin warm to touch. Left foot and leg remains cooler to touch compared to right leg and foot. Right dorsalis pedis pulse strong and regular with palpation. Left dorsalis pedis pulse weak but palpable. Capillary refill less than 3 seconds × 4 extremities. Lungs auscultated for fine inspiratory crackles noted to posterior bilateral lower lobes. Clears with cough. No other adventitious lung sounds noted. No cough noted. Client is voiding clear amber urine but requires bed pan. Urine output documented to be 450 mL. Bowel sounds auscultated × 4 quadrants with abdomen soft and round during palpation. Client complains of nausea, no emesis noted. #16-gauge peripheral venous access device noted right antecubital fossa and infusing Ringer's lactate at 125 mL/hr.
1115h: Orthopedic surgeon consulted.

▶ Select 3 assessment findings that require **immediate** follow-up.

- ☐ Pupillary response
- ☐ Alertness
- ☐ Lung sounds
- ☐ Characteristics of the pulses
- ☐ Pulse oximetry
- ☐ Skin temperature
- ☐ Urine output
- ☐ Pain

▶ Which of the following potential complications is the client at risk of experiencing? **Select all that apply.**

- ☐ Anxiety
- ☐ Infection
- ☐ Reduced perfusion to kidneys
- ☐ Heart failure
- ☐ Fat embolism
- ☐ Depression
- ☐ Nerve damage
- ☐ Compartment syndrome

▶ Complete the following sentence by choosing from the list of options.

The nurse should **first** address the client's ______________.

WORD OPTIONS
Neurological status
Complaints of pain
Nausea
Limited mobility
Respiratory status

▶ For each potential nursing intervention listed, identify whether the intervention is **indicated** or **not indicated** for the care of this client.

POTENTIAL NURSING INTERVENTIONS	INDICATED	NOT INDICATED
Prepare to administer acetaminophen	○	○
Place the affected bone in proper alignment	○	○
Apply ice packs to the affected site of injury	○	○
Maintain splinting of the affected fracture site	○	○
Offer a warm blanket	○	○
Prepare to administer opioid analgesic	○	○
Mark location of pulses to facilitate repeat assessments	○	○

Note: Each row must have one response option selected.

The nurse is caring for a 25-year-old client on the orthopedic unit after surgical intervention.

Progress Notes

1250h: Client transferred to the operating room to be treated with an open reduction of the ankle, followed by traction as part of the treatment regimen.
1518h: Client returned from the postoperative recovery room to the unit after an open reduction and internal fixation of left ankle. Left tibia placed in a soft cast wrapped with gauze. Vital signs: T: 38.2°C (100.8°F); BP: 101/58; P: 87; RR: 16; with pulse oximetry of 92% on 3 L/min of continuous oxygen therapy per nasal prongs. Client presents as easily rousable and offered minimal assistance when transferring from the stretcher to the bed. Client noted to be moving all four extremities independently and required minimal assistance × 1 person when transferring left leg and soft cast. Pupils equal in size at 2 mm and reactive sluggishly to light. Client denies a headache or dizziness with transporting. Client's primary complaint is 8 out of 10 pain on a numerical pain scale in the left ankle, with numbness in the left toes. Left leg and foot remain cooler to touch compared to the right leg and foot. Left toes noted to be warm with capillary refill less than 3 seconds. Left dorsalis pedis pulse required Doppler to auscultate the presence of a pulse. Lungs auscultated for fine inspiratory crackles that do not clear with cough. Client noted to have short, shallow breaths upon return from the operating room. Client placed in semi-Fowler's position. Absent bowel sounds × 4 quadrants. Client reports feeling nauseated. Foley catheter in situ draining clear amber urine. Catheter bag emptied of 750 mL of clear dilute yellow urine.

The nurse has reviewed the Progress Notes at 1250h and 1518h.

The nurse has reviewed the Orders from 1520h.

▶ Highlight the orders the nurse should consider a priority.

Orders

1520h:
- Cefazolin 2.25 g PO q8h
- Administer tetanus toxoid intramuscularly × 1 dose
- 0.9% sodium chloride 100 mL/hr until able to tolerate fluids, then discontinue
- Elevate affected extremity
- Initiate full regular diet immediately
- Consult a dietitian to ensure adequate calcium and protein intake
- Ambulate when ready
- Hydromorphone 2 mg PO q6h prn

The nurse performed the interventions as ordered by the health care provider.

▶ For each assessment finding, identify if the finding indicates that the client's condition has **improved**, has **not changed**, or has **declined**.

ASSESSMENT FINDINGS	IMPROVED	NO CHANGE	DECLINED
T 37.3°C	○	○	○
Pain 10 out 10 on a numerical pain scale	○	○	○
Pulse oximetry 95% on room air	○	○	○
Respiratory 16 breaths per minute	○	○	○
Bowel sounds × 2 quadrants	○	○	○
Complaints of numbness and tingling	○	○	○

Note: Each row must have one response option selected.

Medical-Surgical 21.0

The nurse is caring for a 37-year-old male client on a respiratory unit.

Progress Notes

1100h: Client was seen in the emergency department complaining of shortness of breath even while at rest and increased frequency of ear, nose, throat, and chest infections over the past year. The client was diagnosed with cystic fibrosis at birth. Vital signs: T: 38.2°C (100.8°F); BP: 124/68; P: 114; RR: 20; with pulse oximetry of 92% on room air. Client presents as pleasant, cooperative, alert and oriented to person, place, and time. Gait steady. Shortness of breath has increased over the past 2 days. Pupils are equal in size, measured at 2 mm, and briskly reactive to light. Client denies pain but states that chest feels heavy. S1 and S2 heart sounds; apical heart rate is regular and equals radial pulse. Bilateral radial pulses and bilateral dorsalis pedis pulses are strong × 4. Capillary refill less than 3 seconds. Reduced air entry is noted in right lower lung posteriorly, but clear air entry noted throughout the left lung field. Inspiratory crackles are noted throughout bilateral lung fields. Client complains of dizziness after repeated coughing. If ambulating or driving, client will pull over to finish coughing. Sputum is noted to be purulent, thick, and greenish, with increasing need to cough. At times, sputum was blood-tinged. Client is voiding clear, amber urine. Bowel sounds auscultated × 4 quadrants with abdomen soft and round during palpation. Client denies any nausea or emesis or loss of appetite. Last bowel movement × 2 days ago.

▶ Select the top 3 client findings that would require **immediate** follow-up.

- ☐ Alertness
- ☐ Pupillary response
- ☐ Vertigo
- ☐ Hemoptysis
- ☐ Vital signs
- ☐ Characteristics of the cough

▶ For each client finding, identify whether the finding is consistent with the disease process of pneumonia, atelectasis, or cor pulmonale. Each finding may support more than one disease process.

CLIENT FINDINGS	PNEUMONIA	ATELECTASIS	COR PULMONALE
Crackles with lung auscultation	○	○	○
Weight loss	○	○	○
Pain with inspiration	○	○	○
Febrile	○	○	○
Shortness of breath	○	○	○
Jugular venous distension	○	○	○

Note: Each column must have at least one response option selected.

▶ Complete the following sentence by choosing from the list of word options.

The client is at **highest** risk of developing ______________ (word options 1) as evidenced by ________________ (word options 2).

WORD OPTIONS 1	WORD OPTIONS 2
Failure to thrive	Gastrointestinal assessment
Sepsis	Respiratory assessment
Bowel obstruction	Cardiovascular assessment
Diabetic ketoacidosis	Neurological assessment
Renal failure	Renal assessment

The nurse is caring for a 37-year-old male client on a respiratory unit.

Progress Notes

1100h: Client was seen in the emergency department complaining of shortness of breath even while at rest and increased frequency of ear, nose, throat, and chest infections over the past year. The client was diagnosed with cystic fibrosis at birth. Vital signs: T: 38.2°C (100.8°F); BP: 124/68; P: 114; RR: 20; with pulse oximetry of 92% on room air. Client presents as pleasant, cooperative, alert and oriented to person, place, and time. Gait steady. Shortness of breath has increased over the past 2 days. Pupils are equal in size, measured at 2 mm, and briskly reactive to light. Client denies pain but states that chest feels heavy. S1 and S2 heart sounds; apical heart rate is regular and equals radial pulse. Bilateral radial pulses and bilateral dorsalis pedis pulses are strong × 4. Capillary refill less than 3 seconds. Reduced air entry is noted in right lower lung posteriorly, but clear air entry noted throughout the left lung field. Inspiratory crackles are noted throughout bilateral lung fields. Client complains of dizziness after repeated coughing. If ambulating or driving, client will pull over to finish coughing. Sputum is noted to be purulent, thick, and greenish, with increasing need to cough. At times, sputum was blood-tinged. Client is voiding clear, amber urine. Bowel sounds auscultated × 4 quadrants with abdomen soft and round during palpation. Client denies any nausea or emesis, or loss of appetite. Last bowel movement × 2 days ago.

1622h: Client was found difficult to rouse. Required sternal rub. Client has ++ pallor with pale conjunctiva and palms. Colour grey, skin cool to touch. Vital signs: T: 38.8°C (101.8°F); BP: 85/53; P: 134; RR: 28; with pulse oximetry of 83% on room air. Capillary refill greater than 3 seconds. Health care provider notified.

The nurse has reviewed the Progress Note entries from 1100h and 1622h.

▶ For each potential nursing intervention, identify whether the intervention is **indicated** or **not indicated** for the care of this client.

POTENTIAL NURSING INTERVENTIONS	INDICATED	NOT INDICATED
Plan to perform percussion, vibration, and postural drainage	○	○
Encourage oral fluids	○	○
Place client in reverse Trendelenburg position	○	○
Ambulate client with physiotherapy	○	○
Prepare client for a chest X-ray	○	○
Place client on isolation	○	○

Note: Each row must have one response option selected.

The nurse has received orders from the physician.

▶ Select the actions the nurse should take **first**. **Select all that apply**.

- ☐ Initiate 0.9% sodium chloride (normal saline) 500 mL bolus × 1 then 125 mL/hr
- ☐ Oxygen 0–5 L per nasal prongs to maintain pulse oximetry greater than or equal to 92%
- ☐ Insert an in-dwelling urinary catheter
- ☐ Initiate a regular diet
- ☐ Laboratory tests: ABG, blood cultures
- ☐ Initiate metoprolol 25 mg PO twice a day

The nurse performed the interventions as ordered by the health care provider.

▶ For each assessment finding, identify whether the finding indicates that the client's condition has **improved**, has **not changed**, or has **declined**.

ASSESSMENT FINDINGS	IMPROVED	NOT CHANGED	DECLINED
Posterior lung sounds become clear with auscultation	○	○	○
Expectorating green-tinged sputum only	○	○	○
Absent bowel sounds	○	○	○
Pulse oximetry levels 96% on 3 L/min of oxygen therapy	○	○	○
Respiratory rate 22	○	○	○
Chest X-ray shows atelectasis to right lower lung	○	○	○
Voiding clear, amber urine	○	○	○

Medical-Surgical 22.0

The nurse is caring for a 45-year-old client on a cardiovascular unit.

Progress Notes

1044h: Client presented to the hospital with complaints of fatigue, increased shortness of breath × 1 day with the feeling of a "racing heart." Transferred to the cardiovascular unit. Vital signs: T: 36.9°C (98.4°C); BP: 132/72; P: 155; RR: 22; with pulse oximetry of 95% on room air. Client rouses easily to voice and stimulation, alert and oriented to person, place, time, and situation. Able to follow commands and move all extremities independently, with motor power strong × 4. Denies any pain at present. Client expresses ++ stress at work and not sleeping well × 3 days. Difficult to auscultate S1 and S2 due to rapid, irregular heartbeat. Unable to capture if apical is equal to radial pulse. Bilateral radial pulses strong but irregular to touch. Bilateral dorsalis pedis pulses weak but palpable. Skin warm and dry to touch, no diaphoresis noted. Client denies any chest pain but feels like heart is beating "out of their chest." Jugular venous distension measured at 4 cm. Lungs auscultated for clear air entry throughout. No adventitious breath sounds noted. Client presents with shortness of breath, even at rest, that worsens with minimal exertion. Complains of difficulty catching breath at times and recovery is taking longer over the course of 1 day. Abdomen noted to be round and firm to touch. Active bowel sounds auscultated × 4 quadrants. Client states absence of a bowel movement for 2 days, which is unusual for their routine. Client voids clear amber urine in the toilet independently. Denies any pain, urgency, or burning when voiding. The client's comorbidities include only prediabetes controlled by diet and exercise.

▶ Select 3 of the client findings that require immediate attention.

- ☐ Motor power
- ☐ Stress
- ☐ Jugular venous distension
- ☐ Radial pulse characteristic
- ☐ Shortness of breath
- ☐ Bowel sounds
- ☐ Urine quality

▶ For each client finding listed below, identify whether the finding is consistent with the disease process of right-sided heart failure, atrial fibrillation, or pericarditis. Each finding may support more than one disease process.

CLIENT FINDINGS	RIGHT-SIDED HEART FAILURE	ATRIAL FIBRILLATION	PERICARDITIS
Irregular pulse	○	○	○
Jugular venous distension	○	○	○
"Racing heart"	○	○	○
Shortness of breath	○	○	○
Fatigue	○	○	○

Note: Each column must have at least one response option selected.

▶ Complete the following sentence by choosing from the list of options.

The client is at **highest** risk of developing _____________.

WORD OPTIONS
Sinus bradycardia
Ventricular tachycardia
Atrial fibrillation
Sinus tachycardia
Heart block

The nurse is caring for a 45-year-old client on a cardiovascular unit.

Progress Notes

1200h: An ECG is taken and it confirms arrhythmia. The client is scheduled for a cardioversion. A transesophageal echocardiogram will be completed prior to the cardioversion to rule out any blood clots.

The nurse has reviewed the Progress Notes at 1044h and 1200h.

▶ For each potential nursing intervention, identify whether the intervention is **indicated** or **not indicated** for the care of this client.

POTENTIAL NURSING INTERVENTIONS	INDICATED	NOT INDICATED
Prepare the consent form for the health care provider	○	○
Allow the health care provider to answer all the questions	○	○
Ensure suction is connected and working	○	○
Collect oral pharyngeal airway and bag-valve mask device	○	○
Allow the client to eat a regular diet	○	○
Review policy and procedure	○	○

Note: Each row must have one response option selected.

▶ Which of the following health care orders should the nurse anticipate? **Select all that apply**.

☐ Insert a peripheral venous access device
☐ 0.9% normal saline (sodium chloride) IV to keep vein open
☐ Ensure medications are available for conscious sedation (propofol and midazolam)
☐ Monitor input and output
☐ Complete a chest X-ray post-procedure

The nurse is caring for a 45-year-old client on a cardiovascular unit.

Progress Notes

1205h: Client to remain NPO until procedure.
1640h: Consent was obtained. The client's transesophageal echocardiogram revealed no clots. The cardioversion was successful, returning the client to normal sinus rhythm. Post-procedure vital signs: T: 36.9°C (98.4°F); BP: 105/70; P: 74; RR: 14; with pulse oximetry of 92% on 2 L/min of oxygen per nasal prongs.

The nurse has reviewed the Progress Notes from 1205h and 1640h.

▶ For each assessment finding, identify whether the finding indicates that the client's condition has **improved**, has **not changed**, or has **declined**.

ASSESSMENT FINDINGS	IMPROVED	NO CHANGE	DECLINED
Temperature	○	○	○
Respiratory rate	○	○	○
Heart rate	○	○	○
Rhythm	○	○	○
Pulse oximetry	○	○	○

Note: Each row must have one response option selected.

Medical-Surgical 23.0

The nurse is caring for a 67-year-old client on a general medical unit.

Progress Notes

1100h: Client was admitted to the unit after being taken to the emergency department via emergency medical services (EMS). The client was shopping at the grocery store, became dizzy in the aisle, and collapsed onto the floor. Bystanders rushed to their aid and placed the client in the recovery position until EMS arrived. Client was stable in the emergency department and transferred to the general medical unit. Vital signs: T: 36.9°C (98.4°F); BP: 100/68; P: 67; RR: 16; with pulse oximetry of 94% on room air. Client presents as pleasant, cooperative, alert, and oriented to person, place, and time. Pupils equal in size, measured at 3 mm, and briskly reactive to light. Client denies hitting head on the linoleum in the store. No bruising noted on the client's head. Motor power strong × 4, moves all extremities independently. S1 and S2 heart sounds, apical heart rate regular and equals radial pulse. Bilateral radial pulses and bilateral dorsalis pedis pulses strong × 4. Capillary refill less than 3 seconds. Lungs auscultated for clear air entry throughout posteriorly. No cough noted. Denies chest pain or shortness of breath. Client noted to be small in stature and frail-looking. Quiet bowel sounds auscultated × 4 quadrants with abdomen soft and flat during palpation. Client states having nausea on occasion, with emesis. Reported diarrhea as last bowel movement × 4 days ago. Small amount of stool noted on the gown. Client does not appear to have adequate personal hygiene. Client's urine dark and concentrated with a strong odour. Skin ++dry and cracking with flakes of skin noted in the bed. Client has a Loonie-sized open coccyx wound noted to be crusted, no drainage noted, borders noted to be grey in colour. The client presents with dry lips and cracking where the top and bottom lips meet. No emergency contact provided. Client has no partner, no children. Lives independently at their home. Client is guarded about their social situation.

The nurse has reviewed the Progress Notes at 1100h.

▶ Which of the following findings require **immediate** follow-up? **Select all that apply.**

- ☐ Pupillary size
- ☐ Cognitive status
- ☐ Heart sounds
- ☐ Lung sounds
- ☐ Frail-looking
- ☐ Nausea with emesis
- ☐ Diarrhea × 4 days ago
- ☐ Hygiene
- ☐ Urine characteristics
- ☐ No social supports

▶ From the list below, identify the **most appropriate** word choice to fill in each blank in the following sentence.

The nurse should recognize that the client is potentially experiencing _______________ and _______________.

WORD OPTIONS
Malnutrition
Dysrhythmias
Dehydration
Hypoxemia
Renal failure

The nurse is caring for a 67-year-old client on a general medical unit.

Progress Notes | **Laboratory Results**

0916h: (Emergency Department)

Hemoglobin 140–180 g/L (14–18 g/dL) (male) 120–160 g/L (12–16 g/dL) (female)	80 g/L (8 g/dL)	Sodium 136–145 mmol/L	148 mmol/L
Platelets 150–400 × 10^9/L (150 000–400 000/mm^3)	145 × 10^9/L (145 000/mm^3)	Potassium 3.5–5.1 mmol/L	5.0 mmol/L
White blood cells 3.5–12.0 × 10^9/L (3 500–12 000/mm^3)	6.0 × 10^9/L (60 00/mm^3)	Creatinine 53–106 mcmol/L (male)	
44–97 mcmol/L (female)	110 mcmol/L		
Neutrophils 3.0–5.8 × 10^9/L (3 000–5 800/mm^3)	3.7 × 10^9/L (3 700/mm^3)	Blood urea nitrogen (BUN) 2.9–8.2 mmol/L	8.0 mmol/L
		Blood glucose 4–6 mmol/L	4.2 mmol/L

▶ Complete the following sentence by choosing from the list of options.

The client is at **highest** risk of developing _______________.

WORD OPTIONS
Polycythemia vera
Ventricular dysrhythmias
Seizures
Pneumonia
Weakness
Poor wound healing

▶ For each potential nursing intervention, identify whether the intervention is **indicated** or **not indicated** for the care of this client.

POTENTIAL NURSING INTERVENTIONS	INDICATED	NOT INDICATED
Determine frailty level through use of the Clinical Frailty Scale	○	○
Maintain NPO status	○	○
Request a consult for dietitian	○	○
Identify whether the client is experiencing food insecurity	○	○
Monitor for nausea	○	○
Request a consult for social work	○	○

Note: Each row must have one response option selected.

▶ Select 3 actions the nurse should take.

☐ Record the client's height and weight.
☐ Complete a food diary for the client.
☐ Avoid interrupting the client during meals.
☐ Encourage friends to bring food and to visit during mealtimes.
☐ Plan tasks during mealtimes.
☐ Reduce between-meal nutrition supplements.

▶ For each assessment finding, identify whether the finding indicates that the client's condition has **improved**, has **not changed**, or has **declined**.

ASSESSMENT FINDINGS	IMPROVED	NO CHANGE	DECLINED
Client gains 1.5 kg	○	○	○
Bowel movements become more solid	○	○	○
Client able to choose nutritionally dense food on a budget	○	○	○
Client develops a stage 2 wound on their left scapula	○	○	○
Dizziness persists with standing	○	○	○

Note: Each row must have one response option selected.

Medical-Surgical 24.0

The nurse is caring for a 68-year-old client on the general surgical unit.

Progress Notes

1124h: Client was a direct admission to the unit, accompanied by their partner for further gastrointestinal investigations. The client has had difficulty swallowing fluids and solids × months, but it has grown increasingly worse over the past 2 days. Vital signs: T: 37.6°C (99.7°F); BP: 102/58; P: 87; RR: 22; with pulse oximetry of 96% on room air. Client presents as pleasant and cooperative. Motor power strong × 4 extremities with client ambulating independently. Gait steady. Pupils equal in size and shape, measured at 3 mm, and respond briskly to light. Client denies pain. S1 and S2 heart sounds, apical heart rate regular and equals radial pulse. Bilateral radial pulses palpable, bilateral dorsalis pedis pulses palpable and strong. No edema noted. Capillary refill less than 3 seconds. Bilateral fine inspiratory crackles noted in right and left base lung fields when auscultated posteriorly. Client has a weak cough reflex; coughs when takes in too much fluid at one time. Respirations regular but tachypneic. No indrawing, nasal flaring, or use of accessory muscles noted. Abdomen flat with hyperactive bowel sounds auscultated in all four quadrants. BMI 17.1. Client states nausea on occasion with emesis if able to tolerate food and fluids. Takes sips to avoid emesis. Client states no pain with urination, no frequency or urgency. Urine concentrated when able to void.

The nurse has reviewed the Progress Notes from 1124h.

▶ Highlight the findings below that would require **immediate** follow-up.

Progress Notes

1124h: Client was a direct admission to the unit, accompanied by their partner for further gastrointestinal investigations. The client has had difficulty swallowing fluids and solids × months, but it has grown increasingly worse over the past 2 days. Vital signs: T: 37.6°C (99.7°F); BP: 102/58; P: 87; RR: 22; with pulse oximetry of 96% on room air. Client presents as pleasant and cooperative. Motor power strong × 4 extremities with client ambulating independently. Gait steady. Pupils equal in size and shape, measured at 3 mm, and respond briskly to light. Client denies pain. S1 and S2 heart sounds, apical heart rate regular and equals radial pulse. Bilateral radial pulses palpable, bilateral dorsalis pedis pulses palpable and strong. No edema noted. Capillary refill less than 3 seconds. Bilateral fine inspiratory crackles noted in right and left base lung fields when auscultated posteriorly. Client has a weak cough reflex; coughs when takes in too much fluid at one time. Respirations regular but tachypneic. No indrawing, nasal flaring, or use of accessory muscles noted. Abdomen flat with hyperactive bowel sounds auscultated in all four quadrants. BMI 17.1. Client states nausea on occasion with emesis if able to tolerate food and fluids. Takes sips to avoid emesis. Client states no pain with urination, no frequency or urgency. Urine concentrated when able to void.

▶ Which of the following complications is the client at risk of experiencing? **Select all that apply**.

- ☐ Stroke
- ☐ Dehydration
- ☐ Deep vein thrombosis
- ☐ Bowel obstruction
- ☐ Pneumonia
- ☐ Failure to thrive

▶ Complete the following sentence by choosing from the list of options.

The client is at **highest** risk of developing _____________.

WORD OPTIONS
Gastroesophageal reflux disease
Life-threatening dysrhythmias
Diabetic ketoacidosis
Aspiration pneumonia
Renal failure
Gastrointestinal bleed

▶ For each potential nursing intervention, identify whether the intervention is **indicated** or **not indicated** for the care of this client.

POTENTIAL NURSING INTERVENTIONS	INDICATED	NOT INDICATED
Keep client NPO (nothing by mouth)	○	○
Encourage client to position self in the chair or semi-Fowler's position	○	○
Plan to administer thickened fluids for hydration	○	○
Prepare the client for a barium swallow	○	○
Consult speech-language pathologist	○	○
Ensure mouth swabs are close to the client	○	○
Request an order to insert a peripheral venous access device	○	○

Note: Each row must have one response option selected.

The nurse is caring for a 68-year-old client on the general surgical unit.

Progress Notes	Orders

1357h: Dietitian consulted for client's nutritional status.
1645h: New orders from the health care provider.

Progress Notes	**Orders**

1645h:

- Obtain chest X-ray
- Insert nasogastric tube and initiate tube feeds as per policy
- Obtain a swallowing assessment
- Consult physiotherapy
- Initiate 0.9% normal saline (sodium chloride) at 75 mL/hr
- Heparin subcutaneous as per weight

The nurse has reviewed the Progress Notes at 1357h and the new Orders at 1645h.

▶ Select 2 orders the nurse should perform **immediately**.

☐ Obtain chest X-ray
☐ Insert nasogastric tube and initiate tube feeds as per policy
☐ Obtain a swallowing assessment
☐ Consult physiotherapy
☐ Initiate 0.9% normal saline (sodium chloride) at 75 mL/hr
☐ Heparin subcutaneous as per weight

▶ For each of the statements by the client, identify whether the statement indicates an **understanding** or **no understanding** of the client teaching plan.

CLIENT STATEMENTS	UNDER-STANDING	NO UNDER-STANDING
"I can still take sips of water."	○	○
"I need to perform good mouth care as needed."	○	○
"If the tube falls out, let someone know."	○	○
"I am going to have the tube forever."	○	○
"If I get the tube caught on something, let someone know."	○	○
"I need to check the opening of my nose on both sides for irritation."	○	○

Note: Each row must have one response option selected.

Medical-Surgical 25.0

The nurse is caring for a 28-year-old client in the emergency department.

Progress Notes

1805h: Client was seen in the emergency department complaining of new-onset hemoptysis along with feeling lightheaded and unstable on their feet. Client has been experiencing increased stress at work and was recently diagnosed with headaches, treated with ibuprofen, and peptic ulcer disease, treated with pantoprazole. Vital signs: T: 37.3°C (99.1°F); BP: 106/54; P: 99; RR: 18; with pulse oximetry of 96% on room air. Client presents as pleasant, cooperative, alert and oriented to person, place, and time. Client requires one-person stand-by assist when transferring. Pupils equal in size at 2 mm and briskly reactive to light. Client complains of a headache rated 3 out of 10 on a numerical pain scale. S1 and S2 heart sounds, apical heart rate regular and equals radial pulse. Bilateral radial pulses strong with bilateral dorsalis pedis pulses weak but palpable. Clear air entry noted throughout all lung fields anterior and posterior. Cough noted with blood-tinged expectorant. Hyperactive bowel sounds auscultated × 4 quadrants with abdomen firm and round during palpation. Client noted to have guarding with palpation. Client states feeling nauseated × 1 day with no emesis. Client did not eat any food today due to nausea and did not take pantoprazole. Client states reduced fluid intake due to nausea. Urine noted to be dark and concentrated when client is able to void. Client denies any pain with urination, no frequency or urgency. Peripheral venous access device inserted left antecubital fossa.

▶ Select 4 client findings that require **immediate** follow-up.

- ☐ Pupillary response
- ☐ Blood pressure
- ☐ Cognitive orientation
- ☐ Dorsalis pedis pulses
- ☐ Lung sounds
- ☐ Hemoptysis
- ☐ Bowel sounds
- ☐ Abdomen firm and round
- ☐ Nausea
- ☐ Urine characteristics

▶ For each client finding listed below, identify whether the finding is consistent with the disease process of bowel obstruction, pulmonary embolus, or upper gastrointestinal bleed. Each finding may support more than one disease process.

CLIENT FINDINGS	BOWEL OBSTRUCTION	PULMONARY EMBOLUS	UPPER GASTROINTESTINAL BLEED
Nausea	○	○	○
Hemoptysis	○	○	○
Abdomen firm and round	○	○	○
Loss of appetite	○	○	○

Note: Each column must have at least one response option selected.

▶ Which of the following potential conditions is the client at risk of developing? **Select all that apply.**

- ☐ Gastroesophageal reflux disease
- ☐ Acute renal failure
- ☐ Pneumonia
- ☐ Pulmonary edema
- ☐ Acute myocardial infarction
- ☐ Hemorrhage

The nurse is caring for a 28-year-old client in the emergency department.

Progress Notes | Laboratory Results

2155h: Client rang for assistance complaining of vomit all over the bed. Upon arrival, client was found to have projectile-vomited coffee-ground emesis; client presents grey in colour, reduced perfusion to conjunctiva, pale palms noted. Client presents as lethargic but is able to answer questions and follow commands. Vital signs: T: 37.9°C (100.2°F); BP: 88/52; P: 137; RR: 28; with pulse oximetry of 92% on room air.

The nurse has reviewed the Progress Notes from 2155h and the Laboratory Results from 1900h.

▶ For each potential order, identify whether the intervention is **indicated** or **not indicated** for the care of this client.

Progress Notes	Laboratory Results		
1900h: (Emergency Department)			
Hemoglobin 140–180 g/L (14–18 g/dL) (male) 120–160 g/L (12–16 g/dL) (female)	70 g/L (7 g/dL)	Sodium 136–145 mmol/L	140 mmol/L
Platelets 150–400 × 10^9/L (150 000–400 000/mm³)	150 × 10^9/L (150 000/mm³)	Potassium 3.5–5.1 mmol/L	4.2 mmol/L
White blood cells 3.5–12.0 × 10^9/L (3 500–120 000/mm³)	8.0 × 10^9/L (8 000/mm³)	Creatinine 53–106 mcmol/L (male)	
44–97 mcmol/L (female)	76 mcmol/L		
Neutrophils 3.0–5.8 × 10^9/L (3 000–5 800/mm³)	4.2 × 10^9/L (4 200/mm³)	Blood urea nitrogen (BUN) 2.9–8.2 mmol/L	3.5 mmol/L

POTENTIAL NURSING INTERVENTIONS	INDICATED	NOT INDICATED
Insert another large-bore venous access device	○	○
Packed red blood cells	○	○
Clear fluids diet and advance to regular diet	○	○
Insert a nasogastric tube and attach to low suction	○	○
Chest X-ray	○	○
Insert an in-dwelling Foley catheter	○	○
Initiate Ringer's lactate	○	○

Note: Each row must have one response option selected.

▶ Complete the following sentences by choosing from the list of options.

The nurse should insert a(n)_______________ (word options 1) **first**.

It would be a priority for the nurse to request a prescription for _______________ (word options 2).

WORD OPTIONS 1	WORD OPTIONS 2
Peripheral venous access device	Antiemetic
Nasogastric tube	Proton pump inhibitor
In-dwelling Foley catheter	Antipyretic

The nurse has performed the interventions as ordered by the health care provider for the client.

▶ For each assessment finding, identify whether the finding indicates that the client's condition has **improved**, has **not changed**, or has **declined**.

ASSESSMENT FINDINGS	IMRPOVED	NO CHANGE	DECLINED
BP 110/65	○	○	○
Frank red blood with emesis	○	○	○
Clear amber urine	○	○	○
Dizziness	○	○	○
Alert and communicative	○	○	○

Note: Each row must have one response option selected.

Medical-Surgical 26.0

The nurse is caring for a 28-year-old client on the neurology unit.

Nurses' Notes

1745h: Client was admitted to the unit from the emergency department with unexplained weakness, numbness and tingling in their lower extremities, and severe dehydration 2 days ago. A venous access device system was inserted in the emergency department for rehydration and subsequently saline locked at present. The client's past medical history consists of drug misuse with heroin, although the client states they have been sober and attending Narcotics Anonymous for 2 months; current smoker 1/2 pack per day; and previous admissions for endocarditis. Vital signs: T: 37.1°C (98.8°F); BP: 122/68; P: 76; RR: 18; with pulse oximetry of 98% on room air. Client presents as pleasant, cooperative, alert and oriented to person, place, time, and situation. Gait steadiness has improved since admission. Client denies any dizziness or a headache. Numbness and tingling persists, noticed with toes and fingertips. Client denies any pain, states feeling like "pins and needles." Bilateral pupils equal in shape, measured at 3 mm, and briskly react to light. S1 and S2 heart sounds, apical heart rate regular and equals radial pulse. No peripheral edema noted. Bilateral radial pulses regular and palpable, bilateral dorsalis pedis pulses present and palpable. Skin warm and dry to touch. No diaphoresis noted. Upon auscultation, reduced air entry noted right lower lobe but clear air entry noted throughout left lobe. Abdomen flat, no pain with palpation, bowel sounds auscultated × 4 quadrants. Client denies nausea or emesis. Client states able to void independently in the washroom, denies any pain or urgency with urination.

2055h: Client noted to be off unit, observed to be accompanied by friend, who was pushing the client in a wheelchair. Client indicated they were going for a "smoke break."

2203h: Upon evening rounds, client noted to have returned from being off the unit, sitting alone in their room. Client presents with disorganized speech, slurring words, gait unsteady requiring two-person assist to transfer from wheelchair to the bed. Pupils pinpoint and sluggish to react to light. Skin warm to touch, face flushed, with diaphoresis noted. Client unable to remember why they are in the hospital. Presents as confused. Only oriented to name. Client somnolent, lethargic, and drifts off to sleep easily, requiring physical stimulation to respond. Vital signs: T: 36.9°C (98.4°F); BP: 96/56; P: 58; RR: 14; with pulse oximetry of 92% on room air. Bilateral radial pulses palpable, regular, but slower in rate. No change in auscultation in lung sounds, gastrointestinal assessment. Difficult to assess renal system. Health care provider notified of change in client status.

The nurse has reviewed the Nurses' Notes from 1745h, 2055h, and 2203h.

▶ Select 4 client findings that require **immediate** follow-up.

- ☐ Pupillary response
- ☐ Speech
- ☐ Client orientation
- ☐ Vital signs
- ☐ Lethargy
- ☐ Radial pulses
- ☐ Lung sounds

▶ For each client finding, identify if the finding is consistent with the condition of stroke, traumatic brain injury, or medication ingestion. Each finding may support more than one disease process.

CLIENT FINDINGS	STROKE	TRAUMATIC BRAIN INJURY	MEDICATION INGESTION (OPIOID)
Hypotension	○	○	○
Pinpoint pupils	○	○	○
Altered level of consciousness	○	○	○
Moves extremities independently	○	○	○
Somnolence	○	○	○
Flushed face	○	○	○

Note: Each column must have at least one response option selected.

The nurse is caring for a 28-year-old client on the neurology unit.

Nurses' Notes

2230h: Health care provider reviewed client status. No new orders received.
2315h: Client noted to have shallow respirations mixed with cluster breathing. No response to verbal stimuli. Client moans with initial sternal rub. Neurological assessment completed. Client only opens eyes to painful stimuli, noted to withdraw extremity with painful stimulation, no speech noted. No posturing noted. Glasgow Coma Scale documented at 7. Skin cool and clammy to touch. Vital signs: T: 36.9°C (98.4°F); BP: 85/52; P: 52; RR: 12; with pulse oximetry of 76% on room air.

The nurse has reviewed the Nurses' Notes from 2230h and 2315h.

▶ Complete the following sentence by choosing from the list of options.

The client is at **highest** risk of developing ____________.

WORD OPTIONS
Endocarditis
Ventricular tachycardia
Respiratory distress
Subdural hematoma
Renal failure

▶ For each potential nursing intervention, identify whether the intervention is **indicated** or **not indicated** for the care of this client.

POTENTIAL NURSING INTERVENTIONS	INDICATED	NOT INDICATED
Position the client in the recovery position supported by pillows	○	○
Prepare to call a code blue	○	○
Insert an in-dwelling Foley catheter	○	○
Request an order to initiate oxygen therapy	○	○
Ensure suction is working in the room with a Yankauer suction tip	○	○
Encourage oral fluid intake	○	○
Prepare to administer naloxone	○	○

Note: Each row must have one response option selected.

▶ Highlight the orders the nurse should consider a **priority**.

- Oxygen 1–10 L/min nasal prongs or non-rebreather mask for pulse oximetry greater than 92%
- Insert a second peripheral venous access device
- Naloxone 0.4 mg IM and may be repeated q4min to a maximum of 10 mg
- 0.9% sodium chloride (normal saline) 500 mL IV bolus × 1, reconfirm for a second dose
- Chest X-ray
- Laboratory tests: toxicity screen, electrolytes, creatinine, BUN, arterial blood gas (ABG)
- Methadone 20 mg PO liquid solution
- Monitor input and output
- Regular diet
- Consult social work
- Consult addiction counsellor

▶ For each assessment finding, identify if the finding indicates that the client's condition has **improved**, has **not changed**, or has **declined**.

ASSESSMENT FINDINGS	IMPROVED	NO CHANGE	DECLINED
Client awake and sitting upright	○	○	○
Coarse crackles auscultated throughout bilateral anterior base lung fields	○	○	○
Client on 4 L/min of continuous oxygen per nasal prongs for pulse oximetry of 97%	○	○	○
Respiratory rate 18	○	○	○
T 36.9°C (98.4°F)	○	○	○

Note: Each row must have one response option selected.

Medical-Surgical 27.0

The nurse is caring for a 55-year-old client on the respiratory unit.

Nurses' Notes

1140h: Client presented to the emergency department with chills, lethargy, general malaise, productive cough × 3 days and pain when taking deep breaths. The client denies falling and states they attended their granddaughter's school concert 5 days ago. Transferred to the respiratory unit. Vital signs: T: 38.7°C (101.7°F); BP: 103/68; P: 86; RR: 22; with pulse oximetry of 94% on room air. Client presents to the unit alert and oriented to person, place, time, and situation. Bilateral pupils regular in shape and measured at 2 mm with positive and brisk reaction to light. Motor power strong × 4 with independent movement. Client presents with dizziness when ambulating long distances. Complains of tingling in lips, which is new since coming to the hospital. S1 and S2 heart sounds, apical heart rate regular and equals radial pulse. Bilateral radial pulses palpable and strong. Bilateral dorsalis pedis pulses weak to touch but remain palpable. Skin cool to touch. Client presents with mild shortness of breath, lungs auscultated for coarse inspiratory crackles noted to right lower lobe anteriorly with clear air entry to left lobe. Client denies a sore throat. Abdomen rounded, soft, with active bowel sounds noted × 4 quadrants. Client states they do not feel hungry as it takes energy to stand for long periods. Client complains of a "lump in their throat" and difficulty swallowing water. Client denies any pain when voiding, denies frequency or urgency but reports dark, concentrated urine. Client settled in the room. Allergy wristband applied to left wrist indicating an allergy to penicillin.

1153h: Shift nurse notified unit that they administered an oral dose of amoxicillin to the client in error as it was meant for another client in the next bed to the right while in emergency.

The nurse has reviewed the Nurses' Notes at 1140h, 1153, and 1200h.

▶ For each body system below, identify the findings that require **immediate** follow-up. Each body system may support more than one priority finding.

BODY SYSTEM	PRIORITY FINDINGS
Neurological	○ Client orientation ○ Dizziness ○ Motor power ○ Tingling
Cardiovascular	○ Radial pulse characteristics ○ Heart rate ○ Heart sounds ○ Client perfusion
Respiratory	○ Characteristics of the lung sounds ○ Pulse oximetry ○ Breathing patterns ○ Tripod position
Gastrointestinal	○ Bowel sounds ○ Anorexia ○ Characteristics of swallowing

Note: Each category must have at least one response option chosen.

▶ Which of the following complications is the client at risk of experiencing? **Select all that apply.**

- ☐ Injury from falling
- ☐ Cerebral edema
- ☐ Shunting
- ☐ Hypoxemia
- ☐ Weight loss
- ☐ Mitral valve stenosis
- ☐ Coronary artery constriction

Nurses' Notes

1200h: Client found sitting at the edge of the bed in tripod position over the bedside table. The client presents with indrawing at the clavicle, nasal flaring, and short, shallow breaths. Upon auscultation, an audible wheeze auscultated throughout all lung fields. Client's colour pale with mild cyanosis noted around the lips. Client is able to nod or shake head in response to questions. Remains alert and oriented. Moves all extremities independently. Denies any pain. Bilateral radial pulses regular and tachycardic. Vital signs: T: 38.9°C (102.0°F); BP: 86/52; P:130; RR: 28; with pulse oximetry of 82% on room air.
1204h: Health care provider notified of client's change in status.

▶ Complete the following sentence by choosing from the list of options.

The client is at **highest** risk of developing __________ (word options 1) and ________________ (word options 1) as evidenced by ____________ (word options 2).

WORD OPTIONS 1	WORD OPTIONS 2
Anaphylaxis	Vital signs
Dysrhythmias	Respiratory assessment
Respiratory distress	Cardiovascular assessment
Stroke	Neurological assessment
Renal failure	Renal assessment

▶ For each potential nursing intervention, identify whether the intervention is **indicated** or **not indicated** for the care of this client.

POTENTIAL NURSING INTERVENTIONS	INDICATED	NOT INDICATED
Request an order to administer a bronchodilator	○	○
Prepare an emergency kit with epinephrine	○	○
Encourage oral fluids	○	○
Reposition client in high-Fowler's position	○	○
Request an order to administer oxygen	○	○
Prepare to insert a peripheral venous access device	○	○

Note: Each row must have one response option selected.

The nurse is caring for a 55-year-old client on the respiratory unit.

Nurses' Notes | **Orders**

1208h:
- Initiate oxygen 1–10 L/min via nasal prongs or non-rebreather mask for pulse oximetry greater than 92%
- 0.9% normal saline (sodium chloride) 500 mL IV bolus × 1 then 100 mL/hr
- Insert an in-dwelling Foley catheter
- Laboratory draws: complete blood count, electrolytes, arterial blood gas (ABG), blood cultures
- Computed tomography (CT) chest
- Salbutamol sulphate 2.5 mg nebulizer q4h prn. Monitor heart rate
- Dimenhydrinate 25–50 mg PO/IV q4–6h prn

The nurse has reviewed the Orders at 1208h.

▶ Which of the following orders require the nurse to clarify with the health care provider prior to taking action? **Select all that apply.**

- ☐ Initiate oxygen 1–10 L/min via nasal prongs or non-rebreather mask for pulse oximetry greater than 92%
- ☐ 0.9% normal saline (sodium chloride) 500 mL IV bolus × 1 then 100 mL/hr
- ☐ Insert an in-dwelling Foley catheter
- ☐ Laboratory draws: complete blood count, electrolytes, arterial blood gas (ABG), blood cultures
- ☐ Computed tomography (CT) chest
- ☐ Salbutamol sulphate 2.5 mg nebulizer q4h prn. Monitor heart rate
- ☐ Dimenhydrinate 25–50 mg PO/IV q4–6h prn

▶ For each assessment finding, identify if the finding indicates that the client's condition has **improved**, **not changed**, or **worsened**.

CLIENT FINDINGS	IMPROVED	NOT CHANGED	WORSENED
Respirations 18	○	○	○
T 38.9°C (102.0°F)	○	○	○
Respiration rate to be regular	○	○	○
Colour, pink, well perfused to mucous membranes and palms of hands	○	○	○
No stridor noted	○	○	○
Oxygen therapy 4 L/min	○	○	○

Note: Each row must have one response option selected.

Medical-Surgical 28.0

The nurse is caring for a 57-year-old client on a neurological unit.

Nurses' Notes

0745h: Client presented to the emergency room with complaints of left-sided paralysis, short- term memory loss, and fatigue. Client, who is a police officer, was walking home after a shift and collapsed on the pavement. Client denies hitting head, just lost their balance and fell. They laid on the ground for approximately 5 minutes and walked home without further issue. The client suffered throughout the night with a 9 out of 10 headache based on the numerical rating scale and reported blurry vision this morning. Client reports no previous comorbidities and must maintain physical health due to position. Client transferred to neurology unit for further testing. Vital signs: T: 37.2°C (99.0°F); BP: 143/66; P: 82; RR: 18; pulse oximetry of 97% on room air. Client presents as pleasant, cooperative, alert and oriented to person, place, and time. Partner reported verbal frustration trying to put shoes on prior to coming to the hospital. Motor power strong × right side upper and lower and weak × left upper and lower extremities. Client denies any numbness or tingling. No facial droop noted. Client able to follow all commands with ease. Gait slow but steady. Client noted to take careful steps. Pupils equal in size and shape and reactive to light at 2 mm. Client denies any pain at present but able to feel residual headache from the time of admission labelled at 2 out 10. S1 and S2 heart sounds noted, apical heart rate irregular and equals radial pulse with palpation. Bilateral radial pulses irregular but palpable. Client states that is new but able to feel heart rate in their ears at times off and on × 2 weeks. Bilateral dorsalis pedis pulses noted to be palpable by touch. Skin warm and dry to touch. Capillary refill documented to be less than 3 seconds. Lung sounds clear with auscultation anteriorly and posteriorly. Client states they have experienced mild shortness of breath when walking long distances or up several flights of stairs. They felt they needed more exercise. Active bowel sounds auscultated × 4 quadrants. Client denies nausea or emesis. Appetite unchanged. Denies any pain or increased frequency with voiding.

▶ Which of the following assessment findings require **immediate** follow-up? **Select all that apply.**

- ☐ Pupillary response
- ☐ Shortness of breath
- ☐ Alertness
- ☐ Characteristics of pulses
- ☐ Lung sounds
- ☐ Headache
- ☐ Pulse oximetry
- ☐ Skin temperature
- ☐ Motor power
- ☐ Musculoskeletal weakness

▶ Identify the correct complication from the options below to fill in each blank in the following sentence.

The nurse should recognize that the client potentially experienced a(an) ____________________ prior to admission as a result of untreated ________________.

WORD OPTIONS
Atrial fibrillation
Encephalopathic event
Anginal episode
Headache
Transient ischemic attack (TIA)

▶ Complete the following sentence by choosing from the list of options.

The client is at **highest** risk of developing a(an)_________.

WORD OPTIONS
Subdural hematoma
Pneumonia
Aortic stenosis
Stroke
Heart failure
Acute myocardial infarction

The nurse is caring for a 57-year-old client on a neurological unit.

Nurses' Notes

1003h: Client's partner ran to nurses' station requesting assistance with the client. Client was found to have slurred speech, left-sided hemiparesis with left facial droop, and left-side neglect. Vital signs: T: 37.5°C (99.5°F); BP: 168/86; P: 111; RR: 26; with pulse oximetry of 96% on room air. Right pupil noted to be 5 mm in size and dilated with minimal reaction to light where the left-sided pupil remains 2 mm in size, briskly reactive to light, and comparable to shape from previous assessment. Client shook head when asked if they were in pain. Motor power remains strong × right-side upper and lower extremities with left side noted to have reduced strength from previous assessment. Client remains able to follow commands, with delayed response. Bilateral radial pulses remain irregular with palpation. Skin warm and dry to touch. Capillary refill remains less than 3 seconds. Lungs auscultated for clear air entry throughout all lobes anteriorly and posteriorly. Client visibly in distress with furrowed brows. ++ reassurance provided to client and partner.
1015h: Health care provider notified of change in client's status.

The nurse has reviewed the Nurses' Notes from 1003h and 1015h.

▶ Identify 4 health care orders the nurse should anticipate.

- ☐ Insert a small-bore peripheral venous access device
- ☐ Nasogastric tube and attach to low suction
- ☐ Computed tomography (CT) scan of the brain
- ☐ Social work consult
- ☐ Speech-language pathology consult for swallowing assessment
- ☐ Antiplatelet medication
- ☐ Anticoagulation medication
- ☐ Culture and sensitivity (C&S) for pathogens
- ☐ Complete blood count (CBC), electrolytes, creatinine, BUN, lipid profile, fasting glucose, coagulation panel

▶ For each nursing intervention, identify whether the intervention is **indicated** or **not indicated** for the care of this client.

NURSING INTERVENTIONS	INDICATED	NOT INDICATED
Assess for presence of dysphagia	○	○
Ensure left side of the body is supported by pillows	○	○
Ask open-ended, multiple questions	○	○
Place client on fluid restriction	○	○
Monitor for Cushing's triad	○	○
Assess client's ability to communicate, and choose best tool based on the client's ability	○	○

Note: Each row must have one response option selected.

▶ For each assessment finding, identify if the finding indicates that the client's condition has improved, not changed, or has declined.

ASSESSMENT FINDINGS	IMPROVED	NO CHANGE	DECLINED
BP 130/76 mm Hg	○	○	○
Urinary incontinence requiring frequent toileting	○	○	○
Lungs auscultated for fine inspiratory crackles that clear with cough	○	○	○
Active bowel sounds × 4 quadrants	○	○	○
Client presents as apathetic	○	○	○

Note: Each row must have one response option selected.

Medical-Surgical 29.0

The nurse is caring for a 75-year-old client in the emergency department (ED).

Nurses' Notes

1100h: Client was brought to the ED by emergency medical services (EMS) after their daughter found the client in bed. The client was lethargic, had slurred speech, and unable to follow commands. The daughter reported to EMS that the client had been suffering from a gastrointestinal virus × 3 days prior, consisting of vomiting and diarrhea. The daughter was concerned the client was not responding to their phone calls and went to the client's house to check on their status. The client's past medical history includes type 2 diabetes mellitus (Glucophage 500 mg bid) and hypertension (ramipril 2.5 mg od). Vital signs: T: 37.5°C (99.5°F); BP: 112/52 P: 82 RR: 10; with pulse oximetry of 97% on room air. Client presents as pleasant, cooperative, oriented to person, place, and time when provided stimulation. Falls back to sleep quickly with heavy snoring. Speech clear mostly but incoherent at times and difficult to understand. Obeys all commands when awake. Motor power strong × 4 extremities. Client has remained on the stretcher since admission so unable to assess gait. Bilateral pupils 3 mm in size, equal in shape and briskly reactive to light. Presents with S1 and S2 heart sounds, apical heart rate regular and equal to radial pulse. Bilateral radial pulses and bilateral dorsalis pedis pulses palpable to touch. Skin cool to touch on all four extremities. Dry mucous membranes noted with pallor observed on bilateral palms and conjunctiva. Reduced air entry noted right lower lobe with fine inspiratory crackles noted throughout left lower lobe auscultated anteriorly. Client presents with a nonproductive cough. Client has not voided since admission. Client encouraged to inform staff for additional support. Hyperactive bowel sounds auscultated × 4 quadrants with abdomen flat during palpation. Client states last bowel movement was this morning and associated with emesis consisting of only bile. Client complains of nausea. Zero food intake for 2 days and drinking only diet ginger ale and water. Kidney basin provided. Peripheral venous access device inserted to right forearm and saline locked.

1124h: Unable to obtain blood sugar with glucometer. Reading identified as error on two different machines. Lab to draw blood sugar with other laboratory blood tests.

▶ Identify 4 assessment findings that require **immediate** follow-up.

- ☐ Pupillary size
- ☐ Lethargy
- ☐ Motor power
- ☐ Lung sounds
- ☐ Dorsalis pedis pulses × 2
- ☐ Bowel sounds
- ☐ Nausea
- ☐ Speech pattern
- ☐ Pulse oximetry
- ☐ Anorexia

▶ Which of the following potential complications could the client be at risk of developing? **Select all that apply.**

- ☐ Bowel obstruction
- ☐ Dehydration
- ☐ Heart failure
- ☐ Acute respiratory distress syndrome
- ☐ Hyperglycemia
- ☐ Hypoglycemia
- ☐ Ethanol (ETOH) intoxication

The nurse is caring for a 75-year-old client in the emergency department (ED).

Nurses' Notes | **Laboratory Results**

1145h:			
Hemoglobin 140–180 g/L (14–18 g/dL) (male) 120–160 g/L (12–16 g/dL) (female)	160 g/L (16 g/dL)	Sodium 136–145 mmol/L	132 mmol/L
Platelets 150–400 × 10^9/L (150 000–400 000/mm^3)	225 × 10^9/L (225 000/ mm^3)	Potassium 3.5–5.1 mmol/L	3.1 mmol/L
White blood cells 3.5–12.0 × 10^9/L 3 500–12 000/ mm^3)	7.2 × 10^9/L (7 200/mm^3)	Creatinine 53–106 mcmol/L (male) 44–97 mcmol/L (female)	96 mcmol/L
Neutrophils 3.0–5.8 × 10^9/L (3 000–5 800/ mm^3)	5.0 × 10^9/L (5 000/mm^3)	Blood urea nitrogen (BUN) 2.9–8.2 mmol/L	7.6 mmol/L
Ethanol level (Absent)	Absent	Glucose (random) 3.9–6.1 mmol/L	44 mmol/L (792 mg/dL)
		Ketones (Absent)	(Absent)

The nurse has reviewed the Laboratory Results drawn at 1145h.

▶ Complete the following sentence by choosing from the list of options.

The client is at **highest** risk of developing ____________, ____________, and ____________.

WORD OPTIONS
Stroke
Dysrhythmias
Diabetic ketoacidosis
Hypoxemia
Renal failure
Hyperosmolar hyperglycemia state
Seizures

▶ For each potential nursing intervention, identify whether the intervention is **indicated** or **not indicated** for the care of this client.

POTENTIAL NURSING INTERVENTIONS	INDICATED	NOT INDICATED
Monitoring intake and output	○	○
Encourage independent mobilization	○	○
Frequent vital signs with specific attention to blood pressure	○	○
Prepare the client for cardiac monitoring	○	○
Encourage oral fluid intake	○	○
Allow the client to rest and recover with limited assessments	○	○

Note: Each row must have one response option selected.

The nurse is caring for a 75-year-old client in the emergency department (ED).

Nurses' Notes | Laboratory Results | Orders

1215h: Client continues to be lethargic and somnolent, only opening eyes to visual and physical stimulation. Client presents as oriented to person and place with difficulty remembering time and date. Vital signs: T: 37.5°C (99.5°F); BP: 92/56 P: 97 RR: 14; with pulse oximetry of 95% on room air.

The nurse has reviewed the Nurses' Notes at 1215h and the Orders from 1230h.

▶ Highlight the orders that the nurse should consider a **priority**. **Select all that apply.**

Nurses' Notes	Laboratory Results	Orders	
1145h:			
Hemoglobin 140–180 g/L (14–18 g/dL) (male) 120–160 g/L (12–16 g/dL) (female)	160 g/L (16 g/dL)	Sodium 136–145 mmol/L	132 mmol/L
Platelets 150–400 × 10^9/L (150 000–400 000/mm^3)	225 × 10^9/L (225 000/mm^3)	Potassium 3.5–5.1 mmol/L	3.1 mmol/L
White blood cells 3.5–12.0 × 10^9/L (3 500–12 000/mm^3)	7.2 × 10^9/L (7 200/mm^3)	Creatinine 53–106 mcmol/L (male) 44–97 mcmol/L (female)	96 mcmol/L
Neutrophils 3.0–5.8 × 10^9/L (3 000–5 800/mm^3)	5.0 × 10^9/L (5 000/mm^3)	Blood urea nitrogen (BUN) 2.9–8.2 mmol/L	7.6 mmol/L
Ethanol level (Absent)	Absent	Glucose (random) 3.9–6.1 mmol/L	44 mmol/L (792 mg/dL)
		Ketones (Absent)	Absent

Nurses' Notes	Laboratory Results	Orders

1230h:

- 0.9% (sodium chloride) IV at 500 mL/hr × 4 hours then 250 mL × 4 hours
- Potassium chloride (KCL) 20 mmol/100 mL IV × 2 doses ASAP
- Humulin R IV as per protocol initiating at 0.1 unit/kg/hour once potassium level returns to.3.3 mmol/L
- Place client on a cardiac monitor
- Insert arterial line for closer blood pressure monitoring
- Insert peripheral venous access device for additional fluid administration
- Transfer to ICU for observation and airway management
- Laboratory draws: complete blood count, electrolytes with serum glucose, creatinine, BUN, lipids, troponin q6h
- Point of care testing q30 min to 60 min prn
- Oxygen 2–6 L/min to maintain pulse oximetry greater than or equal to 92%

Orders

- 0.9% (sodium chloride) IV at 500 mL/hr × 4 hours then 250 mL × 4 hours
- Potassium chloride (KCL) 20 mmol/100 mL IV × 2 doses ASAP
- Humulin R IV as per protocol initiating at 0.1 unit/kg/hr once potassium level returns to greater or equal to 3.3 mmol/L
- Place client on a cardiac monitor
- Insert arterial line for closer blood pressure monitoring
- Insert peripheral venous access device for additional fluid administration
- Transfer to ICU for observation and airway management
- Laboratory draws: complete blood count, electrolytes with serum glucose, creatinine, BUN, lipids, troponin q6h
- Point-of-care testing q30 min to 60 min prn
- Oxygen 2–6 L/min to maintain pulse oximetry greater than or equal to 92%

▶ For each assessment finding, identify if the finding indicates that the client's condition has **improved**, has **not changed**, or has **declined**.

ASSESSMENT FINDINGS	IMPROVED	NO CHANGE	DECLINED
Respiratory rate 26	○	○	○
Creatinine 288 mcmol/L	○	○	○
Urine output 35 mL/hr	○	○	○
Heart rate 97	○	○	○
T 38.4°C (101.1°F)	○	○	○
Blood glucose 22 mmol/L	○	○	○

Note: Each row must have one response option selected.

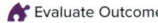

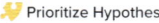

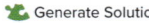

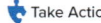

Medical-Surgical 30.0

The nurse is caring for a 72-year-old male client on cardiac unit.

Nurses' Notes

1200h: The client was readmitted to the cardiac unit for further monitoring of chest pain. While shovelling their driveway, the client developed 8 out of 10 chest pain, based on numerical pain scale, diaphoresis, and shortness of breath. Three years ago, the client had an acute myocardial infarction (MI) with angioplasty of the left anterior descending (LAD) coronary artery due to an 85% blockage. The ejection fraction of the left ventricle was documented to be 48% at the time of the acute MI. Client unable to remember subsequent results of their ejection fraction. The client has had no issues since the MI. Vital signs: T: 37.2°C (99.0°F); BP: 100/60; P: 105; RR: 18 at rest and 26 with speaking and ambulation; with pulse oximetry of 96% on room air. The client presents alert and oriented to person, place, and time. Obeys all commands. Motor power strong × 4 peripheral extremities. Client able to ambulate independently without any issue. Client pain free during assessment. The pain subsided en route to the hospital and has not returned since the shovelling. Jugular venous distension noted to be at 6 cm. S1 and S2 cardiac sounds auscultated with a noticeable S3. Bilateral radial pulses palpable and regular. Bilateral dorsalis pedis pulses palpable and regular. Capillary refill documented at less than 3 seconds. Skin warm and dry to touch. Dry mucous membranes noted. Coarse inspiratory crackles auscultated upon anterior assessment with left lower lobe greater than right lower lobe. Client complains of shortness of breath at rest and states, "I feel like I cannot get enough oxygen when I am talking." Dry, nonproductive cough noted. Respiratory rate increases from 18 to 26 when client speaks. No diaphoresis, nausea, or emesis noted. Abdomen soft and flat with palpation, bowel sounds auscultated in all four quadrants. Urinal provided at the bedside in the event the client has to void. Client denies any issue with voiding prior to admission. Client states avoiding drinking excessively due to frequently needing to use the washroom. Denies any pain with voiding, only frequent, small amounts, and often at night. Venous access device inserted into left forearm infusing 0.9% normal saline at 150 mL/hr.

▶ Highlight the client findings that require **immediate** follow-up.

Nurses' Notes

1200h: The client was readmitted to the cardiac unit for further monitoring of chest pain. While shovelling their driveway, the client developed 8 out of 10 chest pain, based on numerical pain scale, diaphoresis, and shortness of breath. Three years ago, the client had an acute myocardial infarction (MI) with angioplasty of the left anterior descending (LAD) coronary artery due to an 85% blockage. The ejection fraction of the left ventricle was documented to be 48% at the time of the acute MI. Client unable to remember subsequent results of their ejection fraction. The client has had no issues since the MI. Vital signs: T: 37.2°C (99.0°F); BP: 100/60; P: 105; RR: 18 at rest and 26 with speaking and ambulation; with pulse oximetry of 96% on room air. The client presents alert and oriented to person, place, and time. Obeys all commands. Motor power strong × 4 peripheral extremities. Client able to ambulate independently without any issue. Client pain free during assessment. The pain subsided en route to the hospital and has not returned since the shovelling. Jugular venous distension noted to be at 6 cm. S1 and S2 cardiac sounds auscultated with a noticeable S3. Bilateral radial pulses palpable and regular. Bilateral dorsalis pedis pulses palpable and regular. Capillary refill documented at less than 3 seconds. Skin warm and dry to touch. Dry mucous membranes noted. Coarse inspiratory crackles auscultated upon anterior assessment with left lower lobe greater than right lower lobe. Client complains of shortness of breath at rest and states, "I feel like I cannot get enough oxygen when I am talking." Dry, nonproductive cough noted. Respiratory rate increases from 18 to 26 when client speaks. No diaphoresis, nausea, or emesis noted. Abdomen soft and flat with palpation, bowel sounds auscultated in all four quadrants. Urinal provided at the bedside in the event the client has to void. Client denies any issue with voiding prior to admission. Client states avoiding drinking excessively due to frequently needing to use the washroom. Denies any pain with voiding, only frequent, small amounts, and often at night. Venous access device inserted into left forearm infusing 0.9% normal saline at 150 mL/hr.

▶ Which of the following complications is the client at risk of developing? **Select all that apply.**

- ☐ Oliguria
- ☐ Pneumonia
- ☐ Pulmonary edema
- ☐ Dysrhythmia
- ☐ Peripheral dependent edema
- ☐ Orthopnea
- ☐ Emesis
- ☐ Fatigue

The nurse is caring for a 72-year-old male client on cardiac unit.

Nurses' Notes

1520h: Nutrition brought to the client. Client found to be ++ short of breath with increased tachypnea, sitting in tripod position, with documented 30 breaths per minute. Client noted to have worse dry, nonproductive cough than upon admission. Vital signs: T: 37.6°C (99.7°F); BP: 128/82; P: 133; with pulse oximetry of 92% on room air. Upon further assessment, coarse crackles auscultated bilateral lower lung fields and inspiratory crackles bilateral upper lung fields, posteriorly and anteriorly.

The nurse has reviewed the Nurse's Notes at 1520h.

▶ Complete the following sentence by choosing from the list of options.

The client is at **highest** risk of developing ____________ (word options 1) as evidenced by the ____________ (word options 2) and ________________ (word options 2).

WORD OPTIONS 1	WORD OPTIONS 2
Anemia	Vital signs
Pulmonary hypertension	Respiratory assessment
Pneumothorax	Cardiovascular assessment
Heart failure	Neurological assessment
Dehydration	Renal assessment

▶ For each potential nursing intervention, identify whether the intervention is **indicated** or **not indicated** for the care of this client.

POTENTIAL NURSING INTERVENTIONS	INDICATED	NOT INDICATED
Request an order to administer a diuretic	○	○
Request an order to administer a 500-mL bolus of an isotonic solution	○	○
Request an order to draw electrolytes, BNP, creatinine, BUN	○	○
Discontinue continuous intravenous fluid infusion	○	○
Request an order to insert a Foley catheter	○	○
Place the client on fluid restriction	○	○

Note: Each row must have one response option selected.

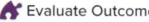

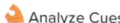

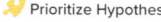

▶ Identify 2 of the following tests that the nurse would expect be ordered for the client.

- ☐ Chest X-ray
- ☐ Arterial blood gas
- ☐ Continuous cardiac monitoring
- ☐ External pacemaker
- ☐ Echocardiogram

▶ For each assessment finding, identify if the finding indicates that the client's condition has improved, not changed, or has declined.

ASSESSMENT FINDINGS	IMPROVED	NO CHANGE	DECLINED
BP 92/58 mm Hg	○	○	○
Urine output 200 mL	○	○	○
ECG showing normal sinus rhythm	○	○	○
Pulse oximetry measured at 92% on room air	○	○	○
Respiratory rate 16	○	○	○

Note: Each row must have one response option selected.

Medical-Surgical 31.0

The nurse is caring for a 16-year-old male client in the emergency department.

Nurses' Notes

0120h: Client arrived at the emergency department accompanied by friends. The client was skateboarding and doing a trick. According to observers, he did not land securely on the board and instead over-rotated, hitting the occipital/right lateral side of his head on the pavement. Unable to determine if the client lost consciousness at the time of the injury because it was dark. Friends reported the client was motionless on the ground and slow to rise. When he did get to his feet, he was unsteady on his feet. Vital signs: T: 37.2°C (99.0°F); BP: 110/74; P: 62; RR: 16; with pulse oximetry of 99% on room air. Client rouses easily with minimal verbal and physical stimulation. Client oriented to person, place, but unsure of the time. The last memory of the night was arriving at the skateboard park. Client is complaining of a headache behind his eyes, rated 4 out of 10 on a numerical pain scale. Pupils equal and slow to react to light at 3 mm. Client complaints of the room spinning when his eyes are open. Prefers to keep eyes closed. Unable to determine if diplopia is present. Client moves all extremities independently. Obeys commands. Motor power strong × 4 extremities. As client is lying with head on the back of the stretcher, postauricular ecchymosis noted on the right side. Glasgow Coma Scale (GCS) 13. S1 and S2 auscultated with no adventitious heart sounds noted. Bilateral radial pulses documented at +2 with bilateral dorsalis pedis pulses +1 and posterior tibial pulses require Doppler but audible. Client denies any chest pain or difficulty breathing but states, "I do not feel right." All lung fields auscultated for clear air entry throughout. Client's abdomen flat and soft. Bowel sounds auscultated × 4 quadrants. Client complains of nausea. Client's parents have been notified. No previous comorbidities.
0145h: Client's mom arrives at the hospital and is provided information about the client's status.

The nurse reviewed the Nurses' Notes from 0120h and 0145h.

▶ Identify the top 4 clinical client findings that would require **immediate** follow-up in the box on the right.

CLIENT FINDINGS
Posterior tibial pulses requiring Doppler for assessment
Lung sounds
Pupillary response
Vertigo
Nausea
Bowel sounds
Postauricular ecchymosis

TOP 4 FINDINGS

▶ Which of the following complications is the client at risk of experiencing? **Select all that apply.**

- ☐ Blindness
- ☐ Changes in consciousness
- ☐ Pulmonary edema
- ☐ Increased cerebral pressure
- ☐ Deafness
- ☐ Hydrocephalus
- ☐ Bleeding

The nurse is caring for a 16-year-old male client in the emergency department.

Nurses' Notes

0214h: Client's mom rang for assistance, requesting a basin as the client began vomiting yellow bile, soiling the sheets. Client stated ++ nauseated and yelled "Turn off the light" when the nurse attempted to turn on the light. Client noted to be slurring speech and responses do not answer questions. Client noted to be more lethargic and somnolent. Pupils remain equal in size at 2 mm and reactive to light but remain sluggish in response. GCS 11. Vital signs: T: 37.7°C (99.9°F); BP: 130/86; P: 96; RR: 22; with pulse oximetry of 93% on room air. Health care provider notified of change in status.

The nurse has reviewed the Nurses' Notes at 0214h.

▶ Complete the following sentence by choosing from the list of options.

The client is at **highest** risk of developing _______________ (word options 1) as evidenced by the client's _______________ (word options 2) and _______________ (word options 2).

WORD OPTIONS 1	WORD OPTIONS 2
Intracranial pressure	Vital signs
Stroke	Headache
Traumatic encephalopathy	Pupillary response
Migraine	Level of consciousness
Meningitis	Emesis

▶ For each potential nursing intervention, identify whether the intervention is **indicated** or **not indicated** for the care of this client.

POTENTIAL NURSING INTERVENTIONS	INDICATED	NOT INDICATED
Assess neurological vital signs every 8 hours	○	○
Prepare to insert two large-bore peripheral venous access devices	○	○
Position the head of the bed in the lowest position for comfort	○	○
Keep the lights dimmed	○	○
Regulate and keep number of visitors at a minimum	○	○
Prepare bolus intravenous fluids	○	○
Prevent shivering by keeping environment's temperature comfortable	○	○

Note: Each row must have one response option selected.

The nurse is caring for a 16-year-old male client in the neurological intensive care unit.

Nurses' Notes | Orders

0245h: The health care provider wrote new orders and requested that the client be transferred to the neurological intensive care unit for further monitoring and intervention if necessary.

Nurses' Notes | **Orders**

- Initiate 3% normal saline (sodium chloride) at 0.5 mL/kg/hr
- Ondansetron 4–8 mg IV q12h prn
- Pantoprazole 40 mg IV od
- Head of the bed (HOB) to remain 30 degrees
- Insert an in-dwelling urethral catheter
- Computed tomography (CT) scan of the head to be completed without contrast
- Neuro vitals q1h × 4 hr and if stable q2h × 4 hr
- Draw ABG now
- Laboratory draws: complete blood count, electrolytes, BUN, creatinine, liver function tests, INR, PTT
- Monitor intake and output
- Blood glucose monitoring q4h
- Sequential compression devices to be applied while client is immobile

The nurse has reviewed the Nurses' Notes at 0245h and the Orders.

▶ Highlight the 4 orders the nurse should perform right away.

Orders

- Initiate 3% normal saline (sodium chloride) at 0.5 mL/kg/hr
- Ondansetron 4–8 mg IV q12h prn
- Pantoprazole 40 mg IV od
- Head of the bed (HOB) to remain 30 degrees
- Insert an in-dwelling urethral catheter
- Computed tomography (CT) scan of the head to be completed without contrast
- Neuro vitals q1h × 4 hr and if stable q2h × 4 hr
- Draw arterial blood gas (ABG) now
- Laboratory draws: complete blood count, electrolytes, BUN, creatinine, liver function tests, INR, PTT
- Monitor intake and output
- Blood glucose monitoring q4h
- Sequential compression devices to be applied while client is immobile

▶ For each assessment finding, identify if the finding indicates that the client's condition has **improved**, has **not changed**, or has **declined**.

ASSESSMENT FINDINGS	IMPROVED	NO CHANGE	DECLINED
Pupils equal and briskly reactive to light at 2 mm	○	○	○
Nausea only, no emesis	○	○	○
Left lower leg increased edema and calf pain	○	○	○
Negative 250 mL shift fluid balance	○	○	○
RR 18	○	○	○

Note: Each row must have one response option selected.

Medical-Surgical 32.0

The nurse is caring for a 31-year-old client in the emergency department.

Nurses' Notes

1752h: The client presents to the emergency department with sharp abdominal pain located in left lower quadrant and right lower quadrant rated 6 out of 10 on a numerical pain scale along with extreme nausea and inability to keep any fluids down × 2 days. The client began semaglutide for weight loss × 3 weeks ago, taking the medication as prescribed, but reports having no bowel movement × 5 days with no flatus × 3 days. The client states the pain is nonradiating and intermittent throughout the night. Vital signs: T: 38.1°C (100.6°F); BP: 133/89; P: 114; RR: 18; with pulse oximetry of 99% on room air. Client presents as pleasant, cooperative, alert and oriented to person, place, and time. Gait steady, denies any dizziness. Bilateral pupils equal in size and shape, measured at 3 mm, and briskly reactive to light. Motor power strong × 4. S1 and S2 heart sounds, apical heart rate regular and equals radial pulse. Bilateral radial pulses and bilateral dorsalis pedis pulses palpable and regular. Skin warm to touch with mild diaphoresis noted due to abdominal pain. Client noted to be taking small, shallow breaths. Colour remains appropriate with no cyanosis noted. Capillary refill less than 3 seconds. No complaints of shortness of breath from the client. Hypoactive bowel sounds identified in all four quadrants with persistent eructation. Abdomen rounded and firm to touch. Tympany noted × 4 quadrants of the abdomen with mild percussion. Complaints of increased pain at 8 out of 10 with percussion. Client states feeling bloated and full despite reduced nutritional intake. Client denies difficulty voiding, no pain, but due to reduced fluid intake, voiding approximately 3 times per day for small amounts.

▶ Highlight the assessment findings that require **immediate** follow-up by the nurse.

Nurses' Notes | Medications

1752h: The client presents to the emergency department with sharp abdominal pain located in left lower quadrant and right lower quadrant rated 6 out of 10 on a numerical pain scale, along with extreme nausea and inability to keep any fluids down × 2 days. The client began semaglutide for weight loss × 3 weeks ago, taking the medication as prescribed, but reports having no bowel movement × 5 days with no flatus × 3 days. The client states the pain is nonradiating and intermittent throughout the night. Vital signs: T: 38.1°C (100.6°F); BP: 133/89; P: 114; RR: 18; with pulse oximetry of 99% on room air. Client presents as pleasant, cooperative, alert and oriented to person, place, and time. Gait steady, denies any dizziness. Bilateral pupils equal in size and shape, measured at 3 mm, and briskly reactive to light. Motor power strong × 4. S1 and S2 heart sounds, apical heart rate regular and equals radial pulse. Bilateral radial pulses and bilateral dorsalis pedis pulses palpable and regular. Skin warm to touch with mild diaphoresis noted due to abdominal pain. Client noted to be taking small, shallow breaths. Colour remains appropriate with no cyanosis noted. Capillary refill less than 3 seconds. No complaints of shortness of breath from the client. Hypoactive bowel sounds identified in bilateral upper quadrants and absent bowel sounds identified in bilateral lower abdominal quadrants with persistent eructation. Abdomen rounded and firm to touch. Tympany noted × 4 quadrants of the abdomen with mild percussion. Complaints of increased pain at 8 out of 10 with percussion. Client states feeling bloated and full despite reduced nutritional intake. Client denies difficulty voiding, no pain, but due to reduced fluid intake, voiding approximately 3 × per day for small amounts.

▶ Which of the following complications is the client at risk of experiencing. **Select all that apply.**

☐ Dehydration
☐ Irregular heart rate
☐ Reduced perfusion to the brain
☐ Anal fissures
☐ Hemorrhoids
☐ *Clostridium difficile*

The nurse is caring for a 31-year-old client in the emergency department.

Nurses' Notes

2200h: The client calls for assistance and is found sitting at the edge of the bed vomiting foul-smelling orange–brown coloured bile and watery emesis. Client states increased pain in the abdomen that is now a 10 out of 10 on a numerical scale. Vital signs: T: 38.8°C (101.8°F); BP: 146/89; P: 129; RR: 24 with pulse oximetry of 94% on room air. Client indicates more noticeable shortness of breath. Abdomen remains distended and firm to touch. Absent bowel sounds noted in all four quadrants. Client's eructation increasing in frequency. Client unable to pass any flatus. Client complaining of nausea despite emesis. No change in cardiovascular assessment. Health care provider notified with change of status.
2220h: Health care provider present and completing a full assessment.

The nurse reviewed the Nurses' Notes from 2200h and 2220h.

▶ Complete the following sentence by choosing from the list of options.

The client is at **highest** risk of developing ____________ (word options 1) as evidenced by ______________ (word options 2).

WORD OPTIONS 1	WORD OPTIONS 2
Renal failure	Absent bowel sounds
Dysrhythmias	Tachypnea
Anorexia	Cardiovascular assessment
Hypoxemia	Poor nutritional intake
Bowel obstruction	Anuria

▶ For each potential order, identify whether the order is **indicated** or **not indicated** for the care of this client.

POTENTIAL ORDERS	INDICATED	NOT INDICATED
Consult general surgery	○	○
Insert a nasogastric tube and attach to low suction	○	○
Transport the client to obtain a chest X-ray	○	○
Laboratory tests: complete blood count, serum electrolytes, amylase, creatinine, and BUN	○	○
Insert an in-dwelling Foley catheter	○	○
Intravenous fluids: dextrose 5% and water preferred solution	○	○

Note: Each row must have one response option selected.

▶ Select 3 actions the nurse should take.

- ☐ Encourage deep breathing and coughing
- ☐ Administer oxycodone/acetaminophen for pain control
- ☐ Monitor for muscle guarding
- ☐ Insert two peripheral venous access devices
- ☐ Initiate bowel protocol

The nurse is caring for a 31-year-old client on a general surgical unit for postoperative care.

Nurses' Notes

2300h: The general surgeon recommended surgical intervention as soon as possible. Client aware of treatment plan.
2333h: Client transported to the operating room.
0445h: Client returned to the general surgical unit with a right lower quadrant ileostomy. Vital signs: T: 37.7°C (99.9°F); BP: 114/65; P: 66; RR: 16; with pulse oximetry of 99% on 2 L/min of oxygen per nasal prongs. Client fatigued but rouses easily to verbal and touch stimulation. Alert and oriented to person, place, and time. Denies any pain, states feeling exhausted. Stoma mildly edematous, brick red in colour, with small amount of blood noted on the stoma. Absent bowel sounds at present. Abdomen distended but soft to touch. In-dwelling Foley catheter in situ draining concentrated urine with 500 mL of urine noted in the drainage bag.

The nurse has reviewed the Nurses' Notes from 2300h, 2333h, and 0445h.

▶ For each assessment finding, identify if the finding indicates that the client's condition has improved, not changed, or has declined.

ASSESSMENT FINDINGS	IMPROVED	NO CHANGE	DECLINED
Stoma brick red in colour postoperatively	○	○	○
Urine output of 500 mL	○	○	○
Temperature: 37.7°C (99.8°F)	○	○	○
Distended abdomen	○	○	○
Fatigue	○	○	○

Note: Each row must have one response option selected.

Medical-Surgical 33.0

The nurse is caring for an 83-year-old client on an internal medical unit.

Nurses' Notes

1717h: Client admitted to the unit after suffering a fall in their independent living facility. The client's neighbour found the client lying on their left side. Client estimated to be lying on the floor for over 7 hours. Previous comorbidities include stress incontinence, mild arthritis in knees, type 2 diabetes mellitus controlled with diet and exercise. Vital signs: T: 37.4°C (99.3°F); BP: 110/72; P: 85; RR: 16; with pulse oximetry of 97% on room air. Client presents as pleasant, cooperative, alert and oriented to person, place, and time. Client denies hitting head when they fell, denies a headache. Bilateral pupils equal in shape, measured at 2 mm, and briskly reactive to light. Motor power strong × 4. Client denies any dizziness. Client complains of feeling muscle soreness, but pain is manageable. Presents with S1 and S2 heart sounds. No adventitious heart sounds noted. Apical pulse regular and equal to right radial pulse, left radial pulse documented as weak but palpable. Right-side upper and bilateral lower extremities noted to be warm to touch. Left upper arm noted to be edematous, measured at 26 cm (10 inches), warm and red to touch with left forearm and left hand cool to touch. Left hand capillary refill 3 seconds whereas all other extremities noted to have capillary refill less than 3 seconds. Bilateral dorsalis pedis pulses and post-tibial pulses noted to be strong. Mucous membranes of the conjunctiva and mouth remain pink in colour and perfused. Anteriorly, right lung fields auscultated for clear air entry with fine inspiratory crackles noted anteriorly to left lower lung. Client encouraged to deep-breathe and cough while in bed. Ambulation encouraged as tolerated. Client denies a cough or shortness of breath. Abdomen flat and soft to touch. Active bowel sounds auscultated throughout all four quadrants. Client voiding clear, concentrated urine. Large purple bruise noted on left shoulder and left hip. Edema noted on left elbow.

▶ Which of the following assessment findings require **immediate** follow-up? **Select all that apply.**

- ☐ Radial pulses
- ☐ Temperature
- ☐ Lung sounds
- ☐ Edema
- ☐ Bruising
- ☐ Mobility
- ☐ Dizziness
- ☐ Skin temperature
- ☐ Bowel sounds

▶ Identify 4 complications the client is at risk of experiencing.

- ☐ Organ damage
- ☐ Limb ischemia
- ☐ Peripheral vascular disease
- ☐ Thrombosis
- ☐ Embolus
- ☐ Pleural effusions

▶ Complete the following sentence by choosing from the list of options.

The client is at **highest** risk of developing __________.

WORD OPTIONS
Respiratory distress
Dysrhythmias
Bowel obstruction
Hypoxemia
Deep vein thrombosis

The nurse is caring for an 83-year-old client on an internal medical unit.

Nurses' Notes

2010h: Client complains of increased pain of left arm, rated 9 out of 10 on a numerical pain scale. Vital signs: T: 38.2°C (100.7°F); BP: 132/82; P: 99; RR: 18; with pulse oximetry of 97% on room air. The left upper arm presents with increased redness and warmth extending from shoulder to mid-forearm, now measured at 30 cm (11 inches). Client states left arm feels heavy. Left hand ++ cool to touch, no radial pulse palpable or auscultated with Doppler. Left hand fingertips cyanotic. Unable to measure capillary refill on left-hand nail beds. No change in assessment from previous assessment on right upper and bilateral lower extremities. Health care provider notified of change in status.

The nurse has reviewed the Nurses' Notes from 2010h.

▶ For each potential nursing intervention, identify whether the intervention is **indicated** or **not indicated** for the care of this client.

POTENTIAL NURSING INTERVENTIONS	INDICATED	NOT INDICATED
Prepare to insert a peripheral venous access device in the left hand	○	○
Encourage ambulation	○	○
Prepare to administer an anticoagulant	○	○
Ensure nasal prongs are available and oxygen is working	○	○
Apply lower extremity venous compression stockings	○	○
Elevate the affected extremity for comfort	○	○
Prepare to transport client for a computed tomography (CT) chest	○	○

Note: Each row must have one response option selected.

▶ Highlight the 3 orders that the nurse should perform **immediately**.

Orders

- Initiate heparin IV per protocol with laboratory draw for INR and PTT 6 hours after starting therapy
- Venous Doppler ultrasound of left upper arm
- Acetaminophen 500–1000 mg PO q4–6h prn
- Laboratory tests: complete blood count, liver function tests, creatinine, BUN, and D-dimer
- Encourage oral fluids
- Regular diet
- Apply sequential compression devices to lower extremities while client is in bed

▶ For each statement made by the client, identify whether the client has **understanding** or **no understanding** of the client teaching provided by the nurse.

CLIENT STATEMENTS	UNDER-STANDING	NO UNDER-STANDING
"I should avoid blowing my nose forcefully."	○	○
"It is best to stay in bed and rest."	○	○
"I need to stop drinking so much water."	○	○
"I should watch not to bump into anything."	○	○
"I will call for help if I notice any bleeding or bruising."	○	○

Note: Each row must have one response option selected.

Medical-Surgical 34.0

The nurse is caring for a 44-year-old male client on an orthopedic unit.

Nurses' Notes

1017h: Client admitted to the unit after experiencing a crushing right lower leg injury as a result of a steel beam falling on him at work. Client has no previous comorbidities. Vital signs: T: 37.7°C (99.9°F); BP: 149/67; P: 80; RR: 18; with pulse oximetry of 97% on room air. Client presents as pleasant, cooperative, alert and oriented to person, place, and time. Bilateral pupils measured at 3 mm and briskly react to light. Client to remain on bed rest with right lower leg elevated on pillows. Complains of vertigo when head of bed is raised from supine to semi-Fowler's position. Client states pain level is 3 out of 10 on a numerical pain scale and tolerable. Denies need for analgesic as he indicates he has a high pain tolerance. Apical pulse regular and equal to radial pulse. Bilateral radial pulses +2 in force with left dorsalis pedis pulse +2 and right dorsalis pedis pulse palpable but weak. Bilateral upper extremities warm to touch with capillary refill less than 3 seconds. Right foot and right lower extremity cool to touch above the site of injury with peripheral edema noted at +2 with no edema noted for left foot and lower extremity. Left foot and lower extremity warm to touch with no peripheral edema. All lung fields anteriorly auscultated for clear air entry. Client encouraged to deep-breath and cough while in bed. Respirations regular and easy at rest. Abdomen flat and soft to touch. Active bowel sounds auscultated throughout all four quadrants. Urinal at client's bedside. Client noted to be voiding clear, amber urine. Client requires one-person assistance to use the washroom to assist with stability.

▶ Identify 4 assessment findings that require **immediate** follow-up?

- ☐ Pedal pulse characteristics
- ☐ Temperature
- ☐ Blood pressure
- ☐ Heart rate
- ☐ Lung sounds
- ☐ Peripheral edema
- ☐ Vertigo
- ☐ Skin temperature characteristics

▶ Which of the following complications is the client at risk of experiencing? **Select all that apply.**

- ☐ Headache
- ☐ Anxiety
- ☐ Impaired motor function
- ☐ Ventilation/perfusion mismatching
- ☐ Increased pain
- ☐ Increased preload
- ☐ Normal capillary refill

The nurse is caring for a 44-year-old male client on an orthopedic unit.

Nurses' Notes | Laboratory Results

1200h: The client states being not hungry and refusing lunch.
1400h: Client reported increased pain to right lower leg. Vital signs: T: 37.9°C (100.2°F); BP: 152/89; P: 96; RR: 22; with pulse oximetry of 94% on room air. Upon assessment, skin increased coolness to touch above the injury than previously documented with a complete loss of right dorsalis pedis pulse, requiring Doppler to locate a pulse, which was present. Right popliteal pulse palpable but weak and right femoral pulse noted to be weak. Capillary refill on right foot documented as greater than 3 seconds. Right lower extremity noted to have +3/+4 peripheral edema and hot to touch. Client indicates numbness and tingling in right foot and indicates pain has increased to 6 out of 10 on a numerical pain scale. Left lower extremity assessment remains unchanged. Clients states they are uncomfortable, scared, and trying to remain calm despite new physiological changes. Denies the need to void.

The nurse has reviewed Nurses' Notes from 1400h and Laboratory Results drawn at 0800h.

▶ Complete the following sentence by choosing from the list of options.

The client is at **highest** risk of developing _____________.

WORD OPTIONS
Hyponatremia
Deep vein thrombosis
Infection
Contractures
Compartment syndrome

Nurses' Notes | **Laboratory Results**

0800h: (Drawn in the Emergency Department Before Transfer)

Test	Result	Test	Result
Hemoglobin 140–180 g/L (14–18 g/dL) (male) 120–160 g/L (12–16 g/dL) (female)	160 g/L (16 g/dL)	Sodium 136–145 mmol/L	136 mmol/L
Platelets 150–400 × 10^9/L (150 000–400 000/mm^3)	650 × 10^9/L (650 000/mm^3)	Potassium 3.5–5.1 mmol/L	5.0 mmol/L
White blood cells 3.5–12.0 × 10^9/L (3 500–12 000/mm^3)	11.0 × 10^9/L (11 000/mm^3)	Creatinine 53–106 mcmol/L (male) 44–97 mcmol/L (female)	260 mcmol/L
Neutrophils 3.0–5.8 × 10^9/L (3 000–5 800/mm^3)	5.0 × 10^9/L (5 000/mm^3)	Blood urea nitrogen (BUN) 2.9–8.2 mmol/L	6.7 mmol/L

▶ For each potential nursing intervention, identify whether the intervention is **indicated** or **not indicated** for the care of this client.

POTENTIAL NURSING INTERVENTIONS	INDICATED	NOT INDICATED
Elevate the client's right lower leg higher than their heart level	○	○
Request an order for analgesic	○	○
Apply cold compresses to the injured area	○	○
Request an order to add creatine kinase to the morning laboratory blood draw	○	○
Measure the size of the right lower extremity	○	○
Add a graduated cylinder to measure urine output	○	○

Note: Each row must have one response option selected.

The nurse is caring for a 44-year-old male client on an orthopedic unit.

Nurses' Notes | Laboratory Results

1412h: The health care provider was notified of the client's symptomatic changes.
1422h: Orthopedic surgery was consulted to assess the client.
1438h: The client is to be taken to the operating room for an emergency fasciotomy and to return postoperatively to the orthopedic unit after the recovery room.

The nurse has reviewed the Nurses' Notes from 1412h, 1422, and 1438h.

▶ Which of the following actions should the nurse take prior to the client being transferred to the operating room? **Select all that apply.**

- ☐ Document the last time the client ate or drank anything
- ☐ Review all medications and inform the surgical team of all medications administered that shift
- ☐ Inform the client's family of impending surgery
- ☐ Ensure goals of care are discussed by the nurse with the client and documented in the chart
- ☐ Provide reassurance to the client to help reduce anxiety
- ☐ Place mark on the client's bilateral lower extremities indicating dorsalis pedis pulses and posterior tibial pulses
- ☐ Ensure the health care provider or orthopedic surgeon has obtained consent for the procedure

▶ For each assessment finding, identify if the finding indicates that the client's condition has improved, not changed, or has declined when he returns from the recovery room.

ASSESSMENT FINDINGS	IMPROVED	NO CHANGE	DECLINED
RR 8	○	○	○
Concentrated, urine output 35 mL/hr	○	○	○
BP 124/74 mm Hg	○	○	○
T 38.9°C (102.0°F)	○	○	○
Client alert and oriented to person, place, and time	○	○	○

Note: Each row must have one response option selected.

Maternal/Birth Parent Health Unfolding Cases

Maternal/Birth Parent Health 1.0

The nurse is caring for a 38-year-old female who is 12 weeks' gestation on the postpartum unit.

Nurses' Notes | Flow Sheet

0800h: Client was admitted to the unit experiencing fatigue and weakness. G1 P0 A0 L0. She states she is unable to keep any food down and she cannot stay awake long enough to eat anything. Vital signs: T: 37.7°C (99.9°F); BP: 100/65; P: 110 RR: 20; with pulse oximetry of 99% on room air. Client alert and oriented × 3, gait steady. Bilateral air entry to posterior lungs noted to be clear with auscultation. Mucous membranes noted to be dry, tenting observed on the back of the client's hand, capillary refill less than 3 seconds, all pulses strong and regular, apical pulses regular and equal to radial, extremities cool to touch. Abdomen soft, flat, no pain with palpation. Client complains of emesis × 3 overnight. Emesis noted in the kidney basin on the bedside table, found to be clear, only bile. Client encouraged to drink fluids to maintain hydration. Client states she is able to void without issue. Pre-pregnancy weight was documented at 70 kg. Current weight: 66 kg. The client has no previous comorbidities.

Nurses' Notes | **Flow Sheet**

Intake and Output	0700	1500h	2300h	0700h
Intake (fluid intake)	100 mL	375 mL	225 mL	125 mL
Output (urine)	90 mL	200 mL	250 mL	75 mL
Output (emesis)	325 mL	300 mL	475 mL	200 mL

▶ Identify the top 3 findings that would require follow-up in the box on the right.

CLIENT FINDINGS
Vital signs
Fatigue
Output
Clear emesis
Dry mucous membranes

TOP 3 FINDINGS

▶ Which of the following complications is the client at risk of experiencing? **Select all that apply.**

- ☐ Gastroenteritis
- ☐ Ectopic pregnancy
- ☐ Hypotension
- ☐ Appendicitis
- ☐ Fluid imbalance

The nurse is caring for a 38-year-old female who is 12 weeks' gestation on the postpartum unit.

Nurses' Notes | Flow Sheet

1025: Client found supine in bed, difficult to rouse, and found with large amount of clear bile, vomitus in the bed. Vital signs: T: 37.7°C (99.9°F); BP: 80/55; P: 130 RR: 12; with pulse oximetry of 92% on room air. Client's peripherals noted to be cool to touch, pulses weak. Health care provider notified.
1030: Orders received from health care provider.

Nurses' Notes | Flow Sheet | **Laboratory Data**

0830h:

Test	Result	Test	Result
Hemoglobin 140–180 g/L (14–18 g/dL) (male) 120–160 g/L (12–16 g/dL) (female)	160 g/L (16 g/dL)	Sodium 136–145 mmol/L	132 mmol/L
Platelets 150–400 × 10^9/L (150 000–400 000/mm^3)	250 × 10^9/L (250 000/mm^3)	Potassium 3.5–5.1 mmol/L	5.0 mmol/L
White blood cells 3.5–12.0 × 10^9/L (3 500–12 000/mm^3)	6.8 × 10^9/L (6 800/mm^3)	Creatinine 53–106 mcmol/L (male) 44–97 mcmol/L (female)	76 mcmol/L
Neutrophils 3.0–5.8 × 10^9/L (3 000–5 800/mm^3)	3 × 10^9/L (3 000/mm^3)	Hematocrit 0.37–0.47	0.52
		Urine analysis	Positive for ketones

The nurse has reviewed the Nurses' Notes from 1025h and new Laboratory Data drawn at 0830h.

▶ Complete the following sentence by choosing from the list of options.

The client is at **highest** risk of developing ____________.

WORD OPTIONS
Acute renal failure
Cerebral edema
Severe dehydration
Pyelonephritis
Syndrome of antidiuretic hormone
Dysrhythmias

▶ For each nursing intervention, click to specify whether the intervention is **indicated** or **not indicated** for the care of this client.

POTENTIAL NURSING INTERVENTIONS	INDICATED	NOT INDICATED
Place client in the side-lying position	○	○
Anticipate blood draws	○	○
Reassure client addressing fears	○	○
Call a code blue	○	○
Apply oxygen	○	○

Note: Each row must have one response option selected.

The nurse has received orders from the physician at 1030h.

▶ Highlight below the 3 orders that the nurse should perform right away.

Orders

1030h:
- Insert an in-dwelling Foley catheter
- Draw an arterial blood gas
- Initiate oxygen therapy when pulse oximetry is less than 90%
- 0.9% sodium chloride (normal saline) 500 mL bolus × 1 then 125 mL/hr
- Insert peripheral intravenous catheter
- Monitor intake and output
- Begin to monitor with the Pregnancy-Unique Quantification of Emesis Scale
- Administer dimenhydrinate 50 mg IVPB q4h
- Administer acetaminophen 500–1 000 mg PO qid
- Consult dietitian

The nurse is caring for a 38-year-old female who is 12 weeks' gestation on the postpartum unit.

Nurses' Notes	Flow Sheet	Laboratory Data

1200h: Client alert and appropriate, sitting in high Fowler's position. Vital signs: T: 37.7°C (99.9°F); BP: 100/75; P: 87 RR: 18; with pulse oximetry of 99% on room air. Nausea improved but client experiencing reduced amounts of emesis since anti-nausea agent administered. Urine output 450 mL of clear amber urine.

The nurse has reviewed the Nurses' Notes at 1200h.

▶ Which of the following assessment data are most indicative that the client's status is improving? **Select all that apply.**

- ☐ Blood pressure
- ☐ Heart rate
- ☐ Pulse oximetry
- ☐ Nausea with emesis
- ☐ Urine output

Maternal/Birth Parent Health 2.0

The nurse is caring for a 17-year-old female who is 28 weeks' gestation in the emergency department.

Nurses' Notes

0900: Client presents with vague symptoms of feeling "unwell" and is accompanied by her mother. Vital signs: T: 36.3°C (97.3°F); BP: 167/96; P: 85; RR: 28; with pulse oximetry of 94% on room air. No previous medical history. Client reports dizziness with occasional double vision and a severe headache. Gait steady with strong motor power. Pupils equal and reactive to light at 2 mm. Client's mother reports her daughter is "puffy all over" with mild pedal edema noted. Client reports occasional shortness of breath with mild chest discomfort when she takes in a breath. Lung auscultated for clear air entry throughout. Client reported seeing small purple dots on her lower extremities but thought she must have accidentally bumped into something. Client reports occasional red spotting in the last week, "about the size of a nickel." Client reports not drinking as much water as usual, with approximately 4–250 mL of water each day. Reports voiding at least four times per day. Fundal height measuring at 28 cm with fetal heart rate measured by Doppler at 152 beats/min. Urine dipstick analysis completed and shows protein in urine (+3).

▶ Identify the top 4 assessment findings that require **immediate** follow-up.

ASSESSMENT FINDINGS
BP: 167/96; P: 85; pulse oximetry 94% on room air
Pupils
Severe headache
Peripheral edema
Protein in urine
Fundal height
Spotting

TOP 4 FINDINGS

▶ Which of the following complications is the client at risk of experiencing? **Select all that apply.**

- ☐ Thrombocytopenia
- ☐ Stroke
- ☐ Acute renal failure
- ☐ Confusion
- ☐ Blurred vision

The nurse is caring for a 17-year-old female who is 28 weeks' gestation in the emergency department.

Nurses' Notes	Laboratory Results

1100h: Client continues to complain of severe headache. Vital signs: T: 36.3°C (97.3°F); BP: 178/99; P: 90; RR: 26; with pulse oximetry of 92% on room air.

The nurse has reviewed the Nurses' Notes from 1100h.

▶ Complete the following sentence by choosing from the list of options.

The client is at **highest** risk for developing _____________ and _____________.

WORD OPTIONS
Eclampsia
Fetal compromise
Postpartum hemorrhage
Placental abruption
Infection
Seizures

Nurses' Notes	**Laboratory Results**		
0800h:			
Hemoglobin 140–180 g/L (14–18 g/dL) (male) 120–160 g/L (12–16 g/dL) (female)	260 g/L (26 g/dL)	Sodium 136–145 mmol/L	140 mmol/L
Platelets 150–400 × 10^9/L (150 000–400 000/mm^3)	75 × 10^9/L (75 000/mm^3)	Potassium 3.5–5.1 mmol/L	4.6 mmol/L
White blood cells 3.5–12.0 × 10^9/L (3 500–12 000/mm^3)	7.0 × 10^9/L (7 000/mm^3)	Creatinine 53–106 mcmol/L (male) 44–97 mcmol/L (female)	60 mcmol/L
Neutrophils 3.0–5.8 × 10^9/L (3 000–5 800/mm^3)	3.0 × 10^9/L (3 000/mm^3)		

▶ For each nursing intervention, click to specify whether the intervention is **indicated** or **not indicated** for the care of this client.

POTENTIAL NURSING INTERVENTIONS	INDICATED	NOT INDICATED
Permit a highly stimulated environment	○	○
Request an order to insert intravenous access (peripheral venous access device)	○	○
Encourage mobility	○	○
Monitor for HELLP syndrome	○	○
Test suction equipment in the room	○	○
Place bed in highest position	○	○

Note: Each row must have one response option selected.

The nurse has received orders from the physician.

▶ Select 2 priority actions most appropriate for the care of this client.

- ☐ Insert an in-dwelling urinary catheter
- ☐ Initiate magnesium sulphate IV loading dose 4 g, then initiate rate at 1 g/hr
- ☐ Apply oxygen 2–4 L/min per nasal prongs to maintain pulse oximetry greater than 90%
- ☐ Administer labetalol IV 2 mg/min
- ☐ Contact all family for family conference

The nurse has performed the two priority interventions as ordered by the physician for the client.

▶ For each assessment finding, click to specify if the finding indicates the client's condition has improved, not changed, or has declined.

ASSESSMENT FINDINGS	IMPROVED	NO CHANGE	DECLINED
BP 145/77	○	○	○
Oliguria	○	○	○
Petechiae	○	○	○
Loss of deep tendon reflexes	○	○	○
Double vision	○	○	○
RR 20	○	○	○

Note: Each row must have one response option selected.

Maternal/Birth Parent Health 3.0

The nurse is caring for a 30-year-old transmasculine client in the community health centre 1 month post-delivery who prefers the pronouns he/him/his.

Discharge Notes	Progress Notes

0400h: Client G1 P1 A0 discharged home after uneventful spontaneous vaginal delivery. Minimal tears noted. No episiotomy required. Newborn had documented Apgars of 7 and 9, weighing 3500 g at delivery and 3425 g at discharge. Newborn nursed well after delivery with no issues noted during postpartum period. Partner present during client's side and for client education. Client will continue to chest feed as he indicated this for his birth and postpartum plan.

Discharge Notes	**Progress Notes**

1330h: Client reported a difficult postpartum experience in hospital. Client reported several staff nurses were disrespectful toward him and unaccepting of transmasculine status and parenthood. He overheard the night nurses laughing at his desire to chest feed his newborn despite a successful latch at delivery. The client was unable to share his fears of not having enough milk and could not ask when he could start lightly binding after delivery. The client has not had chest masculinization surgery, denied taking any hormones while chest feeding, and stopped testosterone 6 months prior to conceiving. Client reported expected associated pregnancy changes related to chest size with ability to express colostrum during hospital time. When client returned home post-discharge, chest feeding became difficult after well-child visit at 1 week post-discharge. Given the hospital experience, he did not seek additional chest feeding support and began binding chest regularly 2 weeks after discharge. Client presents to clinic with swollen and shiny right chest that is tender and warm to touch, sore nipples, and not able to express milk from right chest. Client states fatigue, but he thought this was normal with a newborn, complains of chills, aches. Left chest continues to produce milk and he has been able to feed his child off that chest while also supplementing with formula. He states that he did not know he would feel like he lost his body that he worked so hard to gain and feels like an imposter, knowing he wanted to chest feed but now feels shame that his chest has grown to this size. Vital signs: T: 38.6°C (101.5°F); BP: 120/77; P: 97; RR: 14; with pulse oximetry of 99% on room air. Infant noted to be healthy in appearance. Small milia noted on face. Weight 3700 g, infant feeding without issue, normal bowel movements, minimal jaundice noted during 1-week checkup but resolved with increased feeds and bowel movements.

▶ Which of the following findings require **immediate** follow-up? **Select all that apply.**

- ☐ Disrespectful nursing staff
- ☐ No hormones for several months
- ☐ Expected pregnancy chest changes
- ☐ Started chest binding 2 weeks ago
- ☐ Right chest assessment data
- ☐ Vital signs
- ☐ Feelings of imposter syndrome
- ☐ Newborn weight

▶ For each client finding below, specify if the finding is consistent with the condition of engorgement, plugged duct, or insufficient milk supply. Each finding may support more than one disease finding.

CLIENT FINDINGS	ENGORGEMENT	PLUGGED DUCT	INFECTION
Tender to touch	○	○	○
Fever	○	○	○
Sore nipples	○	○	○
Swollen tissue of left chest	○	○	○

The nurse is caring for a 30-year-old transmasculine client in the community health centre 1 month post-delivery who prefers the pronouns he/him/his.

Discharge Notes	**Progress Notes**

1400h: Client removed chest binding for further assessment. Left chest noted to have several white pearls × 3 on the tip of the nipple, with erythema and swelling noted on left chest. Left chest remains tender to touch. Client reported not listening during final client teaching as he wanted to go home and get away from the nursing staff. Client states feeling indifferent when asked if he wanted to continue chest feeding.

The nurse has reviewed the Progress Notes from 1400h.

▶ Complete the following sentence by choosing from the lists of options.

The client is at **highest** risk of developing _______________.

WORD CHOICES
Insufficient milk supply
Mastitis
Hemorrhage
Newborn rejection
Lack of newborn bonding

▶ For each nursing intervention, click to specify whether the intervention is **indicated** or **not indicated** for the care of this client.

POTENTIAL NURSING INTERVENTIONS	INDICATED	NOT INDICATED
Discuss potential causes of the mastitis	○	○
Confirm chest is best for newborn feeding	○	○
Collaborate with client about the best time to begin wearing chest binders	○	○
Discuss alternate sources of newborn nutrition	○	○

The nurse is caring for a 30-year-old transmasculine client in the community health centre 1 month post-delivery who prefers the pronouns he/him/his.

Discharge Notes	**Progress Notes**

1430h: Client teaching provided to the client and his partner, who was able to join the end of the appointment. The client has expressed a desire to continue to chest feed and supplement feeding with formula. He feels that the connection and bond between parent and newborn is important to him. The client reports feeling like he started chest binding too soon and would start slower binding and monitoring for clinical signs of mastitis.

The nurse has reviewed the Progress Notes from 1430h.

▶ Select 2 actions the nurse should take.

- ☐ Suggest the client purchase lanolin ointment
- ☐ Draw complete blood count, electrolytes
- ☐ Assess latch of the newborn to left chest
- ☐ Encourage the use of cold compresses for milk production
- ☐ Request an order for antibiotic treatment

▶ Identify 4 client sentences that would indicate an **understanding** of the client teaching.

CLIENT STATEMENTS	STATEMENTS BY THE CLIENT THAT DEMONSTRATE UNDERSTANDING
"I should stop chest feeding when it hurts."	
"It is important to maintain hydration."	
"I can use chest binders but gradually increase the time."	
"Nipple pain is normal."	
"Monitor for yeast to develop if the nipple does not heal."	
"We can supplement with formula."	

Maternal/Birth Parent Health 4.0

The nurse is caring for a 40-year-old female client on the postpartum unit.

Nurses' Notes

1500h: Client arrived on unit from recovery room after delivering a healthy newborn via Caesarean birth. Vital signs: T: 37.9°C (100.2°F); BP: 84/52; P: 102; RR: 14; with pulse oximetry of 92% on 2 L/min per nasal prongs. Client noted to be lethargic but rousable with voice and stimulation. Oriented to new environment and able to relay events of the delivery. Client unaware of significant blood loss during delivery, requiring 2 units of packed red blood cells, 3 L Ringers lactate in the operating room (OR) suite for hypotension documented at 77/54. Client presents with pallor, no cyanosis noted, capillary refill less than 3 seconds, with radial pulses × 2 weak but palpable to touch. Peripheral extremities cool to touch, pedal pulses × 2 and post-tibial pulses × 2 weak requiring Doppler but pulses present. Respirations regular and easy at rest. Client requires one-person assist to ambulate to washroom to void without assistance. Urine output noted to be dark, concentrated, and measured at 100 mL. The client's fundus was noted to be boggy during uterine massage and she was unable to expel any clots from the uterus.

▶ Identify the top 4 client findings that would require follow-up.

CLIENT FINDINGS
Vital signs
Age of the client
Characteristics of the fundus
Low urine output
Oxygen requirements
Blood loss

TOP 4 FINDINGS

▶ Which of the following complications is the client **at risk** of experiencing? **Select all that apply.**

- ☐ Pneumosepsis
- ☐ Heparin-induced thrombocytopenia
- ☐ Disseminated intravascular coagulation
- ☐ Acute respiratory distress syndrome
- ☐ Acute renal failure
- ☐ Postpartum hemorrhage

The nurse is caring for a 40-year-old female client on the postpartum unit.

Nurses' Notes

1630h: Client found sitting at the edge of the bed slumped over the bedside table. Vital signs: T: 37.7° C (99.9°F); BP 75/43; HR: 122; RR: 28; with pulse oximetry of 82% on 2 L/min. Upon assessment, client had difficulty answering easy questions but responsive, level of consciousness reduced since previous assessment. Client's breathing appears to be laboured, taking shallow breaths with indrawing noted at the chest wall, nasal flaring. Client expectorating blood-tinged sputum. Client appears to be grey in colour, cool to touch, capillary refill greater than 3 seconds. Bilateral radial pulses rapid but strong × 2, bilateral pedal pulses weak × 2. Skin cool to touch. No urine output noted.

The nurse has reviewed the Nurses' Notes from 1630h.

▶ Complete the following sentence by choosing from the list of options.

The client is at **highest** risk of developing _______________.

WORD CHOICES
Venous thromboembolism
Pulmonary embolism
Dysrhythmias
Acute myocardial infarction
Hemorrhagic shock

The nurse has reviewed the Nurses' Notes from 1500h and 1630h to plan care for this client.

▶ For each potential nursing intervention, specify whether the intervention is **indicated** or **not indicated** for the care of this client. Only one option per row can be selected.

POTENTIAL NURSING INTERVENTIONS	INDICATED	NOT INDICATED
Prepare to increase oxygen per nasal cannula	○	○
Set up the rapid infuser	○	○
Call a code blue	○	○
Request an order to administer blood products	○	○
Request an order to administer crystalloids	○	○

The nurse is caring for a 40-year-old female client on the postpartum unit.

Nurses' Notes | **Laboratory Results**

2300h:			
Hemoglobin 140–180 g/L (14–18 g/dL) (male) 120–160 g/L (12–16 g/dL) (female)	76 g/L (7.6 g/dL)	Sodium 136–145 mmol/L	145 mmol/L
Platelets 150–400 × 10^9/L (150 000–400 000/mm^3)	100 × 10^9/L (100 000/mm^3)	Potassium 3.5–5.1 mmol/L	4.8 mmol/L
White blood cells 3.5–12.0 × 10^9/L (3 500–12 000/mm^3)	9.9 × 10^9/L (9 900/mm^3)	Creatinine 53–106 mcmol/L (male) 44–97 mcmol/L (female)	255 mcmol/L
Neutrophils 3.0–5.8 × 10^9/L (3 000–5 800/mm^3)	5.0 × 10^9/L (5 000/mm^3)		

The nurse has received orders from the health care provider.

▶ Highlight or identify below the orders the nurse should perform right away.

Orders

1645h:
- Insert an in-dwelling urinary catheter
- Administer 0.9% sodium chloride (normal saline) 2 L bolus with rapid infuser
- Spiral computed tomography (CT) to be done in diagnostic imaging
- Insert another large-bore (at least 18 gauge) intravenous catheter
- Apply high-flow nasal prongs and titrate for pulse oximetry of greater than 92%
- Administer 1 unit platelets
- Administer 2 units packed red blood cells now
- Laboratory tests: D-dimer, arterial blood gas (ABG)

The nurse performed the interventions as ordered by the health care provider for the client.

▶ For each assessment finding, identify if the finding indicates that the client's condition has **improved**, has **not changed**, or has **declined**.

ASSESSMENT FINDINGS	IMPROVED	NO CHANGE	DECLINED
Skin cool to touch	○	○	○
BP 90/64	○	○	○
D-dimer result is positive	○	○	○
Urine output 30 mL/hr	○	○	○
Shortness of breath	○	○	○

Maternal/Birth Parent Health 5.0

The nurse is caring for a 46-year-old female client at the outpatient high-risk pregnancy clinic.

Progress Notes

May 12 at 0937h: Client was seen in the clinic for her 36-week appointment. Primary complaint is general malaise × 3 days, just a feeling of being unwell. The client's comorbidities include gestational diabetes mellitus and hypertension prior to pregnancy controlled through diet and exercise. The client presents as G2 T0 P0 A1 L0 with a previous miscarriage documented at 13 weeks. Client is accompanied to the clinic by their partner. Vital signs: T: 36.7°C (98.0°F); BP: 152/96; P: 97; RR: 22; with pulse oximetry of 97% on room air. Client presents with 8 out of 10 headache based on numerical rating scale, without any relief from acetaminophen, complains of blurry vision, denies numbness or tingling in hands or feet. Bilateral pupils equal in size and shape at 2 mm and react briskly to light. Motor power strong × 4 and gait steady with independent ambulation. Client indicates dizziness when rising too fast. Skin warm and dry to touch. Mild edema noted in client's bilateral hands, with wedding rings on left hand noted to be tight. Finger remains warm to touch and capillary refill less than 3 seconds. Bilateral radial pulses bounding and palpable, with apical pulses equal to radial pulses. Bilateral dorsalis pedis pulses palpable and regular to touch. Client denies any chest pain but states able to "feel" heart beating in her head. Client thinks they are silly for even saying that. Upon auscultation, bilateral fine inspiratory crackles noted to anterior bases of lung fields. Client denies any cough and noted to be taking short, shallow breaths. Client states her breathing has become more difficult as the pregnancy has progressed. Client denies any pain with urination, denies changes in frequency. Urine sample collected in the office to complete a urine dipstick. Client indicates no change in appetite, eating healthy but × 2 days feeling nauseated. Fetal heart rate documented at 146 beats per minute. Client referred to the obstetrical unit for further investigation.

▶ Highlight the assessment findings that require **immediate** follow-up.

Progress Notes

May 12 at 0937h: Client was seen in the clinic for their 36-week appointment. Primary complaint is general malaise × 3 days, just a feeling of being unwell. The client's comorbidities include gestational diabetes mellitus and hypertension prior to pregnancy controlled through diet and exercise. The client presents as G2 T0 P0 A1 L0 with a previous miscarriage documented at 13 weeks. Client is accompanied to the clinic with their partner. Vital signs: T: 36.7°C (98.0°F); BP: 152/96; P: 97; RR: 22; with pulse oximetry of 97% on room air. Client presents with 8 out of 10 headache based on numerical rating scale, without any relief from acetaminophen, complains of blurry vision, denies numbness or tingling in hands or feet. Bilateral pupils equal in size and shape at 2 mm and reactive briskly to light. Motor power strong × 4 and gait stead with independent ambulation. Client indicates dizziness when rising too fast. Skin warm and dry to touch. Mild edema noted in client's bilateral hands, with wedding rings on left hand noted to be tight. Finger remains warm to touch and capillary refill less than 3 seconds. Bilateral radial pulses bounding and palpable, with apical pulses equal to radial pulses. Bilateral dorsalis pedis pulses palpable and regular to touch. Client denies any chest pain but states able to "feel" heart beating in her head. Client thinks they are silly for even saying that. Upon auscultation, bilateral fine inspiratory crackles noted to anterior bases of lung fields. Client denies any cough and noted to be taking short, shallow breaths. Client states that their breathing has become more difficult as the pregnancy has progressed. Client denies any pain with urination, denies changes in frequency. Urine sample collected in the office to complete a urine dipstick. Client indicates no change in appetite, eating healthy but × 2 days feeling nauseated. Fetal heart rate documented at 146 beats per minute. Client referred to the obstetrical unit for further investigation.

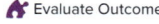

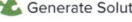

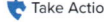

▶ Which of the following potential complications is the client at risk of experiencing? **Select all that apply.**

☐ Blindness
☐ Impaired immunity
☐ Seizures
☐ Venous thrombosis
☐ Leukopenia
☐ Gastritis
☐ Viral stomach infection

▶ Complete the following sentence by choosing from the list of options.

The client is at **highest** risk of developing __________ and __________ (word options 1) with effects to the fetus that may include ______________ (word options 2).

WORD OPTIONS 1	WORD OPTIONS 2
Anemia	Hypoglycemia
Dysrhythmias	Oligohydramnios
Stroke	Increased intrauterine growth
Pneumonia	Placenta previa
Acute renal failure	Hyperglycemia

The nurse is caring for a 46-year-old female client on the antepartum department of the obstetrical floor.

Progress Notes	**Nurses' Notes**	Laboratory Results	Vital Signs

May 12 at 1115h: Client received into care on the antepartum department. Client settled into a bed with external fetal monitor applied for continuous assessment. The client and partner present as anxious and scared given the client's age and the previous miscarriage. The client presents as alert and oriented to person, place, and time. Bilateral pupils equal in size and shape at 3 mm and react briskly to light. Client denies any chest pain. Presents with mild shortness of breath and difficulty catching her breath with longer sentences. Upon auscultation, coarse inspiratory crackles noted to bilateral anterior bases. Client noted to have dry nonproductive cough. Client denies any epigastric pain. Client positioned to be comfortable in the bed. Venous access device initiated and saline locked. Client has not voided upon arrival at the hospital.

The nurse has reviewed the client's Progress Notes from the high-risk clinic, the Nurses' Notes in the antepartum clinic at 1115h, and the Laboratory Results at 1132h.

▶ For each potential nursing intervention, identify whether the intervention is **indicated** or **not indicated** for the care of this client.

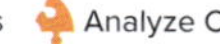

Progress Notes	Nurses' Notes	**Laboratory Results**	Vital Signs
1132h: Hemoglobin 140–180 g/L (14–18 g/dL) (male) 120–160 g/L (12–16 g/dL) (female)	98 g/L (9.8 g/dL)	Sodium 136–145 mmol/L	145 mmol/L
Platelets 150–400 × 10^9/L (150 000–400 000/ mm^3)	45 × 10^9/L (45 000/ mm^3)	Potassium 3.5–5.1 mmol/L	4.9 mmol/L
White blood cells 3.5–12.0 × 10^9/L (3 500–12 000/mm^3)	14 × 10^9/L (14 000/ mm^3)	Creatinine 53–106 mcmol/L (male) 44–97 mcmol/L (female)	186 mcmol/L
Neutrophils 3.0–5.8 × 10^9/L (3 000–5 800/ mm^3)	6.5 × 10^9/L (6 500/ mm^3)	Blood urea nitrogen (BUN) 2.9–8.2 mmol/L	8.0 mmol/L
Aspartate aminotransferase (AST) 0–35 U/L	82 U/L	PT (INR) 0.9–1.1	1.0
		PTT 60–70 seconds	66 seconds
Alanine aminotransferase (ALT) 35–55 g/L	77 g/L (7.7 g/dL)	Urine for protein 0—negative Trace—trace +1—0.3 g/L +2—1.0 g/L +3—3.0 g/L +4—more than 10 g/L	+2–1.0 g/L

Progress Notes	Nurses' Notes	Laboratory Results	**Vital Signs**

	1115h:	**1130h:**
T	36.9°C (98.4°F)	37.1°C (98.8°F)
P	108	115
RR	24	24
BP	164/112	168/116
Pulse oximetry reading	97% on room air	88% on room air

POTENTIAL NURSING INTERVENTIONS	INDICATED	NOT INDICATED
Ensure the client is isolated from family	○	○
Prepare to insert a nasogastric tube to minimize movement	○	○
Create a nonstimulating and quiet environment	○	○
Evaluate deep tendon reflexes at baseline assessment	○	○
Instruct the client to remain on strict bed rest	○	○
Limit fluid intake	○	○
Ensure all safety equipment such as suction and oxygen are available	○	○

Note: Each row must have one response option selected.

The nurse has reviewed the Nurses' Notes at 1115h, the Laboratory Results from 1132h, and the Vital Signs taken at 1115h and 1130h.

▶ Identify the 4 orders the nurse should consider a **priority**.

- ☐ Initiate magnesium infusion with a loading dose of 4 g followed by 1 g/hr IV
- ☐ Administer labetalol 100 mg PO to be taken twice a day
- ☐ Continuous external fetal monitoring
- ☐ Labs to draw q6h: complete blood count, electrolytes, creatinine, PT (INR), PTT, AST, ALT
- ☐ Ensure calcium gluconate is available
- ☐ Oxygen therapy 6 L/min (50% oxygen) for 1 hr then reassess
- ☐ Use a urine collection hat placed in the toilet
- ☐ Monitor input and output × 48 hr

▶ For each assessment finding, identify if the finding indicates that the client's condition has **improved**, has **not changed**, or has **declined**.

ASSESSMENT FINDINGS	IMPROVED	NO CHANGE	DECLINED
Client noted to be indrawing and having difficulty speaking	○	○	○
BP 135/85	○	○	○
Urine clear and measured at 170 mL/hr	○	○	○
Client presents with emesis ,50 mL of bile	○	○	○
Bilateral pupils equal in size and shape at 3 mm and react briskly to light	○	○	○

Note: Each row must have one response option selected.

Maternal/Birth Parent Health 6.0

The nurse on a postpartum unit is caring for a 42-year-old female client.

Nurse's Notes

1145h: The client was admitted to the postpartum unit after delivering a baby 25 minutes ago with Apgars of 7 at 1 minute and 9 at 5 minutes, through a forceps delivery. The newborn is currently in the nursery. The client, G1 T1 P0 A0 L1, experienced pre-eclampsia at the end of her pregnancy, prompting the need for induced labour. Vital signs: T: 38.2°C (100.8°F); BP: 90/60; P: 135; RR: 24; with pulse oximetry of 90% on room air. The client presents with lethargy, is difficult to rouse with verbal and physical stimulation. When awake, client obeys all commands, motor power strong × bilateral upper and lower extremities. Pupils measured at 2 mm, symmetrical in round shape, and react briskly to light. Client noted to return back asleep quickly after verbal or physical stimulation. S1 and S2 noted with no adventitious heart sounds auscultated. Apical pulse equals radial pulse. The client presents with pale conjunctiva with reduced perfusion noted on bilateral palms. Bilateral radial pulses bounding, regular and bilateral dorsalis pedis pulses noted to be weak but palpable. Capillary refill measured at 3 seconds. Skin cool to touch. Client denies chest pain but comments on feeling fast heart rate. Upon auscultation right lower base anterior lung sound noted to have fine inspiratory crackles that do not clear with cough. Left lung auscultated for clear air entry. Client taking rapid, shallow breaths without full lung expansion. Client does not complain about any shortness of breath, just fatigue. Nasal flaring noted prior to moving the client from the stretcher to the bed with minimal assistance. Client's lips mildly cyanotic. Oxygen at 2 L/min per nasal prongs applied as per intrapartum orders. The client's fundus noted to be boggy, not firm, and unable to expel any clots from the uterus with massage. Second-degree perineal tear noted with well-approximated stitches and repair. The client has not voided yet after delivery due to quick discharge from intrapartum to postpartum unit. The client is accompanied to the postpartum unit with her partner.

The nurse reviewed the Nurses' Notes from 1145h.

▶ Which of the following client findings require **immediate** follow-up? **Select all that apply.**

- ☐ Newborn's Apgars
- ☐ Episiotomy site
- ☐ Pallor
- ☐ Pupillary response
- ☐ Palpitations
- ☐ Nasal flaring
- ☐ Skin temperature
- ☐ Uterine characteristics
- ☐ Cyanosis
- ☐ Lung sounds

▶ Identify 2 complications the client is at risk of developing.

- ☐ Hypoxemia
- ☐ Anuria
- ☐ Respiratory acidosis
- ☐ Deep vein thrombosis
- ☐ Cerebral edema
- ☐ Anoxia
- ☐ Bleeding

The nurse on a postpartum unit is caring for a 42-year-old female client.

Nurse's Notes | Laboratory Results

1215h: Client found sitting at the edge of the bed in a tripod position over the bedside table. Client is short of breath, unable to speak in full sentences, indrawing noted at chest wall, with consistent nasal flaring as previously observed. Coarse crackles auscultated in right lower and middle lobe anteriorly with productive cough. Client presents ashen in colour. Capillary refill greater than 3 seconds and fingertips noted to be cyanotic with increasing cyanosis around the lips. Client complains of pain with inspiration and feeling lightheaded. Bilateral radial pulses remain palpable but weak and bilateral dorsalis pedis pulses remain weak but palpable. Shadowing noted on the client's episiotomy sutures. Fundus remains boggy and unable to firm up or expel clots even with fundal massage. Vital signs: T: 38.2°C (100.8°F); BP: 80/40; P: 139; RR: 32; pulse oximetry reading 75% on 2 L/min of oxygen per nasal prongs.
1220h: Health care provider notified of client status.

The nurse reviewed the Nurses' Notes from 1215h and 1220h and Laboratory Results at 1200h.

▶ Complete the following sentence by choosing from the list of options.

The client is at **highest** risk of developing ____________.

WORD OPTIONS
Infection
Dysrhythmias
Anorexia
Subdural hematoma
Amniotic fluid embolism

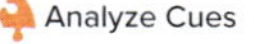
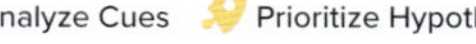
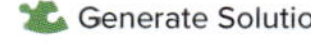
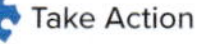
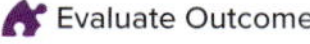
Recognize Cues · Analyze Cues · Prioritize Hypothesis · Generate Solutions · Take Action · Evaluate Outcomes

Nurse's Notes | **Laboratory Results**

1200h:			
Hemoglobin 140–180 g/L (14–18 g/dL) (male) 120–160 g/L (12–16 g/dL) (female)	67 g/L (6.7 g/dL)	Sodium 136–145 mmol/L	144 mmol/L
Platelets 150–400 × 10^9/L (150 000–400 000/mm^3)	44 × 10^9/L (44 000/mm^3)	Potassium 3.5–5.1 mmol/L	4.4 mmol/L
White blood cells 3.5–12.0 × 10^9/L (3 500–12 000/mm^3)	10 × 10^9/L (10 000/mm^3)	Creatinine 53–106 mcmol/L (male) 44–97 mcmol/L (female)	272 mcmol/L
Neutrophils 3.0–5.8 × 10^9/L (3 000–5 800/mm^3)	4.6 × 10^9/L (4 600/mm^3)	Blood urea nitrogen (BUN) 2.9–8.2 mmol/L	9.4 mmol/L

▶ For each potential nursing intervention, click to specify whether the intervention is **indicated** or **not indicated** for the care of this client.

POTENTIAL NURSING INTERVENTIONS	INDICATED	NOT INDICATED
Prepare to increase oxygen delivery or add a non-rebreather mask	○	○
Place client in semi-Fowler's position	○	○
Encourage rest for the client	○	○
Request an order to administer blood products	○	○
Provide emotional support to the client and partner	○	○
Request an order to administer hypertonic intravenous solutions	○	○

Note: Each row must have one response option selected.

The nurse has received orders from the physician.

▶ Highlight below the 4 orders the nurse should perform right away.

Orders

1220:
- Insert an in-dwelling urinary catheter
- Administer 0.9% sodium chloride (normal saline) 500 mL bolus × 1
- Spiral computed tomography (CT) to be done in diagnostic imaging
- Insert another large-bore (at least 18 gauge) peripheral venous access device
- Apply non-rebreather mask at 10 L/min and titrate for a pulse oximetry of greater than 92%
- Contact the blood bank and administer 2 units packed red blood cells ASAP
- Laboratory tests: complete blood count, electrolytes, PTT, INR, type and cross-match, repeat D-dimer, arterial blood gas

▶ For each new assessment finding, click to specify if the finding indicates the client's condition has **improved**, has **not changed**, or has **declined**.

ASSESSMENT FINDINGS	IMPROVED	NO CHANGE	DECLINED
RR 16	○	○	○
Urine output of 75 mL/hr	○	○	○
Pedal pulses found with Doppler	○	○	○
Ashen colour	○	○	○
BP 97/54 mm Hg	○	○	○
Fundus firms up with massage	○	○	○

Note: Each row must have one response option selected.

Pediatric Unfolding Cases

Pediatrics 1.0

The nurse is caring for a 19-year-old client (they/them) and their newborn on the postpartum unit.

Nurses' Notes

1115h: Client and newborn presented to the unit 1 hour after an uneventful delivery. Newborn Apgar's were documented at 7 and 9 with birth weight at 3750 g. Client able to void post-delivery with one-person assist. Newborn nursed within 20 minutes of delivery, but documentation indicated new parent had difficulty with obtaining a good latch for the newborn and gave up prior to admission to unit. Skin-to-skin contact recommended between new parent and newborn during feeding in the future. Client received no medical prenatal care prior to delivery of newborn as they hid the pregnancy from their parents. Client requesting assistance with position and determining proper latch during nursing, "I know I want to breastfeed my baby." Client assisted into semi-reclining position with newborn lying prone, skin-to-skin on bare chest. Newborn latched well onto nipple. New parent commended on attempting different positions to find which one best supports their newborn.
1128h: Called to bedside by client stating, "my baby is blue, my baby is blue!" Upon further assessment, axillary temperature 37.0°C (98.6°F), newborn moves all four extremities independent with appropriate tone, bilateral symmetrical features, and soft, flat anterior fontanel. Systolic murmur noted with rhythm regular and strong. Respiratory rate noted to be 67 breaths per minute with nasal flaring and equal chest expansion.

▶ Which of the following assessment findings would be most concerning for the nurse? **Select all that apply.**

☐ Apgars
☐ Birth weight
☐ Cyanosis
☐ Soft fontanel
☐ Systolic murmur
☐ Heart rhythm
☐ Respiratory rate
☐ Nasal flaring

▶ Complete the following sentence by choosing from the list of options.

The client is at **highest** risk of developing ______________ as a complication.

WORD OPTIONS
Fluid imbalance
Low pulse oximetry level
Hypothermia
Bleeding
High blood sugar

▶ Identify the correct word choices from below to fill in the blanks in the following sentence.

The client is at **highest** risk of developing ______________ (word options 1) as evidenced by the client's ______________ (word options 2).

WORD OPTIONS 1	WORD OPTIONS 2
Croup	Vital signs
Aspiration pneumonia	Respiratory assessment
Bacterial endocarditis	Nutritional assessment
Tet spell	Parent to newborn connection

The nurse is caring for a 19-year-old client (they/them) and their newborn on the postpartum unit.

Nurses' Notes | Diagnostic Results

1130h: Health care provider notified of change in newborn status. Orders received to send newborn to diagnostic interventions for an echocardiogram.

The nurse has reviewed the Nurses' Notes from 1130h and Diagnostic Results from 1245h.

▶ For each potential nursing intervention, specify whether the intervention is **indicated** or **not indicated** for the care of this client.

Nurses' Notes | **Diagnostic Results**

1245h:

Summary:
Normal LV size with decreased wall function
Normal RV size with normal wall function
Mitral valve regurgitation noted with large ventricular septal defect identified
Mild to moderate pulmonic stenosis identified
Large overriding aorta noted in size
Due to significant size of the ventricular septal defect and narrowing of the pulmonic stenosis, there is a left-to-right shunt of blood flow.

Interpretation:
A noncomplex complete transthoracic echocardiogram was performed. Fair study quality. There is indication that the newborn has a congenital heart defect called tetralogy of Fallot. Further investigations are warranted.

POTENTIAL NURSING INTERVENTIONS	INDICATED	NOT INDICATED
Prepare the newborn for a chest X-ray	○	○
Encourage bottle feeding	○	○
Give the family space to deal with new diagnosis	○	○
Monitor pulse oximetry on the newborn	○	○

Given the newborn's condition, neonatal general surgery was consulted. It was determined the newborn will require surgery within the year to correct the congenital heart defects.

▶ Select 2 actions the nurse should take.

- ☐ Prepare the newborn for surgery now
- ☐ Suggest meditation and yoga for coping
- ☐ Request a consult social work
- ☐ Contact the client's parents
- ☐ Provide client teaching about newborn heart failure

The nurse has reviewed the Nurses' Notes from 1130h and Diagnostic Results from 1245h and is aware of the impending surgical plan for the newborn upon discharge.

▶ For each of the statements made by the client, click to specify whether the statement indicates an **understanding** or **no understanding** of the discharge teaching provided.

CLIENT STATEMENTS	UNDER-STANDING	NO UNDER-STANDING
"I will need to notify the surgical team if the baby is not gaining weight."	○	○
"If the baby turns blue, I need to put the baby against my chest with the knees up. I think you call it a knee–chest position."	○	○
"Seizures do not run in my family so I do not think it would happen with the baby."	○	○
"I have called my best friend who is going to stay with me and help with the baby."	○	○
"If I see the baby is working hard to breath, I will call the nurse on call."	○	○

Pediatrics 2.0

The nurse in the emergency department (ED) is caring for a 3-year-old client.

Nurses' Notes | Vital Signs

1845h: Client arrived at ED accompanied by birth parents. Parents indicated client had low-grade fever all day and was lethargic. Parents felt client had a virus, administered children's acetaminophen (160 mg/5 mL × 1 dose) at 1200h, and encouraged fluid hydration by giving child almond milk and water; client vomits from cow's milk and has been drinking almond milk for 1 year. Client fell asleep on couch at approximately 1620h and parents found client with increased full-body stiffness, eyes open and deviating upward, and unresponsive to voice or physical stimulation. Parents brought child to ED, who presents sitting on birth parent's lap resting head against upper chest. Client found to move all four extremities independently, able to follow commands and squeeze fingers moderately. Pupils equal in size at 2 mm and bilateral reaction to light. Heart rate regular and strong auscultated at the apical site. Skin warm and dry to touch. Lungs auscultated for bilateral clear air entry throughout anterior and posterior. Client has not eaten any food today, only drank almond milk and water. Bowel sounds remain hypoactive × 4. Parents estimate fluid intake at 700 mL of almond milk and 700 mL of water. Client has voided once today a small amount.

Nurses' Notes | **Vital Signs**

Emergency Department
1845h:

T	38.4°C (101.1°F)
P	112
RR	24
BP	95/60
Pulse oximetry reading	98% on room air

▶ Highlight the findings that would require **immediate** follow-up.

Nurses' Notes | Vital Signs

1845h: Client arrived at ED accompanied by birth parents. Parents indicated client had low-grade fever all day and was lethargic. Parents felt client had a virus, administered children's acetaminophen (160 mg/5 mL × 1 dose) at 1200h, and encouraged fluid hydration by giving child almond milk and water; client vomits from cow's milk and has been drinking almond milk for 1 year. Client fell asleep on couch at approximately 1620h and parents found client with increased full-body stiffness, eyes open and deviating upward, and unresponsive to voice or physical stimulation. Parents brought child to ED, who presents sitting on birth parent's lap resting head against upper chest. Client found to move all four extremities independently, able to follow commands and squeeze fingers moderately. Pupils equal in size at 2 mm and bilateral reaction to light. Heart rate regular and strong auscultated at the apical site. Skin warm and dry to touch. Lungs auscultated for bilateral clear air entry throughout anterior and posterior. Client has not eaten any food today, only drank almond milk and water. Bowel sounds remain hypoactive × 4. Parents estimate fluid intake at 700 mL of almond milk and 700 mL of water. Client has voided once today a small amount.

The nurse has reviewed the Nurses' Notes at 1845h and the Vital Signs at 1845h.

▶ Which of the following complications is the client at risk of experiencing? **Select all that apply.**

- ☐ Fluid imbalance
- ☐ Leukocytosis
- ☐ Confusion
- ☐ Dysrhythmias
- ☐ Bowel obstruction

Nurses' Notes | **Vital Signs**

1845h: Emergency Department	
T	38.4° C (101.1°F)
P	112
RR	24
BP	95/60
Pulse oximetry reading	98% on room air

The nurse in the emergency department (ED) is caring for a 3-year-old client.

Nurses' Notes | Vital Signs | **Laboratory Results**

1900h: Emergency Department			
Hemoglobin 95–140 g/L (14–18 g/dL) (male) 120–160 g/L (12–16 g/dL) (female)	110 g/L (11 g/dL)	Sodium 136–145 mmol/L	127 mmol/L
Platelets 150–400 × 10^9/L (150 000–400 000/mm^3)	267 × 10^9/L (267 000/mm^3)	Potassium 3.5–5.1 mmol/L	4.5 mmol/L
White blood cells 3. 3.5–12.0 × 10^9/L (3 500–12 000/mm^3)	8.9 × 10^9/L (8 900/mm^3)	Creatinine 53–106 mcmol/L (male) 44–97 mcmol/L (female)	50 mcmol/L
Neutrophils 3.0–5.8 × 10^9/L (3 000–5 800/mm^3)	5.2 × 10^9/L (5 200/mm^3)	Blood urea nitrogen (BUN) 2.9–8.2 mmol/L	3.2 mmol/L

The nurse has reviewed the Laboratory Results at 1900h.

▶ Complete the following sentence by choosing from the lists of options.

The client is at **highest** risk of developing ____________ (word options 1) as evidenced by ________________ (word options 2).

WORD OPTIONS 1	WORD OPTIONS 2
Shaken baby syndrome	Hemoglobin level
Bacterial meningitis	White blood cell level
Seizure disorder	Sodium level
Hydrocephalus	Potassium level

▶ For each potential order, identify whether the intervention is **indicated** or **not indicated** for the client.

POTENTIAL ORDERS	INDICATED	NOT INDICATED
Computed tomography (CT) head	○	○
Hypotonic intravenous fluids	○	○
Chest X-ray	○	○
Pulse oximetry	○	○
Packed red blood cells	○	○
Anticonvulsant medication	○	○

Note: Each row must have one response option selected.

▶ Which of the following 3 actions should the nurse take **immediately**?

- ☐ Initiate 3% normal saline at a rate of 3 mL/kg
- ☐ Social work consult
- ☐ Encourage oral intake of food
- ☐ Document general observation of seizure
- ☐ Remove harmful objects around the client
- ☐ Restrain child

The nurse has initiated the interventions as ordered by the health care provider for the client.

▶ For each assessment finding, identify if the finding indicates that the client's condition has **improved**, has **not changed**, or has **declined**.

ASSESSMENT FINDINGS	IMPROVED	NO CHANGE	DECLINED
New blood draw with sodium at 137 mmol/L	○	○	○
Emesis	○	○	○
Client sitting upright reading a book	○	○	○
No further seizure activity	○	○	○

Note: Each row must have one response option selected.

Pediatrics 3.0

The nurse is caring for a 16-year-old male client in the emergency department (ED).

Nurses' Notes

0018h: Client presented to the ED via emergency medical services (EMS) with a left lateral/posterior back stab wound after a presumed gang altercation. Client denies any comorbidities. Vital signs: T: 37.7°C (99.9°F); BP: 100/74; P: 115; RR: 22; with pulse oximetry of 90% on room air. Client presents as alert and oriented, pleasant, and cooperative. Client rates pain 4 out of 10 on a numerical pain scale but observed to grimace with movement or change in position. Motor power × 4 extremities strong and independent. Client obeys commands. Steady gait noted. Significant diminished air entry noted on left lower lung posterior and anterior chest wall. Symmetrical chest wall movement noted. No adventitious breath sounds noted anterior or posterior when lungs auscultated. Client taking shallow breaths at rest with increased depth with minimal ambulation. Client noted to have dry mucous membranes, conjunctiva pale in colour. Radial pulses weak × 2, bilateral dorsalis pedis pulses weak and post-tibial pulses require Doppler. Bilateral lower extremities cool to touch with bilateral upper extremities warm and dry to touch. Client complaining of nausea. Denies previous emesis. Urinal at the bedside, no urine noted. Stab wound covered with an abdominal pad dressing × 2 pads and 4 × 4 gauze, secured to the skin with Mefix tape, noted to be saturated with sanguineous drainage. Constant ooze noted. A #18 peripheral intravenous catheter inserted to the right antecubital site.

▶ Which of the following findings require **immediate** follow-up? **Select all that apply.**

- ☐ Mucous membranes
- ☐ Urine output
- ☐ Lung sounds
- ☐ Vital signs
- ☐ Dressing
- ☐ Nausea
- ☐ Pain
- ☐ Skin temperature

▶ Complete the following sentence by choosing from the word choices below to fill in each blank.

The nurse should recognize that the client is potentially experiencing complications of ______________ and ______________.

WORD CHOICES
Anuria
Bleeding
Dizziness
Petechiae
Infection
Impaired gas exchange

▶ Complete the following sentence by choosing from the list of options.

The client is at **highest** risk of developing ______________.

WORD CHOICES
Pneumonia
Deep vein thrombosis
Kidney failure
Dysrhythmia
Acute anemia
Thrombocytopenia

The nurse is caring for a 16-year-old male client in the emergency department (ED).

Nurses' Notes | Laboratory Results

0330h: Laboratory in to draw blood for required tests. Client rouses easily, speech appropriate, complaining of being tired. Vital signs: T: 37.9°C (100.2°F); BP: 92/68; P: 117; RR: 24; with pulse oximetry of 89% on room air but increases with deep breathing for a pulse oximetry of 91%.
0430h: The parents are at the client's bedside and called for assistance. Vital signs: T: 37.8°C (100.0°F); BP: 80/54; P: 135; RR: 26; with pulse oximetry of 84% on room air. Client noted to have increased lethargy and fatigue but remains rousable with physical stimulation. Speech remains appropriate. Client states pain is 7 out of 10 on a numerical rating scale. Client presents with increased pallor. Bilateral dorsalis pedis pulses present with the use of Doppler. Client noted to have shortness of breath at rest with an increased respiratory rate of 30 breaths per minute with minimal change of position in bed or minimal exertion. Breath sounds remain unchanged from previous assessment. Hypoactive bowel sounds auscultated × 4. Concentrated urine of 220 mL noted in the urinal. Health care provider notified of client status.

Nurses' Notes | **Laboratory Results**

0330h:

Test	Result	Test	Result
Hemoglobin 140–180 g/L (14–18 g/dL) (male) 120–160 g/L (12–16 g/dL) (female)	77 g/L (7.7 g/dL)	Sodium 136–145 mmol/L	145 mmol/L
Platelets 150–400 × 10^9/L (150 000–400 000/mm^3)	300 × 10^9/L (300 000/mm^3)	Potassium 3.5–5.1 mmol/L	5.0 mmol/L
White blood cells 3.5–12.0 × 10^9/L (3 500–12 000/mm^3)	10.5 × 10^9/L (10 500/mm^3)	Creatinine 53–106 mcmol/L (male) 44–97 mcmol/L (female)	55 mcmol/L
Neutrophils 3.0–5.8 × 10^9/L (3 000–5 800/mm^3)	5.2 × 10^9/L (5 200/mm^3)	Blood urea nitrogen (BUN) 2.9–8.2 mmol/L	3.0 mmol/L
Type and screen	AB positive		

The nurse has reviewed the Nurses' Notes at 0330h and 0430h and Laboratory Results from 0330h.

▶ For each nursing intervention, identify whether the intervention is **indicated** or **not indicated** for the care of this client.

POTENTIAL NURSING INTERVENTIONS	INDICATED	NOT INDICATED
Request an order to initiate oxygen therapy	○	○
Prepare to insert an in-dwelling urinary catheter	○	○
Encourage oral fluid intake	○	○
Request an order to insert a second peripheral venous access device	○	○
Prepare the rapid fluid infuser	○	○
Inform the client they will be receiving albumin, a blood product	○	○

Note: Each row must have one response option selected.

The nurse has received orders from the health care provider.

▶ Identify below the 3 orders the nurse should perform right away.

- ☐ Monitor intake and output
- ☐ 0.9% sodium chloride (normal saline) 500 mL IV bolus × 1 then reassess BP
- ☐ Transfuse 1 unit of packed red blood cells (PRBC) ASAP
- ☐ Chest X-ray
- ☐ Oxygen therapy 0–6 L to maintain peripheral oximetry greater than 92%
- ☐ Administer hydromorphone 10 mg IV for pain every 1–4 hr

The nurse performed the interventions as ordered by the health care provider for the client.

▶ For each assessment finding, identify if the finding indicates that the client's condition has **improved**, has **not changed**, or has **declined**.

ASSESSMENT FINDINGS	IMPROVED	NO CHANGE	DECLINED
Pulse oximetry reading 93%	○	○	○
Dressing changes required every 1 hour	○	○	○
Pale mucous membranes	○	○	○
Dorsalis pedis pulses palpable	○	○	○
BP 102/75	○	○	○

Note: Each row must have one response option selected.

Pediatrics 4.0

The nurse is caring for a 7-year-old client in the pediatric emergency department.

Progress Notes

2032h: Client was brought to the emergency department by both parents with complaints of lethargy, fever, headache all day unrelieved with analgesic, nausea, and vomiting. The parents thought their child was just tired after a sleepover at a friend's house the night before, but the child's headache and listlessness got worse throughout the day. The client is unvaccinated. Vital signs: T: 38.7°C (101.7°F); BP: 102/68; P: 92; RR: 18; with pulse oximetry of 98% on room air. Client presents as agitated from being at the hospital, irritable when assessed, swatting at the use of a stethoscope, then falls back asleep quickly after being touched. Client able to move extremities independently × 4, even when asleep. Client moans in pain when light is turned on, so dim lighting used during assessments. Difficult to assess pupillary response to light and assess size and shape. Client presents with stiffness and is unable to put chin to their chest without drawing up bilateral knees. S1 and S2 heart sounds, apical heart rate regular and equals radial pulse. Bilateral radial pulses regular and palpable. Lips are cracked, tongue noted to be dry. Clear air entry noted throughout all lung fields. No shortness of breath noted. Active bowel sounds auscultated × 4 quadrants with abdomen soft and round during palpation. Emesis basin present due to client retching with clear bile. Client has not eaten any food today. Client has not voided yet upon arrival at the hospital. Peripheral venous access devices inserted right and left antecubital fossa.

▶ Select 5 findings that require **immediate** follow-up.

- ☐ Temperature
- ☐ Photophobia
- ☐ Stiff neck
- ☐ Listlessness
- ☐ Bowel sounds
- ☐ Lack of appetite
- ☐ Emesis
- ☐ Urine output

▶ For each client finding, identify whether the finding is consistent with the disease process of migraine, gastroenteritis, or bacterial meningitis. Each finding may support more than one disease process.

CLIENT FINDINGS	MIGRAINE	GASTROENTERITIS	BACTERIAL MENINGITIS
Fever	○	○	○
Lethargy	○	○	○
Neck stiffness	○	○	○
Headache	○	○	○
Nausea	○	○	○
Emesis	○	○	○

Note: Each column must have at least one response option selected.

▶ Complete the following sentence by choosing from the list of options.

The client is at **highest** risk of developing _______________ and _______________.

WORD OPTIONS
Increased intracranial pressure
Dysrhythmias
Seizure
Cardiomyopathy
Weight gain

The nurse is caring for a 7-year-old client in the pediatric emergency department.

Progress Notes

2205h: Called to the client's room by the parent. The client is difficult to rouse. Pupils sluggish to respond to light with left pupil measured at 4 mm and right pupil measured at 2 mm. Client's breathing altered and client is noted to be taking short, shallow breaths. Client unable to answer questions correctly, providing slurred speech. Unable to follow commands. Noted to projectile vomit while assessing the client. Vital signs: T: 39.7°C (103.5°F); BP: 124/62; P: 62; RR: 22; with pulse oximetry of 86% on room air. Health care provider notified of changes in client status.

The nurse has reviewed the Progress Notes from 2205h.

▶ For each potential nursing intervention, identify whether the intervention is **indicated** or **not indicated** for the care of this client.

POTENTIAL NURSING INTERVENTIONS	INDICATED	NOT INDICATED
Reposition the client in high-Fowler's position	○	○
Prepare client for a lumbar puncture	○	○
Place the client on contact isolation	○	○
Ensure suction is working properly	○	○
Provide reassurance to the parents	○	○

Note: Each row must have one response option selected.

The nurse has reviewed the Orders from 2220h.

▶ Highlight the 4 orders that the nurse should consider a priority.

Orders

2220h:
- Acetaminophen for temperature greater than 38.5°C (101.3°F)
- Strict monitoring of input and output
- Initiate broad-spectrum cephalosporin (Ceftriaxone)
- Phenytoin to be administered per peripheral venous access device
- Initiate oxygen therapy at 2 L/min to 6 L/min to achieve pulse oximetry greater than 92%
- Laboratory tests: blood cultures, electrolytes, glucose, complete blood count, coagulation profile
- Computed tomography (CT) head
- Keep head of the bed elevated to 45-degree angle
- Minimize stimulation in the room, lights dimmed

The orders were implemented by the nurse.

▶ For each assessment finding, identify whether the finding indicates that the client's condition has **improved**, has **not changed**, or has **declined**.

ASSESSMENT FINDINGS	IMPROVED	NO CHANGE	DECLINED
Client requests a popsicle	○	○	○
T 39.7°C (103.5°F)	○	○	○
Respirations become regular with good lung expansion	○	○	○
Hemiparesis	○	○	○
Nauseated with emesis	○	○	○

Note: Each row must have one response option selected.

Pediatrics 5.0

The nurse is caring for a 2-month-old infant on the general medicine pediatric unit.

Nurses' Notes

1115h: Client's birth parent brought the infant to the emergency department with pallor and wet-sounding cough, absent of a fever. Pregnancy and delivery were unremarkable. Vital signs: T: 37.2°C (99.0°F); BP: 114/62 (upper extremities) and 80/50 (lower extremities); P: 145; RR: 50; with pulse oximetry of 92% on room air. Bilateral upper extremities and trunk warm to touch with bounding brachial pulses noted bilateral upper arms. Bilateral lower extremities noted to be cool to touch and weak bilateral femoral pulses. S1 and S2 heart sounds auscultated with an S3 present. Systolic murmur auscultated at the left sternal border. Fine inspiratory crackles auscultated throughout all lung fields anteriorly. Abdomen rounded but soft. Client having regular bowel movements and soiled diapers despite difficulty feeding. Infant was chest fed until a week ago and now nutrition is obtained through formula. The parent became concerned when the infant became diaphoretic and the respiratory rate increased. Client's weight at last well-baby checkup was in the 50th percentile and currently in the 15th percentile, despite change to formula. A peripheral venous access device was inserted and intravenous fluids initiated for hydration. The birth parent, a refugee, did not receive any prenatal care or ultrasound for assessment. Upon discharge from the hospital, minimal social resources were in place for a new parent speaking English as a second language.
1230h: Parent called for assistance. Client presents with cyanotic lips and fingertips with shrill, high-pitched cry. Vital signs: T: 37.2°C (99.0°F); P: 165; RR: 64; with pulse oximetry of 80% on room air. Bilateral pupils small in size but reactive to light. Murmur persists with an audible S3 present. Petechiae noted on lower extremities that were not present during initial assessment. Health care provider was notified.

The nurse has reviewed the Nurses' Notes at 1115h and 1230h.

▶ Identify the top 4 client findings that would require **immediate** follow-up.

- ☐ Temperature
- ☐ Abnormal heart sounds
- ☐ Bilateral upper extremities warm, bilateral lower extremities cool
- ☐ Cyanotic lips
- ☐ Discontinuation of chest feeding
- ☐ Characteristics of the cry
- ☐ Weight

▶ Which of the following complications is the client at risk of developing? **Select all that apply.**

- ☐ Impaired renal perfusion
- ☐ Peripheral edema
- ☐ Increased intracranial pressure
- ☐ Impaired gas exchange
- ☐ Delayed gastric emptying
- ☐ Respiratory infection
- ☐ Reduced cardiac output

▶ Complete the following sentence by choosing from the list of options.

The client is at **highest** risk of developing ___________ as a result of ___________.

WORD OPTIONS
Anemia
Dysrhythmias
Stroke
Hypoxemia
Renal failure
Coarctation of the aorta

▶ For each potential diagnostic intervention, identify whether the intervention is **indicated** or **not indicated** for the care of this client.

POTENTIAL INTERVENTIONS	INDICATED	NOT INDICATED
Doll's head manoeuvre	○	○
Computed tomography (CT) of the head	○	○
Cardiac electrocardiography (ECG)	○	○
Magnetic resonance imaging (MRI)	○	○
Chest X-ray	○	○
Cardiac echocardiography	○	○

Note: Each row must have one response option selected.

The nurse is caring for a 2-month-old infant on the general medicine pediatric unit.

Nurses' Notes | Diagnostic Results

1245h: Pediatric thoracic surgeon consulted for further assessment. A transthoracic echocardiogram ordered to be completed for assessment and oxygen to be applied via non-rebreather mask to maintain pulse oximetry at 95%.
1300h: Pediatric thoracic surgeon present during the transthoracic echocardiogram. Parents informed of treatment plan and surgical repair intervention. All questions answered and consent signed. Client to be prepped for repair of coarctation of the aorta. Parents informed of the plan.
1900h: Client returned from the recovery room.

Nurses' Notes | **Diagnostic Results**

1258h: Echocardiogram Report
The client presents with symptoms associated with coarctation of the aorta. There is consistent narrowing of the postductal type with an approximation of 0.5 cm in size and confirmation of the diagnosis of coarctation of the aorta.

The nurse has reviewed the Nurses' Notes from 1245h, 1300h, and 1900h and Diagnostic Results from 1258h.

▶ Highlight the priority nursing action(s) the nurse should take when caring for this client postoperatively.

- Ensure the client's hospital bed is prepared for the parent
- Check that all safety equipment is working, such as suction and oxygen flow meter
- Obtain baseline vital signs upon return to the unit
- Outline any bleeding on the dressing with a pen and document finding
- Monitor for pain by observing for rigidity or thrashing, crying, lowered brows

▶ Which of the following outcomes would the nurse consider a **decline** in the client's status upon returning to the unit. Each nursing action may support more than one priority finding.

BODY SYSTEM	NEW ASSESSMENT FINDINGS
Neurological	○ Sunken fontanel ○ Moves all four extremities independently ○ Requires q2h pain medication ○ Temperature 38.9°C (102.0°F)
Cardiovascular	○ Capillary refill greater than 4 seconds ○ Heart rate 170 ○ S1 and S2 heart sounds only ○ Client extremities cool to touch × 4
Respiratory	○ Fine inspiratory crackles ○ Pulse oximetry measured at 97% on 3 L/min by mask ○ Respiratory rate 68 ○ No cyanosis noted
Gastrointestinal	○ 3% weight loss since last known weight ○ Decreased tear production ○ Desire to take formula from bottle

Note: Each category must have at least one response option chosen.

Pediatrics 6.0

The nurse is caring for a 4-year-old client on a general pediatric medical unit.

Nurses' Notes | History and Physical

1000h: Client admitted to general pediatric medical unit as a direct admission after being seen by the family physician at 0830h same day. Client awoke with a temperature of 38.5°C (101.3°F), sore throat, and painful swallowing this morning. Client was able to take sips of fluids and ate popsicles at home. Health care provider decided to admit the client as further observation was warranted.
1050h: Client presents with increased irritability, restlessness, and difficulty finding comfortable position. Both parents are present for emotional support for client.

The nurse has reviewed the Nurses' Notes from 1000h and 1050h as well as the History and Physical at 1000h.

▶ Which of the following assessment findings require **immediate** follow-up? **Select all that apply**.

- ☐ Pupillary response
- ☐ Alertness
- ☐ Pain with swallowing
- ☐ Lung sound characteristics
- ☐ Pulses
- ☐ Pulse oximetry
- ☐ Respiratory breathing pattern characteristics

Nurses' Notes | **History and Physical**

1000h:

Body System	**Findings**
Neurological	Alert and oriented to person, place, and time. Cooperative, obeys commands. Denies headache. Complains of feeling "cold." Bilateral pupils briskly react to light. Gait steady but provided assistance from parents with ambulation. Primarily sitting on parent's lap in the bed. Generalized feeling unwell.
Cardiovascular	Bilateral upper and lower extremities warm and dry to touch with palms of hands noted to be cool to touch. Capillary refill less than 3 seconds. Bilateral radial pulses palpable and weak. Bilateral dorsalis pedis pulses palpable and weak. T: 38.7°C (101.7°F); BP: 101/62; P: 99; RR: 22; with pulse oximetry of 92% on room air.
Pulmonary	Client noted to be taking shallow breaths and avoiding swallowing. Client reports sore throat that hurts to drink or when eating popsicles. Quiet, clear air entry auscultated in all anterior lung fields. No cough noted. No stridor noted. No use of accessory muscles.
Gastrointestinal	Abdomen round and flat. No pain with palpation. Client denies feeling hungry. The parent reports no bowel movement noted × 2 days.

▶ For each client finding, identify if the finding is consistent with the disease process of pneumonia, acute epiglottitis, or respiratory syncytial virus. Each finding may support more than one disease process.

CLIENT FINDINGS	PNEUMONIA	ACUTE EPIGLOTTITIS	RESPIRATORY SYNCYTIAL VIRUS
Fever	○	○	○
Shallow breaths	○	○	○
Sore throat	○	○	○
Restlessness	○	○	○
Lack of cough	○	○	○
Clear air entry	○	○	○

Note: Each column must have at least one response option selected.

The nurse is caring for a 4-year-old client on a general pediatric medical unit.

Nurses' Notes | History and Physical

1200h: Client's parents rang for assistance. Client noted to have nasal flaring with the use of suprasternal and substernal accessory muscles. Client found sitting upright and forward at the edge of the bed, leaning over the bedside table, drooling clear sputum. Client presents with pallor, and skin cool to touch × 4 extremities. Lips noted to be cyanotic. Capillary refill remains at less than 3 seconds. No adventitious breath sounds auscultated in the anterior lung fields. Audible stridor noted with breathing. Vital signs: T: 38.7°C (101.7°F); BP: 97/57; P: 102; RR: 26; with pulse oximetry of 86% on room air. Health care provider notified of change of status.

▶ Complete the following sentence by choosing from the list of options.

The client is at **highest** risk of developing _______________ (word options 1) as evidenced by _______________ (word options 2) and _______________ (word options 2).

WORD OPTIONS 1	WORD OPTIONS 2
Epistaxis	Drooling
Atrophic glossitis	Pallor
Foreign body aspiration	Lung sounds
Respiratory distress	Capillary refill
Pneumothorax	Nasal flaring
Candidiasis	Leaning over the bedside table

▶ For each potential nursing intervention, identify whether the intervention is **indicated** or **not indicated** for the care of this client.

POTENTIAL NURSING INTERVENTIONS	INDICATED	NOT INDICATED
Place the client in Trendelenburg position	○	○
Ensure the difficult airway cart is present	○	○
Encourage oral fluid intake	○	○
Ensure suction is working correctly	○	○
Prepare to insert a peripheral venous access device	○	○
Ensure the client has a regular diet ordered	○	○

Note: Each row must have one response option selected.

▶ Select 4 orders the nurse should perform right away.
- ☐ Initiate humidified oxygen therapy at 2–6 L/min to maintain pulse oximetry greater than 95%
- ☐ Ceftriaxone 25 mg/kg IV q12h
- ☐ 0.9% normal saline (sodium chloride) 50 mL/hr
- ☐ Transfer to pediatric intensive care unit for close monitoring
- ☐ Monitor intake and output
- ☐ Vital signs q4h and prn

▶ Which of the following assessment findings indicate improvement in the client's overall status? **Select all that apply.**
- ☐ Temperature 37.9°C (100.2°F)
- ☐ Client watching a movie on their parent's lap and laughing
- ☐ Able to eat a popsicle without complaining of sore throat
- ☐ Client has voided 250 mL in 8 hours since IV fluids initiated
- ☐ Respiratory rate 16 breaths per minute on 4 L of continuous oxygen via nasal prongs

Mental Health Unfolding Cases

Mental Health 1.0

The nurse is caring for a 33-year-old male client in the emergency department.

Admission Notes

2138h: Police department called to scene and found client wandering streets, barefoot, disheveled, poor hygiene, with no identification. Emergency medical service (EMS) were contacted to assess client. Client stated to EMS, "I need help. I can't sleep or eat; I can't seem to take care of my kids and I'm all they have." The client added more information: "I lost my job as a cook in a local restaurant 6 months ago because of the COVID-19 pandemic and cannot find another job. It's been really hard paying for food, not to mention the rent. I am going to be evicted. Where are my kids and I going to go? I feel so hopeless; what kind of a parent can't care for their children?" Client reports type 2 diabetes mellitus comorbidities treated by diet and exercise. Overall, client appears to be in good health. Client is appropriate, alert and oriented to person, place, and time, moves all extremities independently, no weakness noted. Chest remains clear upon air entry, client denies any chest pain, S1, S2 auscultated with no additional abnormal heart sounds noted. Client reports losing weight, approximately 2 kilograms in the last week, due to loss of appetite. Denies any suicidal ideation, "I could never do that to my children." Bilateral bottom of feet assessed and noted to have four toonie-sized excoriated open areas with dried blood. No drainage noted.

▶ Highlight below or write down on a separate piece of paper the findings that require **immediate** follow-up.

Admission Notes

2138h: Police department called to scene and found client wandering streets, barefoot, disheveled, poor hygiene, with no identification. Emergency medical service (EMS) were contacted to assess client. Client stated to EMS, "I need help. I can't sleep or eat; I can't seem to take care of my kids and I'm all they have." The client added more information: "I lost my job as a cook in a local restaurant 6 months ago because of the COVID-19 pandemic and cannot find another job. It's been really hard paying for food, not to mention the rent. I am going to be evicted. Where are my kids and I going to go? I feel so hopeless; what kind of a parent can't care for their children?" Client reports anxiety, type 2 diabetes mellitus as comorbidities treated by diet and exercise. Overall, client appears to be in good health. Client is appropriate, alert and oriented to person, place, and time, moves all extremities independently, no weakness noted. Chest remains clear upon air entry, client denies any chest pain, S1, S2 auscultated with no additional abnormal heart sounds noted. Client reports losing weight, approximately 2 kilograms in the last week due to loss of appetite. Denies any suicidal ideation, "I could never do that to my children." Bilateral bottom of feet assessed and noted to have four toonie-sized excoriated open areas with dried blood. No drainage noted.

▶ For each client finding below, click to specify if the finding is consistent with the disease process of acute anxiety, major depressive disorder, or bipolar disorder. Each finding may support more than one disease process.

CLIENT FINDINGS OR STATEMENTS	ANXIETY	DEPRESSION	BIPOLAR DISORDER
"I can't eat or sleep."	○	○	○
Client found wandering and disheveled	○	○	○
"I feel helpless."	○	○	○
Possibility of eviction	○	○	○
Denies suicidal ideation	○	○	○

▶ Choose the **most likely** options for the information missing from the statement below by selecting from the lists of options provided.

The client's is at **highest** risk of developing _______ (word options 1) as evidenced by the client's stated ______ (word options 2).

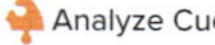 Recognize Cues 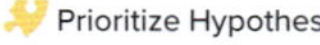 Analyze Cues 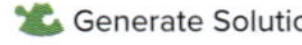 Prioritize Hypothesis 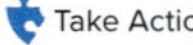 Generate Solutions 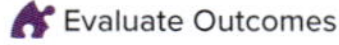 Take Action Evaluate Outcomes

WORD OPTIONS 1	WORD OPTIONS 2
Acute anxiety	Feelings of hopelessness
Suicidal ideation	Loss of employment
Major depressive disorder	Insomnia and loss of appetite
Impaired health	Fear of possible homelessness

The nurse is caring for a 33-year-old male client on the mental health unit.

Admission Notes | Nurses' Notes | Orders

2330h: Client is transferred to the mental health unit for further observation.

Admission Notes | **Nurses' Notes** | Orders

2342h: Client received into care from the emergency department visibly upset, with a flat affect, crying, and inconsolable to verbal stimuli. Vital signs: T: 36.4°C (97.5°F); BP: 120/84; P: 82; RR: 14; with pulse oximetry of 92% on room air.
2352h: Lorazepam 1 mg SL × 1 dose administered as ordered
0149h: Client reported suicidal thoughts, not only taking his life but also those of his children. He did not know what else to do. He planned on doing it last night but decided to go for a walk instead. He was unfortunately mugged, physically assaulted, and lost his shoes in the scuffle. He thinks being found by the police and EMS is a blessing. He needed help, he just did not know where to turn.

Admission Notes | Nurses' Notes | **Orders**

2350h:
•Lorazepam 1 mg SL × 1 dose
•Escitalopram 10 mg PO od
•Engage in unit group focused on problem solving
•Suicide precautions per hospital policy
•Complete blood count (CBC)
•Glycosylated hemoglobin (HbA_{1c}) level
•Urinalysis
•Point-of-care glucose finger stick daily in morning
•Daily weights

The nurse has reviewed the Nurses' Notes at 2342h, 2352h, and 0149h as well as the Orders at 2350h.

▶ Which of the following nursing care plans would be **most appropriate** for this client? **Select all that apply.**
- ☐ Client will be able to accurately describe rationale for prescribed antidepressant medication
- ☐ Client will collaborate on determining treatment goals
- ☐ Client will be able to accurately describe rationale for precautions that will be implemented for client safety
- ☐ Client will verbalize importance of attending unit-centred problem-solving group sessions
- ☐ Client with utilize extended periods of alone time for self-reflection
- ☐ Client will snack frequently on high-carbohydrate foods to supplement diet and manage weight loss

▶ Complete the following sentence by choosing from the list of nursing intervention options.
The nurse's **first** action should be to ____________.

NURSING INTERVENTIONS
Provide medication education regarding monoamine oxidase inhibitors (MAOIs)
Assess client frequently for need to institute one-on-one observation
Evaluate client's understanding of the signs of hypoglycemia
Assure client that the typical coarse of medication therapy for depression lasts 3 to 6 months

The nurse is caring for a 33-year-old male client on the mental health unit.

Admission Notes | **Nurses' Notes** | Orders

7 days from admission: Client has participated in group sessions, began oral antidepressant medication, and will continue attending as outpatient. Discharge instructions provided.

The nurse reviews the Nurses' Notes 7 days from admission.

▶ Identify which of the following statements by the client indicates an **understanding** or **no understanding** of discharge instructions.

CLIENT STATEMENTS	UNDERSTANDING	NO UNDERSTANDING
"I need to keep my appointments with the clinic, so I won't get depressed again."	○	○
"I'll call the clinic's hot line immediately if I start having suicidal thoughts."	○	○
I'll need an electroencephalogram (EEG) done regularly."	○	○
"The stress will go away as soon as I get a job."	○	○

Mental Health 2.0

The nurse is caring for a 54-year-old female client admitted to a general medical unit.

Nurses' Notes

1000h: Client was brought to the emergency department (ED) by her partner due to confusion, unstable gait with frequent falls, slurring of words, and difficulty tending to activities of daily living (ADLs) independently, leading to a failure to thrive. The client has a history of alcohol use disorder (30 years +), depression, hypertension, seizures, and type 2 diabetes mellitus. Vital signs: T: 37.8°C (100.0°F); BP: 150/90; P: 122; RR: 28; with pulse oximetry of 92% on room air. Upon assessment on the unit, client presents as confused, unable to remember name and reason for being at the hospital, unable to follow commands as simple as sitting at edge of the bed. Motor power strong × 4. Client attempts to leave room despite several redirect attempts, gait remains unstable with independent mobility. Bed alarm placed with four side rails applied. PEARL 3 mm, client denies pain, bilateral hand tremors noted. Client's breathing noted to be tachypneic but not laboured, clear air entry throughout all lung fields, no cough noted. Skin flushed and diaphoretic to touch, capillary refill is less than 3 seconds, S1 S2 heart sounds, no abnormal heart sounds auscultated, denies chest pain. Client has not requested to void. Will continue to monitor urine output. Partner reports that client has not taken in much fluid or nutrition × 24 hours. Last known drink of alcohol was approximately 12 hours ago.

▶ Identify the top 4 client findings that would require **immediate** follow-up.

CLIENT FINDINGS
Vital signs
Unable to follow commands
Unstable gait
Hand tremors
Low urine output
Last known drink of alcohol 12 hours ago
Tachypnea

TOP 4 FINDINGS

▶ Which of the following complications is the client at risk of experiencing? **Select all that apply.**

☐ Heart failure
☐ Pneumonia
☐ Seizures
☐ Delirium
☐ Respiratory depression
☐ Dysrhythmias
☐ Pulmonary embolus
☐ Diabetic ketoacidosis

The nurse is caring for a 54-year-old female client admitted to a general medical unit.

Nurses' Notes | **Laboratory Results**

1000h: (Drawn in ED)

Hemoglobin 140–180 g/L (14–18 g/dL) (male) 120–160 g/L (12–16 g/dL) (female)	85 g/L (8.5 g/dL)	Sodium 136–145 mmol/L	154 mmol/L
Platelets 150–400 × 10^9/L (150 000–400 000/mm^3)	90 × 10^9/L (90 000/mm^3)	Potassium 3.5–5.1 mmol/L	5,8 mmol/L
White blood cells 3.5–12.0 × 10^9/L (3 500–12 000/ mm^3)	6.8 × 10^9/L (6 800/mm^3)	Creatinine 53–106 mcmol/L (male) 44–97 mcmol/L (female)	187 mcmol/L
		Blood glucose	6.2 mmol/L

The nurse has reviewed the Laboratory Results from 1000h.

▶ Complete the following sentence by choosing from the list of options.

The client is at **highest** risk of developing ___________ (word options 1) as evidenced by the ___________ (word options 2).

WORD OPTIONS 1	WORD OPTIONS 2
Stroke	Potassium level
Deep vein thrombosis	Sodium level
Infection	Platelet level
Grand mal seizures	White blood cell count level

The nurse is caring for a 54-year-old female client admitted to a general medical unit.

Nurses' Notes | Laboratory Results

1225h: Client heard screaming out, "Get away from me! Stop touching me." During assessment the nurse observed the client swatting at their arm and hiding under the blanket.

The nurse has reviewed the Nurses' Notes from 1000h and 1225h and is planning care for the client.

▶ For each potential nursing intervention, identify whether the intervention is **indicated** or **not indicated** for the care of this client.

POTENTIAL NURSING INTERVENTIONS	INDICATED	NOT INDICATED
Prepare the client for Foley catheter insertion	○	○
Reorient client to the environment	○	○
Prepare to administer an opioid	○	○
Contact a family member to sit with the client	○	○
Request an order to insert a peripheral IV	○	○

The nurse has received orders from the health care provider.

▶ Select 3 orders that the nurse should perform right away.

- ☐ Administer lorazepam 1–2 mg SL × 1 dose now, then as per Clinical Institute Withdrawal Assessment for Alcohol–Revised (CIWA-AR) protocol
- ☐ Place client in bilateral wrist restraints
- ☐ Initiate 0.9% sodium chloride (normal saline) at 75 mL/hr
- ☐ Prepare for cardioversion
- ☐ Continue to monitor vital signs
- ☐ Client to remain NPO
- ☐ Administer Resonium calcium 15 g PO × 1
- ☐ Initiate CIWA-AR protocol

The nurse is caring for a 54-year-old female client admitted to a general medical unit.

Nurses' Notes | Laboratory Results

1230h: Lorazepam 2 mg SL given as per orders. Will continue to monitor client as per CIWA-AR protocol.
1330h: Client found lethargic and difficult to rouse, requiring sternal rub. GCS 10. Client pale and skin cool to touch. Bilateral radial pulses weak × 2, bilateral pedal pulses weak × 2. Vital signs: T: 38.5°C (101.3°F); BP: 88/60; P: 135; RR: 32; with pulse oximetry of 81% on room air. Oxygen applied to client at 3 L/min per nasal prongs to achieve pulse oximetry of 93%. Health care provider contacted. Client assessed for an unwitnessed tonic-clonic seizure. Will continue to monitor client status.
1345h: Client assessed after unwitnessed tonic-clonic seizure. Client noted to open eyes to nurse entering room, alert and oriented to person, place, and time. Able to follow commands. Motor power strong × 4 extremities. Pupils equal and reactive to light at 3 mm. Client speech clear and appropriate. No agitation noted. Skin colour noted to be warm and perfused to touch. Capillary refill less than 3 seconds. Radial pulses strong and regular × bilateral radials, bilateral pedal pulses strong × 2. Respirations regular and easy at rest. Vital signs: T: 38.2°C (100.8°F); BP: 92/66; P: 104; RR: 24; with pulse oximetry of 95% on 3 L/nasal prongs.

The nurse performed the interventions as ordered by the health care provider for the client. The nurse reviewed the Nurses' Notes from 1230h, 1330h, and 1345h.

▶ For each assessment finding, specify if the finding indicates that the client's condition has **improved**, has **not changed**, or has **declined**.

ASSESSMENT FINDINGS	IMPROVED	NO CHANGE	DECLINED
RR 24	○	○	○
BP 92/66	○	○	○
Speech clear and appropriate	○	○	○
Oxygen level at 3 L/min per nasal prongs	○	○	○
Skin perfused	○	○	○

Note: Each row must have one response option selected.

Mental Health 3.0

The nurse is caring for a 78-year-old female client on a cardiology unit.

Nurses' Notes

2010h: Client arrived on the internal medicine unit dehydrated due to a gastrointestinal illness that included nausea and vomiting for 3 days and required cardiovascular monitoring. Past medical history includes bipolar illness, diagnosed at 52 years old and managed with lithium. Vital signs: T: 36.8°C (101.5°F); BP: 92/55; P: 57; RR: 22; with pulse oximetry of 90% on room air. Client presents with scattered thoughts, does not understand reason for admission, and does not know the date or time. Client states season is summer when the month is currently March. Small tremor noted on right hand, will continue to monitor. Pupils noted to be 3 mm, equal in size, and react briskly to light. Client reports a "pounding heart" but denies chest pain, skin cool to touch. Bilateral radial pulses palpable but weak. Capillary refill less than 3 seconds. Mucous membranes dry. Chest auscultated for bilateral clear air entry posterior and anterior. Abdomen flat and soft. Bowel sounds auscultated in all four quadrants. Kidney basin presented to client in the event of emesis. None noted since arriving on the unit. Client complaining of feeling thirsty.

▶ Which of the following findings require **immediate** follow-up? **Select all that apply.**

- ☐ Gastrointestinal presentation
- ☐ Client orientation
- ☐ Tremor
- ☐ "Pounding heart"
- ☐ Cardiovascular perfusion
- ☐ Mucous membranes
- ☐ Thirsty

The nurse is caring for a 78-year-old female client on a cardiology unit.

Nurses' Notes | **Laboratory Results**

1900h: (Drawn in Emergency Department)

Hemoglobin 140–180 g/L (14–18 g/dL) (male) 120–160 g/L (12–16 g/dL) (female)	110 g/L (11 g/dL)	Sodium 136–145 mmol/L	130 mmol/L
Platelets 150–400 × 10^9/L (150 000–400 000/mm^3)	220 × 10^9/L (220 000/ mm^3)	Potassium 3.5–5.1 mmol/L	5.5 mmol/L
White blood cells 3.5–12.0 × 10^9/L (3 500–12 000/ mm^3)	6.4 × 10^9/L (6 400/mm^3)	Creatinine 53–106 mcmol/L (male)	
44–97 mcmol/L (female)	350 mcmol/L		
		Blood glucose	4.4 mmol/L
		Lithium level 0.6–1.2 mEq/L	2.17 mEq/L

The nurse reviews the Laboratory Results at 1900h.

▶ Identify the most appropriate word choice from below to fill in the blank in the following sentence.

The nurse should recognize that the client is potentially experiencing symptoms associated with _______________.

WORD CHOICES
Stroke
Myocardial infarction
Lithium toxicity
A urinary tract infection
Sepsis inflammatory response syndrome
Hypoglycemia

The nurse reviews all information.

▶ Complete the following sentence by choosing from the lists of options.

The client is at **highest** risk of developing _______________ (word options 1) as evidenced by the client's _______________ (word options 2).

WORD OPTIONS 1	WORD OPTIONS 2
Muscle weakness	Right hand tremor
Pulmonary embolism	Sodium level
Cardiogenic shock	Need for cardiac monitoring
Convulsions	Respiratory rate

▶ For each body system below, click to specify the potential nursing interventions that would be appropriate for the care of this client. Each body system may support more than one potential nursing intervention.

BODY SYSTEM	POTENTIAL NURSING INTERVENTIONS
Neurological	O Sensory exam every 4 hours O Monitor level of consciousness O Seizure protocols
Cardiovascular	O Vitals signs every 4 hours or more if needed O Monitor cardiovascular rhythm for ventricular tachycardia O Insert arterial line
Renal	O Monitor output O Request 24-hour urine collection O Urine test strip every morning

The nurse is caring for a 78-year-old female client on a cardiology unit.

Nurses' Notes | Laboratory Results

2215h: During evening hygiene care, client noted to have tonic-clonic seizure that lasted for 22 seconds. No evacuation of bowels of bladder. Client placed in recovery position and noted to be taking small breaths. Pupils measured at 3 mm, equal and brisk to light. Vital signs: T: 36.8°C (98.2°F); BP: 86/57; P: 55; RR: 28; with pulse oximetry of 82% on room air. Oxygen applied at 2 L/min per nasal prongs. Client opens eyes to command. Health care provider notified
2217h: Vital signs: T: 37.3°C (99.1°F); BP: 90/55; P: 57; RR: 20; with pulse oximetry of 93% on 2 L/min per nasal prongs.
2230h: Vital signs: T: 37.0°C (98.6°F); BP: 86/52; P: 52; RR: 20; with pulse oximetry of 93% on 2 L/min per nasal prongs. Client more awake, responsive. Oriented to person, place, and time. Client noted to be lethargic but more alert.

The nurse has reviewed the Nurses' Notes from 2215h, 2217h, and 2230h.

The nurse has received orders from the health care provider.

▶ Select 3 actions the nurse should perform right away.

☐ Initiate a large-bore peripheral intravenous catheter
☐ Administer 3% sodium chloride (normal saline) at 25 mL/hr
☐ Laboratory tests: CBC, electrolytes, lithium level, type and cross-match
☐ Prepare client for a computed tomography (CT) head
☐ Insert Foley catheter

The nurse is caring for a 78-year-old female client on a cardiology unit.

Nurses' Notes | Laboratory Results

0600h: Client slept through the night. Aroused easily when vitals were required. No further seizure activity noted. Vital signs: T: 37.0°C (98.6°F); BP: 99/62; P: 59; RR: 18; with pulse oximetry of 97% on room air. Tremor of right hand remains. Client reports feeling of nausea but only able to wretch, no emesis. Client states feeling better.

Nurses' Notes | **Laboratory Results**

1900h: (Drawn in Emergency Department)			
Hemoglobin 140–180 g/L (14–18 g/dL) (male) 120–160 g/L (12–16 g/dL) (female)	110 g/L (11 g/dL)	Sodium 136–145 mmol/L	130 mmol/L
Platelets 150–400 × 10^9/L (150 000–400 000/mm^3)	220 × 10^9/L (220 000/mm^3)	Potassium 3.5–5.1 mmol/L	5.5 mmol/L
White blood cells 3.5–12.0 × 10^9/L (3 500–12 000/mm^3)	6.4 × 10^9/L (6 400/mm^3)	Creatinine 53–106 mcmol/L (male) 44–97 mcmol/L (female)	350 mcmol/L
		Blood glucose	4.4 mmol/L
		Lithium level 0.6–1.2 mEq/L	2.17 mEq/L
0600h:			
Hemoglobin 140–180 g/L (14–18 g/dL) (male) 120–160 g/L (12–16 g/dL) (female)	99 g/L (9.9 g/dL)	Sodium 136–145 mmol/L	135 mmol/L
Platelets 150–400 × 10^9/L (150 000–400 000/mm^3)	200 × 10^9/L (200 000/mm^3)	Potassium 3.5–5.1 mmol/L	5.0 mmol/L
White blood cells 3.5–12.0 × 10^9/L (3 500–12 000/mm^3)	6.0 × 10^9/L (6 000/mm^3)	Creatinine 53–106 mcmol/L (male) 44–97 mcmol/L (female)	320 mcmol/L
		Blood glucose	5.2 mmol/L

The nurse reviewed the Nurses' Notes from 0600h and Laboratory Results from 0600h.

▶ For each assessment finding, specify if the finding indicates that the client's condition has improved, not changed, or has declined.

ASSESSMENT FINDINGS	IMPROVED	NO CHANGE	DECLINED
Nausea	○	○	○
Blood pressure	○	○	○
Hemoglobin	○	○	○
Oxygen level	○	○	○
Skin perfused	○	○	○

Note: Each row must have one response option selected.

Mental Health 4.0

The nurse is caring for a 20-year-old male client on the mental health unit.

Nurses' Notes | History and Physical

2010h: Client arrived at the emergency department via emergency medical services (EMS) after the police were called to locate the client. The client was found running along the river without any shoes in December yelling, "I have to get away. Help! Help! They are after me!" The client is an out-of-province local university student living in a bachelor unit in residence on campus. Because COVID-19 precautions had been lifted, the client attended an on-campus party the night he was found, where he smoked cannabis. He reports being a regular cannabis user. The client's parents contacted the unit after being notified by a third party. They said the client is an introvert who does not associate with many people and found it unusual he smoked cannabis. The client has a limited social circle. In high school he said he was romantically involved with a girl who was adamant she barely knew him and obtained a restraining order against the client. Vital signs: T: 37.7°C (99.9°F); BP: 122/60; P: 76; RR: 18; with pulse oximetry of 98% on room air. Client was uneasy, noted to look at opening of the door several times during assessment. Client states, "I know they will come back for me. They will find me." Writer reassured client no one was in the doorway and that there is security in the hospital for safety. Client repeated "security in the hospital for safety."

Nurses' Notes | **History and Physical**

Body System	Findings
Neurological	Client presents with flat affect. Found rearranging towels in the bathroom and placed within perfect distance on the counter. Denies hearing voices but adamant people were chasing him: "I know they will come for me. They will find me." States he does not shower. Client presents as disheveled as noted by his dirty clothes and uncombed hair. Client reports the shower in his apartment is broken. States he has thought about ending his life, has sent texts about this to his family and knows that when he decides to do it things will be better for everyone. He reports not feeling like doing anything, losing motivation.
Pulmonary	Bilateral fine inspiratory crackles auscultated posteriorly. Dry cough noted.
Cardiovascular	Client states he feels his heart is racing and can hear it pounding in his head. No edema noted. Pulses noted to be bilaterally strong in radials. Mucous membranes dry.
Gastrointestinal	Client presents with lower normal body weight. States he is not eating for fear "they will poison him." He has not told anyone but feels safe now.
Renal	Client has not voided since arrival at hospital. Smell of urine noted on clothes.

▶ Highlight findings from the History and Physical that require **immediate** follow-up.

Body System	Findings
Neurological	Client presents with flat affect. Found rearranging towels in the bathroom and placed within perfect distance on the counter. Denies hearing voices but adamant people were chasing him: "I know they will come for me. They will find me." States he does not shower. Client presents as disheveled as noted by his dirty clothes and uncombed hair. Client reports the shower in his apartment is broken. States he has thought about ending his life, has sent texts about this to his family and knows that when he decides to do it things will be better for everyone. He reports not feeling like doing anything, losing motivation.
Pulmonary	Bilateral fine inspiratory crackles auscultated posteriorly. Dry cough noted.
Cardiovascular	Client states he feels his heart is racing and can hear it pounding in his head. No edema noted. Pulses noted to be bilaterally strong in radials. Mucous membranes dry.
Gastrointestinal	Client presents with lower normal body weight. States he is not eating for fear "they will poison him." He has not told anyone but feels safe now.
Renal	Client has not voided since arrival at hospital. Smell of urine noted on clothes.

▶ Select 2 potential complications that this client is at risk of experiencing.

- ☐ Ventricular dysrhythmias
- ☐ Hypotension
- ☐ Pleural effusion
- ☐ Acute renal failure
- ☐ Hypertension

▶ Complete the following sentence by choosing from the list of options.

The nurse should recognize that the client is potentially experiencing ____________________ (word options 1) due to symptoms of ____________________ (word options 2).

WORD OPTIONS 1	WORD OPTIONS 2
Generalized anxiety disorder	Suicidal ideation
Mania	Isolation
Post-traumatic stress disorder	Persecution
Addictions	Motivation
Psychosis	Hallucinations (olfactory)

The nurse is caring for a 20-year-old male client on the mental health unit.

Nurses' Notes	History and Physical	Laboratory Results

21000h:			
Hemoglobin 140–180 g/L (14–18 g/dL) (male) 120–160 g/L (12–16 g/dL) (female)	130 g/L (13 g/dL)	Sodium 136–145 mmol/L	148 mmol/L
Platelets 150–400 × 10^9/L (150 000–400 000/mm^3)	253 × 10^9/L (253 000/mm^3)	Potassium 3.5–5.1 mmol/L	5.5 mmol/L
White blood cells 3.5–12.0 × 10^9/L (3 500–12 000/mm^3)	9.9 × 10^9/L (9 900/mm^3)	Creatinine 53–106 mcmol/L (male) 44–97 mcmol/L (female)	187 mcmol/L
Neutrophils 3.0–5.8 × 10^9/L (3 000–5 800/mm^3)	5.6 × 10^9/L (5 600/mm^3)	Blood glucose	10.2 mmol/L

▶ For each body system below, specify the potential nursing intervention that would be appropriate for the care of this client. Each body system may support more than one potential nursing intervention.

BODY SYSTEM	POTENTIAL NURSING INTERVENTIONS
Neurological	○ Administer atypical antipsychotics, such as olanzapine ○ Encourage therapeutic group therapy ○ Promote sleep–wake cycle
Cardiovascular	○ Encourage oral intake of fluids ○ Administer sodium polystyrene sulfonate powder (Resonium) (or Patiromer) ○ Monitor for atrial fibrillation
Gastrointestinal	○ Encourage small meals and packaged foods such as crackers or peanut butter ○ Allow sugar drinks such as carbonated beverages ○ Encourage client to eat in his room

▶ Which of the following actions should the nurse take? **Select all that apply.**

- ☐ Request an order for sodium polystyrene sulfonate powder (Resonium) (or Patiromer)
- ☐ Administer antipsychotic medication, olanzapine
- ☐ Initiate 0.9% sodium chloride per peripheral intravenous catheter
- ☐ Prepare client to join group therapy activities
- ☐ Connect the client to continuous cardiac monitoring
- ☐ Insert a Foley urinary catheter.

The nurse is caring for a 20-year-old male client on the mental health unit.

Nurses' Notes	History and Physical	Laboratory Results

3 weeks later: Discharge summary: Client was admitted for psychosis as evidenced by delusional thinking related to schizophrenia and exuberated due to cannabis use. The client was brought to the emergency department by police. The client had attended a party where he smoked cannabis and later believed that he was being chased and was in danger of being harmed. The client attended a rave because he thought that he could avoid being found in a large crowd.
Potassium levels returned to normal and presently are at 4.3 mmol/L. Client is willing to take olanzapine 10 mg orally bid as prescribed. Client aware that he needs to avoid alcohol and illicit drug use. Client's psychotic symptoms have diminished, and he no longer responds to delusions of people chasing him. Client attends to hygiene every other day. Denies suicidal ideation and denies thoughts of self-harm. Client recognizes the need for continued medication and the benefits of attending a weekly support group to manage positive and negative symptoms of schizophrenia, develop healthy coping strategies to reduce stress, and build positive relationships. Client teaching provided on these aspects of the treatment plan.

The nurse reviews the discharge summary.

▶ For each of the statements made by the client, click to specify whether the statement indicates an **understanding** or **no understanding** of the discharge teaching provided.

CLIENT STATEMENTS	UNDER-STANDING	NO UNDER-STANDING
"I need to keep my regular appointments with my psychiatrist."	○	○
"I will have to withdraw from school to avoid stress."	○	○
"It is ok if I miss a dose. I can take it when I remember."	○	○
"If I do everything right, I can cure my illness."	○	○
"Attending outpatient group therapy is important for me to feel connected to other people."	○	○

8 Let's Practise Stand-Alone Case Studies

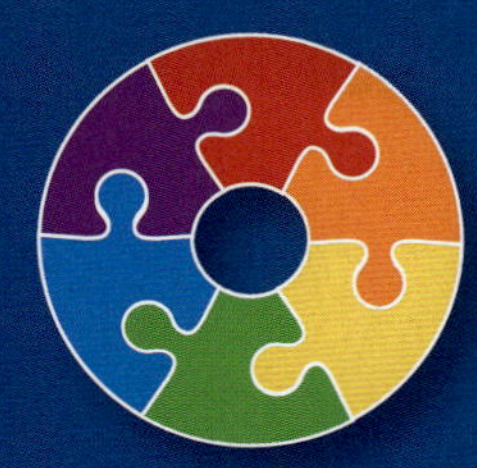

The following stand-alone case studies will cover content from medical-surgical topics as well as those from maternity/postpartum, pediatrics, and mental health. As you practise these case studies and review the answers, identify not only your strengths but also your gaps in knowledge related to content. As you work through the practise cases, you will recognize areas of the cognitive steps that may be strengths and those that require more practice. Remember, a bow-tie case study is designed to assess the test writer's understanding of each level of the cognitive steps (recognizing cues, analyzing those cues, developing a hypothesis, generating a solution or plan of care, taking action, and evaluating client outcomes). A trend case study is a narrative that occurs over time and may or may not include the primary diagnosis. It may include only one Next Generation NCLEX® item type question. Make notes about your own strengths and areas for improvement, then make a plan to work on these gaps. The answer key to these cases is in Chapter 10.

Medical-Surgical Bow-tie Cases

Medical-Surgical 1.0

The nurse is caring for a 19-year-old client in a community-based sexual health clinic.

Progress Notes

1000h: Client presents to the community sexual health clinic with complaints of voiding several times per hour, sharp, burning sensation when starting to void, chills, and a generalized feeling of unwell × 2 days. Client indicates they are in a monogamous same-sex relationship for 1 month which now includes intercourse. No previous comorbidities and currently only taking birth control pill to regulate menstruation. Vital signs: T: 38.5°C (101.3°F); BP: 120/77; P: 75; RR: 14; with pulse oximetry of 99% on room air. Client presents alert and oriented to person, place, and time. Pleasant during assessment and expresses anxiety about what could be wrong. Denies any chest pain, no shortness of breath. Peripheral pulses palpable and strong, no peripheral edema noted, capillary refill less than 3 seconds. Client reports an urgent sensation to void and has been incontinent at times trying to make it to the washroom. Client reports embarrassment with being incontinent. They have reduced their oral intake so as "not to have an accident."

The nurse is reviewing the client's assessment data to prepare the client's plan of care.

▶ Complete the diagram by identifying from the choices below to specify what condition the client is most likely experiencing, 2 actions the nurse should take to address that condition, and 2 parameters the nurse should monitor to assess the client's progress.

Action to Take	Condition Most Likely Experiencing	Parameter to Monitor
Action to Take		Parameter to Monitor

Action to Take	Potential Condition	Parameters to Monitor
Insert a urinary catheter	Renal failure	Fluid intake balance
Provide a requisition to collect a urine specimen for urinalysis	Stress incontinence	Temperature
Encourage oral cranberry juice intake	Urinary tract infection	Heart rate
Request an order for antibiotic therapy	Urinary retention	Urine colour
Prepare the client for a bladder scan		Pulse oximetry

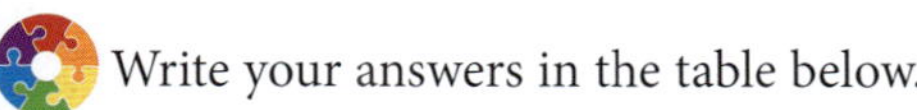

Write your answers in the table below.

Action to Take	Condition Most Likely Experiencing	Parameter to Monitor
Action to Take		Parameter to Monitor

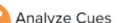

Medical-Surgical 2.0

The nurse is caring for a 92-year-old male client on a medical unit awaiting long-term care placement.

Nurses' Notes	Vital Signs	Medications

0424h: Client rang for assistance and nurse found client on the floor beside the bed. The client states he was getting up to use the washroom, felt like the room was spinning upon standing, became incontinent of urine, slipped on the urine, then slid down the side of the bed. The client presents alert and oriented to person place, time, and situation. Denies hitting head on any portion of the bed or floor and denies losing consciousness at any time. Denies any pain at present. Pupils equal and reactive to light at 2 mm. Moving all four extremities independently with motor power strong. Client was able to assist with standing and denies any pain at present. Client denies any chest pain, shortness of breath, or palpitations. Client assisted to washroom and cleaned of urine, his linens changed, and client repositioned in bed. The client's past medical history includes hypertension, benign prostate hyperplasia, dyslipidemia, coronary artery disease with myocardial infarction in 2002.

Nurses' Notes	**Vital Signs**	Medications

	1600h	**2300h**	**0424h**
T	36.7°C (98.0°F)	37.0°C (98.6°F)	36.9°C (98.4°F)
P	84—regular	76—regular	62—regular
RR	16	18	16
BP	110/76	108/72	88/52
Pulse oximetry reading	96% on room air	95% on room air	96% on room air

Nurses' Notes	Vital Signs	**Medications**

Furosemide (loop diuretic) 20 mg PO twice a day
Metoprolol (beta blocker) 50 mg PO twice a day
Ramipril (angiotensin converting enzyme inhibitor) 2.5 mg PO once a day
Lipitor (HMG-CoA reductase inhibitor) 40 mg PO once a day

The nurse is reviewing the client's assessment data to prepare the client's plan of care.

▶ Complete the diagram by identifying from the choices below to specify what condition the client is most likely experiencing, 2 actions the nurse should take to address that condition, and 2 parameters the nurse should monitor to assess the client's progress.

Action to Take	Condition Most Likely Experiencing	Parameter to Monitor
Action to Take		Parameter to Monitor

Action to Take	Potential Condition	Parameters to Monitor
Administer oxygen at 2 L/min via nasal cannula	Traumatic head injury	Blood pressure
Provide a urinal at the bedside	Atrial fibrillation	Temperature
Discuss with the health care provider the dosages and times of medications	Urinary tract infection (UTI)	Pulse oximetry
Request an order for antibiotic therapy	Postural hypotension	Urine output
Call a code blue		Pain

Write your answers in the table below.

Action to Take	Condition Most Likely Experiencing	Parameter to Monitor
Action to Take		Parameter to Monitor

Medical-Surgical 3.0

The nurse is caring for a 16-year-old client on a pediatric general medical unit.

Nurses' Notes

0924h: Client presents to the unit with diarrhea and failure to thrive. Previous comorbidities include cerebral palsy with bilateral contractures noted on wrists, elbows, and hips and a percutaneous endoscopic gastrostomy (PEG) tube in situ for nutrition. Vital signs: T: 37.3°C (99.1°F); BP: 112/64; P:109; RR: 24; with pulse oximetry of 90% on room air. On assessment, client presents as nonverbal but opens eyes to voice and tracks with eyes. Client is unable to follow commands but moves all extremities independently in the bed. Pupils equal and reactive to light. Skin cool to touch with dry mucous membranes noted. Pulses bounding, strong and regular. Apical = radial pulse. Client's breathing noted to be tachypneic, with fine crackles in bilateral lower lungs with minimal cough reflex. Client positioned in high-Fowler's position. Foley catheter in situ as client is incontinent of urine. Dark, concentrated urine noted in the Foley bag with 250 mL documented from 8-hour night shift. Client presents as cachectic with lower body weight. Client to receive tube feeds as per dietitian's caloric requirements for basal metabolic rate through PEG tube and pill form medications to be crushed and administered as per institution policy. Skin around tube site noted to have mild excoriation but is dry and intact. No open areas noted.

The nurse is reviewing the client's assessment data to prepare the client's plan of care.

▶ Complete the diagram by identifying from the choices below to specify what condition the client is most likely experiencing, 2 actions the nurse should take to address that condition, and 2 parameters the nurse should monitor to assess the client's progress.

Action to Take	Condition Most Likely Experiencing	Parameter to Monitor
Action to Take		Parameter to Monitor

Action to Take	Potential Condition	Parameters to Monitor
Administer oxygen at 2 L/min via nasal cannula	Aspiration pneumonia	Heart rate
Request an order to insert a peripheral venous access device	Hypertension	Temperature
Place patient in semi-Fowler's position during tube feeds	Dehydration	Skin breakdown
Request an order to administer intravenous fluids	Diabetes	Urine output
Prepare the client for a chest X-ray		Pain

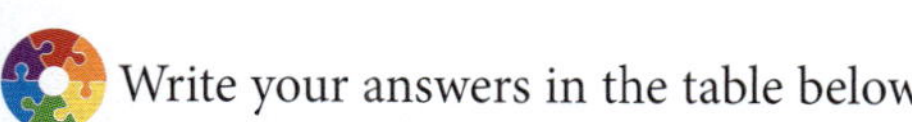
Write your answers in the table below.

Action to Take	Condition Most Likely Experiencing	Parameter to Monitor
Action to Take		Parameter to Monitor

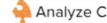

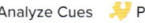

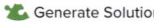

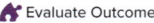

Medical-Surgical 4.0

The nurse is caring for a 55-year-old female client on a general surgical unit.

Nurses' Notes

1044h: Client returned from the recovery room after a breast reconstruction post–bilateral mastectomy 6 months ago under general anaesthetic. Vital signs: T: 37.9°C (100.2°F); BP: 99/60; P: 102; RR: 14; with pulse oximetry of 92% on 3 L/min per nasal prongs. Client rouses easily to voice and stimulation. Able to follow commands and move all extremities independently. Denies pain at present but states generalized discomfort. Pupils equal and reactive to light at 2 mm. Client presents with a regular bilateral radial pulse. Apical = radial. Bilateral dorsalis pedis pulses strong. Skin warm and dry to touch, no diaphoresis noted. Client denies any chest pain. Fine inspiratory crackles auscultated to bilateral lung fields. Clear air entry noted to bilateral upper lungs. Respirations regular and easy at rest. No cough noted. Abdomen soft with hypoactive bowel sounds noted in right lower quadrant and left lower quadrant fields. Client denies nausea, not passing flatus or eructation. Client has not voided yet and does not feel urgency yet. Peripheral venous access device in left forearm with 0.9% normal saline infusing at 100 mL/hr. Incision covered by dry dressings with Jackson-Pratt drains noted on each side draining blood. Jackson-Pratt emptied of 25 mL on the left side and 20 mL on the right side.

1300h: Client assisted to the washroom to void. Denies any dizziness. Encouraged to perform deep-breathing and coughing exercises every hour. Denies any chest pain. Lung sounds remain unchanged.

0800h (Postoperative day 1/POD1): During assessment, client presents as feeling chilled and pale. Vital signs: T: 38.5°C (101.3°F); BP: 110/72; P: 84; RR: 22; with pulse oximetry of 93% on 4 L/min per nasal prongs. Productive cough noted during assessment with coarse crackles auscultated throughout bilateral lung bases, with fine inspiratory crackles auscultated bilateral upper bases. Client denies chest pain but is feeling short of breath with ambulation. Client noted to be using accessory muscles for breathing.

The nurse is reviewing the client's assessment data to prepare the client's plan of care.

▶ Complete the diagram by identifying from the choices below to specify what condition the client is most likely experiencing, 2 actions the nurse should take to address that condition, and 2 parameters the nurse should monitor to assess the client's progress.

Action to Take	Condition Most Likely Experiencing	Parameter to Monitor
Action to Take		Parameter to Monitor

Action to Take	Potential Condition	Parameters to Monitor
Request an order for antibiotic therapy	Pneumonia	Cardiovascular status
Request a consult from physiotherapy	Hypotension	Neurological status
Prepare to increase oxygen level	Stroke	Temperature
Prepare the client for computed tomography (CT) of the head	Acute myocardial infarction	Gastrointestinal status
Prepare the client for a chest X-ray		Respiratory status

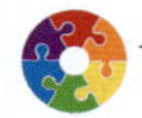
Write your answers in the table below.

Action to Take	Condition Most Likely Experiencing	Parameter to Monitor
Action to Take		Parameter to Monitor

Medical-Surgical 5.0

The nurse is caring for a 79-year-old client on a cardiovascular unit.

Nurses' Notes

1044h: Client presented to the emergency department with complaints of fatigue, shortness of breath with minimal exertion, and palpitations. Vital signs: T: 36.8°C (98.2°F); BP: 122/77; P: 136; RR: 22; with pulse oximetry of 93% on room air. Client rouses easily to voice and stimulation. Able to follow commands and move all extremities independently. Denies any pain at present. Client expresses extreme fatigue and not sleeping during the night. Client presents with an irregular bilateral radial pulse palpable and strong at 136. It is difficult to capture if apical is equal to radial pulse given the speed of the pulse. Bilateral radial pulses strong but irregular to touch. Bilateral dorsalis pedis pulses strong. Skin warm and dry to touch, no diaphoresis noted. Client denies any chest pain but feels warm. Lungs auscultated for clear air entry throughout. No adventitious breath sounds noted. Client presents with shortness of breath with minimal exertion in the room. Complains of difficulty catching breath at times but able to recover with rest. Abdomen noted to be rounded and firm to touch. Bowel sounds auscultated × 4 quadrants. Client states absence of a bowel movement for 2 days, which is unusual for their routine. Client voids clear amber urine in the toilet independently. Denies any pain, urgency, or burning when voiding. The client's comorbidities include only prediabetes controlled by diet and exercise.

The nurse is reviewing the client's assessment data to prepare the client's plan of care.

▶ Complete the diagram by identifying from the choices below to specify what condition the client is most likely experiencing, 2 actions the nurse should take to address that condition, and 2 parameters the nurse should monitor to assess the client's progress.

Action to Take	Condition Most Likely Experiencing	Parameter to Monitor
Action to Take		Parameter to Monitor

Action to Take	Potential Condition	Parameters to Monitor
Request an order for an antidysrhythmia medication	Atrial fibrillation	Urine output
Request a consult from the dietitian	Bradycardia	Pulse oximetry
Prepare to apply oxygen via nasal cannula	Tachycardia	Respiratory rate
Prepare the client for an electrocardiogram	Pneumonia	Heart rate
Prepare the client for a chest X-ray		Temperature

Write your answers in the table below.

Action to Take	Condition Most Likely Experiencing	Parameter to Monitor
Action to Take		Parameter to Monitor

Medical-Surgical 6.0

The nurse is caring for an 88-year-old client on a general medical unit.

Nurses' Notes

1342h: Client presented to the emergency department with complaints of weakness and noted confusion by client's daughter. Vital signs: T: 37.8°C (100.0°F); BP: 89/57; P: 122; RR: 24; with pulse oximetry of 95% on room air. Residential staff indicated client had developed a gastrointestinal illness accompanied by several bouts of emesis over the past 2 days. Client rouses easily to voice and tactile stimulation. Daughter informed staff that prior to the emergency department, the client was trying to "pick apples off the tree" as they had done as a child and grab "fruit" in the air. Client is able to follow simple commands and move all extremities independently but requires one-person stand-by assistance during ambulation. Client denies any pain at present. Primary complaint is extreme fatigue and weakness. Client complains of palpitations with bursts of a racing heart while at rest. Bilateral radial pulses palpable and regular during assessment. Bilateral dorsalis pedis pulses palpable but weak to touch. Skin cool to touch with capillary refill noted to be greater than 3 seconds on bilateral toes. Mucous membranes noted to be pale. Skin warm and dry to touch, no diaphoresis noted. Client denies any chest pain at present. Lungs auscultated for clear air entry throughout all lung fields with no adventitious breath sounds noted. Client presents with tachypnea but denies dyspnea with ambulation. Abdomen noted to be flat and soft to touch. Client cannot remember the last time they ate or drank anything. Bowel sounds loud and auscultated × 4 quadrants. When client was assisted to the commode, they voided approximately 250 mL of concentrated amber urine. Client denies any pain, urgency, or burning when voiding. The client's comorbidities include hypertension and type 2 diabetes mellitus. A peripheral venous access device was initiated in the right antecubital fossa and saline locked for use.

The nurse is reviewing the client's assessment data to prepare the client's plan of care.

▶ Complete the diagram by identifying from the choices below to specify what condition the client is most likely experiencing, 2 actions the nurse should take to address that condition, and 2 parameters the nurse should monitor to assess the client's progress.

Action to Take	Condition Most Likely Experiencing	Parameter to Monitor
Action to Take		Parameter to Monitor

Action to Take	Potential Condition	Parameters to Monitor
Administer a diuretic	Atrial fibrillation	Temperature
Request an order to administer a fluid bolus intravenously	Pneumonia	Pulse oximetry
Request an order to draw electrolytes blood work (sodium and potassium)	Dehydration	Blood pressure
Consult psychiatry for confusion	Dementia	Urine output
Request an order to insert a Foley catheter		Continuous electrocardiogram (ECG) monitoring

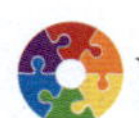

Write your answers in the table below.

Action to Take	Condition Most Likely Experiencing	Parameter to Monitor
Action to Take		Parameter to Monitor

Medical-Surgical 7.0

The nurse is caring for a 22-year-old client in the emergency department (ED).

Nurses' Notes

0124h: Client was brought to the ED via emergency medical services (EMS) after being extricated from a car in a motor vehicle accident and impaled by glass in the abdomen after their car hit a guard rail head on due to black ice and winter driving conditions. The client presented to the ED in a c-spine collar but alert and oriented to person, place, and time. Vital signs: T: 36.8°C (98.2°F); BP: 110/77; P: 102; RR: 20; with pulse oximetry of 93% on room air. The client denies hitting head on the steering wheel. Bilateral pupils measured at 2 mm, equal in size, with brisk reaction to light. Client denies a headache, able to move all four extremities independently and follows commands. Denies any numbness or tingling. Remains in c-spine precautions until a CT head can be completed and precautions removed. Client denies any chest pain. Capillary refill less than 3 seconds. Skin warm and dry to touch. Bilateral lung fields auscultated for fine inspiratory crackles noted only at the bases. Client remains well perfused, no cyanosis noted. Client expressed fear of the situation. Denies any shortness of breath. Left upper abdomen quadrant noted to have large 5-cm wound where glass from the windshield impaled the client at the time of the accident. Glass shard removed and area cleansed as per protocol, stitches required, area dressed with dry gauze and abdominal pads, secured with tape. Foley catheter inserted and draining clear amber urine. Bilateral peripheral venous access devices inserted with Ringer's lactate infusing at 100 mL/hr.

0214h: Client taken for CT head. C-spine precautions removed.

0317h: Nurse called to the client's room. Client expressed feeling lightheaded and weak. Vital signs: T: 37.4°C (99.3°F); BP: 82/57; P: 122; RR: 22; with pulse oximetry of 94% on room air. Nurse noted frank red blood on the sheets with the left upper abdomen wound saturated. Client states they had a coughing spell and felt a "pop." Health care provider notified and orders received to type and cross-match but to administer 1 unit packed red blood cells, O-negative, ASAP.

0325h: O-negative received from the blood bank. Vital signs: T: 37.3°C (99.1°F); BP: 80/53; P: 129; RR: 24; with pulse oximetry of 92% on room air. Blood transfusion initiated.

0330h: T: 37.3°C (99.1°F); BP: 81/54; P: 130; RR: 28; with pulse oximetry of 92% on room air. Client states feeling "fidgety," cannot sit still and feels like they cannot catch their breath. Complains of scratchy throat, with audible expiratory wheeze auscultated on lung fields. Client develops stridor.

The nurse is reviewing the client's assessment data to prepare the client's plan of care.

▶ Complete the diagram by identifying from the choices below to specify what condition the client is most likely experiencing, 2 actions the nurse should take to address that condition, and 2 parameters the nurse should monitor to assess the client's progress.

Action to Take	Condition Most Likely Experiencing	Parameter to Monitor
Action to Take		Parameter to Monitor

Action to Take	Potential Condition	Parameters to Monitor
Stop the transfusion immediately	Sepsis	Respiratory rate
Request an order to administer a narcotic for pain	Spinal cord injury	Bowel sounds
Prepare to administer epinephrine	Hypovolemia	Blood pressure
Obtain blood cultures	Anaphylaxis	Urine output
Prepare client for a chest X-ray		Capillary refill

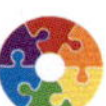 Write your answers in the table below.

Action to Take	Condition Most Likely Experiencing	Parameter to Monitor
Action to Take		Parameter to Monitor

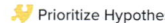

Medical-Surgical 8.0

The nurse is caring for a 73-year-old male client on the renal unit.

Nurses' Notes

1050h: Client was admitted to the unit for urine retention and subsequent diagnostic testing. The client explained he had been waking up several times throughout the night to void and is exhausted. Denies any pain with voiding. No complaints of chills. Expresses difficulty starting to void but then notices a small stream of urine and never feels like the blader is completely empty. Throughout the night and the day he feels a sense of urgency to void, and there have been times he has "dribbled," which is very embarrassing. Client denies any discharge or smell in the urine. The client denies any headache, independently walks around the unit with steady gait. Motor power strong × 4 extremities. Denies any numbness or tingling. No complaints of chest pain. Respirations regular and easy at rest with clear air entry throughout all lung fields. Vital signs: T: 37.2°C (99.0°F); BP: 128/64; P: 72; RR: 16; with pulse oximetry of 99% on room air. The client's previous comorbidities include hypertension. He is in a monogamous relationship with his partner of 40 years, a retired police officer.

The nurse is reviewing the client's assessment data to prepare the client's plan of care.

▶ Complete the diagram by identifying from the choices below to specify what condition the client is most likely experiencing, 2 actions the nurse should take to address that condition, and 2 parameters the nurse should monitor to assess the client's progress.

Action to Take	Condition Most Likely Experiencing	Parameter to Monitor
Action to Take		Parameter to Monitor

Action to Take	Potential Condition	Parameters to Monitor
Prepare to insert a Foley catheter	Urinary tract infection	Respiratory rate
Request an order to administer an antibiotic	Gonorrhea	Volume of urine in the bladder
Encourage oral fluids	Kidney stones	Temperature
Obtain a urine sample for culture and sensitivity	Benign prostate hyperplasia	Intake and output
Prepare the client for a transurethral resection of the prostate (TURP)		Capillary refill

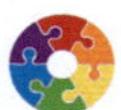
Write your answers in the table below.

Action to Take	Condition Most Likely Experiencing	Parameter to Monitor
Action to Take		Parameter to Monitor

Medical-Surgical 9.0

The nurse is caring for a 35-year-old client in the emergency department (ED).

Nurses' Notes

1843h: Client was brought to the ED accompanied by their partner with complaints of abdominal pain, chills, and generalized feeling of being unwell. Vital signs: T: 38.7°C (101.7°F); BP: 133/72; P: 87; RR: 18; with pulse oximetry of 96% on room air. Upon further assessment, the client presents as alert and oriented to person, place, and time. Walks independently without assistance, motor power strong × 4 extremities. Denies any numbness and tingling. Client's conjunctiva pink and perfused. Capillary refill less than 3 seconds. Fine inspiratory crackles auscultated anteriorly to bilateral lung fields that clear with a cough. Client denies difficulty breathing, no shortness of breath noted, no use of accessory muscles. Abdomen rounded and firm to touch. Hyperactive bowel sounds auscultated to left lower quadrant of the abdomen, with adequate bowel sounds noted in remaining three quadrants. Colostomy in left upper quadrant. Client states they developed severe ulcerative colitis in their late teens and early 20s, prompting the intervention. A permanent colostomy was surgically created 3 years ago. The skin under the flange noted to be pink and excoriated with multiple areas of skin breakdown. Serous, yellow-tinged purulent drainage noted under the skin barrier wafer. Client states they have not been as diligent about cleaning under the flange since arrival of a new 1-month-old baby, which is the couple's first child together. The client reports extreme exhaustion. Client denies emesis or nausea. The client drains the colostomy pouch 3 to 4 times per day. The stoma has not changed colour and remains pink with healthy tissue. No necrotic areas noted. Client denies any issue with voiding. No pain, urgency, or frequency noted.

The nurse is reviewing the client's assessment data to prepare the client's plan of care.

▶ Complete the diagram by identifying from the choices below to specify what condition the client is most likely experiencing, 2 actions the nurse should take to address that condition, and 2 parameters the nurse should monitor to assess the client's progress.

Action to Take	Condition Most Likely Experiencing	Parameter to Monitor
Action to Take		Parameter to Monitor

Action to Take	Potential Condition	Parameters to Monitor
Administer a cleansing enema	Skin infection	Respiratory rate
Prepare client for a chest X-ray	Pneumonia	Bowel sounds
Clean the skin by the stoma with sterile normal saline	Urinary tract infection	Temperature
Change wafer of the two-piece ostomy system	Gastrointestinal illness	Urine output
Collect a culture and sensitivity sample of the purulent drainage		Wound discharge

 Write your answers in the table below.

Action to Take	Condition Most Likely Experiencing	Parameter to Monitor
Action to Take		Parameter to Monitor

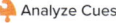

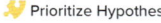

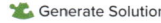

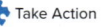

Medical-Surgical 10.0

The nurse is caring for a 94-year-old client on the general medical unit.

Nurses' Notes

1436h: Client was admitted to the unit for observation from the long-term care (LTC) facility with increasing generalized weakness and apathetic mood for several weeks. The staff at the LTC facility indicated the client's best friend in the facility had recently passed away and the client has become more withdrawn, not willing to participate in activities or attend meals with other residents. Vital signs: T: 38.1°C (100.6°F); BP: 92/65; P: 96 RR: 16; with pulse oximetry of 94% on room air. Client is pleasant and cooperative, presents as alert and oriented to person, place, time, and situation. Client requires two-person assist with the commode when needing to use the washroom. Client moves all four extremities independently but slowly and carefully. Client expressed they are scared of falling as they get dizzy with movement. Client denies any pain or numbness and tingling. Presents with pallor, pale conjunctiva and palms of their hands. Capillary refill is sluggish but less than 3 seconds. Skin cool to touch. Client indicates feeling cold most of the day. Bilateral radial pulses palpated to be regular and equal to apical rate. Bilateral dorsalis pedis pulses palpable but weak to touch. No adventitious heart sounds auscultated. Lungs auscultated for fine inspiratory crackles throughout all lung fields that remain present even after a cough. Client denies shortness of breath or chest pain. Respirations regular and easy at rest. Client indicates feeling tired and requests to rest. Abdomen flat with bowel sounds auscultated in all four quadrants. Client presents as cachectic and malnourished. Client denies a bowel movement for days but does not feel hungry. Bony prominences showed redness as noted on bilateral scapular shoulder blades and bilateral heels. A 5 cm by 3 cm stage 3 coccyx wound noted with slough in the middle of the wound, bone borders noted to be grey with reduced perfusion as they do not blanch with palpation. Client states they do not feel the wound and requests that staff not move them as they want to be left alone. Braeden skin assessment complete and documented at 9 (severe risk). Client denies suicidal ideation or homicidal intent to harm others. Past medical history includes hypertension, rheumatoid arthritis, peripheral venous disease, type 2 diabetes mellitus.

The nurse is reviewing the client's assessment data to prepare the client's plan of care.

▶ Complete the diagram by identifying from the choices below to specify what condition the client is most likely experiencing, 2 actions the nurse should take to address that condition, and 2 parameters the nurse should monitor to assess the client's progress.

Action to Take	Condition Most Likely Experiencing	Parameter to Monitor
Action to Take		Parameter to Monitor

Action to Take	Potential Condition	Parameters to Monitor
Insert a nasogastric tube	Dysrhythmia	Heart rate
Request a consult for wound specialists	Pneumonia	Bowel sounds
Reposition client to reduce pressure on coccyx	Constipation	Affect
Request to insert a peripheral venous device	Skin infection	Range of motion
Prepare to administer an intravenous antibiotic		Skin integrity

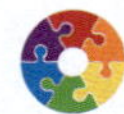
Write your answers in the table below.

Action to Take	Condition Most Likely Experiencing	Parameter to Monitor
Action to Take		Parameter to Monitor

Medical-Surgical 11.0

The nurse is caring for a 34-year-old client in the emergency department (ED).

Progress Notes

1554h: Client presented to the ED via emergency medical services (EMS). This unhoused client was found by an urban mobile outreach team during regular safe checks, covered with garbage bags during freezing winter temperatures. Vital signs: T: 34.8°C (94.6°F); BP: 102/754; P: 54; RR: 12; and unable to obtain pulse oximetry due to coolness of skin. Client presents alert and oriented to person and place, but is unable to determine time, date, month, or year. Speech is slow and slurred. Client denies pain. Excessive shivering noted. Pupils equal and react briskly to light, measured at 2 mm. No irregularity in shape identified. Gait is unsteady, client requires two-person assist. Client denies any dizziness. Skin cool to touch, palms light in colour, with paleness of conjunctiva noted. Bilateral radial pulses regular and weak, but palpable. Bilateral dorsalis pedis pulses and posterior tibial pulses unable to be palpated and required Doppler. Capillary refill greater than 3 seconds. Shallow, quiet breaths noted. Fine bilateral lower lobe inspiratory crackles auscultated posteriorly. Abdomen flat and soft with hypoactive bowel sounds auscultated × 4 quadrants. Client denies need to void at present time. A peripheral venous access device was inserted into the left antecubital fossa and infusing warmed fluids.

The nurse is reviewing the client's assessment data to prepare the client's plan of care.

▶ Complete the diagram by identifying from the choices below to specify what condition the client is most likely experiencing, 2 actions the nurse should take to address that condition, and 2 parameters the nurse should monitor to assess the client's progress.

Action to Take		Parameter to Monitor
Action to Take	Condition Most Likely Experiencing	Parameter to Monitor

Action to Take	Potential Condition	Parameters to Monitor
Remove the client's wet clothing	Hypertension	Urine output
Obtain a blood sugar	Hyperthermia	Temperature
Administer antipyretic	Hypotension	Blood pressure
Connect the client to a cardiac monitor	Hypothermia	Dysrhythmias
Call a code blue		Pain

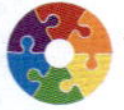

Write your answers in the table below.

Action to Take	Condition Most Likely Experiencing	Parameter to Monitor
Action to Take		Parameter to Monitor

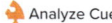

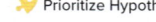

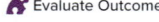

Medical-Surgical 12.0

The nurse is caring for a 28-year-old client in the emergency department (ED).

Progress Notes

2256h: Client presented to the ED with primary complaint of a headache. The client detailed the abrupt start of a headache around 1900h but the headache progressed to a pain level rated 10 out of 10 on a numerical pain scale. The client is accompanied by their partner. Vital signs: T: 37.2°C (99.0°F); BP 210/125; P: 108; RR 22; with pulse oximetry of 97% on room air. The client presents with double vision (diplopia), unsteady gait, and slurred speech at times. Client reports these are new symptoms. No previous comorbidities. Recreational drug user of cocaine with last dose at 1700h after work. Client presents alert and oriented to person, place, and time. Pupils equal in size and briskly reactive to light, measured at 3 mm. Gait remains unsteady only because client cannot stop clutching their head. Client denies any chest pain but feels "fluttering" in chest with ambulation. Skin is warm and flushed to touch. Diaphoresis noted. Bilateral radial pulses bounding. Apical = radial. Client states mild shortness of breath, even at rest. Lungs auscultated for coarse crackles noted posterior bilateral bases. Denies any cough. Client reports voiding less frequently because of a reduction in oral intake. Abdomen soft and rounded. Client indicates ++ nausea with emesis. Bowel sounds active and auscultated in all four quadrants.

The nurse is reviewing the client's assessment data to prepare the client's plan of care.

▶ Complete the diagram by identifying from the choices below to specify what condition the client is most likely experiencing, 2 actions the nurse should take to address that condition, and 2 parameters the nurse should monitor to assess the client's progress.

Action to Take	Condition Most Likely Experiencing	Parameter to Monitor
Action to Take		Parameter to Monitor

Action to Take	Potential Condition	Parameters to Monitor
Prepare to insert a peripheral venous access device	Hypertensive emergency	Blood sugar
Obtain a blood sugar	Pulmonary embolus	Temperature
Administer antihypertensive	Stroke	Blood pressure
Prepare the client for a chest X-ray	Acute myocardial infarction	Pupillary size and reaction
Call a code blue		Pain

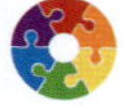
Write your answers in the table below.

Action to Take	Condition Most Likely Experiencing	Parameter to Monitor
Action to Take		Parameter to Monitor

Medical-Surgical 13.0

The nurse is caring for a 66-year-old client in the emergency department (ED).

Progress Notes

1044h: Client presented to the ED with complaints of fatigue, shortness of breath with minimal exertion, and palpitations described as a "fluttering or racing heart" in their chest × 1 day. The shortness of breath has increased, prompting the visit to the ED. Vital signs: T: 36.8°C (98.2°F); BP: 122/77; P:156; RR: 24; with pulse oximetry of 95% on room air. Client rouses easily to voice and stimulation. Client is alert and oriented to person, place, and time; is able to follow commands and move all extremities independently. Motor power strong × 4 extremities. Client denies any pain, numbness, or tingling at present. Client expresses extreme fatigue and is not sleeping during the night due to the racing heart. Unable to settle. Client presents with an irregular bilateral radial pulse palpable and strong at 156. It is difficult to capture if apical is equal to radial pulse, given the speed of the pulse. Bilateral dorsalis pedis pulses strong with palpable posterior bilateral tibial pulses. Skin warm and dry to touch, with client feeling flushed. Denies any chest pain. Lungs auscultated for clear air entry throughout. No adventitious breath sounds noted. Client presents with shortness of breath with minimal exertion when walking about the room. Complains of difficulty catching breath at times but is able to recover with rest. Abdomen noted to be rounded and firm to touch. Bowel sounds auscultated × 4 quadrants. Client states absence of a bowel movement for 2 days, which is unusual for their routine. Denies any nausea or emesis. Client voids clear amber urine in the toilet independently. Denies any pain, urgency, or burning when voiding. The client's comorbidities include only prediabetes controlled by diet and exercise. Client states they have never had this feeling before.

The nurse is reviewing the client's assessment data to prepare the client's plan of care.

▶ Complete the diagram by identifying from the choices below to specify what condition the client is most likely experiencing, 2 actions the nurse should take to address that condition, and 2 parameters the nurse should monitor to assess the client's progress.

Action to Take	Condition Most Likely Experiencing	Parameter to Monitor
Action to Take		Parameter to Monitor

Action to Take	Potential Condition	Parameters to Monitor
Request a consult from the dietitian	Atrial fibrillation	Clinical manifestations of a stroke
Prepare the client for a cardioversion	Bradycardia	Pulse oximetry
Apply oxygen via nasal cannula	Tachycardia	Urine output
Obtain an electrocardiogram	Pneumonia	Heart rate
Prepare the client for a chest X-ray		Temperature

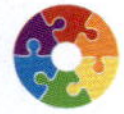

Write your answers in the table below.

Action to Take	Condition Most Likely Experiencing	Parameter to Monitor
Action to Take		Parameter to Monitor

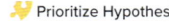

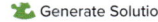

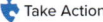

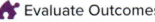

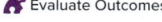

Medical-Surgical 14.0

The nurse is caring for a 62-year-old male client on the internal medicine unit.

Nurses' Notes | History and Physical

1012h: The client presented to the emergency department accompanied by their partner. Primary complaints of extreme fatigue, palpitations, and shortness of breath precipitated the need for further assessment. T: 37.9°C; BP: 96/60 mm Hg; HR: 117; RR: 28; with pulse oximetry of 86% on room air.

Nurses' Notes | **History and Physical**

1012h:	
Neurological	Alert and oriented to person, place, time, and situation. Cooperative, obeys commands. Motor power strong × 4. Gait steady. Denies headache, double vision, or dizziness. Denies any pain.
Cardiovascular	Skin cool and dry to the touch. Capillary refill less than 3 seconds. Jugular venous distension (JVD) noted at 3 cm. Bilateral radial pulses are strong and irregular. The client complains of feeling a fast heart rate in the chest at rest, then disappearing. Denies any chest pain but feels a "fluttering" in the left upper chest wall. S1, S2 auscultated and accompanied by an S3, no S4. Bilateral dorsalis pedis pulses strong. Posterior tibial pulses × 2 are weak but palpable. +1 Non-pitting peripheral edema was noted in the bilateral lower extremities.
Pulmonary	Shortness of breath with minimal exertion. Coarse crackles were noted to the left lower lobe, with fine crackles noted to the right lower lobe. No cyanosis was noted. No use of accessory muscles was noted. The client is taking short, shallow breaths. Nonproductive cough noted.
Gastrointestinal	Abdomen flat, no pain with palpation. Normal bowel sounds noted × 4 quadrants. The client states they have not felt hungry × 24 hours but otherwise their habits have been unchanged.
Renal	Urinal at the bedside with a concentrated small amount urine. Despite drinking fluids and feeling thirsty, the client has not voided many times in the past 24 hours.
Psychosocial	Married, CEO of a company with over 500 employees in an urban centre. Past medical history: type 2 diabetes diagnosed 3 years ago controlled with oral hypoglycemic agents, coronary artery disease with acute myocardial infarction 10 years ago with percutaneous coronary intervention (PCI) to distal RCA and CABG × 2 vessels—LAD and circumflex. Acute renal failure (ARF) post-CABG.

The nurse is reviewing the client's assessment data to prepare the client's plan of care.

▶ Complete the diagram by identifying from the choices below to specify what condition the client is most likely experiencing, 2 actions the nurse should take to address that condition, and 2 parameters the nurse should monitor to assess the client's progress.

Action to Take	Condition Most Likely Experiencing	Parameter to Monitor
Action to Take		Parameter to Monitor

Action to Take	Potential Condition	Parameters to Monitor
Prepare the client for a chest X-ray	Tricuspid valve regurgitation	Changes in jugular venous distension
Request an order to administer furosemide	Pericardial effusion	Temperature
Request an order to administer 0.9% sodium chloride bolus × 500 mL × 1	Cardiomyopathy	Continuous electrocardiogram (ECG) monitoring for dysrhythmias
Restrict the client's activity	Chronic pericarditis	Urine output
Request an order to initiate oxygen therapy		Weight

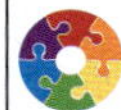
Write your answers in the table below.

Action to Take	Condition Most Likely Experiencing	Parameter to Monitor
Action to Take		Parameter to Monitor

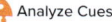

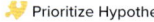

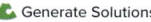

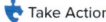

Medical-Surgical 15.0

The nurse is caring for a 24-year-old client in a community health centre.

Progress Notes

1225h: Client presented to the health centre complaining of anterior left upper arm pain. Client indicates they received a hepatitis B vaccine 1 day ago and woke up feeling chilled, but their left arm was painful to move and ++ warm. Vital signs: T: 38.3°C (100.9°F); BP: 110/60; P: 104; RR: 20; with pulse oximetry of 90% on room air. Upon assessment, client is alert and oriented to person, place, and time. Denies any chest pain at present. Capillary refill less than 3 seconds. Overall mucous membranes are pink with adequate perfusion. Lungs auscultated for clear bilateral air entry throughout, no adventitious breath sounds noted. Client's abdomen is flat with bowel sounds auscultated × 4 quadrants. Client voiding independently in the washroom. Back of left arm is noted to have a hot, tender, swollen, and red area approximately 2 cm in diameter where client received vaccine injection.

1600h: Client rang for nursing assistance complaining of increased pain in the back of the left arm. Further assessment reveals that redness has increased in size to 8 cm wide, as compared to previous assessment, with client complaining of chills and feeling unwell. Client denies any chest pain, palpitations, remains well perfused to mucous membranes, and clear air entry noted to bilateral lung fields. Health care provider notified of change in status. Awaiting further orders.

The nurse is reviewing the client's assessment data to prepare the client's plan of care.

▶ Complete the diagram by identifying from the choices below to specify what condition the client is most likely experiencing, 2 actions the nurse should take to address that condition, and 2 parameters the nurse should monitor to assess the client's progress.

Action to Take	Condition Most Likely Experiencing	Parameter to Monitor
Action to Take		Parameter to Monitor

Action to Take	Potential Condition	Parameters to Monitor
Obtain titre levels	Chicken pox	Gangrene
Prepare client for a chest X-ray	Cellulitis	Pain level
Request antibiotic therapy	Herpes zoster	Temperature
Apply moist heat and elevate	Psoriasis	Redness borders decreasing in size
Collect a culture and sensitivity sample of the purulent drainage		Wound discharge

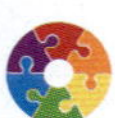

Write your answers in the table below.

Action to Take	Condition Most Likely Experiencing	Parameter to Monitor
Action to Take		Parameter to Monitor

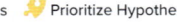

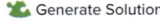

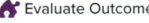

Medical-Surgical 16.0

The nurse is caring for a 49-year-old female client on a respiratory unit.

Nurses' Notes

1044h: Client was transferred to the unit from Intensive Care Unit (ICU) and an initial diagnosis of pneumosepsis 14 days ago. The client required intubation and ventilatory support for 10 days with a tracheostomy inserted on day 8 without issue. The client's oxygenation has been supported by a trach cradle with reducing oxygen therapy now at 30% fiO_2. Client requires increased rehabilitation and mobility to improve strength. Vital signs: T: 37.7°C (99.9°F); BP: 102/54; P: 72; RR: 16; with pulse oximetry of 96% on 30% fiO_2 humidified air via trach cradle. Client alert and oriented to person, place, and time and is pleasant and cooperative with all commands. Client moves independently in the bed and requires one-person assist during mobility to the washroom with a two-wheeled walker. Client only began mobilizing 1 day prior to transfer to the respiratory unit. Pupils equal and briskly reactive to light at 2 mm. Presents with S1 and S2, no adventitious heart sounds auscultated. Apical heart rate regular and equals radial pulse. Bilateral radial pulses remain strong, regular, and palpable. Bilateral dorsalis pedis pulses and posterior tibial pulses noted to be weak but palpable. Capillary refill less than 3 seconds. Skin cool to touch. Redness and mild swelling noted on the posterior side of the left calf. Client stated completing dorsi planter and dorsi flexion exercises in bed. Complains of discomfort with ambulation. Fine inspiratory crackles located in bilateral lower lobes when lungs auscultated posteriorly. Client unable to expectorate sputum independently and requires suction catheter. Tracheostomy attached with ties and a trach dressing. No drainage noted on the dressing. Abdomen round and soft to touch. Bowel sounds auscultated × 4 quadrants. Client voiding independently. Client has been ordered sequential compression devices to wear when in bed.

1155h: Client rang for assistance. Noted to be coughing and requesting to be suctioned. Wall suction dialed to low level, preoxygenation provided prior to suction. Client required five passes to clear a thick mucus plug streaked with frank red blood. Client noted to be coughing ++ with blood being expectorated. Coarse crackles auscultated throughout all lung fields posteriorly. Client noted to have increased respirations post-suction with a respiratory rate of 24 noted. Pulse oximetry was 86% on 30% fiO_2 humidified air via trach cradle. Client complaining of pain with inspiration. Chest expansion noted to be symmetrical. Health care provider notified.

The nurse is reviewing the client's assessment data to prepare the client's plan of care.

▶ Complete the diagram by identifying from the choices below to specify what condition the client is most likely experiencing, 2 actions the nurse should take to address that condition, and 2 parameters the nurse should monitor to assess the client's progress.

Action to Take	Condition Most Likely Experiencing	Parameter to Monitor
Action to Take		Parameter to Monitor

Action to Take	Potential Condition	Parameters to Monitor
Request an order for antibiotic therapy	Pneumonia	aPTT and INR levels
Prepare to initiate anticoagulant therapy (IV heparin)	Pulmonary embolus	Urine output
Prepare to increase oxygen level	Pleural effusion	Temperature
Increase suction pressure	Pneumothorax	Chest pain
Prepare the client for a computed tomography (CT) scan		Pulse oximetry

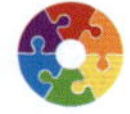

Write your answers in the table below.

Action to Take	Condition Most Likely Experiencing	Parameter to Monitor
Action to Take		Parameter to Monitor

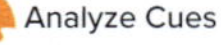
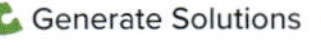

Recognize Cues · Analyze Cues · Prioritize Hypothesis · Generate Solutions · Take Action · Evaluate Outcomes

Maternal/Birthing Parent Health Bow-Tie Cases

Maternal/Birthing Parent Health 1.0

The nurse is caring for a 25-year-old female in the outpatient women's health clinic.

Admission Notes | History and Physical

1115h: Client arrived with primary complaints of a recurrent sore throat and lethargy that has persisted off and on for the past month. Vital signs: T: 38.2°C (100.8°F); BP: 110/66; P: 72; RR: 16; with pulse oximetry of 99% on room air.

Admission Notes | **History and Physical**

1115h

Neurological	Alert and oriented × person, place, time, and situation, pleasant, gait steady, denies headache but has experienced headache in the past
Pulmonary	Chest clear with auscultation, respirations regular and easy at rest
Cardiovascular	Denies any chest pain, no diaphoresis, pulses regular
Gastrointestinal	Abdomen soft, rounded, no pain with palpation, bowel sounds × 4
Genitourinary	Client states she has not noticed bleeding after intercourse and no abnormal vaginal discharge noticed. No issues with voiding, denies pain
Integumentary	Client feels several warts by her vagina that are pink-grey in colour but not itchy. She had one wart 2 months ago but thought it was nothing and it went away. She has developed a rash on the palms of her hands and feet but denies pruritis.
Psychosocial	Client has been in a stable relationship with her partner for 3 months. She has recently started a new job after graduating with her master's in business administration.

The nurse is reviewing the client's assessment data to prepare the client's plan of care.

▶ Complete the diagram by identifying from the choices below to specify what condition the client is most likely experiencing, 2 actions the nurse should take to address that condition, and 2 parameters the nurse should monitor to assess the client's progress.

Action to Take	Condition Most Likely Experiencing	Parameter to Monitor
Action to Take		Parameter to Monitor

Action to Take	Potential Condition	Parameters to Monitor
Screen for other sexually transmitted infections	Chlamydia	Educate client to practise abstinence until treatment is complete
Collect blood cultures	Gonorrhea	Systemic responses such as blood pressure
Do not report infection	Syphilis	Recognize triggers for stress
Review nontreponemal and treponemal results	Herpes simplex virus	Discuss diet associated with rash
Ensure client's partners are not contacted		Jarisch-Herxheimer reactions

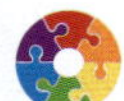 Write your answers in the table below.

Action to Take	Condition Most Likely Experiencing	Parameter to Monitor
Action to Take		Parameter to Monitor

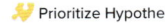

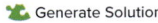

Maternal/Birthing Parent Health 2.0

The nurse is caring for a 35-year-old non-binary client in the emergency department (ED) who is 18 weeks' gestation.

Nurses' Notes

1000h: The client discovered a large amount of blood staining their sheets and developed severe abdominal cramping described as 8 out of 10 on a 1-to-10 numerical pain scale that persisted for approximately 5 minutes then resolved to a low, dull pain rated at 3 out of 10. The client required their partner's assistance walking to the car and noticed constant bleeding requiring a pad and extra protection on the car seat. Vital signs: T: 37.9°C (100.2°F); BP: 110/66; P: 80; RR: 16; with pulse oximetry of 99% on room air. The client presents as lethargic, concerned, and anxious about the pregnancy. They state that they stopped microdosing testosterone 6 months ago to try and get pregnant. The bleeding is scary for them and their partner. The client's lung sounds are clear with no adventitious air entry noted. Pulses are strong. No fetal heart rate noted with use of Doppler. Client denies having any pain or cramping at present.

The nurse is reviewing the client's assessment data to prepare the client's plan of care.

▶ Complete the diagram by identifying from the choices below to specify what condition the client is most likely experiencing, 2 actions the nurse should take to address that condition, and 2 parameters the nurse should monitor to assess the client's progress.

Action to Take	Condition Most Likely Experiencing	Parameter to Monitor
Action to Take		Parameter to Monitor

Actions to Take	Potential Conditions	Parameters to Monitor
Prepare the client for dilation and curettage	Placenta abruption	Temperature
Administer oxytocin	Incomplete spontaneous abortion	Signs associated with hemorrhage
Leave the client and their partner alone	Placenta previa	Extreme fluid shifts
Prepare for laboratory draw of complete blood count, electrolytes, and coagulation	Postpartum hemorrhage	Signs of an ileus
Insert Foley catheter		Initiate support group

Write your answers in the table below.

Action to Take	Condition Most Likely Experiencing	Parameter to Monitor
Action to Take		Parameter to Monitor

Maternal/Birthing Parent Health 3.0

The nurse is caring for a 25-year-old female client on the postpartum unit who has delivered her first baby.

Progress Notes

0124h: Client presented to the labour and delivery unit in active labour as a G1 P1 A0 L1. Pregnancy was unremarkable but client had a prolonged labour. Client delivered a 4 200 g baby boy requiring a forceps delivery and a 10-cm (4-inch) episiotomy repaired tear. Client transferred to the postpartum unit. Vital signs: T: 36.8°C (98.2°F); BP: 110/77; P: 102; RR: 20; with pulse oximetry of 93% on room air. The client presented alert and oriented to person, place, and time. Able to assist with transfer, but complained of dizziness when transferring from stretcher to bed. Bilateral pupils measured at 2 mm, equal in size, and have brisk reaction to light. Client able to move all four extremities independently and follows commands. Denies any numbness and tingling. S1 and S2 auscultated to be regular. No adventitious heart sounds noted. Client denies any chest pain. Capillary refill less than 3 seconds. Skin cool to touch. No diaphoresis noted. Client states she is cold. Client presents as pale with pale conjunctiva. Bilateral lung fields auscultated for fine inspiratory crackles noted only at the bases. No cyanosis noted. Denies any shortness of breath. Client's fundus boggy expelling large, golf ball–size clots when massaged. Lochia rubra consists of bright red flow. Bilateral peripheral venous access devices located right and left forearms, saline locked.

0210h: Client assisted to the washroom where they became unsteady. Client had difficulty voiding despite feeling need to void. Client assisted back to bed. Client states she is exhausted. Bladder scanner revealed approximately 175 mL of urine in the bladder.

0317h: Nurse called to the client's room. Client states feeling lightheaded, weak, wondering what is happening, and she is scared. Vital signs: T: 37.4°C (99.3°F); BP: 82/57; P: 132; RR: 26; with pulse oximetry of 86% on room air. Nurse noted frank red blood on the sheets, fundus remains boggy, with bright red lochia. Client noted respirations rapid and shallow. Health care provider notified.

The nurse is reviewing the client's assessment data to prepare the client's plan of care.

▶ Complete the diagram by identifying from the choices below to specify what condition the client is most likely experiencing, 2 actions the nurse should take to address that condition, and 2 parameters the nurse should monitor to assess the client's progress.

Action to Take	Condition Most Likely Experiencing	Parameter to Monitor
Action to Take		Parameter to Monitor

Action to Take	Potential Condition	Parameters to Monitor
Prepare to administer an intravenous fluid bolus	Post-delivery infection	Pulse oximetry
Request an order to administer an antibiotic	Pulmonary embolus	Gait
Initiate oxygen therapy	Postpartum hemorrhage	Blood pressure
Obtain blood cultures	Dehydration	Urine output
Prepare client for a chest X-ray		Capillary refill

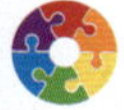 Write your answers in the table below.

Action to Take	Condition Most Likely Experiencing	Parameter to Monitor
Action to Take		Parameter to Monitor

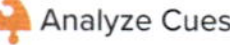 Recognize Cues 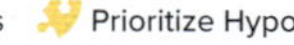 Analyze Cues 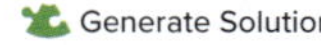 Prioritize Hypothesis 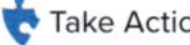 Generate Solutions  Take Action Evaluate Outcomes

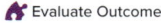

Pediatrics Bow-Tie Cases

Pediatric 1.0

The nurse is caring for a 5-week-old infant in the neonatal intensive care unit (NICU).

Nurses' Notes

0210h: Infant presented to emergency department at 2330h with laboured respirations, abdominal retractions, nasal flaring, wet sounding cough, and pallor. Infant admitted to the NICU for closer observation. Vital signs: T: 38.3°C (100.9°F) axillary; P: 162; RR: 68; pulse oximetry: 88%; weight: 4 000 g. Client presents as pale, no cyanosis noted. Heart rate tachycardic but regular with apical auscultation. Lungs auscultated with bilateral expiratory wheezing noted in right lower to middle lobe and left lower lobe. Diminished air entry noted to left lower lobe as compared to right lower lobe. Conjunctiva noted to be pale in colour when assessed. Birth parents accompanied client to the hospital, concerned. State they had been at a birthday party a week ago and it was the infant's first time around their friends. They feel horrible that they let this happen to their child. They indicate the infant was nursing less than a few days ago and they had to wake up the infant during feeding.

0350h: Birth parents called nurse to the room as they suspected infant was not breathing at times. Apneic episodes notified. Health care provider notified of change in status.

The nurse is reviewing the client's assessment data to prepare the client's plan of care.

▶ Complete the diagram by identifying from the choices below to specify what condition the client is most likely experiencing, 2 actions the nurse should take to address that condition, and 2 parameters the nurse should monitor to assess the client's progress.

Action to Take	Condition Most Likely Experiencing	Parameter to Monitor
Action to Take		Parameter to Monitor

Actions to Take	Potential Conditions	Parameters to Monitor
Initiate peripheral venous access	Asthma	Pulse oximetry
Administer humidified oxygen	Croup	Bowel sounds
Insert Foley catheter	Foreign body aspiration	Meeting developmental milestones
Prepare to administer diuretics	Respiratory syncytial virus (RSV)	Number of wet diapers
Obtain nasal sample for antigen detection		Barking cough

Write your answers in the table below.

Action to Take	Condition Most Likely Experiencing	Parameter to Monitor
Action to Take		Parameter to Monitor

Pediatric 2.0

The nurse is caring for a 4-year-old female client in the pediatric emergency department (ED).

Progress Notes

1000h: Client presented to the ED accompanied by a parent with a primary complaint of frequent voiding and drinking excessive amounts of water. The parent reports the client has been having more urinary accidents during the night. Upon assessment, the client noted to have tenting on the back of the hand with dry mucous membranes in the conjunctiva. The client presents as underweight despite the parent indicating the client eats frequently. Sweet, fruit-smelling breath noted with shallow breaths. The parent indicates the client has normal bowel movements and denies any pain or burning with voiding. The client is up to date on their vaccinations.

The nurse is reviewing the client's assessment data to prepare the client's plan of care.

▶ Complete the diagram by identifying from the choices below to specify what condition the client is most likely experiencing, 2 actions the nurse should take to address that condition, and 2 parameters the nurse should monitor to assess the client's progress.

Action to Take	Condition Most Likely Experiencing	Parameter to Monitor
Action to Take		Parameter to Monitor

Action to Take	Potential Condition	Parameters to Monitor
Prepare to insert a peripheral venous access device	Congenital heart defect	Glycated hemoglobin (hemoglobin A_1c)
Collect a urinalysis sample	Failure to thrive	Temperature
Request an order for antibiotic therapy	Urinary tract infection	Weight loss
Collect a blood specimen for glucose monitoring	Diabetic ketoacidosis	Ketones in urine
Prepare the client for a cardiology consult		Diet

Write your answers in the table below.

Action to Take	Condition Most Likely Experiencing	Parameter to Monitor
Action to Take		Parameter to Monitor

Mental Health Bow-Tie Cases

Mental Health 1.0

The nurse in a community clinic is seeing both new parents for their 4-month-old's well-child visit.

Nurses' Notes

1300h: Infant daughter accompanied to clinic by mother and father. Infant taking breast well, no concerns noted with eating and sleep habits. Infant meeting growth milestones with appropriate social interaction to those around infant. No concerns regarding weight, height, and head circumference. When parents are asked how they are coping with a newborn infant, mother states she is tired and still recovering from intensive care stay. Upon further inquiry, mother informs nurse she had uterine atony after the delivery and began to hemorrhage with a drop in blood pressure and unresponsiveness, requiring rapid administration of blood products and short-term intubation and ventilatory support. The father of the infant witnessed the ordeal and states, "I felt helpless watching her bleed onto the floor. She was a crumpled mess. I could not do anything to help her." The nurse further inquired as to coping now of both parents. The mother indicates having a strong support network to assist with the newborn. The father states he has nightmares of that moment when she became unresponsive, he cannot sleep, he does not want to leave her side, fearing he could lose her, but he has to because he needs to support his family. Nobody is aware of his fears as he does not want to burden anyone while his wife is being an amazing mom to their daughter. He states he is sure these feelings will pass as he is currently taking sertraline, a selective serotonin reuptake inhibitor (SSRI), for depression.

The nurse is reviewing the client's assessment data to prepare the client's plan of care.

▶ Complete the diagram by identifying from the choices below to specify what condition the client is most likely experiencing, 2 actions the nurse should take to address that condition, and 2 parameters the nurse should monitor to assess the client's progress.

Action to Take	Condition Most Likely Experiencing	Parameter to Monitor
Action to Take		Parameter to Monitor

Action to Take	Potential Conditions	Parameters to Monitor
Consult clinic nurse practitioner	Anxiety	Use of drugs or alcohol for coping
Say, "these concerns are normal after a delivery"	Post-traumatic stress disorder (PTSD)	Participation in group therapy sessions
Request an order to administer lorazepam in the clinic	Postpartum depression	Suicidal ideation
Talk with the client of concern about coping strategies	Dissociative identity disorder	Use of sick time
Contact a crisis nurse as family is not coping well at all		Hypertension

Write your answers in the table below.

Action to Take	Condition Most Likely Experiencing	Parameter to Monitor
Action to Take		Parameter to Monitor

Mental Health 2.0

The nurse is caring for a 36-year-old male client in an outpatient community mental health program.

Progress Notes

May 26: Client attended outpatient community mental health program and reveals a complicated past. He was abandoned by his mother at the age of 8 years old and fell into the foster system, never being adopted or having a family of his own. He said, "I did not realize what love was until I became a parent 5 years ago. I try to be happy, but I cannot seem to find it. I get angry at my partner quickly for silly things. When I come home from work the house is a mess and she does not work. I take my frustration out on her. I see that after the fight, but at the time, I explode at her. I have hit her in the past. Several times. She does not deserve that. I scare her. I scare my son. I want to be a better father. I am trying, but it doesn't seem to be helping. That is why I am here. It is court ordered to attend these sessions because of my anger. I cannot keep a job. I bounce from one job to another. I know I need to support my family. I will not do what my mother did to me. I feel helpless most times." Client states that he uses cannabis recreationally approximately 3 to 5 times per week and drinks approximately 26 ounces (768 mL) of whiskey on the weekend. They have used the food bank several times a month for the last 6 months. Client was overheard commenting on the clothing of the unit clerk: "She flirted with him when he walked in, and he would have no problem getting her into bed." Client was reprimanded immediately for that type of inappropriate language, and he denied saying anything to the other group member despite being heard by writer.

The nurse is reviewing the client's assessment data to prepare the client's plan of care.

▶ Complete the diagram by identifying from the choices below to specify what condition the client is most likely experiencing, 2 actions the nurse should take to address that condition, and 2 parameters the nurse should monitor to assess the client's progress.

Action to Take	Condition Most Likely Experiencing	Parameter to Monitor
Action to Take		Parameter to Monitor

Action to Take	Potential Conditions	Parameters to Monitor
Assess risk for suicide	Borderline personality disorder	Family group therapy progress
Administer valium (anticonvulsant)	Avoidant personality disorder	Effectiveness of mindfulness and relaxation techniques
Avoid being "too nice" to client	Schizotypal personality disorder	Effectiveness of mindfulness and relaxation techniques
Initiate peripheral intravenous	Narcissistic personality disorder	Improvement to emotional expressiveness
Initiate therapeutic relationship with client		Depression

Write your answers in the table below.

Action to Take	Condition Most Likely Experiencing	Parameter to Monitor
Action to Take		Parameter to Monitor

Mental Health 3.0

The nurse is caring for a 22-year-old female client on an inpatient mental health unit.

Nurses' Notes | Laboratory Results

1300h: Client was brought to the emergency department (ED) by her friend after she was found lying on the floor of the washroom in the gym. She is currently in her final year of an undergraduate program, lives with a roommate (the person who brought her to the hospital) as she is out-of-province and hopes to write the Law School Admission Test (LSAT) and apply for law school. The ED ruled out a head injury, but she is being admitted for further assessment. The client was recently seen in the ED 2 weeks ago with complaints of palpitations and trouble "catching her breath," but the symptoms were ruled as stress related. The client has no other comorbidities. Vital signs: T: 35.7°C (96.2°F); BP: 87/50; P: 102; RR: 18; with pulse oximetry of 98% on room air. Client presents with inadequate body weight, motor power strong × 4 extremities. Client reports working out to compete in a body building competition in a few months. Client is alert and oriented to person, place and time. She is cooperative and pleasant and obeys all commands. Chest clear with air entry through all lobes anteriorly and posteriorly. Respirations regular and easy at rest but client noted to take short, shallow respirations. Client denies chest pain but reports feeling heaviness in her chest while working out that decreases with rest. Lanugo noted on client's back. Client reports feeling chilled but afebrile. Client noted to have sunken eyes, tenting on the back of the hand, and pale inner canthus when pulled down. Abdomen bloated with borborygmus, despite presenting as flat and cachectic. Client states she has not had a bowel movement for 5 days. Client has not voided yet upon admission. Denies wanting to harm herself.

Nurses' Notes | **Laboratory Results**

1330h:

Test	Result	Test	Result
Hemoglobin 140–180 g/L (14–18 g/dL) (male) 120–160 g/L (12–16 g/dL) (female)	76 g/L (7.6 g/dL)	Sodium 136–145 mmol/L	133 mmol/L
Platelets 150–400 × 10^9/L	90 × 10^9/L	Potassium 3.5–5.1 mmol/L	2.6 mmol/L
White blood cells 3.5–12.0 × 10^9/L	5.0 × 10^9/L (5 000/mm^3)	Creatinine 53–106 mcmol/L	255 mcmol/L
Neutrophils 3.0–5.8 × 10^9/L	3.2 × 10^9/L (3 200/mm^3)	Blood urea nitrogen (BUN) 2.9–8.2 mmol/L	7.6 mmol/L
		Blood glucose (random) 3.9–6.1 mmol/L	3.5 mmol/L

The nurse is reviewing the client's assessment data to prepare the client's plan of care.

▶ Complete the diagram by identifying from the choices below to specify what condition the client is most likely experiencing, 2 actions the nurse should take to address that condition, and 2 parameters the nurse should monitor to assess the client's progress.

Action to Take	Condition Most Likely Experiencing	Parameter to Monitor
Action to Take		Parameter to Monitor

Action to Take	Potential Conditions	Parameters to Monitor
Request an order to administer potassium 10 mEq/50 mL D_5W via peripheral intravenous catheter	Anorexia nervosa	Amenorrhea
Insert nasogastric tube for parenteral nutrition	Bulimia nervosa	Seizure protocols
Complete arterial blood gas draw	Binge eating disorder	Suicidal ideation
Establish therapeutic boundaries	Eating disorder not otherwise specified	Polycythemia vera
Initiate oxygen therapy		Ventricular tachycardia

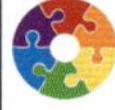

Write your answers in the table below.

Action to Take	Condition Most Likely Experiencing	Parameter to Monitor
Action to Take		Parameter to Monitor

Mental Health 4.0

The nurse is caring for a 78-year-old female client on a home care visit.

Nurses' Notes

0800h: Home care visit required to provide wound care. Client fell while getting out of the shower 2 weeks ago, fractured left hip, requiring surgical intervention. As a result, the client developed osteomyelitis, suffered a lengthy hospital stay, and only returned home 2 days ago but requires daily hip dressings. Vital signs: T: 37.3°C; BP: 110/72 mm Hg; HR: 76; RR: 14; with pulse oximetry of 96% on room air. Client presents as detached and withdrawn; many photos of family, children, and grandchildren noted in the room. Client alert and oriented to person, place, and time. States pain of 2 out of 10 on numerical pain scale; pain subsides with taking acetaminophen tablets. Last dose was at breakfast (0730h) when she took 1 000 mg. Usual pain medication regiment is 1 000 mg every 12 hours with adequate pain relief. Client reports difficulty sleeping since coming home, waking with nightmares she cannot remember. She requires a nap in the afternoon. Gait steady; carpet low level and client using four-wheeled walker with breaks until stability increases. Client's breathing regular and easy at rest. Denies any discomfort with respirations, chest pain, or palpitations. Client's skin warm and dry to touch. Pulses palpable and strong × bilateral radials, posterior tibial and dorsalis pedis. Capillary refill less than 3 seconds. Abdomen flat with hyperactive bowel sounds auscultated throughout all fields. Client reports no bowel movement since arriving home. Voiding without issues. Wound edges pink and blanch with minimal pressure. Wound bed remains present with slough, but healthy granulation is noted. Serosanguinous drainage noted on the dressing. Wound remains deep. Client reports feeling less energy since discharge, denies any visitors, since her family lives out of the city. She has a grown son and daughter, both married, and two grandchildren. There have been several phone calls from friends and family, but she has stopped answering as they make her exhausted. Client reports being a widower and without a partner since 2020. Partner died in a motor vehicle accident. Client presents with poor hygiene, states she is in the same clothes she wore when she left the hospital 2 days ago. Client's home noted to be unkempt with many papers from the time she was in hospital at the door, dishes in the sink, and a large bottle of vodka on the counter. Client reports not leaving her home since being discharged and looks forward to the home care nurse visits.

The nurse is reviewing the client's assessment data to prepare the client's plan of care.

▶ Complete the diagram by identifying from the choices below to specify what condition the client is most likely experiencing, 2 actions the nurse should take to address that condition, and 2 parameters the nurse should monitor to assess the client's progress.

Action to Take		Parameter to Monitor
Action to Take	Condition Most Likely Experiencing	Parameter to Monitor

Action to Take	Potential Condition	Parameters to Monitor
Request an order for hydromorphone 1 mg	Chronic osteomyelitis	Suicidal ideation
Complete a geriatric depression scale screening tool	Post-traumatic stress disorder	Temperature
Request an order to administer intravenous antibiotics	Depression	Alcohol consumption
Contact the client's daughter	Generalized anxiety disorder	Reduced pain
Prepare to consult psychiatry		Reduced use of mobility aids

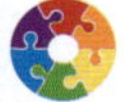
Write your answers in the table below.

Action to Take	Condition Most Likely Experiencing	Parameter to Monitor
Action to Take		Parameter to Monitor

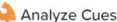

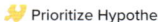

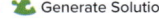

Medical-Surgical Trend Cases

Medical-Surgical 1.0

The nurse is caring for a 57-year-old client on a general medical unit.

Nurses' Notes | Laboratory Results

01153h: The client presented to the emergency department (ED) with 5 days of diarrhea at home prior to seeking care. Client was recently taking oral antibiotic therapy (ciprofloxacin) for pneumonia; diarrhea started after the prescribed antibiotics had been stopped. Vital signs: T: 38.2°C (100.8°F); BP: 90/67; P: 105; RR: 18; with pulse oximetry of 98% on room air. Client alert and oriented to person place and time, obeys all commands, motor power strong × 4 with independent mobility and steady gait noted when up to the washroom. Client presents as pale, skin cool to touch, denies chest pain, dry mucous membranes and tenting noted during assessment of skin turgor. Bilateral radial pulses strong with strong dorsalis pedis pulses × 2. Lungs auscultated for clear air entry throughout. Abdomen flat with borborygmus noted with auscultation. Client complains of mild cramping after frequent bowel movements. Client indicates 4 out of 10 abdominal pain on a numerical pain scale. Client has not voided yet. Skin red and excoriated on coccyx. No open areas noted.

1500h: Client remains lethargic, difficult to rouse. Vital signs: T: 38.5°C (101.3°F); BP: 88/62; P: 118; RR: 22; with pulse oximetry of 92% on room air. Client returned from the washroom and stool collected for assessment. Stool noted to be loose, watery with mucus, and foul smelling. Health care provider notified.

Nurses' Notes | **Laboratory Results**

Laboratory Test and Normal Reference Range	1500h
Clostridium difficile Negative	Positive

The nurse has reviewed the Nurses' Note entries from 1153h and 1500h and is planning care for the client.

▶ For each potential nursing intervention, click to specify whether the intervention is **indicated** or **not indicated** for the care of the client.

POTENTIAL NURSING INTERVENTIONS	INDICATED	NOT INDICATED
Prepare client for chest X-ray	○	○
Initiate isolation protocols	○	○
Request a full-fibre diet from dietary	○	○
Request an order to initiate intravenous fluids	○	○
Apply barrier cream to coccyx	○	○
Administer laxatives as per bowel protocol	○	○
Request a cart with personal protective equipment such as gowns and gloves	○	○

Note: Each row must have one response option selected.

Medical-Surgical 2.0

The nurse is caring for a 60-year-old client in the emergency department (ED).

Nurses' Notes | Vital Signs

1340h: Client presented to the ED, accompanied by their partner, with complaints of a headache rated 8 out of 10 on a numerical pain scale, double vision (diplopia), unsteady gait, and feeling flushed. Client reports these are new symptoms. The client reports having difficulty sleeping at night over the past few weeks, sometimes requiring a nap in the afternoon, with dizziness at times. Client presents alert and oriented to person, place, and time. Pupils equal and reactive to light measured at 3 mm. No irregularity in shape identified. Gait steady. Client denies any chest pain but feels "fluttering" in chest during light exercise, skin warm and flushed to touch. Diaphoresis noted despite client feeling chilled. Bilateral radial pulses regular but fast. Apical = radial. No shortness of breath noted. Lungs clear with auscultation, no adventitious breath sounds noted. Denies any cough. Client reports voiding less frequently due to a reduction in oral intake. Abdomen soft and rounded. Bowel sounds auscultated in all four quadrants. Client states they are the president of a large national company with 1 000 employees and the company is in a financial loss.

Nurses' Notes | **Vital Signs**

	1340h	1530h	1700h	2200h
T	37.3°C (99.1°F)	37.7°C (99.9°F)	37.4°C (99.3°F)	37.5°C (99.5°F)
P	108	100	85	77
RR	22	16	18	18
BP	165/87	153/85	159/80	144/81
Pulse oximetry reading	97% on room air	94% on 2 L/min per nasal prongs		

The nurse has reviewed the Nurses' Notes at 1340h and the Vital Signs table.

▶ Complete the following sentence by choosing from the list of options.

The client is at **highest** risk of developing ____________________ (word options 1) as evidenced by the client's ____________________ (word options 2) and ____________________ (word options 2)

WORD OPTIONS 1	WORD OPTIONS 2
Hyperthermia	Renal assessment
Hypernatremia	Respiratory assessment
Hypertension	Vital signs
Hypoxemia	Neurological assessment
Hyperemesis	Cardiovascular assessment

Medical-Surgical 3.0

The nurse is caring for an 83-year-old male client in the emergency department (ED).

Nurses' Notes | Diagnostic Results

1622h: Client presented to the ED accompanied by his daughter. Client's daughter reported to triage that she found him on the floor, holding his left arm close to his body. He told her that he missed the chair when he went to sit down and found himself on the floor. Vital signs: T: 37.6°C (99.7°F); BP: 126/68; P: 92; RR: 18; with pulse oximetry of 96% on room air. Upon initial assessment, daughter remained in the room answering questions for the client. Daughter received a work phone call and assessment initiated at that time. Client states, "She talks for me a lot." Upon full assessment, client opens eyes to speech, obeys all commands, denies a headache, pupils equal and reactive to light and measuring 2 mm. Motor power strong × 3 extremities with left hand grip weak to moderate. Client reports lower arm pain at 4 out of 10 on a numerical pain scale. Capillary refill less than 3 seconds on bilateral upper and lower nail beds. Client noted to be diaphoretic. Denies any chest pain. Bilateral radial pulses palpable and strong and regular × 2. Bilateral dorsalis pedis pulses strong. Skin warm and dry to touch. Respirations regular and easy at rest. Lung fields clear upon auscultation. Urinal at bedside to monitor urine output. Previous medical history includes type 2 diabetes mellitus, rheumatoid arthritis requiring use of a cane. Client scheduled for X-rays of his left lower arm.

1745h: The nurse assisted the health care provider in applying a fibreglass cast to client's left forearm.

1855h: Client to be transferred to orthopedic unit for observation and geriatric assessment. Social work consulted for assessment of living situation.

2145h: Client admitted to orthopedic unit. Upon intake assessment, admitting nurse noted client's left hand +4 edematous with knuckles and skin on the top of hand coming out of cast. Capillary refill greater than 3 seconds on the left-hand fingertips, skin cool to touch, with pallor noted on the palm. The client complains of mild numbness in left-hand fingertips and 8 out of 10 pain on numerical scale, with minimal movement. Fingers noted to be edematous, and client reports "tightness." T: 37.8°C (100.0°F); BP: 136/72; P: 102; RR: 22; with pulse oximetry of 97% on room air. Health care provider was notified.

Nurses' Notes | **Diagnostic Results**

1650h: Left humerus demonstrates an acute transverse closed fracture of the proximal humeral metadiaphysis. There is medial displacement of the distal fracture fragment. Multiple bone fragments identified.

The nurse has reviewed the Nurses' Notes at 1622h, 1745h, 1855h, and 2145h and Diagnostic Results at 1650h.

▶ For each potential nursing intervention, identify whether the intervention is **indicated** or **not indicated** for the client.

POTENTIAL NURSING INTERVENTIONS	INDICATED	NOT INDICATED
Prepare to insert an 18-gauge peripheral venous access device	○	○
Monitor urine output	○	○
Prepare the client for an ultrasound	○	○
Request an order for an analgesic	○	○
Prepare to draw laboratory tests: electrolytes, creatinine kinase, creatinine, BUN	○	○
Administer sodium chloride per venous access device	○	○
Elevate the forearm on pillows	○	○

Note: Each row must have one response option selected.

Medical-Surgical 4.0

The nurse is caring for a 24-year-old client on a cardiology unit.

Nurses' Notes

1225h: Client presented to the unit with chest pain and shortness of breath as a result of ingesting oral stimulants (i.e., Red Bull) while studying for an exam. Client is a student at the local university. Vital signs: T: 36.9°C (98.4°F); BP: 120/80; P: 83; RR: 16; with pulse oximetry of 98% on room air. Upon assessment, client alert and oriented to person, place, and time. Denies any chest pain at present. Capillary refill less than 3 seconds. Colour pink with adequate perfusion to mucous membranes. Lungs auscultated for clear bilateral air entry throughout, no adventitious breath sounds noted. Client's abdomen flat with bowel sounds auscultated × 4 quadrants. Client voiding independently in the washroom. Back of left arm noted to have a hot, tender, swollen, and red area approximately 2 cm in diameter, where client received heparin subcutaneous injection in the emergency department. Client states it is tender with movement.

1600h: Client rang for nursing assistance complaining of increased pain in the back of the left arm. Upon further assessment, redness has increased in size to 8 cm wide as compared to previous assessment, with client complaining of chills and feeling unwell. Vital signs: T: 38.3°C (100.9°F); BP: 110/60; P: 104; RR: 20; with pulse oximetry of 90% on room air. Client continues to deny chest pain; no palpitations noted. Client remains well perfused to mucous membranes, and clear air entry noted to bilateral lung fields. Health care provider notified of change in status. Awaiting further orders.

The nurse has reviewed the Nurses' Notes at 1225h and 1600h.

▶ Identify the correct word from the options below to complete the sentence.

The nurse should recognize that the client is potentially experiencing ________________.

WORD OPTIONS
Hypertension
Cellulitis
Pneumonia
Diabetes
Heart failure

Medical-Surgical 5.0

The nurse is caring for a 66-year-old male client in the emergency department who developed urosepsis from a cystoscopy now requiring antibiotic therapy.

Nurses' Notes | Intake and Output

1000: The client presents with chills, malaise, and difficulty voiding. Vital signs: T: 38.5°C (101.3°F); BP: 90/54; P: 118; RR: 22; with pulse oximetry of 91% on room air. Upon assessment, the mucous membranes were pale, and tenting occurred when the skin was pinched. The client denies any pain. Peripheral venous access device inserted left antecubital. Urinal at the bedside.

1400h: The client presents as confused and irritable. Vital signs: T: 38.9°C (102.0°F); BP: 84/49; P: 125; RR: 24; with pulse oximetry of 90% on room air. Client complains of chills and pain in bilateral flank area.

1800h: The client remains confused and is now disoriented. Vital signs: T: 38.9°C (102.0°F); BP: 88/52; P: 130; RR: 26; with pulse oximetry of 87% on room air.

Nurses' Notes | **Intake and Output**

Intake and Output	1000h	1400h	1800h
Intake	Piperacillin/ Tazobactum 2.25 g (100 mL) 0.9% normal saline at 125 mL/hr (continuous)	0.9% normal saline 500 mL bolus	Piperacillin/ Tazobactum 2.25 g (100 mL) 0.9% normal saline at 125 mL/hr (continuous)
Output	Admission	400 mL	250 mL

The nurse has reviewed the Nurses' Notes from 1000h, 1400h, and 1800h, as well as the Intake and Output data from 1000h, 1400h, 1800h.

▶ Select 2 actions the nurse should take.

- ☐ Request an order to insert a Foley catheter
- ☐ Check the client's temperature every 1 hr
- ☐ Contact the client's clergy for last rites
- ☐ Initiate oxygen therapy at 2 L/min per nasal prongs
- ☐ Draw laboratory samples: complete blood count, electrolytes, troponin, blood cultures

Medical-Surgical 6.0

The nurse is caring for a 19-year-old male client in the emergency department (ED) being assessed for a left axilla stab wound.

Nurses' Notes

2200h: The client reports increased shortness of breath and pleuritic chest pain rated 8 out of 10 on numerical pain scale. Vital signs: T: 38.0°C (100.4° F); BP: 110/64; P: 108; RR: 20; with pulse oximetry of 90% on room air. A gauze dressing secured on all four sides was applied by emergency medical services prior to arrival in the ED. Dressing noted to have shadowing of dark red blood the size of a pea. Client sitting in high-Fowler's position for comfort.

2345h: The client called the nurse to the room with difficulty breathing. The nurse noted asymmetrical breathing with bilateral inspiration and expiration. Absent breath sounds noted over entire left lung. Nonproductive cough noted. Client's colour noted to be grey with diaphoresis. Vital signs: T: 38.0°C (100.4°F); BP: 92/60; P: 125; RR: 26; with pulse oximetry of 88% on room air.

2348h: Health care provider notified of change in status. Chest X-ray ordered and chest tube to be inserted.

2352h: Client presents as confused, unable to follow simple commands. Client noted to be indrawing at the rib cage, nasal flaring, and found in the tripod position over the bedside table. Tracheal deviation noted to be drifting toward the right. Vital signs: T: 38.3°C (100.9°F); BP: 88/56; P: 139; RR: 28; with pulse oximetry of 76% on room air.

2355h: Code blue called.

The nurse has reviewed the Nurses' Notes at 2200h, 2345h, 2348h, and 2352h.

▶ Select the 4 client findings that require **immediate** follow-up.

- ☐ Gauze dressing secured on all four sides
- ☐ Dressing with dark red shadowing of blood
- ☐ Asymmetrical breathing
- ☐ Diaphoresis
- ☐ Indrawing and nasal flaring
- ☐ Tracheal deviation
- ☐ Temperature

Medical-Surgical 7.0

The nurse is caring for an 85-year-old client on the medical unit admitted with dehydration.

Nurses' Notes

1300h: The client was brought to the hospital after a ground-level fall after being found in their residence apartment. The client had recently recovered from a gastrointestinal viral illness 1 day before the fall. The client denies hitting their head and presented to the emergency department with dizziness and unstable gait. Vital signs: T: 37.7°C (99.9°F); BP: 102/54; P: 102; RR: 16; with pulse oximetry of 95% on room air. Client alert and oriented to person, place, and time. Answers questions appropriately. Pupils equal and reactive briskly to light at 2 mm. Bilateral radial pulses regular and strong with palpation × 2. Bilateral dorsalis pedis pulses strong and palpable × 2. Capillary refill less than 3 seconds. Denies any chest pain. Tenting noted inside of the forearm. Mucous membranes noted to be dry. Lungs clear with auscultation anteriorly and posteriorly. Abdomen tender with palpation but soft. Bowel sounds auscultated in all four quadrants. Client has not voided yet, encouraged to ring with assistance. Venous access device inserted into right hand infusing 0.9% normal saline at 75 mL/hr.

1350h: Client rang for the nurse with complaints of right arm pain. Upon assessment, right arm noted to be edematous, warm to touch, with limited range of motion. Right elbow noted to be edematous as well. Venous access device does not flush. Redness, blanching, and discomfort noted at the site.

The nurse reviews the Nurses' Notes at 1300h and 1350h.

▶ Which of the following assessment findings require **immediate** follow-up? **Select all that apply**.

- ☐ Pupillary response to light
- ☐ Orientation to person, place, and time
- ☐ Oliguria
- ☐ Bowel sounds
- ☐ Interstitial peripheral venous access device

Medical-Surgical 8.0

The nurse is caring for a 72-year-old male client on the cardiac unit.

Nurses' Notes

1200h: The client was admitted to the cardiac unit for further monitoring of chest pain. While shovelling their driveway, the client developed 8 out of 10 chest pain as based on a numerical pain scale, diaphoresis, and shortness of breath. Vital signs: T: 37.2°C (99.0°F); BP: 122/75; P: 88; RR: 18; with pulse oximetry of 98% on room air. The client presents alert and oriented to person, place, and time. Obeys all commands. Motor power strong × 4 peripheral extremities. Client able to ambulate independently without any issue. Client pain free during assessment. The pain subsided en route to the hospital and has not returned since the shovelling. Inspiratory crackles auscultated to bilateral lung field bases. Client denies any shortness of breath. No diaphoresis, nausea, or emesis noted. Capillary refill documented at less than 3 seconds. Abdomen soft, with bowel sounds auscultated in all four quadrants. Urinal provided at the bedside in the event client has to void. Client denies any issue with voiding prior to admission. Venous access device inserted into left forearm infusing 0.9% normal saline at 50 mL/hr with heparin intravenously to be initiated. The client had an acute myocardial infarction (MI) with angioplasty of the left anterior descending coronary artery due to an 85% blockage 3 years before this admission. The ejection fraction of the left ventricle was documented as 48% at the time of the acute MI 3 years ago.

1300h: Nutrition brought to the client. Client found to be short of breath with increased tachypnea, sitting in tripod position, with documented 26 breaths per minute. Client noted to have dry nonproductive cough. Vital signs: T: 37.6°C (99.7°F); BP: 128/82; P: 91; with pulse oximetry of 92% on room air. Upon further assessment, coarse crackles auscultated in bilateral lower lung fields and inspiratory crackles in bilateral upper lung fields, posteriorly and anteriorly. Peripheral venous access device remains in situ with 0.9% normal saline infusing at 250 mL/hr.

The nurse reviews the Nurses' Notes at 1200h and 1300h.

▶ Complete the following sentence by choosing from the list of options.

The client is at **highest** risk of developing ______________ (word options 1) as evidenced by the client's ______________ (word options 2).

WORD OPTIONS 1	WORD OPTIONS 2
Pneumonia	Gastrointestinal assessment
Pleuritis	Respiratory assessment
Pleural effusion	Cardiovascular assessment
Pulmonary edema	Neurological assessment
Pericarditis	Renal assessment

Medical-Surgical 9.0

The nurse is caring for a 49-year-old client in the emergency department (ED)

Nurses' Notes | Vital Signs

1824h: Client presented to the ED via emergency medical services (EMS). The client miscalculated how the temperature would affect their body while playing golf in Palm Springs on vacation. The client became confused and disoriented on the course, ++ diaphoretic, and ++ flushed. EMS was contacted and met the golfers on the course. Vital signs listed in the table below. Client presents alert and oriented to person and place but unable to determine time, date, month, or year. Client has difficulty staying awake and is lying on the stretcher with head backward and eyes closed. Client denies pain. Pupils 5 mm in size but equal. Difficult to determine reactivity to light as pupillary size is large compared to the iris. No irregularity in shape identified. Gait unsteady, requiring one-person stand-by assist. Client denies any dizziness. Client's clothing wet from diaphoresis. Hospital gown provided to client. Skin colour presents as ashen and grey as noticed in the conjunctiva and palms of the hands. Bilateral radial pulses regular, strong in sensation, and bounding. Bilateral dorsalis pedis pulses and posterior tibial pulses bounding. Capillary refill less than 3 seconds. Client noted to be taking quick, fast, shallow breaths. Abdomen flat and soft with hypoactive bowel sounds auscultated × 4 quadrants. Client complaining of nausea with vomiting clear bile of approximately 150 mL into a kidney basin. Client denies need to void at present time. A peripheral venous access device was inserted into the left antecubital fossa and infusing 0.9% sodium chloride at 150 mL/hr.

Nurses' Notes | **Vital Signs**

	1824h	1902h	1930h	2005h
T	39.8°C (104.6°F)	39.9°C (103.8°F)	39.7°C (103.5°F)	39.9°C (103.8°F)
P	148	152	143	149
RR	28	32	30	34
BP	77/52	85/52	82/58	97/64
Pulse oximetry reading	Unable to obtain	Unable to obtain	92% on room air	95% on room air

The nurse has reviewed the Nurses' Notes at 1824h and the Vital Signs table.

▶ Complete the following sentence by choosing from the list of options.

The nurse should recognize that the client is potentially experiencing __________________(word options 1) and __________________ (word options 1) as evidenced by the __________________ (word options 2) __________________ (word options 2).

WORD OPTIONS 1	WORD OPTIONS 2
Hyperthermia	Bowel sounds
Hypothermia	Respiratory rate
Hypertension	Temperature
Hypotension	Pupillary response
Hyperglycemia	Blood pressure
Hypoglycemia	Bilateral radial pulses

Medical-Surgical 10.0

The nurse is caring for a 29-year-old female client in a low-risk outpatient pregnancy clinic connected to a hospital.

Progress Notes

Prenatal Visit Week 16: Client presents to the clinic for her routine checkup, accompanied by partner. The client states she is experiencing extreme fatigue and nausea requiring her to stay in bed and take several days off work. Vital signs: T: 37.4°C (99.3°F); BP: 126/62; P: 88; RR: 18; with pulse oximetry of 99% on room air. Client presents alert and oriented, pale in colour as noted by reduced perfusion to the conjunctiva and pallor on bilateral palms. Tenting noted on the back of the hand. Client states she is only drinking 2 L of water every day. She cannot stay awake. Client encouraged to drink more fluids and eat foods that do not exacerbate nausea. Fetal heart auscultated with Doppler at 137 beats per minute.

Prenatal Visit Week 20: Client presents to the clinic for routine checkup without any support person. Client indicates there was a breakup of the relationship and the other birth parent has moved out. Client states nausea has improved since the last visit but states she is voiding several times per hour, with a sharp, burning sensation when starting to void, chills, and a generalized feeling of being unwell × 2 days. Vital signs: T: 38.0°C (100.4°F); BP: 98/57; P: 124; RR: 22; with pulse oximetry of 95% on room air. Client denies increasing water intake and with the stress of the breakup in the relationship, the client often forgets to drink fluids. Fetal heart auscultated with Doppler at 142 beats per minute. Urine specimen collected in the clinic. Urine dipstick analysis demonstrated positive for leukocytes and traces of blood. Health care provider prescribed nitrofurantoin (Microdantin).

Prenatal Visit Week 21: Client presents to the clinic with complaints of voiding several times per hour, with a sharp, burning sensation when starting to void, chills, now accompanied by flank pain described as 6 out of 10 on numerical pain scale, increased nausea and vomiting. Vital signs: T: 38.5°C (101.3°F); BP: 110/62; P: 130 RR: 22; with pulse oximetry of 92% on room air. Client states she was unable to afford the prescription. Fetal heart auscultated with Doppler at 150 beats per minute. Health care provider notified.

The nurse has reviewed the Progress Notes from Prenatal Visits Weeks 16, 20, and 21.

▶ Select 3 actions the nurse should the nurse take **immediately.**

- ☐ Provide the client with antibiotic samples to treat infection
- ☐ Initiate social work support for the client
- ☐ Consult mental health resources
- ☐ Instruct the client to go directly to the hospital for further assessment
- ☐ Assess the client to see if she is experiencing any uterine cramping or preterm labour
- ☐ Provide education to the client about how to avoid reoccurrence of an infection

Medical-Surgical 11.0

The nurse is caring for a 45-year-old female client on a general surgical unit.

Progress Notes

1130h: Client returned from the recovery room after a breast reconstruction under general anaesthetic as a result of left-sided mastectomy 6 months ago after discovering a malignant mass. Vital signs: T: 37.9°C (100.2°F); BP: 99/60; P: 102; RR: 12; with pulse oximetry of 92% on 3 L/min per nasal prongs. Client rouses easily to voice and stimulation. Alert and oriented to person, place, and time. Client is able to follow commands and move all extremities independently. Denies any pain at present, but states generalized discomfort. Pupils equal and reactive to light at 2 mm. Client presents with a regular bilateral radial pulse. Apical = radial. Bilateral dorsalis pedis pulses strong. Skin warm and dry to touch, no diaphoresis noted. Client denies any chest pain. Fine inspiratory crackles auscultated to bilateral lung fields. Clear air entry noted to bilateral upper lungs. Respirations regular and easy at rest. No cough noted. Abdomen soft with hypoactive bowel sounds noted in right lower quadrant and left lower quadrant fields. No bowel sounds in bilateral upper quadrants. Client denies nausea, not passing flatus or eructation. Client has not voided yet and does not feel urgency yet. Peripheral venous access device noted in left forearm with 0.9% normal saline infusing at 100 mL/hr. Incision covered by dry dressings with Jackson-Pratt drains noted on each side draining blood. Jackson-Pratt emptied for 25 mL on the left side and 20 mL on the right side.

1540h: Client assisted up to the washroom to void. Denies any dizziness. Encouraged to perform deep-breathing and coughing exercises every hour. Denies any chest pain. Lung sounds remain unchanged.

2005h: Client complaining of discomfort from surgery but indicates pain is manageable. Denies any analgesic. Client encouraged to maintain deep-breathing and coughing even with discomfort.

0730h (Postoperative day 1/POD1): During assessment, client presents as feeling chilled and pale. Presents alert and oriented to person, place, and time. No confusion noted. Vital signs: T: 38.5°C (101.3°F); BP: 110/72; P: 127; RR: 26; with pulse oximetry of 88% on 4 L/min per nasal prongs. Productive cough noted during assessment with coarse crackles auscultated throughout bilateral lung bases and fine inspiratory crackles auscultated bilateral upper bases. Expectorating yellow-tinged sputum. Client denies chest pain but is feeling short of breath with ambulation. Client is noted to be using accessory muscles for breathing, with nasal flaring. Client states pain in thorax with inspiration. S1, S2 heart sounds. Bilateral radial pulses strong and regular with palpation. Bilateral dorsalis pedis pulses are weak. No adventitious heart sounds auscultated. Skin cool to touch. No diaphoresis noted. Abdomen soft with active bowel sounds noted × 4 quadrants. Client denies nausea or emesis.

The nurse has reviewed the Progress Notes from 1130h, 1540h, 2005, and 0730h.

▶ Which of the following assessment findings require **immediate** follow-up? **Select all that apply.**

- ☐ Pallor
- ☐ Alertness
- ☐ Bowel sounds
- ☐ Lung sounds
- ☐ Pulses
- ☐ Pulse oximetry
- ☐ Skin temperature
- ☐ Accessory muscles

Medical-Surgical 12.0

The nurse is caring for an 83-year-old male client on the renal unit.

Progress Notes

1050h: Client was admitted to the unit for mild confusion and urinary retention. The client states having to void several times throughout the day and night and becoming exhausted. Complains of feeling chilled × 2 days, dysuria, and lower back pain × 3 days. Vital signs: T: 38.1°C (100.6°F); BP: 110/64; P: 77; RR: 18; with pulse oximetry of 94% on room air. Client presents as pleasant, cooperative, alert and oriented to person, place, and time. Gait steady, denies any dizziness. Pupils equal in size and shape, measured at 2 mm and briskly reactive to light. S1 and S2 heart sounds, apical heart rate regular and equals radial pulse. Bilateral radial pulses palpable, regular, and strong. Client denies any chest pain. Clear air entry noted throughout all lung fields. Respirations regular and easy at rest. Client denies a cough, shortness of breath. Abdomen round and soft. No pain with palpation. Bowel sounds active throughout all four quadrants. Client noted to have incontinence through briefs. Client states he feels a sense of urgency to void and there have been times he has "dribbled," which is very embarrassing. Urinal placed at the bedside. The client's previous comorbidities include mild hypertension controlled with diet. Client lives independently in a residential facility. Client to have urodynamic scan in the morning.

1300h: Client found by a nursing attendant wandering the hallways, unable to locate his hospital room. Client states he went for a walk and forgot which room he was admitted to. Client oriented to person, place, and time. Says he feels silly for not remembering his room number. Urine found in the urinal with a strong odour; dark, concentrated urine measured at 150 mL.

1600h: Client found voiding in the waste basket in the room. Says he could not find the urinal at the bedside and felt an urgency to void. Client oriented to person, place, and time. Vital signs: T: 38.6°C (101.5°F); BP: 99/62; P: 96; RR: 20; with pulse oximetry of 94% on room air. Health care provider notified of changes in behaviour and vital signs.

1630h: Client started on antibiotic therapy.

The nurse reviewed the Progress Notes from 1050h, 1300h, 1600h, and 1630h. All actions carried out by the nurse.

▶ For each assessment finding, identify whether the finding indicates that the client's condition has **improved, not changed,** or **has declined**.

ASSESSMENT FINDINGS	IMPROVED	NO CHANGE	DECLINED
Temperature 37.2°C (98.9°F)	○	○	○
Concentrated urine	○	○	○
Denies dysuria	○	○	○
"Dribbling" incontinence noted	○	○	○
Strong odour	○	○	○
Blood pressure 92/62	○	○	○

Note: Each row must have one response option selected.

Medical-Surgical 13.0

The nurse is caring for a 55-year-old client in the emergency department (ED).

Progress Notes

1843h: Client was brought to the ED accompanied by their partner with complaints of abdominal pain, chills, and generalized feeling of being unwell. Vital signs: T: 38.5°C (101.3°F); BP: 136/74; P: 92; RR: 18; with pulse oximetry of 96% on room air. Upon further assessment, the client presents as alert and oriented to person, place, time, and situation. Walks independently without assistance; motor power strong × 4 extremities. Denies any numbness and tingling. Client's conjunctiva are pink and perfused. Capillary refill less than 3 seconds. Fine inspiratory crackles auscultated anteriorly to bilateral lung fields that clear with a cough. Client denies difficulty breathing, no shortness of breath noted, no use of accessory muscles. Abdomen rounded and firm to touch. Hyperactive bowel sounds auscultated to left lower quadrant of the abdomen, with adequate bowel sounds noted in remaining three quadrants. Colostomy noted in left upper quadrant. Client states they developed severe ulcerative colitis in their late teens and early 20s, prompting the need for this intervention. A permanent colostomy was surgically created 3 years ago. The skin under the flange is pink and excoriated, with multiple areas of skin breakdown noted. Serous, yellow-tinged purulent drainage is noted under the skin barrier wafer. Client denies emesis or nausea. The client drains the colostomy pouch 3 to 4 times per day. The stoma has not changed colour and has remained pink with healthy tissue. There were no necrotic areas noted. Client denies any issue with voiding. No pain, no urgency, no frequency noted.

2120h: Client rang for assistance complaining of increased abdominal pain and was noted to be bleeding at the stoma site. There is concern that there will be contamination at the site now that the skin has broken. Health care provider notified.

The nurse has reviewed the Progress Notes at 1843h and 2120h.

▶ Complete the following sentence by choosing from the list of options.

The client is at **highest** risk of developing

____________________.

WORD OPTIONS
Sepsis
Pneumonia
Urinary tract infection
Gastrointestinal illness
Bowel obstruction

Medical-Surgical 14.0

The nurse is caring for a 19-year-old male client in the emergency department being assessed for a left axilla stab wound.

Nurses' Notes

2200h: The client reports increased shortness of breath and pleuritic chest pain rated 8 out of 10 on a numerical pain scale. Vital signs: T: 38.0°C (100.4°F); BP: 110/64; P: 108; RR: 20; with pulse oximetry of 90% on room air. A gauze dressing secured on all four sides was applied by the emergency medical services before arriving in the emergency department. Dressing noted to have shadowing of dark red blood the size of a pea. Client is sitting in high-Fowler's position for comfort.

2345h: The client called the nurse to the room with difficulty breathing. The nurse noted asymmetrical breathing noted with bilateral inspiration and expiration. Absent breath sounds noted over entire left lung. Nonproductive cough noted. Client's colour noted to be grey with diaphoresis. Vital signs: T: 38.0°C (100.4°F); BP: 92/60; P: 125; RR: 26; with pulse oximetry of 88% on room air.

2348h: Health care provider notified of change in status. Chest X-ray ordered and chest tube to be inserted.

2352h: Client presents as confused, unable to follow simple commands. Client noted to be indrawing at the rib cage, nasal flaring, and found in the tripod position over the bedside table. Tracheal deviation noted to be drifting towards the right. Vital signs: T: 38.3°C (100.9°F); BP: 88/56; P: 139; RR: 28; with pulse oximetry of 76% on room air.

2355h: Code blue called.

The nurse has reviewed the Nurses' Notes at 2200h, 2345h, 2348h, and 2352h.

▶ Complete the following sentence by choosing from the list of options.

The client is at **highest** risk of developing _______________ .

WORD OPTIONS
Pneumonia
Pulmonary embolism
Pleural effusion
Pulmonary edema
Tension pneumothorax

Medical-Surgical 15.0

The nurse is caring for a 72-year-old client in the respiratory unit.

Nurses' Notes

2140h: Client presented to the emergency department with exacerbation of chronic obstructive pulmonary disease (COPD). Client indicates a recent pneumonia treated with antibiotic therapy that exacerbated dyspnea and increased work of breathing. Client presents to the unit alert and oriented to person, place, and time. Denies any pain or chest pain. Continues to exhibit shortness of breath, lungs auscultated for inspiratory and expiratory wheeze throughout all lung fields, client noted to have nonproductive cough. Reports significant weight loss over the past year due to COPD progressing. Vital signs: T: 37.7°C (99.9°F); BP: 123/68; P: 90; RR: 24; with pulse oximetry of 92% on room air. Client settled in the room. Allergy wristband applied indicating an allergy to penicillin.

0030h: Client found sitting at the edge of the bed in tripod position gasping for air. Audible wheeze and stridor noted. Client's colour pale with cyanosis noted around their lips and fingertips. Vital signs: T: 37.9°C (100.2°F); BP: 142/94; P:130; RR: 28; with pulse oximetry of 82% on room air. Code blue activated.

0033h: Code team arrived on the unit.

0035h: Shift nurse notified unit they administered an oral dose of amoxicillin to the client in error; it was meant to be the client's roommate's medication.

0100h: The client was administered a bronchodilator and epinephrine (adrenalin) during the code blue. No intubation necessary. Vital signs: T: 37.7°C (99.9°F); BP: 110/76; P:87; RR: 18; with pulse oximetry of 93% on 4 L/min per nasal prongs. Client's respirations regular and easy. No further stridor or wheeze noted. Client's colour pink with capillary refill less than 3 seconds. Client states they are exhausted.

The nurse has reviewed the Nurses' Notes at 2140h, 0030h, 0033h, and 0100h.

▶ For each assessment finding, identify if the finding indicates that the client's condition has **improved, not changed,** or **worsened**.

CLIENT FINDINGS	IMPROVED	NO CHANGE	WORSENED
Respirations 18	○	○	○
T 37.9°C (100.2°F)	○	○	○
Respiration rate to be regular	○	○	○
Colour pink	○	○	○
No stridor noted	○	○	○
Oxygen therapy 4 L/min	○	○	○

Note: Each row must have one response option selected.

Medical-Surgical 16.0

The nurse is caring for an 85-year-old client on the medical unit admitted with dehydration.

Nurses' Notes

1300h: The client was brought to the hospital after a ground-level fall after being found in their residence apartment. The client was recovering from a gastrointestinal viral illness 1 day before the fall. The client denies hitting their head and presented to the emergency department with dizziness and unstable gait. Vital signs: T: 37.7°C (99.9°F); BP: 102/54; P: 102; RR: 16; with pulse oximetry of 95% on room air. Client alert and oriented to person, place, and time. Answers questions appropriately. Pupils equal and reactive briskly to light at 2 mm. Bilateral radial pulses regular and strong with palpation × 2. Bilateral dorsalis pedis pulses strong and palpable × 2. Capillary refill less than 3 seconds. Denies any chest pain. Tenting noted inside of the forearm. Mucous membranes noted to be dry. Lungs clear with auscultation anteriorly and posteriorly. Abdomen tender with palpation but soft. Bowel sounds auscultated in all four quadrants. Client has not voided yet. Encouraged to ring with assistance. Venous access device inserted into right hand infusing 0.9% normal saline at 125 mL/hr.

1900h: Client ambulating to the washroom with one-person stand-by assistance. Gait steady. Voiding large amounts of dilute urine. Client concerned they will be awake most of the night. Lungs auscultated for fine to coarse inspiratory crackles to right lower lobe posteriorly and right middle lobe. Orders received from health care provider to reduce continuous intravenous rate to keep vein open.

2250h: Client rang for the nurse with complaints of right arm pain. Upon assessment, right forearm noted to be edematous, warm to touch, with redness along the course of the vein pathway. The venous wall in the right forearm noted to be rigid and cord-like. Venous access device sluggish to flushing. Client complains of increased pain at the insertion site.

The nurse reviews the Nurses' Notes at 1300h, 1900, and 2250h.

▶ Complete the following sentence by choosing from the list of options.

The client is at **highest** risk of developing ________________.

WORD OPTIONS
Infiltration
Extravasation
Valvular obstruction
Phlebitis
Catheter obstruction from clot

Maternal/Birthing Parent Health Trend Cases

Maternal/Birthing Parent Health 1.0

The nurse is caring for a 37-year-old client who is 24 weeks' gestation in the outpatient obstetrics clinic.

Progress Notes | Laboratory Results

July 12: Client presents to clinic for maternal assessment follow-up. Past medical history includes polycystic ovary syndrome, body mass index (BMI) 31. Vital signs: T: 36.9°C (98.4°F); BP: 122/67; P: 74; RR: 18; with pulse oximetry of 99% on room air. Client presents as pleasant and cooperative, excited for the birth of their first child. Client reports mild nausea, usually in the afternoon, that settles with lemon tea. No emesis. Complains of increased thirst but denies any pain with voiding. Temperatures have been seasonally high and hot. Client denies air conditioning and is increasingly feeling high temperatures. Client is scheduled for routine screening for gestational diabetes in a few weeks, will re-evaluate possible risk for needing treatment with health care provider. External fetal heart rate with Doppler 155 beats per minute. Client measures 26 cm.

July 28: Client presents to clinic for review of laboratory results and maternal assessment follow-up. Vital signs: T: 37.1°C (98.8°F); BP: 116/72; P: 77; RR: 18; with pulse oximetry of 96% on room air. Client placed on a diabetic diet, encouraged to increase exercise activity, and teaching provided regarding monitoring of blood sugars with a glucose-monitoring device. Client encouraged to keep a diary to track glucose levels before the next visit to determine if medications are warranted.

Progress Notes | **Laboratory Results**

July 22	Result
Oral Glucose Tolerance* Fasting: <5.8 mmol/L 1 hour: <10.5 mmol/L 2 hour: <9.1 mmol/L 3 hour: <8.0 mmol/L	Fasting: 8.8 mmol/L 1 hour: 11.9 mmol/L 2 hour: 9.6 mmol/L 3 hour: 7.9 mmol/L

*Gestational diabetes diagnosis warranted if two or more of the following are greater than normal levels.

The nurse has reviewed the Progress Notes from July 12 and July 28 and the Laboratory Results from July 22.

▶ Which of the following statements by the client indicate an **understanding** or **no understanding** of the treatment plan?

CLIENT STATEMENTS	UNDER-STANDING	NO UNDER-STANDING
"My grandpa has diabetes; I can use his medications."	○	○
"I was trying to lose weight before getting pregnant and I want to continue walking."	○	○
"I should test my blood sugar before driving."	○	○
"I already eat healthy, so I do not have to make any dietary changes."	○	○
"Controlling my blood sugar helps reduce complications for my baby."	○	○

Note: Each row must have one response option selected.

Maternal/Birthing Parent Health 2.0

The nurse is caring for a 29-year-old female, 33 weeks' gestation, in the emergency department (ED).

Nurses' Notes

1800h: Client arrived at ED with primary complaints of severe left lower leg pain with edema that started approximately 12 hours ago, progressively worsening throughout the day. Client is unable to walk without the aid of her partner for additional support. Client states she fell on the last three stairs when doing laundry yesterday, denied any injury except sore muscles in lower back. She rested throughout the day with her legs elevated. Vital signs: T: 37.3°C (99.1°F); BP: 122/75; P: 90; RR: 18; with pulse oximetry of 94% on room air. Client is alert and oriented to person, place, and time. Speech is clear and appropriate. Motor power strong, gait steady, left lower leg pain described as 8 on a numerical pain scale of 1 to 10 when required to walk, and then described as 5 when at rest. Lung sounds clear with auscultation, no adventitious sounds noted. Respirations regular and easy at rest. Client denies shortness of breath or chest pain. Apical pulse regular. Left lower leg and calf swollen, red, and warm to touch. Dorsalis pedis pulse on left and right foot palpable and strong. Bilateral feet cool to touch. Capillary refill less than 3 seconds. Left leg measured at 35.7 cm. Client denies any difficulty voiding. Fetal heart rate (FHR) 130 beats per minute (bpm). Client denies any change in movement with the fetus, remains active with more than six movements in 2 hours noted throughout the day.

2200h: Client rang for assistance complaining of shortness of breath and pain with inspiration. Vital signs: T: 37.8°C (100.4°F); BP: 138/85; P: 114; RR: 26; with pulse oximetry of 85% on room air. Client noted to have laboured respirations. Lungs auscultated for wheezing breath sounds over left lower lobe. Oxygen applied at 2 L/min per physician's standing order to maintain pulse oximetry greater than 90%. Left lower leg redness noted to increase from left calf to left thigh with increased edema. Left dorsalis pedis pulse palpated to be weak and thready with capillary refill greater than 3 seconds. ED physician notified. FHR 120 bpm and external fetal monitor applied to the client.

The nurse has reviewed the Nurses' Notes at 1800h and 2200h.

▶ Complete the following sentence by choosing from the lists of options.

The client is at **highest** risk of developing a(an) ____________________ (options 1) as evidenced by the client's ________________________ (options 2).

WORD OPTIONS 1	WORD OPTIONS 2
Pleural effusion	Left dorsalis pedis pulse
Pulmonary edema	Laboured respirations
Pulmonary embolus	Left lower leg redness plus edema
Cardiac tamponade	Capillary refill assessment
Acute myocardial infarction	Characteristics of voiding

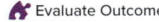

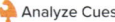

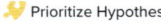

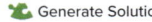

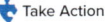

Maternal/Birthing Parent Health 3.0

The nurse is caring for a 23-year-old female in the women's clinic.

Nurses' Notes

May 2: Client requesting information about menstruation. Client states her period has been sporadic over the past year and she feels embarrassed to ask her male family doctor anything about gynecological issues. Client reports she started menstruating at 15 years old without any irregularities but recognizes her cycle at 42 to 50 days. Vital signs: BP: 102/66; P: 77; RR: 16; with pulse oximetry of 99% on room air. Client denies exhaustion or fatigue, speech is clear and appropriate, no chills or extreme changes in temperature. Client noted to be well perfused, voiding well, intake of 4–6 L/day; mild acne noted on client's face, client reports occasional blemish. BMI: 17; height: 165 cm. Information provided about contraception and pregnancy given irregular cycle. Client encouraged to track menstruation on a calendar. Client denies taking any medications.

July 10: Client returned to the clinic concerned that there was something wrong with her. She indicates she has not menstruated since April. Vital signs: BP: 100/62; P: 56 (irregular); RR: 16; with pulse oximetry of 99% on room air. She states she currently does not have a regular partner. She has not engaged in sexual activity since February and she practised safe sex. Speech is clear and appropriate. Complains of occasional dizziness. Client presents as pale with capillary refill sluggish but less than 3 seconds. Chest clear with auscultation. Client reports she is preparing for a national long-distance running competition. BMI: 14; Height: 165 cm. Client denies taking any medications.

The nurse has reviewed the Nurses' Notes from May 2 and July 10.

▶ For each nursing intervention, identify whether the intervention is **indicated** or **not indicated** for the care of the client.

POTENTIAL NURSING INTERVENTIONS	INDICATED	NOT INDICATED
Collect urine sample	○	○
Draw arterial blood gas	○	○
Recommend consultation with a dietitian	○	○
Speak to the client's coach	○	○
Suggest oral contraception	○	○

Note: Each row must have one response option selected.

Pediatrics Trend Cases

Pediatric 1.0

The nurse is caring for a 12-year-old client on the general inpatient pediatric medical unit.

Admission Notes | Nurses' Notes

1124h: Client was brought to the emergency department accompanied by their parent. The client, who is nonverbal, living with a developmental delay and known dysphagia, presented with shortness of breath, skin warm to touch, and increased irritability. The parent observed the client had developed tachypnea and became increasingly warm to touch since last evening. The parent did not have a thermometer to check temperature. Vital signs: T: 38.6°C (101.5°F); BP: 110/79; P: 90; RR: 26; with pulse oximetry of 93% on room air. Upon assessment, the client grimaces with mild painful stimuli, bilateral pupils are equal in size and shape and react briskly to light. Bilateral upper and lower peripheral extremities noted to have contractures. No skin breakdown noted. Regular bilateral radial pulses palpated with weaker but palpable dorsalis pedis pulses noted. Client presents with pale extremities, which is unchanged according to baseline, with flushed face noted. Bilateral fine inspiratory crackles noted in lung fields when auscultated posteriorly. Client has a weak cough reflex. Respirations regular but tachypneic. No indrawing, nasal flaring, or use of accessory muscles noted. Abdomen flat with bowel sounds auscultated in all four quadrants. PEG tube in situ left upper/middle side of abdomen. Skin around tube noted to be pink, with no breakdown or discharge noted. Client receives tube feeds four times a day: 0800h, 1200h, 1600h, and 2000h. Foley catheter in situ draining clear amber urine.

1245h: The client transferred from the emergency department to the general inpatient pediatric medical unit.

Admission Notes | **Nurses' Notes**

1257h: The client arrived on the unit in clear respiratory distress. Vital signs: T: 38.9°C (102.0°F); BP: 101/60 P: 104; RR: 30; with pulse oximetry of 88% on room air. The client was noted to be using abdominal accessory muscles and taking small, shallow breaths. The client noted to have foul-smelling oral secretions. Health care provider notified of change in status.

The nurse has reviewed the Admission Notes from the emergency department at 1124h and 1245h and the Nurses' Notes at 1257h.

▶ For each potential nursing intervention, specify whether the intervention is **indicated** or **not indicated** for the care of the client.

POTENTIAL NURSING INTERVENTIONS	INDICATED	NOT INDICATED
Offer oral fluids to the client	○	○
Request an order to insert a peripheral venous access device	○	○
Prepare to initiate oxygen therapy	○	○
Initiate tube feeds to maintain regular schedule	○	○
Prepare to take the client for a chest X-ray	○	○
Place the client in high-Fowler's position	○	○

Note: Each row must have one response option selected.

Pediatric 2.0

The nurse is caring for a 4-year-old client in the emergency department (ED).

Nurses' Notes

1740h: The client is brought to the ED via emergency medical services (EMS) after suffering a scald burn after the client dropped approximately 250 mL of boiling water onto their torso and rib cage. The parents were cooking dinner, turned their backs, and discovered the client had gotten a chair to "help cook dinner." The client presents with moderate partial-thickness burns across upper chest. The skin presents as mottled with pink, red serous filled blisters and erythemal edema. Total body surface area documented to be approximately 13%. Sensitive to touch and exposure to air. Vital signs: T: 37.9°C (100.2°F); BP: 110/66; P: 99; RR: 20; with pulse oximetry of 99%. Respirations regular at rest. Lungs auscultated for clear air entry throughout. No stridor noted. Client whimpering, without shirt, sitting on the lap of birth parent. Analgesic provided for comfort. Oxygen at 100% via mask applied. No peripheral intravenous was initiated by EMS.

1915h: Client found in tripod position, drooling, lips edematous and shiny. Vital signs: T: 38.1°C (100.5°F); BP: 88/50; P: 102; RR: 22; with pulse oximetry of 87%. Health care provider notified of change in client status.

The nurse has reviewed the Nurses' Notes from 1740h and 1915h.

▶ Which of the following actions should the nurse take immediately? **Select all that apply.**

- ☐ Initiate fluids through large-bore peripheral venous access device
- ☐ Call a code blue
- ☐ Provide ice chips to the client
- ☐ Draw an arterial blood gas
- ☐ Ask the client's parents to leave the room while the doctor completes the assessment
- ☐ Initiate antibiotic therapy
- ☐ Monitor urine output
- ☐ Draw CBC, electrolytes, and BUN

Mental Health

Mental Health 1.0

The school nurse is assessing a 14-year-old male client in the clinic office, which is attached to a community health care facility.

Progress Notes

April 17, 0800h: Client was brought to the clinic office after engaging in a fight with another youth prior to the start of school. The client reports to the nurse he has attention-deficit/hyperactivity disorder (ADHD) and does not always make the best decisions. He said, "I try to do right but I get so angry. I hit first, think later. I know I am in big trouble." The client has minimal bruising to his right knuckles and minor scratch marks on his lower arms. No other visible wounds noted. A note was sent with the client to take home that the school nurse assessed the student after the fight. Vital signs: T: 36.7°C (98.0°F); BP: 152/68; P: 98; RR: 16; with pulse oximetry of 98% on room air.

April 19, 1400h: School nurse follow-up with client today. Client reports his mom made him see a health care provider for his ADHD. He said, "She is sick of my behaviour, my poor grades, and staying up all hours of the night." The client presented the school nurse with a prescription for Biphentin 30 mg per day as per the parent's request to have on the client's health file. Vital signs: T: 36.5°C (97.7°F); BP: 144/75; P: 87; RR: 14; with pulse oximetry of 99% on room air.

April 30, 1000h: School nurse was called to outside social area and found client standing on the picnic table yelling out to the student body he was the King of France and for everyone to bow down to him. With encouragement, the client was convinced to return to the clinic area where he continued to proclaim his royal blood. Vital signs: T: 38.4°C (101.1°F); BP: 146/60; P: 95; RR: 26; with pulse oximetry of 92% on room air. Client indicated he felt a racing heart with skips and that he noticed small pinpoint, purple bruising on his legs, which must mean his royal blood is showing up for everyone to see. The client's parent was notified of incident and will come to school to pick up the client for further assessment.

The nurse reviews the Progress Notes dated April 17, April 19, and April 30.

▶ Complete the following sentence by choosing from the list of options.

The nurse should recognize that the client is potentially experiencing ____________ (option 1) and ____________ (option 1) as evidenced by ____________ (option 2) and ____________ (option 2).

WORD OPTIONS 1	WORD OPTIONS 2
Aggressive behaviour	Temperature: 38.4°C (101.1°F)
Raynaud's phenomenon	Viral respiratory infection
Thrombocytopenia	Bradycardia
Anemia	Small pinpoint, purple bruising
Leukopenia	Client proclaiming King of France status
Adverse event from medication	Tachycardia
Serotonin syndrome	Fatigue

Mental Health 2.0

The nurse is caring for a 16-year-old female client in the emergency department (ED).

Nurses' Notes

1000h: Client was brought into the ED by emergency medical services (EMS). EMS was called to the scene by the police after finding client unconscious in an alley of an area known for unhouse youth. Upon assessment, vital signs: T: 38.8°C (101.8°F); BP: 135/70; P: 142; RR: 22; with pulse oximetry of 98% on room air. She is alert and oriented to person, place, and time. Pupils equal and reactive to light at 2 mm. Client obeys all commands with motor power strong × 4 extremities and gait steady when walking. She denies any dizziness or pain but complains of sensitivity to light. Restlessness and anxiousness noted with inability to remain still. Client noted to have regular respirations. Clear air entry bilateral posterior lungs upon auscultation. She presents well perfused, capillary refill less than 3 seconds, pulses strong. No peripheral edema noted. No complaints of palpitations. Abdomen round but soft. Active bowel sounds × 4 quadrants. Bruising noted on the left flank side of torso. Bruising purple in colour, and area approximately the size of a cantaloupe. Client voiding independently. No voiced complaints. Bruising noted on bilateral upper arms approximately 3 cm in size each. There are five on each upper arm and one on the anterior side of the upper arm, approximately 3 cm in diameter. Small burns noted on the client's upper thigh. Burns approximately 1 cm in size, five in total. Skin red, noted to be warm to touch, with wound bed noted to have slough. Small amount of serous drainage noted on her pants from the burn marks.

1200h: Client found unresponsive and difficult to rouse. Vital signs: T: 39.3°C (102.7°F); BP: 190/60; P: 58; RR: 26; with pulse oximetry of 82% on room air. Pupils sluggish to light bilaterally with left pupil noted to be 3 mm in size and right pupil noted to be 6 mm in size. Client unable to follow commands, grunting to sternal rub only. Client noted to have irregular respirations. Oxygen applied per nasal prongs at 2 L/min. Will continue to monitor. Health care provider notified for immediate assessment.

The nurse has reviewed the Nurses' Notes from 1000h and 1200h.

▶ Which of the complications is the client at risk of experiencing? **Select all that apply.**

- ☐ Leukopenia
- ☐ Sepsis
- ☐ Stroke
- ☐ Pulmonary embolism
- ☐ Increased intracranial pressure

Mental Health 3.0

The nurse is caring for a 23-year-old female client admitted to a general medical unit.

Progress Notes | History and Physical

1328h: Client admitted to unit for further assessment of generalized anxiety disorder that has been encroaching on the client's personal life. Client found to engage in hot showers several times per day due to increased anxiety. Family supports the hot showers and states client is difficult to manage otherwise. No new triggers were identified at the time of admission to initiate this change in behaviour. The client started taking showers in high school for anxiety, but family noticed the client is taking up to eight hot showers per day.

1630h: Client found in the bathroom under the hot shower by nurse. Requested to leave the washroom. Client refused initially but with additional support and verbal motivation, client turned off the shower. The client was assessed, and large open areas were noted on the client's upper back. Two areas the size of a bagel, approximately 10 cm in diameter, were noted, with one on the left upper shoulder and one on the right shoulder below the scapula. Inside the wounds, the skin is red, but does not blanch, the edges are pale in colour with minimal perfusion noted. Health care provider notified.

2100h: Blisters noted on large scald burned areas × 2. Both burns contain serous fluid with large intact sacs. Unable to assess for blanching. Patient denies pain at present but will continue to monitor. Vital signs: T: 38.8°C (101.8°F); BP: 86/55; P: 95; RR: 16; with pulse oximetry of 98% on room air.

Progress Notes | **History and Physical**

1328h

Body System	Findings
Neurological	Alert and oriented × 3; obeys all commands; denies any pain; PEARL 2 mm; motor power strong × 4 extremities. Client complains of headache but relieved in the shower
Pulmonary	Vital signs: 18 at rest and 30 with anxiety; respirations regular and easy at rest but RR increases with increased anxiety and requires guidance to control breathing; pulse oximetry 98% on room air; no cough noted; no sputum
Cardiovascular	Vital signs: BP 110/54 and pulse 66 at rest but BP 140/86 pulse 122 with anxiety; capillary refill less than 3 seconds, pulses regular and strong; S1 and S2 auscultated, no S3 or S4; client experiences dizziness when standing in the shower for long periods, requires a bench to sit
Gastrointestinal	Bowel sounds auscultated × 4 quadrants; patient reports 6 kg (15 lb) weight loss over past month; anorexia; no emesis, passing flatus, bowel movements daily
Genitourinary	Client voided 500 mL of clear, concentrated urine
Integumentary	Client observed to pick at skin when not in the shower; open areas noted on client's forearms, underside of fingers closest to palm of hand; scabs formed in some areas with continued skin breakdown noted in areas not under clothes; client to call nurse when she feels need to shower again to further assess client's body
Immunological	Vital signs: T: 38.5°C (101.3°F)
Psychosocial	Client becomes anxious several times per day and states, "The hot water makes me feel like I can relax. There is no world. There is no pain. I don't have to hear my mother say what a mess-up I am. The hot shower is the only thing that makes me feel better." Client's parent states client remains living at home, unable to hold down a job or attend postsecondary school because of increased anxiety over the years, barely leaves the house, has few friends and support systems, and will throw items in the house, breaking picture frames and doors, making holes in walls when family prevents client from taking hot showers.

The nurse has reviewed the Progress Notes from 1328h, 1630h, and 2100h and the History and Physical from 1328h.

▶ For each potential nursing intervention, identify whether the intervention is **indicated** or **not indicated** for the care of this client.

POTENTIAL NURSING INTERVENTIONS	INDICATED	NOT INDICATED
Draw blood cultures	○	○
Request chest X-ray	○	○
Nurse asks client, "Can you identify what happens before you feel you need to take a hot shower?"	○	○
Monitor for septic shock	○	○
Request an order to insert a peripheral venous access device	○	○
Stay with the client	○	○
Call security when the client attempts to take a shower again	○	○
Group therapy will produce better results than cognitive-behavioural therapy	○	○
Anticipate an order for lorazepam	○	○

Note: Each row must have one response option selected.

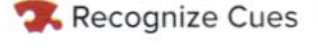 Recognize Cues 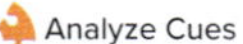 Analyze Cues 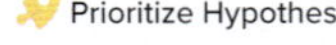 Prioritize Hypothesis 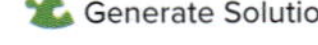 Generate Solutions 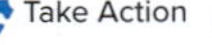 Take Action Evaluate Outcomes

Mental Health 4.0

The nurse is caring for a 68-year-old client in an outpatient cancer clinic.

Nurses' Notes | Progress Notes

1000h: Client was seen in the outpatient cancer clinic for review of a diagnostic biopsy which indicated the client was no longer in remission. Prognosis was provided to the client, no further treatment was appropriate, and client encouraged to make end-of-life arrangements. Client was very teary with news and visibly upset. No support person was with client during the visit as all family members were working and unable to take a day off. The news was unexpected and the client stated, "I thought things were getting better and the treatment was working. I was hopeful that I was going to meet my grandchildren. How am I going to tell my family this news? What do I say? What do I do now?" The client begins to sob uncontrollably.

1045h: Patient to be transferred to the emergency department for further assessment. Unable to console client. May require further medical assistance.

Nurses' Notes | **Progress Notes**

1115h: Client admitted to the emergency department following receiving devastating news in the outpatient clinic. Client continues to be weeping and unable to speak. Vital signs: T: 36.7°C (98.0°F); BP: 110/76; P: 77; RR: 22; with pulse oximetry of 94% on room air. Client notified family.

The nurse has reviewed the Nurses' Notes from 1000h and 1045h and the Progress Notes from 1115h.

▶ Complete the following sentence by choosing from the lists of options.

The client is at **highest** risk of developing _______________ (option 1) as evidenced by _______________ (option 2) and _______________ (option 2) and _______________ (option 2).

WORD OPTIONS 1	WORD OPTIONS 2
Anticipatory grief	No support person
Complicated grief	"How am I going to tell my family this news?
Disenfranchised grief	Unable to speak
Prolonged grief	Weeping

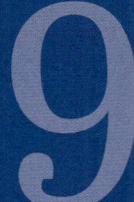

Answers and Rationales for Unfolding Case Studies

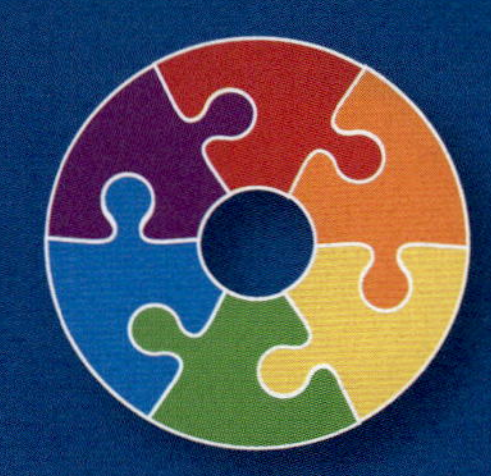

Medical-Surgical Cases

Medical-Surgical 1.0 (Cardiovascular)

Answer 1.1

History & Physical | Nurses' Notes | Vital Signs

1400h:

Body System	Findings
Neurological	Alert and orientated to person, place, time, and situation. Cooperative, obeys commands, moves all four extremities independently, gait steady.
Cardiovascular	Client was a direct admit to the unit with a "fast heartbeat" so strong that the client reports it felt like his heart was going to beat out of his chest.
Pulmonary	Complaints of shortness of breath at rest that worsens with any physical activity. Reports lack of energy most of the day.
Renal	Client denies any issue with voiding. Urinal at bedside and client encouraged to use.
Psychosocial	No previous cardiac history. Past medical history includes previous COVID-19 infection 7 months ago, prediabetes, body mass index (BMI) 37.

History & Physical | **Nurses' Notes** | Vital Signs

1420h: Client was directly admitted to the unit for further follow-up. Client denies headache or any pain. Pupils equal and reactive to light at 3 mm. Motor power strong × 4. S1 and S2 noted, no S3 or S4 auscultated. Client denies chest pain but can feel his heart beating fast, even at rest when he is not doing anything physically active. Client noted to be well perfused, mucous membranes pink, and client well hydrated. Apical = radial pulses × 2, noted to be irregular but strong. Lungs clear with auscultation, no adventitious breath sounds noted.

History and Physical | Nurses' Notes | **Vital Signs**

	1415h:
T	36.9°C (98.4°F)
P	155
RR	26
BP	132/77
Pulse oximetry reading	97% on room air

Rationale: The client is experiencing an irregular, fast heartbeat that is compromising his respiratory system, making him feel short of breath, even at rest, with lethargy. This indicates that the left ventricle cannot pump adequately to provide the client with enough oxygenated blood to be delivered to the systemic system. This fast, irregular heart rate requires additional electrical stimulation from the heart's conduction system to stimulate the myocardium of the ventricle to contract, leading to systole and eventually providing cardiac output.

NCJMM Step: Recognize Cues
Reference: Tyerman & Cobbett (2023), pp. 858–859.

Answer 1.2

- ☐ Venous thrombosis
- ✔ Pulmonary embolism
- ✔ Stroke
- ☐ Peripheral arterial disease
- ☐ Atherosclerosis
- ☐ Cardiac tamponade
- ☐ Pleural effusion

Rationale: The client has an irregular heartbeat that has been untreated with anticoagulation as this is a new issue. Clots can form in the atriums due to static blood flow. Where the clot can develop determines the type of issue the client may have. For example, if a clot forms in the right atrium and travels through the pulmonary vasculature, the client will develop a pulmonary embolism; if a clot forms in the left atrium, as the blood is ejected from the left ventricle, there is a possibility that it could travel to the brain and cause a stroke. A venous thrombosis will not occur from an irregular heartbeat producing a clot as the venous system involves blood returning to the heart. Peripheral arterial disease is not a possible issue for this client as this occurs when there is thickening of the artery walls that progressively narrows the arteries of the upper and lower extremities. An irregular heartbeat does not contribute to the formation of atherosclerosis, which is characterized by deposits of lipids within the intima of the artery. Cardiac tamponade develops as fluid accumulates in the pericardial sac, causing an increase in intrapericardial pressure and producing compression of the heart. A pleural effusion is fluid that accumulates in the pleural space and has no connection to an irregular heartbeat.

NCJMM Step: Analyze Cues
Reference: Tyerman & Cobbett (2023), pp. 618–620 (pleural effusion), 622–624 (pulmonary embolism), 899 (peripheral artery disease), 914–919 (venous thromboembolism), 858–859 (atrial fibrillation), 878 (cardiac tamponade), 1490–1492 (stroke).

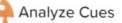

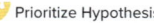

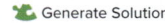

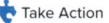

Answer 1.3

The nurse should **first** address the client's **heart rhythm**.

Rationale: The irregular heart rhythm is the cause of the shortness of breath and the difficulty the left ventricle is having to produce enough blood to sustain an adequate cardiac output. The client's blood pressure is stable at presentation; however, there is a possibility the client could become hypotensive. Once the rhythm returns to a normal, regular rhythm, the client will feel better. Addressing that will be the priority for the nurse. The heart sounds were documented as S1 and S2 with no adventitious heart sounds such as S3 or S4 auscultated. This indicates that despite an irregular heartbeat, the primary conduction remains intact with re-entry beats in the AV node. It is important to monitor the urine output for this client; however, the client denies any issue with voiding. Once the heart rhythm is stabilized, the shortness of breath will diminish, and the client will return to normal respiration. The previous COVID-19 diagnosis could be a contributing factor to the irregular heartbeat; however, this is not a priority for the nurse at this time. The client has a steady gait, which does not require follow-up.

NCJMM Step: Prioritize Hypothesis
Reference: Tyerman & Cobbett (2023), pp. 858–859 (atrial fibrillation).

Answer 1.4

POTENTIAL NURSING INTERVENTIONS	INDICATED	NOT INDICATED
Place the client in the tripod position	○	✔
Prepare to apply oxygen	○	✔
Prepare to administer metoprolol	✔	○
Consult spiritual care	○	✔
Provide reassurance to the client	✔	○
Insert venous access device	✔	○

Rationale: Medications used for rate control include beta-adrenergic medications, such as metoprolol, and calcium channel blockers, such as diltiazem. Metoprolol can be administered through intravenous access and can be pushed if the client is monitored and the nurse is certified to administer intravenous push medications. Providing reassurance to the client is important as the experience of not being able to catch their breath can cause feelings of anxiety, only increasing respirations. A venous access site will be necessary to administer metoprolol and other fluids if necessary. The tripod position is recommended for clients with chronic obstructive pulmonary disease to increase respiratory surface area and enhance gas exchange. Consulting religious preferences is not indicated at this time. Oxygen is not required as the client is maintaining pulse oximetry at 92%, which is adequate despite atrial fibrillation.

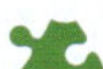
NCJMM Step: Generate Solutions
Reference: Tyerman & Cobbett (2023), pp. 858–859 (atrial fibrillation).

Answer 1.5

- ✔ Assist with a transesophageal echocardiogram (TEE)
- ☐ Administer anticoagulation
- ✔ Consult respiratory therapy to monitor airway
- ☐ Keep suction outside of the room in case it is needed
- ☐ Place the client in the recovery position for the cardioversion
- ☐ Draw up paralytic to administer

Rationale: A TEE should be performed before the cardioversion to rule out clots in the atria. If a cardioversion proceeds without first ruling out whether clots are present or not, the client has a high risk of having a stroke. Respiratory therapy is on site to provide airway support and monitor pulse oximetry. They will apply a mask to the client to enable the highest oxygen support without intubation or other supportive measures. The client will be on his side for the TEE and then placed on his back for the cardioversion. This position provides a better angle from which to move the camera and identify if there are clots in the atria. Placing the client on his back for the cardioversion enables better adherence of the pads to the skin to deliver a hands-off discharge. Anticoagulation should only be administered if the client has been in atrial fibrillation for longer than 48 hours and then maintained for 3 to 4 weeks to prevent clots from forming. The client will be placed in the recovery position for the TEE, not the cardioversion. Sedation will be administered to the client, but not a paralytic. This would inhibit any respiratory movement, and the client would require intubation and ventilatory support. This order should be clarified with the health care provider.

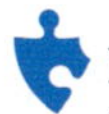
NCJMM Step: Take Action
Reference: Tyerman & Cobbett (2023), pp. 858–859 (atrial fibrillation).

Answer 1.6

CLIENT STATEMENTS	UNDER-STANDING	NO UNDER-STANDING
"I have taken *Ginkgo biloba* before, so there is no issue taking it now, right?"	○	✔
"I will call 9-1-1 if I experience sudden numbness or inability to speak."	✔	○
"I have a big project that needs to be dealt with today. I can return back to work."	○	✔
"I am to rest if my heart feels like it is racing and monitor if it slows down by feeling my pulse."	✔	○
"My partner can drive me home today."	✔	○

Rationale: Moving forward, all medications should be discussed with the client's health care provider. During follow-up, over-the-counter medications and herbal remedies should be reviewed for potential adverse effects if medications have been ordered. After a cardioversion, an identified clot may still have dislodged in the heart, even after a TEE. It is important to inform clients and their families of the signs and symptoms of a stroke. After a cardioversion, clients may be unsteady and fatigued. It is recommended clients not drive or return back to work for 24 hours until the effects from the sedation medication have worn off. It is important to show the client how to feel for his own pulse so that if his heart should race again, he can determine if the rhythm is regular or irregular and seek medical attention as necessary. Discharge teaching is very important after a cardioversion for the client and family to understand what is and what is not allowed.

NCJMM Step: Evaluate Outcomes
Reference: Healthwise Staff (2023).

Medical-Surgical 2.0 (Cardiovascular)

Answer 2.1

- ☐ Lung sounds
- ☐ Heart sounds
- ✔ Nausea
- ✔ Chest pain
- ✔ Vital signs
- ✔ ECG findings
- ☐ Urine drainage

Rationale: The client is presenting with classic acute coronary syndrome clinical manifestations. The diaphoresis is associated with a sympathetic response in relation to the chest pain. The nausea is associated with the location of the coronary blockage or where spasm is occurring. The chest pain indicates that there is a plaque rupture in the coronary arteries, leading to blockage of blood flow to the myocardium. Vital signs indicate that the client's left ventricle is compromised as the cardiac output has been reduced and, therefore, the blood pressure is decreased. To compensate, the client's heart rate will increase to accommodate for the lower blood pressure. The client is tachypneic as a result of the low blood pressure. Despite the myocardium having less oxygenated blood, the body is also having less oxygenated blood. ECG findings indicate that the client's ventricle is being affected during diastole, which is shown by the ST elevation in the anterior leads. Cardiac compromise on the anterior leads indicates a left ventricular pump issue with possible coronary artery spasm or blockage.

NCJMM Step: Recognize Cues
Reference: Tyerman & Cobbett (2023), pp. 751–772, 1406–1407.

Answer 2.2

CLIENT FINDINGS	UNSTABLE ANGINA	INFECTIVE ENDOCARDITIS	CARDIAC TAMPONADE
Hypotension	○	○	✔
Chest pain	✔	✔	○
ST changes	✔	○	✔
Nausea	✔	○	○
Tachypnea	○	✔	✔
Afebrile	✔	○	○

Rationale: Angina occurs when coronary arteries become blocked or develop a spasm. Clients who present with unstable angina present with fatigue, shortness of breath, indigestion, and anxiety. Anginal pain has progressed rapidly in the past few hours, days, or weeks, culminating in pain at rest. ST changes may include flipped T waves, indicating ischemic changes have occurred. Clients may present with nausea if the blockage is located in the left anterior descending coronary artery or circumflex. Hypotension may occur if the left ventricle is unable to pump effectively due to coronary artery blockage or spasm. Infective endocarditis is an infection of the heart values of the endocardial surface of the heart. It typically presents with a low-grade fever, weakness, malaise, fatigue, and anorexia. Arthralgias, myalgias, back pain, abdominal discomfort, weight loss, headache, and clubbing of fingers may occur. Clients may also present with splinter hemorrhages, new or changing murmurs, and heart failure. Cardiac tamponade is a condition in which fluid accumulates in the pericardial sac, causing increased intrapericardial pressure and producing compression of the heart. Clients develop tachypnea, tachycardia, and decreased cardiac output. The neck veins are distended due to increased jugular venous pressure and pulsus paradoxus. Pulsus paradoxus is a decrease in systolic blood pressure with inspiration. ST changes may occur as the left ventricle is compromised, and there can be changes to the amount of oxygen being delivered to the myocardium due to the compression.

NCJMM Step: Analyze Cues
Reference: Tyerman & Cobbett (2023), pp. 751–772, 804–808 (angina), 872–884 (infective endocarditis), 878 (cardiac tamponade).

Answer 2.3

The client is at highest risk of developing **acute myocardial infarction** as evidenced by the client's **cardiovascular assessment**.

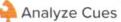

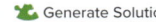

Rationale: Based on the objective and subjective cardiovascular assessment data of chest pain that feels like an elephant is sitting on the client's chest, diaphoresis, nausea, ST changes on the ECG, and a drop in blood pressure post–surgical procedure indicates the client is at highest risk for an acute myocardial infarction. Further blood work including a troponin or creatine-kinase MB (CKMB) would confirm the hypothesis. The client's highest risk is not dysrhythmias, as the client's heart rate is regular, although documented as tachycardia. The client is not at risk for any atrial dysrhythmias and there is no indication of ventricular dysrhythmias. The client is afebrile, and there are no adventitious lung sounds such as wheezing or crackles to identify if pneumonia was the issue. Hypoxemia and respiratory failure are always a possible consideration if the client should develop cardiogenic shock; however, at the presentation, the client is most at risk for an acute myocardial infarction.

NCJMM Step: Prioritize Hypothesis
Reference: Tyerman & Cobbett (2023), pp. 796–828.

Answer 2.4

POTENTIAL ORDERS	INDICATED	NOT INDICATED
Initiate low-molecular weight heparin (LMWH)	○	✔
Apply oxygen 0–5 L/min per nasal prongs to maintain pulse oximetry greater than 92%	✔	○
Initiate a nitroglycerine infusion	○	✔
Prepare the client for an angiogram immediately	○	✔
Discontinue the continuous bladder irrigation	○	✔
Transfer client to Coronary Care Unit	✔	○
Administer dimenhydrinate	✔	○

Rationale: For a client who has just undergone a surgical procedure, tight control of anticoagulation is necessary. The heparin medication of choice would be unfractionated heparin per the venous access device. In the event the client is bleeding from the TURP, the heparin can be stopped until the clotting cascade corrects itself and then restarted when it is safe. With subcutaneous LMWH, it is more difficult to control bleeding after the medication is administered. An order of oxygen therapy is necessary when the client is struggling to maintain adequate systemic oxygenation. This would offer supportive measures to the client. The client is stable and could be given nitroglycerin sublingual (SL) rather than through the intravenous route. The client will go for an angiogram to determine the next steps for the plan of care. If the client continues to have chest pain, then emergent angiography may be done; however, at this time, this order is not indicated. The continuous bladder irrigation would continue as ordered by Urology. The nurses in Cardiology will continue to monitor for clots or changes in the colour of the urine. If the urine output is frank red in colour, the health care provider will be notified to determine the next steps with the anticoagulant therapy. The client will be transferred to the Coronary Care Unit to monitor this client since they are newly postoperative. Managing the cardiac care will take priority over the urological procedure.

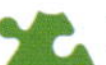

NCJMM Step: Generate Solutions
Reference: Tyerman & Cobbett (2023), pp. 796–828.

Answer 2.5

- ✔ Discontinue unfractionated heparin IV prior to going to the angiogram catheter suite
- ☐ Contact the client's spouse to join us at the angiogram suite
- ✔ Initiate nitroglycerine IV to achieve pain-free status for the client
- ✔ Apply oxygen at 2 L/min to achieve pulse oximetry above 92%
- ☐ Provide sips of water
- ✔ Mark dorsalis pedis and post-tibialis pulses on right and left feet and ankles

Rationale: Unfractionated heparin IV should not be infusing before the angiogram as this may cause further bleeding and instability in the coronary vessel. The heparin IV can be safely stopped 4 to 6 hours before a procedure as the half-life is short, but the nurse must follow institutional policy. The client continues to have chest pain that is not relieved by SL nitroglycerine spray. The goal for a cardiac client with unstable plaque is to achieve pain-free status. The IV nitroglycerine can be monitored and titrated according to the client's status and hemodynamic presentation. The client's pulse oximetry is low, indicating oxygen is needed to support systemic tissues. All pulses are marked on the client if the interventional cardiologist performs a femoral approach. Monitoring the pulses after the procedure is imperative to identify if a hematoma forms. There would not be time to contact the spouse, and visitors are not allowed in angiogram suites. The client is to be NPO before the procedure. Usually, with a booked angiogram, clients are NPO from midnight. Sips of fluids cannot be given in the event there is an emergency and the client requires intubation.

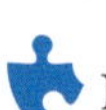

NCJMM Step: Take Action
Reference: Tyerman & Cobbett (2023), pp. 796–828.

Answer 2.6

CLIENT STATEMENTS	UNDERSTANDING	NO UNDERSTANDING
"I am going to have to follow the DASH diet now."	✔	○
"My wife and I are going to need to speak with a counsellor about our intimate life."	✔	○
"I need to drive myself to the foodbank where I volunteer. My next shift is in a couple of days."	○	✔
"I cannot wait to sit up in a couple of hours."	○	✔
"I can participate in exercise programs."	✔	○

Rationale: When clients are discharged, the DASH (**d**ietary **a**pproaches to **s**topping **h**ypertension) diet is recommended to reduce sodium intake. After a heart attack, reducing the workload of the heart is imperative for healing time. The client is aware of erectile dysfunction after a TURP has been conducted. The client learns that for a successful TURP, sensitive nerve endings are affected, and clients may not be able to get an erection after this procedure. Maintaining a healthy relationship with open communication is promoted. After a client undergoes a percutaneous coronary intervention (PCI), there is no driving for 30 days. The cardiac muscle is unstable, and the client may have dysrhythmias for several days after the procedure. When a client has a femoral approach, the client must lie flat on their back for 6 hours to avoid disturbing the clot that has formed after the sheath was removed. This could initiate bleeding or a hematoma to form, obstructing blood flow to the lower extremities. The gradual introduction of exercise programs is encouraged post–myocardial infarction. Many urban centres in Canada have exercise programs with dietitians recommended to cardiac clients.

NCJMM Step: Evaluate Outcomes
References: Heart & Stroke Foundation of Canada. (2024); Tyerman & Cobbett (2023), pp. 818–827.

Medical-Surgical 3.0 (Cardiovascular/Renal)

Answer 3.1

- ☐ Pupillary response
- ✔ Oliguria
- ☐ Headache
- ✔ Lung sounds
- ☐ Diarrhea
- ✔ Vertigo
- ☐ Pulses

Rationale: The client presents with oliguria, fine crackles auscultated in the lung fields, low blood pressure, tachycardia, pitting edema, and vertigo (postural hypotension) when the head of the bed is raised, indicating a low systemic volume state. There is reduced blood flow and filtration of the kidneys, likely due to the gastrointestinal virus and the inability to consume food and fluids orally. These three areas require immediate attention as the inability to find a solution could result in prolonged renal failure, impaired gas exchange, and possibly a type 2 acute myocardial infarction, as the left ventricle ejection fraction was documented at 43%. The pupils are reactive appropriately to light. It is important to ensure pupillary response since the client has a bruise on his temple. The client reports a mild headache, but gas exchange and heart function are more important assessment findings. Although the diarrhea is contributing to the reduced systemic circulatory volume, it is not an immediate finding that requires attention. The pulses are to be monitored as they indicate poor systemic blood flow.

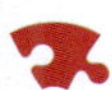
NCJMM Step: Recognize Cues
References: Power-Kean et al. (2023), p. 120; Tyerman & Cobbett (2023), p. 211.

Answer 3.2

CLIENT FINDINGS	ACUTE SUBDURAL HEMATOMA	DEHYDRATION	PULMONARY EDEMA
Headache	✔	✔	○
Drowsiness	✔	✔	○
Fine crackles	○	○	✔
S1, S2 no S3 or S4	✔	✔	○
Shortness of breath	○	✔	✔
Oliguria	○	✔	○

Rationale: Since the client was found on the floor by the residential staff, there is a possibility the client could develop an acute subdural hematoma. The client presents with a mild headache and drowsiness, which are all clinical manifestations of an acute subdural hematoma. The client does present as alert and orientated and obeys commands without agitation or confusion. It would be imperative to monitor for a subdural hematoma or chronic subdural hematoma throughout as a precaution; however, the client does not currently present with these symptoms. The clinical manifestations associated with dehydration include headache, drowsiness, shortness of breath, and oliguria, which can be associated with low systemic blood flow due to the gastrointestinal virus. Although fine crackles are auscultated with shortness of breath, the possibility of pulmonary edema is low as the client still has adequate blood pressure despite tachycardia.

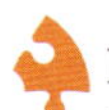
NCJMM Step: Analyze Cues
Reference: Power-Kean et al. (2023), pp. 120 (dehydration), 385 (subdural hematoma), 678 (pulmonary edema).

Answer 3.3

The client is at highest risk of developing **acute kidney injury**.

Rationale: Acute kidney injury occurs as a result of ischemic damage to the renal tubular epithelial cells due to dehydration and hypovolemia. With this client, the persistent diarrhea and vomiting for several days have depleted water and electrolytes, leaving reduced blood flow to the kidneys, causing an acute kidney injury. As a person ages, the number of nephrons decreases, and an older adult is less able to tolerate dehydration and excessive volume overloads. This situation leads to oxidative stress and inflammation. The client would demonstrate more significant signs of a hemorrhagic stroke if an acute subdural hematoma had developed. All older adults should be monitored for acute and chronic subdural hematomas, as a small bleed can occur. The client does not present with facial drooping, otorrhea, or paresis. As with all older adults, there is a risk of dysrhythmias, especially with a client who is not voiding; however, the client is not presenting with any chest pain, palpitations, jugular venous distension, or any other symptoms associated with dysrhythmias. Despite being found on the floor, the client can move his extremities bilaterally and has no complaints of musculoskeletal pain.

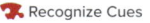

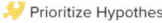

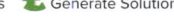

NCJMM Step: Prioritize Hypothesis
Reference: Power-Kean et al. (2023), pp. 728, 744–745 (acute kidney injury).

Answer 3.4

POTENTIAL NURSING INTERVENTIONS	INDICATED	NOT INDICATED
Place the crash cart outside of the room in the event of a code blue	○	✔
Request an order to administer intravenous (IV) fluids continuously	✔	○
Perform a bladder scan	✔	○
Prepare the client for chest X-ray	○	✔
Administer cardiac medications previously ordered prior to hospital admission	○	✔
Request a regular diet tray be delivered to the unit	○	✔
Place the bed in the lowest position with the brakes on	✔	○

Rationale: The client presents with hyperkalemia, given the poor renal function. It is not appropriate to place the crash cart outside the client's hospital room in the event of a cardiac event. The client will be monitored closely. The client's blood pressure decreased from admission to the ED to admission to the Internal Medicine Unit, which should have created a sympathetic response. The client's condition remains hemodynamically challenged, and the administration of external fluids is required. The client could benefit from additional continuous intravenous fluids to return to an adequate replacement of lost volume due to gastrointestinal viral illness. Encouraging oral fluids will be supplemental, but it will take time to adjust the systemic volume and increase the client's blood pressure. It is within the nurses' scope to perform a bladder scan to indicate the amount of urine in the bladder. Given the client's abdominal pain, there may be additional volume in the client's bladder from the fluid bolus administered in the ED. Crackles are present in the client's lung bases; however, there is no indication the client is experiencing pneumonia (no fever) or other condition, such as pulmonary edema, as the presentation is only fine crackles, and the client denies any change in breathing pattern despite low pulse oximetry levels. The client's blood pressure has decreased from arrival at the hospital; therefore, administering evening medications could further decrease the blood pressure, placing the client in a hemodynamically unstable situation where there is not sufficient intravascular volume to accommodate the demands of the heart. The client has not eaten solid food for several days. Initiating a regular diet would be difficult for the stomach to digest and absorb. It would be recommended that the client's diet be started with clear fluids and advanced as tolerated to a regular diet. The client's sodium levels are high, likely due to the dehydration and bolus of 0.9% sodium chloride. The client's seizure threshold is unknown; therefore, maintaining a safe environment for the client is important. The bed should be placed in the lowest position and with brakes on.

NCJMM Step: Generate Solutions
Reference: Tyerman & Cobbett (2023), pp. 1185–1186.

Answer 3.5

- ✔ Initiate 0.45% sodium chloride at 100 mL/hr
- ✔ Perform an in-and-out catheter × 1 then monitor urine output
- ☐ Administer a narcotic analgesic as needed
- ☐ Draw laboratory tests: type and cross-match, arterial blood gas (ABG)
- ✔ Apply oxygen starting at 2 L/min per nasal prongs to maintain pulse oximetry greater than 92%.

Rationale: The client requires additional intravenous solutions to replace fluids lost due to the gastrointestinal viral illness. 0.45% sodium chloride is to be administered due to the high sodium levels in the blood. An in-and-out catheter may be necessary because of benign prostate hyperplasia. The client's larger prostate and inflammatory state may result in retained urine. Perfusion of the kidneys may result in electrolyte disturbances reverting back to normal levels. The client's pulse oximetry was low, requiring oxygenation. This client compensates for the lower oxygen levels by increasing respiratory rate slightly. The administration of a lower level of oxygen will assist with determining respiratory status. Administering a narcotic analgesic for the abdominal pain may precipitate a further decrease in the client's blood pressure. The client is not anemic and does not require additional blood products or ABG to be drawn.

NCJMM Step: Take Action
Reference: Tyerman & Cobbett (2023), pp. 1185–1186.

Answer 3.6

0630h: The client was found confused, no oxygen per nasal prongs on, and searching for the door to the washroom, trying to push the IV pole through the door in the hallway. Client redirected and assisted to the toilet and voided concentrated, foul-smelling urine. Identified correctly person, place, and time but slow in response. Pupillary response sluggish with right pupil documented at 2 mm in size and left pupil 4 mm in size. Client denies a headache, chest pain, or difficulty breathing. Indicates relief after voiding. Client repositioned back to the bed and oxygen reapplied at 2 L/min. Vital signs: T: 38.0°C (100.4°F); BP: 92/57; P: 122; RR: 20; with pulse oximetry of 92% on 2 L/min per nasal prongs.

Rationale: It is important to follow up with a change in neurological status. The client exhibited confusion and was found wandering. There is no report of any instability in gait, as the client was able to get from the bed to the washroom independently and with an IV pole. The client voided concentrated, foul-smelling urine, which is a change in status from the previous entry at 0215h. There is now a change in pupillary response, as well as size. The client is also now exhibiting a fever. Given the client's confusion, increase in temperature, and change in urine, further investigation is required to rule out a bleed in the brain; additional laboratory values, including blood cultures and a urine culture and sensitivity will need to be investigated. Older adults are at increased risk of developing a further infection on top of the acute kidney injury. They also have a blunted febrile response to an infection. Further investigation is warranted in this situation. Although the blood pressure has improved with administration of intravenous fluid, continuing to monitor hemodynamic status is important because this client remains hypotensive (less than 95/60).

NCJMM Step: Evaluate Outcomes
Reference: Tyerman & Cobbett (2023), pp. 1185–1186.

Medical-Surgical 4.0 (Respiratory)

Answer 4.1

- ✔ Confusion
- ☐ Unsteady gait
- ✔ Irregular breathing with snorting
- ☐ Pale fingertips
- ☐ Frailty
- ☐ Malnourished
- ☐ Yellow-coloured sclera
- ✔ Fever
- ☐ Lung sounds
- ☐ Pupillary response
- ☐ Hypoactive bowel sounds
- ☐ Use of Doppler for bilateral posterior tibial pulses

Rationale: The client's confusion presentation requires further follow-up to identify if the client did not have a chronic hematoma or hepatic encephalopathy. The pupils are equal and reactive to light, which is normal during assessment. Irregular breathing upon admission is concerning, which could be associated with alcohol poisoning. Protecting the airway would be important to monitor if the client is difficult to rouse. A low-grade fever is concerning and should be monitored, given the narrative of the client's presentation and being found in a puddle of emesis. Immediate follow-up requires further assessment of airway, breathing, and circulation. An unsteady gait is concerning, and the client is at risk of falling; however, four side rails are in place to maintain safety for the client. Pale fingertips are an important finding but not an immediate finding. This indicates poor perfusion, but the capillary refill lasts less than 3 seconds. If this should change and be greater than 3 seconds, then the client finding becomes more relevant. The client's frailty will affect her recovery; however, is not a recommended finding for immediate follow-up. Malnourished and petite frame are concerning for healing and recovery. A client's lack of muscle will continue to minimize recovery and healing. Yellow sclera indicates liver dysfunction; however, at this point, it is a contributing finding, not something that requires immediate attention. Fine inspiratory crackles do not require immediate follow-up as this finding does not seem to be impeding gas exchange and could be related to the position in which the client was found when EMS entered the home. The respiratory rate is in the 20's and the pulse oximetry is at 93% on room air. Coarse crackles would be more immediate. The pupillary response is equal but sluggish. Without knowing the toxicology report, the pupils may be sluggish despite something to monitor. Hypoactive bowel sounds indicate that the gas is moving through the colon, albeit slowly. The use of Doppler to auscultate the posterior tibial pulses indicates a weaker pulse moving through the lower extremity. The fact that bilateral dorsalis pedis pulses were palpable is an indication that this client finding does not require immediate follow-up.

NCJMM Step: Recognize Cues
Reference: Jarvis et al. (2024), pp. 457–501, 698–758.

Answer 4.2

CLIENT FINDINGS	CIRRHOSIS	SUBDURAL HEMATOMA	PNEUMONIA
Confusion	✔	✔	○
Irregular breathing	○	✔	✔
Fever	○	○	✔
Yellow-coloured sclera	✔	○	○
Fine inspiratory crackles	○	○	✔

Rationale: Liver cirrhosis has a gradual onset. Confusion may occur in clients when their ammonia levels begin to elevate. Even though the abdomen is documented to be distended and hard, it is a likely indicator of ascites. The client also presents with jaundiced sclera, indicating an advanced disease process. The client may present with tachypnea due to the distended abdomen; however, this client presents with irregular breathing. Subdural hematomas can form easily in older adults. At this point, it is unclear if the client hit her head. Confusion can occur when a client experiences a subdural hematoma. The client is also difficult to rouse and may be somnolent. If the intracranial pressure becomes high, irregular breathing may occur. There is no fever, yellow sclera, or fine inspiratory crackles associated with a subdural hematoma. This client presents with a low-grade fever, but given the age of the client, it would be classified as a fever; irregular breathing pattern could be a result of fluid in the lungs leading to fine inspiratory crackles in the bases, identifying pulmonary congestion. Confusion is not associated with complications associated with pneumonia. The sclera would not be yellow in a client with pneumonia.

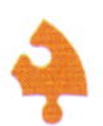
NCJMM Step: Analyze Cues
Reference: Tyerman & Cobbett (2023), pp. 1093 (cirrhosis), 1468–1469 (subdural hematoma), 590–596 (pneumonia).

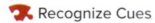

Answer 4.3

The client is at highest risk of developing **respiratory failure.**

Rationale: Given the client presentation, the most likely condition the client is experiencing is aspiration pneumonia. This usually develops within 48 to 72 hours as a secondary event. It is known as chemical (noninfectious) pneumonitis. The client presents with petechiae and purpura, indicating lower levels of platelets, which in turn indicate a risk of bleeding; however, the primary presentation is related to the airway and not bleeding. The client presents with regular pulses with no indication of irregularity, minimizing the risk of dysrhythmias. The client presents with fine crackles as well as a fever, indicating an infective process is occurring, eliminating heart failure as the highest risk to develop. Despite not voiding yet upon presentation, the client's clinical symptoms are not congruent with a risk of renal failure.

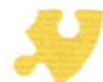

NCJMM Step: Prioritize Hypothesis
Reference: Tyerman & Cobbett (2023), pp. 590–596 (pneumonia), 829–848 (heart failure), 849–871 (dysrhythmias), 1093 (thrombocytopenia), 1103 (renal failure), 1753–1773 (respiratory failure).

Answer 4.4

POTENTIAL NURSING INTERVENTIONS	INDICATED	NOT INDICATED
Prepare the client for a chest X-ray and spiral computed topography (CT)	○	✔
Check pupillary response	✔	○
Call a code blue	✔	○
Contact the client's family	○	✔
Request an order to administer an intravenous fluid bolus	✔	○
Review the client's allergies	○	✔

Rationale: Based on the client's laboratory values, the client either has a dysrhythmia or a pulmonary embolus. Either way, an unresponsive client requires immediate intervention to protect the airway and maintain circulation. Pupillary response would be checked to identify neurological assessment and to query if the client may have had a stroke, too. A code blue will be called as the client is unresponsive. The carotid pulse is weak and thready; therefore, the client requires further advanced life support. Additional supportive measures are required as the client's blood pressure has decreased to critically abnormal levels. To ensure appropriate circulation, initiating intravenous fluids would be necessary and warranted. The client would go for a spiral CT and a chest X-ray given the potential aspiration pneumonia and positive D-dimer; however, the client's status is unstable. Contacting the client's family would be appropriate, but it can be done by a colleague.

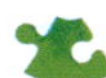

NCJMM Step: Generate Solutions
Reference: Tyerman & Cobbett (2023), pp. 1774–1780.

Answer 4.5

- ☐ Place the client in Trendelenburg position
- ☐ Request an order to administer sodium polystyrene sulfonate (Kayexalate) or sodium zirconium cyclosilicate powder (Lokelma)
- ✔ Perform chest compressions
- ☐ Connect the client to an external pacemaker
- ✔ Prepare for rapid defibrillation
- ☐ Manage temperature regulation

Rationale: The client is in a cardiac code blue situation. Performing chest compressions and preparing for rapid defibrillation is the most appropriate nursing action. If the nurse places the client in Trendelenburg position, it would be difficult to perform adequate chest compressions. The administration of Kayexalate or Lokelma will take time to minimize the potassium level. If high, insulin can be used to reduce potassium levels. The client should be connected to an external defibrillator, not to an external pacemaker. Managing temperature is important when hypothermia is part of the client's narrative. Reduction in temperature requires careful warming of the body's core temperature.

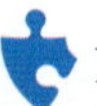

NCJMM Step: Take Action
Reference: Tyerman & Cobbett (2023), pp. 1774–1781.

Answer 4.6

TOP 4 CLIENT FINDINGS
Weakening pulse
Palliative sedation is required more frequently
"Guppy breathing"
Incontinent

Rationale: Monitoring for end-of-life clinical manifestations is important for client and family care. Symptom management to reduce suffering is imperative to address concerns associated with the dying process. Dying is a multisystem process. Supporting clients and families by identifying and explaining these changes provides holistic care. As the heart weakens, the pulse becomes weaker for palpation. End-of-life hallucinations can occur as the body begins to shut down, requiring sedation to help the client remain calm. Sedation is only necessary to reduce anxiety for the client and not to assist with oversedation. "Guppy breathing" occurs as bilateral hemispheric brain dysfunction begins to occur, reducing signals from the brain to the lungs to breathe in relation to the amount of carbon dioxide. Renal dysfunction occurs when the brain cannot provide appropriate signals to the bladder. Bladder tone begins to decrease over time. As the body begins to reduce cardiac output, the skin will be cool to touch, not warm to touch. The client's inability to protect their airway with a gag reflex indicates brainstem dysfunction as the brain slowly reduces in function.

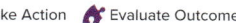

NCJMM Step: Evaluate Outcomes
Reference: Tyerman & Cobbett (2023), pp. 201–203.

Medical-Surgical 5.0 (Respiratory)

Answer 5.1

- ✔ Sputum
- ✔ Hoarseness
- ☐ Vital signs
- ☐ Bilateral mastectomy 1 year ago
- ☐ Gait
- ☐ Heart sounds
- ✔ Atelectasis
- ✔ Pain

Rationale: New-onset hemoptysis, nonproductive, dry cough, hoarseness, atelectasis, and pulmonary pain are all concerning and should be followed up immediately. Other potential causes of the respiratory presentation must be considered and ruled out. If a client presents with hemoptysis, the client could have a bleed from the nasal, oral, or esophagus area, or there is bleeding elsewhere in the lung, which is abnormal and could have grave indications for impaired gas exchange. Hoarseness could indicate something benign if presented in isolation; however, when presented with other respiratory symptoms, hoarseness typically is associated with cancers. Atelectasis is the condition of shrunk alveoli or an entire lung due to an obstruction, compression of the lung, or lack of surfactant, and the alveoli collapse. Atelectasis indicates no air entry is occurring, which prevents appropriate gas exchange and oxygenation for the rest of the body. Pain upon inspiration is not abnormal. The client does not complain of chest pain, is not diaphoretic, or nauseated, which are typical symptoms associated with an acute myocardial infarction. Further investigation is necessary. The vital signs do not indicate any impaired gas exchange or hemodynamic shifts at the moment, so the client presents as stable. The news of her previous mastectomy is something to consider with the presentation of information; however, it is not a piece of data that requires immediate follow-up. Although the client reported dizziness at the time of admission, there was no indication that unsteady gait was a problem during the assessment. The client presents with normal heart sounds. Hemoptysis is an abnormal presentation, as are atelectasis and pain with inspiration. These clinical manifestations would need further investigation as gas exchange may be affected.

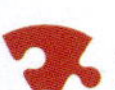
NCJMM Step: Recognize Cues
Reference: Tyerman & Cobbett (2023), pp. 544–566.

Answer 5.2

CLIENT FINDINGS	PNEUMONIA	PULMONARY EMBOLUS	LUNG CANCER
Hemoptysis	○	✔	✔
Atelectasis	✔	○	✔
Pleural pain	✔	✔	✔
Voice hoarseness	○	○	✔
Shortness of breath	✔	✔	✔
Afebrile	○	○	✔

Rationale: Clients who present with pneumonia will present with sudden onset of fever, chills, a productive cough with purulent sputum, and pleuritic chest pain. Consolidation may present as dullness and crackles with lung auscultation. Atelectasis and shortness of breath are complications of pneumonia that can occur with the progression of the illness and the client becoming compromised. Hemoptysis and bleeding in the airway or alveoli are not associated with pneumonia, as the bacteria manifest as purulent sputum. Voice hoarseness is not associated with cases of pneumonia as the bacteria are contained in the alveoli. Finally, a client with a bacterial infection will present with a fever, not afebrile as in this clinical situation. A client who presents with pulmonary embolus experiences hemoptysis from the increased pressure in the pulmonary vasculature due to a blockage of the pulmonary artery and rupture of the vein. As a pulmonary embolus is associated with the pulmonary vasculature, airways are not compromised. Clients may experience pleuritic pain as the lung tissue distal to the blockage is deprived of blood required for gas exchange. Voice hoarseness is not associated with a pulmonary embolus given the location of the block. Owing to a reduction in blood supply to lung tissue due to the block, shortness of breath occurs as the body compensates for the reduced oxygen-rich blood. A fever may or may not accompany a pulmonary embolus. A fever develops when the clot originates from the leg, causing an inflammatory response to be initiated. A client with lung cancer may present with all symptoms presented by the client. The concern for the health care provider is the previous breast cancer diagnosis with double mastectomy. Lung metastasis is common for breast cancer survivors and requires continual monitoring post-recovery from initial breast cancer diagnosis. The most significant symptom often first reported is a persistent cough that may produce sputum, which is blood-tinged due to bleeding from the malignancy. Hemoptysis is typically a latent symptom. Hoarseness occurs as a result of involvement of the recurrent laryngeal nerve. Shortness of breath occurs as the malignancy compromises gas exchange from the pulmonary vasculature to the lung tissue. Pleural pain is often associated with the location of the mass. It is important to address the possible conditions that may be the cause of the clinical presentation.

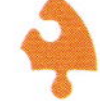
NCJMM Step: Analyze Cues
Reference: Tyerman & Cobbett (2023), pp. 589–595 (pneumonia), 603–609 (lung cancer), 622–624 (pulmonary edema).

Answer 5.3

The client is at highest risk of developing **anemia** and **hypoxemia** as evidenced by the **respiratory assessment**.

Rationale: Given the hemoptysis and obvious signs of bleeding and low hemoglobin, the client is at risk of developing anemia. The client is at risk for hypoxemia due to the location of the mass and the high probability of continued impaired gas exchange. Currently, the client is stable with a RR of

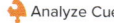

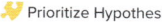

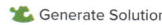

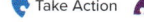

26 and a pulse oximetry of 92% on room air; however, the client may require, oxygenation and even other life-supportive measures if her condition continues to deteriorate. The client is at risk for anorexia as the mass has been located at the base of the esophagus, but that is not a priority condition to consider at this time. Airway, breathing, and circulation are priority complications arising from this condition. The client should be monitored for dysrhythmias, given the location of the mass; however, the potassium remains at a normal level at this time. The client is voiding without issue, so the development of renal failure is minimized. The client's respiratory assessment is evidence of the impending issues ahead for the client. The vital signs are stable despite a RR of 26, which will be monitored, but the pulse oximetry is 92% on room air, so the client is compensating at the time of presentation. Currently, the client is alert and orientated to person, place, and time; however, if the client becomes hypoxemic, her level of consciousness and appropriateness for person, place, and time may become impaired. The renal system is not at risk as the client is voiding, and there is still a stable blood pressure, indicating appropriate flow to the kidneys.

NCJMM Step: Prioritize Hypothesis
References: Tyerman & Cobbett (2023), pp. 603–609 (lung cancer).

Answer 5.4

☐ Contact client's partner with new diagnosis
✔ Encourage exercise and a healthy lifestyle
☐ Collaborate with client about end-of-life care
☐ Request an order to consult for dietitian
✔ Be authentically available to the client and family
✔ Assess client needs for counselling and additional resources

Rationale: It is easy to think about the next medical steps, such as chemotherapy, radiation, or other procedures, but creating a plan of care for the client's psychosocial needs is important when a potential diagnosis of a malignant mass is up for consideration. The nurse should address the psychosocial needs of the client by encouraging exercise and a healthy lifestyle. Maintaining exercise and a healthy lifestyle reminds the client and family that despite a possible diagnosis of malignancy, there is life to be lived. Exercise and promotion of a healthy lifestyle may assist with coping strategies. To facilitate the development of a hopeful, realistic attitude about a re-emergence of cancer, the nurse should be authentically available for discussion with the client and family, especially during difficult times. Establishing a therapeutic relationship based on trust and confidence will allow for open, honest discussions. Addressing the client's ability to cope with stressful events is important. Despite a previous diagnosis of breast cancer, the return of a possible malignant mass opens the door to new treatments and a shift in thinking moving forward. It is not the nurse's responsibility to contact the client's partner without the client's knowledge. This is news that needs to occur between both partners. An end-of-life care discussion may be warranted at some point; however, the diagnosis has not been confirmed. A dietitian consult may be necessary during treatment as an altered taste sensation can occur, affecting nutritional quality and weight.

NCJMM Step: Generates Hypothesis
Reference: Tyerman & Cobbett (2023), pp. 335–339 (management of cancer), 603–609 (lung cancer).

Answer 5.5

Orders
0730h:
- Ensure patency of #18 g peripheral venous access device
- Obtain sputum sample
- Initiate 0.9% sodium chloride (normal saline) 100 mL/hr
- Administer lorazepam 0.5 mg SL prior to the procedure
- Consult physiotherapy
- Consult social work
- Regular diet

Rationale: Prior to a lung biopsy, the client must have a large-bore peripheral venous access device inserted with fluids running prior to the procedure. In the event of an emergency, the IV fluids are already initiated, which saves time, plus the client is NPO and will require hydration for the procedure. Sedation will be given prior to the procedure, which could decrease the client's blood pressure due to a vasodilation physiological response. The client expressed anxiety in the night but was calmed with reassurance and nurses' presence. Administering antianxiety medication in the event of increased anxiety will assist the client throughout the procedure. Obtaining a sputum sample is not a priority before being taken for the lung biopsy. All consults and diet can be initiated when the client returns to the unit and can eat or drink.

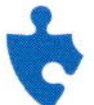
NCJMM Step: Take Action
Reference: Tyerman & Cobbett (2023), pp. 335–339 (management of cancer), 603–609 (lung cancer).

Answer 5.6

ASSESSMENT FINDINGS	IMPROVED	NO CHANGE	DECLINED
Lethargy with sternal rub	○	○	✔
RR 12	✔	○	○
0.9% sodium chloride 200 mL/hr	○	○	✔
BP 116/68	✔	○	○
Hemoptysis	○	✔	○

Rationale: The client will return to the unit lethargic post-sedation for the procedure. Lethargy is expected; however, if the nurse must perform a sternal rub to stimulate the client, that indicates a decline in status. The client's respiratory function must be closely followed. A respiratory rate of 12 is an improvement from the pre-procedure vital signs. Venous access fluids running at 200 mL per hour indicate the client's blood pressure decreased during the procedure, and the fluids are to maintain circulatory volume. Reassessment would be required to check the client's blood pressure. The blood pressure is stable and improved from pre-procedure vital signs. It is likely a result of the intravenous fluids. The client persists with hemoptysis, which is an unchanged finding.

NCJMM Step: Evaluate Outcomes
Reference: Tyerman & Cobbett (2023), pp. 335–339 (management of cancer), 603–609 (lung cancer), Nursing Care Plan 30.2 found on Evolve website (Nursing Care Plan: Thoracotomy).

Medical-Surgical 6.0 (Gastrointestinal)

Answer 6.1

- ✔ Temperature
- ☐ Blood pressure
- ☐ Pulse oximetry
- ☐ Heart sounds
- ☐ Mucous membranes
- ✔ Abdominal pain
- ☐ Diaphoresis
- ✔ Constipation
- ☐ Body mass index (BMI)

Rationale: The client presents with a fever, which may indicate an infection and must be monitored. A fever is a normal physiological inflammatory response activated by the body's defence mechanisms. Any pain is considered abnormal and requires immediate attention. The client has not had a bowel movement for several days, which indicates a dysfunction in the gastrointestinal system. The blood pressure is elevated above normal but does not require immediate attention as it is in relation to the pain. The client is able to maintain adequate blood saturation and systemic delivery of oxygen-rich blood. The client is not experiencing any adventitious heart sounds requiring further investigation. S1 and S2 are normal sounds auscultated by the opening and closing of valves in the heart. The client reports difficulty maintaining oral intake; however, the mucous membranes remain pink, indicating hydration is adequate. If there is a change in fluid status, assessment of mucous membranes, regardless of skin colour, indicates a hydration issue for the client. When a client's heart rate and blood pressure are elevated, the client may experience diaphoresis. The opposite physiological response would be chills, which the client presented to the ED with as a complaint. Diaphoresis is an indicator of cardiac instability if chest pain is present. This client is not experiencing chest pain. Although the client's BMI is high, this is not an assessment detail that requires immediate attention. It is important to consider the client's overall health status. Clients with ulcerative colitis experience bloody diarrhea and lower abdominal cramping associated with diarrhea, which is inconsistent with this client's presentation. Appendicitis is an inflammation of the appendix that presents as anorexia, nausea, and vomiting with pain and guarding in the right lower quadrant, with elevated white blood cells (WBCs) and a fever. This would be a plausible hypothesis; however, the pain is located in the left lower quadrant, which eliminates this possibility.

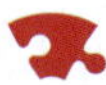
NCJMM Step: Recognize Cues
Reference: Tyerman & Cobbett (2023), pp. 931–950.

Answer 6.2

The nurse should recognize that the client is potentially experiencing a(an) **infection** based on the **gastrointestinal assessment**.

Rationale: When completing a head-to-toe assessment, it is important to determine what is of concern, what is an immediate concern, and what is a critical concern. The gastrointestinal (GI) assessment indicates the client is experiencing cramping, abdominal pain that places him in the fetal position, and constipation. This presentation of GI symptoms are more concerning than those of all other systems. The cardiovascular assessment, including blood pressure (BP) and pulse, is concerning as this is a response to what is happening with the GI system. The client is not experiencing any chest pain; therefore, the increase in BP and pulse are not related to a cardiac issue. A bowel obstruction is a consideration as the client presents with crampy abdominal pain and 4 days without a bowel movement. However, the client presentation that eliminates this as a potential complication would be the fact the client continues to pass flatus. The client is not dehydrated, as evidenced by the adequate, albeit higher, BP and pulse, and the pink mucous membranes. The client presents with a regular heart rhythm, so the chance of a dysrhythmia with only the information provided could not happen. The client has not experienced any blood with emesis, plus the hemodynamic status remains stable. The only primary system of concern is the GI system as identified by the GI assessment.

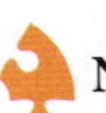
NCJMM Step: Analyze Cues
Reference: Tyerman & Cobbett (2023), pp. 931–950.

Answer 6.3

The client is at highest risk of developing **diverticulitis.**

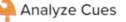

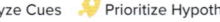

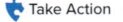

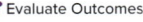

Rationale: The clinical presentation of crampy abdominal pain located in the left lower quadrant, constipation, guarding with palpation, elevated WBC and neutropenia count in the lab values, and a fever indicate diverticulitis. Similar clinical manifestations are associated with gastroenteritis, which include nausea, emesis, abdominal cramping, fever, and increased WBC counts; however, these clients tend to have diarrhea, not constipation. Gastroesophageal reflux disease is an upper GI condition that presents with heartburn, wheezing, coughing, sore throat, hoarseness, nausea, and bloating related to the regurgitation of gastric contents. Peptic ulcer disease is also an upper GI condition. The client may present with burning or cramplike pain located in the mid-epigastric region beneath the xiphoid process. This client is experiencing pain in the left lower quadrant. Knowing the clinical manifestations associated with an upper GI condition as compared to a lower GI condition will assist in determining what the primary issue is for the client.

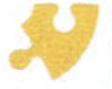
NCJMM Step: Prioritize Hypothesis
Reference: Tyerman & Cobbett (2023), pp. 1002–1003 (gastroesophageal reflux disease), 1020–1023 (peptic ulcer disease), 1048–1049 (appendicitis), 1050 (gastroenteritis), 1051 (ulcerative colitis), 1072–1074 (diverticulitis).

Answer 6.4

POTENTIAL NURSING INTERVENTIONS	INDICATED	NOT INDICATED
Place client in Trendelenburg position	✔	○
Prepare to apply non-rebreather mask to client	○	✔
Request an order for STAT antibiotic therapy	✔	○
Request an order to administer an intravenous fluid bolus	✔	○
Offer the client oral fluids	○	✔

Rationale: The client is bleeding and hemodynamically unstable. Diverticular bleeding is the most common cause of lower GI bleeding. Placing the client in Trendelenburg position will increase venous return to the heart and allow for improved cardiac output and blood pressure. The client should have nasal prongs applied with a pulse oximetry of 84% on room air before a non-rebreather mask is applied. This would be more comfortable for the client. If the client continues to decompensate, an appropriate action would be to move to a mask when the client cannot maintain systemic oxygenation. This client should have antibiotics initiated for the diverticulitis as a complication has developed. The client requires intravenous fluid bolus over oral fluids. This treatment will improve circulatory volume and stabilize hemodynamic status. Oral fluids are allowed only after an acute attack subsides.

NCJMM Step: Generate Solutions
Reference: Tyerman & Cobbett (2023), pp. 1072–1073.

Answer 6.5

- ✔ Cefazolin 2 g, IV, q8h
- ✔ 0.9% sodium chloride (normal saline) 500 mL IV bolus once
- ☐ Consult general surgery
- ☐ Consult dietitian
- ✔ Draw laboratory tests: complete blood count (CBC), urinalysis
- ☐ Insert an additional peripheral venous access device
- ✔ Oxygen at 0–5 L per nasal prongs to maintain pulse oximetry greater than 92%

Rationale: The client requires initiation of high-dose first-generation cephalosporins. The client's diverticulitis has progressed to a lower GI bleed and the client will need to be monitored for further hemodynamic instability. A bolus of isotonic solution is initiated in an attempt to correct the hemodynamic instability. After the client has had a bleeding episode, it is important to monitor the client's hemoglobin and correct any anemia with blood products. General surgery will be consulted but this is not a priority nursing action at this time. Dietary will be consulted as well, as the client's diet will change to high fibre. Oxygen is applied to maintain pulse oximetry greater than 92% to allow for systemic oxygenation.

NCJMM Step: Take Action
Reference: Tyerman & Cobbett (2023), pp. 1072–1073.

Answer 6.6

ASSESSMENT FINDINGS	IMPROVED	NOT CHANGED	DECLINED
Hemoglobin 69 g/L (6.9 g/dL)	○	○	✔
P 102	✔	○	○
One-person assistance for mobility	○	✔	○
Skin warm and dry to touch	✔	○	○
BP 98/60	✔	○	○
T 38.0°C (99.9°F)	✔	○	○

Rationale: The client's bleeding has reduced the hemoglobin levels, indicating a decline from the 1145h blood work. With the bolus, the pulse and BP have improved, indicating an improvement in the hemodynamic system. The client's fever has improved from the IV antibiotics as well. The bleeding may require additional monitoring, including additional vital signs, laboratory blood work, and physical support if the client ambulates. Given the lower hemoglobin level, the client requires one-person assist with ambulation, which has been unchanged since finding the client on the floor.

NCJMM Step: Evaluate Outcomes
Reference: Tyerman & Cobbett (2023), pp. 1072–1073.

Medical-Surgical 7.0 (Gastrointestinal)

Answer 7.1

Nurses' Notes

1100h: Client arrived on the unit post–gastric bypass surgery through the Roux-en-Y gastric bypass procedure. Previous comorbidities include coronary artery disease, type 2 diabetes mellitus controlled with metformin and repaglinide, hypertension but controlled with ramipril, and dyslipidemia controlled by rosuvastatin. Client presented with a BMI of 39. Vital signs: T: 37.4°C (99.3°F); BP: 98/68; P: 90; RR: 16; with pulse oximetry of 92% on 4 L/min of oxygen. Client presents as pleasant, cooperative, lethargic postanaesthetic but rouses easily and orientated to person, place, and time. Client denies any pain or discomfort. Pupils equal and reactive to light at 3 mm. Denies a headache or dizziness. Client presents with S1 and S2 heart sounds, no adventitious heart sounds noted. Apical equals radial pulse. Bilateral radial pulses strong with bilateral dorsalis pedis pulses noted to be weak. Lower extremities' skin cool to touch. Capillary refill less than 3 seconds. Fine inspiratory crackles noted to bilateral lung bases with upper airway wheezing noted. No shortness of breath or distress noted. Client reports feeling thirsty but reminded of NPO. In-dwelling Foley catheter draining clear amber urine. Approximately 400 mL emptied from drainage device. Bowel sounds auscultated × right and left upper quadrants only with absent bowel sounds noted to right lower quadrant and left lower quadrant. Client is not passing any flatus. Abdomen rounded and soft with palpation. Client arrived with intermittent pneumatic compression device going. Peripheral venous access device noted in left antecubital.

Rationale: Initial postoperative care focuses on assessment for cardiopulmonary complications, thrombus formation, anastomotic leaks, and electrolyte imbalances. Upon returning to the unit, the client's initial blood pressure is low and must be monitored closely. The client's hemodynamic status is imperative to maintain adequate flow to the surgical area. The client requires additional oxygen support to maintain pulse oximetry above 92%. If the oxygen requirements continue to increase, the client may require additional supportive measures to maintain proper systemic oxygenation. Fine inspiratory crackles could be related to surgical positioning; however, crackles may indicate additional fluid in the bases, leading to possible infection. The client does not have a fever at present, but this must be monitored. The upper airways present with a wheeze, which is indicative of narrowing of the airways. The client's lack of bowel sounds to the bilateral lower abdomen area will need to be followed up as the client is not passing any flatus.

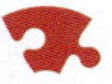

NCJMM Step: Recognize Cues
Reference: Tyerman & Cobbett (2023), pp. 984–989.

Answer 7.2

- ☐ Dehydration
- ☐ Bowel obstruction
- ✔ Respiratory failure
- ✔ Electrolyte imbalances
- ✔ Venous thromboembolism
- ✔ Bleeding
- ✔ Anastomotic leak
- ☐ Pulmonary embolism
- ☐ Malabsorption
- ✔ Dumping syndrome

Rationale: Early complications associated with gastric bypass surgery include cardiorespiratory complications. The client is at risk for rapid oxygen desaturation, as the body stores anaesthetic agents in the adipose tissue. Clients are at risk for resedation. With the reduction in stomach size, clients are at risk for electrolyte imbalances. Routine blood work is important to monitor for these imbalances. Clients postoperative are at risk of developing venous thromboembolisms in their lower extremities. This client returned from the operating room with intermittent sequential compression stockings on. As a result of the procedure, hemorrhage can occur at the surgical site and clients can become anemic and hemodynamically unstable. The hemoglobin level is monitored to determine if the client is bleeding internally and abdominal pain levels are assessed. Anastomotic leak is the most common complication associated with bariatric surgery. Clients will experience abdominal pain, tachycardia, and a fever. Dumping syndrome occurs when gastric contents empty too rapidly into the small intestine, overwhelming its ability to digest nutrients. Often, sugary foods can exacerbate early dumping syndrome. The client is receiving intravenous fluids, so hydration is maintained in the hospital. This is not an early complication of bariatric surgery. A pulmonary embolism must have a clot arrive at the pulmonary vasculature. A venous thromboembolism must develop first; therefore, this is not considered an early complication. Malabsorption is a consideration for clients when they are discharged home; however, malabsorption is not considered an early complication while in hospital but is monitored over time.

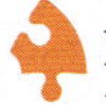

NCJMM Step: Analyze Cues
Reference: Tyerman & Cobbett (2023), pp. 984–989.

Answer 7.3

The client is at highest risk of developing **anastomotic leak**.

Rationale: Anastomotic leak is one of the most common issues related to postoperative care for gastric bypass clients. Early leaks can occur in 1 to 3 days, moderate leaks in 4 to 7 days, and late leaks in up to or after day 8 post-surgery. The client is at increased risk for mortality the longer gastric contents leak into the abdomen. The WBC count is beginning to be elevated with a normal physiological pyretic response. Although the client is experiencing shoulder pain, a consideration of a myocardial infarction is warranted. The troponin level remains normal at this time but should be repeated to confirm the pain was unrelated to anything cardiac. The client is not bleeding, as the hemoglobin and platelet levels remain normal. Dumping syndrome is very common post–bariatric surgery; however, the client did not eat anything presurgery and does not present with nausea, diarrhea, emesis, weakness, or dizziness related to the food ingested. The client's respiratory rate increased in alignment with the abdominal pain and anastomotic leak. A client can progress to shock and should be monitored; however, at the time of the scenario, the client was not experiencing respiratory distress. Compartment syndrome is a condition in which swelling and increased pressure within a limited space reduce capillary perfusion. Clients present with increased work of breathing and ventilation–perfusion inequality due to increased pressure on the diaphragm.

NCJMM Step: Prioritize Hypothesis
Reference: Tyerman & Cobbett (2023), pp. 811–812 (acute myocardial infarction), 986–988 (bypass surgery/anastomotic leak), 1031 (dumping syndrome), 1052 (hemorrhage), 1623–1624 (compartment syndrome), 1746 (respiratory status/shock).

Answer 7.4

POTENTIAL NURSING INTERVENTIONS	INDICATED	NOT INDICATED
Place the client in Trendelenburg position	○	✔
Prepare the client for endoscopy	✔	○
Request an order to insert an additional venous access device	✔	○
Offer oral fluids	○	✔
Increase oxygen delivery	○	✔

Rationale: The client will need to return to the operating room for a full repair. An endoscopy will allow for the placement of a tube to drain the leaking contents until a full surgical procedure can occur to repair the leak. If this is not done, the client can go septic. Inserting another venous access device will enable the administration of medications and IV fluids. The client's head of bed should be at least 35 to 40 degrees to reduce abdominal pressure and increase tidal flow. The balance will be to improve hemodynamic stability, reduce risk of shock, and reduce pressure on the surgical site. The client should be NPO until the surgical procedure can occur to repair the anastomosis leak. The client's oxygen status, although low at 90%, is sufficient at this time. If the pulse oximetry reading should decrease, then considering the application of oxygen would be warranted. Recommending that the client take deep breaths will assist with full lung expansion and improve gas exchange without adding oxygen therapy.

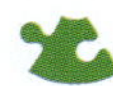

NCJMM Step: Generate Solutions
Reference: Tyerman & Cobbett (2023), pp. 1729–1752 (shock), 1753–1773 (respiratory failure/ARDS).

Answer 7.5

- ✔ Insert an in-dwelling urethral Foley catheter
- ✔ Initiate cefazolin 2 g IV q8h starting now
- ☐ Consult dietitian
- ✔ Administer 0.9% sodium chloride (normal saline) 500 mL bolus × 1
- ☐ Apply oxygen 0–5 L per nasal prongs to maintain pulse oximetry greater than 90%
- ☐ Consult physiotherapy
- ☐ Administer an opiate

Rationale: Monitoring and treating the client for shock is the priority. Inserting a Foley catheter will enable medical staff to monitor fluid status. IV antibiotics are necessary to reduce mortality from the leaking from the surgical site. Cefazolin 2g is broad enough to start and, if necessary, can be discontinued and another antibiotic ordered. The client's blood pressure is low and requires IV fluid administration. Given the client's history, this will reduce the workload of the heart and prevent a possible heart attack. Consulting dietary and physiotherapy is important, just not at 0430h. Oxygen is warranted if the pulse oximetry is below 90% and, currently, the client's gas exchange is stable. Administering an opiate would be an appropriate action only if the blood pressure could handle the vasodilation. Until the blood pressure increases, holding off on administering an analgesic is warranted.

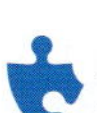

NCJMM Step: Take Action
Reference: Tyerman & Cobbett (2023), pp. 1729–1752 (shock), 1753–1773 (respiratory failure/ARDS).

Answer 7.6

ASSESSMENT FINDINGS	IMPROVED	NO CHANGE	WORSENED
BP 101/60	✔	○	○
Fine inspiratory crackles bilateral lung bases	○	✔	○
Client reports nausea with smell of food	○	○	✔
Afebrile	✔	○	○

Rationale: Administration of fluids and antibiotics, plus temporary repair of the leak, assisted in reversing early shock from developing. Fine inspiratory crackles remain unchanged from the original presentation. This adventitious sound is benign as it never developed into anything further, such as pneumonia. After bariatric surgery, clients will need to determine which foods are tolerable and which foods cause an aversion. Typically, 10 to 14 days post–surgical procedure, clients may begin to eat pureed or soft foods with vitamin supplementation. They can typically transition to solid foods 4 to 6 weeks after surgery. The clients may require additional protein and iron supplements if they become anemic. Learning to eat correctly is part of client teaching upon discharge, requiring follow-up and management of client care after the surgical procedure is complete.

NCJMM Step: Evaluate Outcomes
Reference: Tyerman & Cobbett (2023), pp. 988–989.

Medical-Surgical 8.0 (Gastrointestinal)

Answer 8.1

- ✔ Mucous membranes
- ☐ Urine output
- ☐ Lung sounds
- ✔ Vital signs
- ☐ Cardiac rhythm
- ☐ Motor power
- ☐ Headache
- ✔ Bowel movements

Rationale: Dry mucous membranes indicate dehydration in relation to the lower blood pressure and tachycardia the client is experiencing. The client presents with clinical manifestations of dehydration. This is a sign to consider in monitoring fluid status. It is imperative to monitor vital signs with this client as he presents with a fever on top of low blood pressure accompanied by tachycardia. The client may develop hypovolemia as there is no way to know the degree of fluid loss with the several bouts of diarrhea over the past 2 weeks. The client reports ~12 bowel movements on the day of presenting to the ED. This is extreme and requires further follow-up. The urine output is not concerning at this time, as the bladder scanner revealed only 250 mL of urine. Monitoring the urine output with the infusion is an important nursing consideration but not an assessment detail that requires follow-up at the moment. The lung sounds are clear anteriorly and posteriorly. The cardiac rhythm is tachycardic but regular. It is something to monitor along with vital signs, but the rhythm is not an urgent follow-up issue. The client experiencing a headache is concerning; however, at a pain level of only 2/10, with dry mucous membranes, this could be related to dehydration.

NCJMM Step: Recognize Cues
References: Power Kean et al. (2023), p. 120.

Answer 8.2

CLIENT FINDINGS	GASTRO-ENTERITIS	INFLAMMATORY BOWEL DISEASE	CELIAC DISEASE
Febrile	✔	✔	○
Constipation	○	✔	✔
Dry mucous membranes	✔	✔	✔
Weight loss	○	✔	✔
Frequent bowel movements	✔	✔	✔
Abdominal cramping	✔	✔	✔
Nausea	✔	○	○

Rationale: Clients with gastrointestinal (GI) illness present with frequent bowel movements, abdominal cramping, nausea, and fever and may present with vomiting. Gastroenteritis usually results from a virus, bacteria, or a parasite. Clients may also have increased WBC counts, with blood or mucus in the stool. Older clients may become dehydrated, and fluid status should be monitored. Inflammatory bowel disease can either present with ulcerative colitis (UC) or Crohn's disease (CD). UC is associated with diarrhea and severe abdominal pain that can progress to cramping. When determining if the client has mild, moderate, or severe UC, the determining factor is the presence of a fever, weight loss, anemia, tachycardia, and dehydration. A client may have 10 to 20 bowel movements per day and associated with bloody stool with mucus. The difference between UC and CD is the presence of bloody diarrhea and the frequency of diarrhea, which is less or may not be present in a client with CD. Because of the frequent bowel movements, dehydration can occur with either UC or CD. Weight loss, frequent bowel movements, constipation, and abdominal cramping occur with UC and CD. Celiac disease is typically diagnosed in infancy or childhood. The client may present with diarrhea, abdominal pain and distension, vomiting, anorexia, and constipation only when there is the ingestion of gluten.

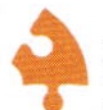
NCJMM Step: Analyze Cues
References: Tyerman & Cobbett (2023), pp. 1050 (gastroenteritis), 1051 (ulcerative colitis), 1059 (celiac disease); Power Kean et al., (2023), pp. 899 (ulcerative colitis), 934 (celiac disease).

Answer 8.3

The client is at highest risk of developing **ulcerative colitis**.

Rationale: Based on the client's presentation of GI symptoms, the client is at risk for an exacerbation of ulcerative colitis, or in this case, a first-time diagnosis. The frequent bowel movements greater than 10; the fever, which could indicate a perforation (severe UC); cramping; blood with purulent stool; weight loss; and symptoms of dehydration are consistent with UC. The symptoms are not completely consistent with Crohn's disease, as there is no tendency for a fever. There is no part of the narrative to explain a gluten sensitivity or intolerance. The client has had several bouts of diarrhea per day over a 2-week period and presents with dehydration. The client does not have gastritis or symptoms consistent with peptic ulcer disease.

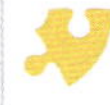
NCJMM Step: Prioritize Hypothesis
Reference: Power Kean et al. (2023), pp. 893 (peptic ulcer disease), 888 (gastroesophageal reflux disease), 899 (UC/CD), 934 (celiac disease).

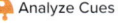

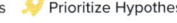

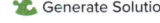

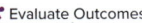

Answer 8.4

POTENTIAL NURSING INTERVENTIONS	INDICATED	NOT INDICATED
Request an order to initiate oxygen therapy	✔	○
Prepare to insert an in-dwelling urinary catheter	○	✔
Encourage oral fluid intake	○	✔
Request an order to insert a second peripheral venous access device	✔	○
Draw laboratory tests: CBC, electrolytes, type and screen/ cross-match,	○	✔
Inform the client they will be receiving AB-negative blood product ASAP	○	✔
Prepare to initiate a 500-mL intravenous bolus of 0.9% normal saline × 1 then reassess blood pressure	✔	○
Prepare to call a code blue	○	✔
Prepare to administer infliximab (Remicade) within the next 30 minutes	○	✔
Consult general surgery for possible colostomy	✔	○

Rationale: Given the severe inflammatory state of the colon, the client has developed a hemorrhage and a lower GI bleed. This is an emergency situation requiring a focus on airway, breathing, and circulation. The client's pulse oximetry is only 81%, requiring supplemental oxygen support. Inserting a Foley catheter at this moment would not be a focus. Once the client is stable, monitoring the urine output would be appropriate, but it is not indicated at this time. The client requires fluids to correct the fluid shift. Administering an intravenous fluid bolus would be more appropriate than encouraging oral intake of fluids. The client is hypotensive and symptomatic, requiring administration of blood products given the soaking of the sheets and blood pressure. The client would require AB-positive or O-negative blood ASAP, not AB-negative. If this was the only blood product on hand, then the client would receive this blood type and then manage antibodies at a subsequent transfusion. With the fever, the bleeding, and the hypotension, the client has likely ruptured the colon, leading to a hypovolemic/shock situation. Blood work does not need to be redrawn as the baseline was already drawn. The 2330h blood work indicates a lower hemoglobin. With the blood on the bed, blood administration and fluid resuscitation would be appropriate. A second peripheral venous access device would be prudent to administer the blood products at the same time while the bolus is infusing. A code blue is not needed at this time as the client can communicate and does not require intubation or defibrillation. If the client's status deteriorates, then a code blue may be necessary to identify the baseline of the client.

A biologic, such as infliximab (Remicade), would be an appropriate drug of choice for this client; however, this is an emergent time requiring a focus on airway, breathing, and circulation. General surgery is a correct indication in this situation. Further investigation is required.

NCJMM Step: Generate Solutions
References: Tyerman & Cobbett (2023), pp. 1054–1056; Sealock & Seneviratne (2021), pp. 881–882.

Answer 8.5

Identify which of the following nursing actions the nurse should take: **monitor stoma viability** and **replace stoma and nasogastric tube output with an isotonic IV solution**.

Rationale: Postoperatively, it is important to monitor the stoma for viability. The stoma should present as pink, rose to brick red; there should be mild to moderate edema; and a small amount of bleeding is considered normal due to the vascularity. A stoma that is pale pink indicates anemia; blanching or dark red to purple in colour indicates inadequate blood supply and moderate to severe edema (obstruction); and a moderate to large amount of bleeding may indicate a coagulation factor deficiency, trauma to the stoma, or a lower GI bleed. Due to the fluid and electrolyte shift postoperatively, it is important to replace any fluid losses to maintain intravascular volume for blood pressure, cardiac output, and electrolytes. A stoma should be rested for 72 hours until the inflammatory process has reduced and the stoma is working to reduce waste. The client will be NPO until the surgeon deems the stoma ready for use. At that time, the client's diet will be clear fluids, then advanced to a more appropriate diet for the client. In some cases, a colostomy may be permanent; however, providing this information for the client immediately after surgery is not appropriate and does not comprise holistic nursing care.

NCJMM Step: Take Action
Reference: Tyerman & Cobbett (2023), pp. 1070–1072, Table 45.34.

Answer 8.6

CLIENT FINDINGS	IMPROVED	NO CHANGE	DECLINED
Pulse oximetry reading 98% on room air	✔	○	○
Stoma dark red with moderate amount of bleeding noted	○	○	✔
Conjunctiva pale and perfused	✔	○	○
Dorsalis pedis pulses weak × 2	○	✔	○
Bowel sounds hypoactive × 4 quadrants 12 hr after the procedure	✔	○	○

Rationale: The client's oxygenation status has improved with the removal of nasal prongs and the client breathing on room air. A stoma that is dark red with moderate bleeding requires further assessment by the surgical team. The client's conjunctiva × 2 present as pale but perfused indicates improved sufficient blood flow and hydration; however, bilateral dorsalis pedis pulses remain weak × 2, which is similar to status at the time of admission. Hypoactive bowel sounds remain a positive indicator for gastric motility, starting in the colon and auscultated throughout all quadrants.

NCJMM Step: Evaluate Outcomes
Reference: Tyerman & Cobbett (2023), pp. 1070–1072, Table 45.34.

Medical-Surgical 9.0 (Renal)

Answer 9.1

Nurses' Notes

1100h: Client presented to the ED with complaints of urgency, frequency, dysuria, left-sided flank pain rated 8 out of 10 on numerical rating scale, and costovertebral tenderness. Client has vomited × 3 this a.m. with emesis consisting of yellow bile. Client was previously camping with friends × 2 days and needed to return due to the pain. Vital signs: T: 39.0°C (102.2°F); BP: 135/82; P: 122; RR: 22; with pulse oximetry of 99% on room air. Upon general assessment, client noted to have "tenting," dry mucous membranes as documented by the conjunctiva. Client reports camping was hot and he did not consume appropriate hydration during the camping trip. He is alert and appropriate, orientated to person, place, and time. Cooperative and follows commands. S1, S2, no extra heart sounds noted. Skin is cool with diaphoresis noted. Denies any chest pain. Capillary refill noted to be less than 3 seconds. Lung sounds clear. Moderate to severe left-sided flank pain that increased this morning prompted visit to the ED. Client reports not being able to get warm and feeling chilled for the last 12 hours. He cannot remember the last time he voided. Client denies any previous pertinent medical history.

Rationale: The client is presenting with a fever, chills, urgency, frequency, and dysuria, which may indicate a possible bacterial infection or viral infection, likely coming from the renal system. Left-sided flank pain plus costovertebral tenderness requires immediate follow-up as the renal system is likely involved. The emesis may indicate a gastrointestinal (GI) viral illness; however, since he cannot remember the last time he voided, he may be at risk for dehydration. Since he is experiencing emesis, his blood pressure may become compromised. At this point, his vitals remain stable. He is already dehydrated, evidenced by the "tenting" and dry mucous membranes.

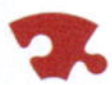
NCJMM Step: Recognize Cues
Reference: Tyerman & Cobbett (2023), pp. 1148, 1156–1158, 1167.

Answer 9.2

- ☐ Urinary tract infection
- ☐ Gastrointestinal viral illness
- ✔ Fluid imbalance
- ✔ Dysrhythmias
- ✔ Acute kidney failure
- ☐ Lower back injury

Rationale: The primary consideration for complications with this client would be associated with the cardiovascular and renal systems. Given the "tenting" and dry mucous membranes, the client is at risk for dehydration and fluid imbalance, which could contribute to acute kidney injury. The lack of urinary output for several hours is concerning because his body remains hemodynamically stable given his age. Without any urinary output, the client is at risk of developing life-threatening dysrhythmias, likely ventricular tachycardia or ventricular fibrillation. The client is not at risk for a urinary tract infection as the symptom presentation is beyond dysuria, frequency, and urgency. The extension of left-sided flank pain with costovertebral pain indicates the cause may be higher. With a urinary tract infection, the client will present with a low-grade fever with chills. This client has presented with a more severe symptom presentation. If the client only presented with emesis, a viral GI illness could be a likely result; however, the client has more than one GI symptom. Although the pain is in the lower back region, an injury is an unlikely cause. The client has no previous comorbidities and reported no injury during the camping trip.

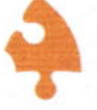
NCJMM Step: Analyze Cues
Reference: Tyerman & Cobbett (2023), pp. 1148, 1156–1158, 1167.

Answer 9.3

The client is at highest risk of developing **pyelonephritis**.

Rationale: The client presents with fever, chills, dysuria, vomiting, and flank and costovertebral pain, all of which point to pyelonephritis. The urinalysis confirmed there were leukocytes and trace amounts of hematuria and was positive for nitrates. The abdominal ultrasound indicates kidney stones are present. When the client went camping and was not hydrated enough, the stones, which were likely starting to develop before the trip, grew in size and blocked the ureter and part of the kidney. The kidney stones were the cause of the pyelonephritis. Presentation of bladder cancer includes a large amount of hematuria. Pyelonephritis and bladder cancer share the clinical manifestations of dysuria, frequency, and urgency. Interstitial cystitis is a chronic, painful, inflammatory disease of the bladder. The stones were noted in the kidney. A stricture is an abnormal temporary or permanent narrowing of the lumen in the ureter or the urethra. Clinical manifestations would be diminished force of the urinary stream, spraying, or split urine stream. The client may report feelings of not emptying the bladder completely. Clients often report a history of urinary tract infections. Glomerulonephritis is an immune-related inflammation of the glomeruli characterized by proteinuria, hematuria, decreased urine production, and edema. These clients present afebrile, but this client has a documented fever.

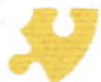

NCJMM Step: Prioritize Hypothesis
Reference: Tyerman & Cobbett (2023), pp. 1148–1149 (pyelonephritis), 1152–1153 (glomerulonephritis), 1155–1159 (renal calculi), 1160–1161 (strictures), 1164–1165 (bladder cancer).

Answer 9.4

POTENTIAL ORDERS	INDICATED	NOT INDICATED
Administration of pain medication	✔	○
Initiate lactated Ringer's at 200 mL/hr	○	✔
Draw CBC, electrolytes, PTT, INR, blood cultures	✔	○
Consult Urology	✔	○
Administer ibuprofen	○	✔
Initiate broad-spectrum antibiotics	✔	○

Rationale: Pain medication would be appropriate for this client, with opiates likely to be ordered. Morphine would cause vasodilation and smooth muscle relaxation of the kidney and bladder. Blood work would need to be drawn to identify the bacteria to apply antibiotic coverage for the client while the kidney stones are being resolved. Urology would be consulted to confirm the stones and determine an appropriate plan of care. The client is in considerable pain and has developed clinical symptoms closely aligned with urosepsis. It would be necessary to break up the stones quickly to improve blood flow to the kidney and enable filtration. Broad-spectrum antibiotics, such as ampicillin or vancomycin, would be started until the infection has resolved. The client has a high probability of developing urosepsis. Intravenous fluids would be ordered and at a high rate; however, lactated Ringer's would not be the intravenous fluid of choice with the high degree of potassium in the fluid. A better choice would be an isotonic solution such as 0.9% sodium chloride until electrolytes can be drawn and the potassium level known. The addition of potassium to a client who is not voiding puts the client at risk of developing dysrhythmias. Acetaminophen, not ibuprofen, would be chosen to alleviate the fever.

NCJMM Step: Generate Solutions
Reference: Tyerman & Cobbett (2023), pp. 1148–1149 (pyelonephritis), 1155–1159 (renal calculi).

Answer 9.5

- ✔ Prepare client for lithotripsy
- ☐ Insert a Foley catheter
- ☐ Monitor blood glucose
- ✔ Initiate 0.9% sodium chloride at 200 mL/hr
- ✔ Monitor urine output

Rationale: Once the client's kidney stones have been broken up, he will pass the fragments, and with antibiotic therapy, the pyelonephritis will resolve. Lithotripsy involves the use of sound waves to break renal stones into small particles that can be eliminated from the urinary tract. The client should have 0.9% sodium chloride administered to maintain proper hydration and blood flow for the kidneys. The dehydration initiated the stone formation. The kidneys will need additional blood flow to remove particles after the lithotripsy is completed. An isotonic solution that does not increase potassium levels would be more appropriate. Once the stones are broken into smaller particles, it is important to monitor renal output. When there is a resolved obstruction, the body can have a diuretic phase due to the buildup of urine. There may be hemodynamic shifts, which require careful monitoring of the client's urine output, as well as vital signs.

NCJMM Step: Take Action
Reference: Tyerman & Cobbett (2023), pp. 1148–1149 (pyelonephritis), 1155–1159 (renal calculi).

Answer 9.6

CLIENT STATEMENTS	UNDER-STANDING	NO UNDER-STANDING
"Drinking more hydrating fluids such as water would have helped prevent the stones from forming"	✔	○
"I am healed now and do not have to monitor urine output."	○	✔
"Until the stones completely pass, I should remain on bed rest."	○	✔
"I have more information about which foods contributed to the stone developing along with lower fluid intake."	✔	○
"I can adequately control the pain with acetaminophen."	○	✔

Rationale: The client understands that inadequate hydration contributed to stone formation, along with diet. Foods rich in purines and oxalates may have contributed to stone formation before a weekend camping trip with limited hydration. Clients will need to continue to monitor urine output even upon discharge. Clients should produce approximately 2 L per day or urine output and to drink approximately 2 000 to 2 200 mL per day. If the client has a demanding job or exercises, then fluid intake should be increased. This will help prevent future stones from forming. Ambulation is recommended for the client to assist in moving the stones from the kidney and ureters down to the bladder and urethra. Bed rest would only prolong the passing of the fragmented stones. Typically, these clients are provided opiates to assist with relaxing the smooth muscle, reducing the constriction around the stone as it passes, and pain management.

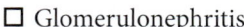

NCJMM Step: Evaluate Outcomes
Reference: Tyerman & Cobbett (2023), pp. 1155–1159 (renal calculi).

Medical-Surgical 10.0 (Renal)

Answer 10.1

Nurses' Notes

1100h: Client was seen in the emergency department complaining of lower abdominal discomfort rated 4 out of 10 on a numerical rating scale, found to be incontinent of urine in the hallway of the long-term care facility. He was trying to find the bathroom in his room and became disoriented. Client presents with a past medical history of coronary artery disease with PCI to LAD in 1995, benign prostate hyperplasia, chronic obstructive pulmonary disease (COPD), and left hip fracture due to frequent falls. Client accompanied by adult child. Vital signs: T: 38.3°C (100.9°F); BP: 143/86; P: 86; RR: 18; with pulse oximetry of 92% on room air. Client presents as pleasant, cooperative, alert and orientated to person, place, and time. No confusion noted while on Urology but he was placed in a room close to the nurses' station. Gait steady, denies any dizziness, but requires one-person assist for support only. S1 and S2 auscultated with S3, apical heart rate regular and equals radial pulse. Crackles auscultated in bilateral lower lung fields increasing to right middle lobe. Respirations regular and easy at rest. Client encouraged to use urinal at bedside when he is able to void. Client reports the urge to void but cannot, has to get up several times in the night to void, and he is exhausted. There is some discomfort when he starts to void but diminishes with stream. Bowel sounds auscultated × 4 quadrants with abdomen soft and round during palpation.

Rationale: The client presents with lower abdominal pain, which could be related to an infection, bladder issue, kidney stones, or prostate. The disorientation and increased fever may be related to a urinary tract infection. The client presents with hypertension, as a result of the lower abdominal discomfort or inability to void. The S3 and crackles indicate higher volume in the left ventricle, possibly leading to pulmonary edema. S3 is an abnormal heart sound that is often associated with increased preload of the left ventricle and with heart failure. These findings could be related to the previous PCI to the LAD or a renal condition. If not treated, the client could develop increased respiratory rates, difficulty with oxygenation, and hemodynamic instability. The client is experiencing the urgency to void as well as nocturia. Exhaustion could be leading to the confusion.

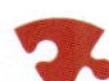
NCJMM Step: Recognize Cues
Reference: Tyerman & Cobbett (2023), pp. 1121–1142 (renal assessment).

Answer 10.2

- ✔ Dehydration
- ☐ Leukopenia
- ✔ Incontinence
- ☐ Glomerulonephritis
- ✔ Distended bladder
- ✔ Hypertension
- ✔ Peripheral edema
- ☐ Syndrome of inappropriate antidiuretic hormone (SIADH)

Rationale: If a client cannot void despite feeling the urge to void, they may choose to reduce oral intake of fluid, leading to dehydration. With dehydration, the client's blood pressure can fall, the kidney will not be perfused, and this could lead to an acute kidney injury. When the client is unable to void, there is an increased risk for overflow incontinence, which occurs when the pressure of urine in an overfull bladder overcomes sphincter control and the client will dribble after voiding. The client is unable to fully empty his bladder. With chronic delayed bladder emptying, complications include hydronephrosis (distension of the pelvis and the calyces of the kidney by urine that cannot flow through the ureter to the bladder); pyelonephritis, not glomerulonephritis; and bladder damage. The client could experience a distended bladder with urinary retention, which could lead to acute kidney injury, urinary tract infections, or even urosepsis. Hypertension occurs when there is volume expansion and activation of the renin–angiotensin–aldosterone system. Although rare, it is a complication for clients with distended bladders to experience pain. Peripheral edema is a consequence of the body's inability to excrete volume. SIADH is an endocrine disorder of impaired water excretion typically caused by head trauma, psychosis, medications, brain tumours, or metabolic disorders. This client does not present with an endocrine disorder.

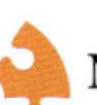
NCJMM Step: Analyze Cues
Reference: Tyerman & Cobbett (2023), pp. 1121–1142 (renal assessment), 1165–1168 (urinary retention/incontinence), 1402–1403 (benign prostate hyperplasia), 1240–1241 (SIADH).

Answer 10.3

The client is at highest risk of developing **urosepsis** and **dysrhythmias**.

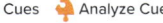

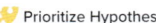

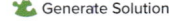

Rationale: This client is unable to empty his bladder because of his benign prostate hyperplasia. He presents with nocturia, urgency, lower abdominal discomfort, and incontinence. These conditions allow for bacteria to grow in his bladder and can lead to, at best, a urinary tract infection and, in the worst-case scenario, urosepsis. When the client does not empty his bladder, he is at risk for hyperkalemia, which could lead to life-threatening dysrhythmias such as ventricular tachycardia or ventricular fibrillation, or worse, sudden cardiac death. The higher levels of potassium lead to cardiac cellular instability, causing excitability. The client may not feel like eating with an extended bladder due to urinary retention, but this is not the highest priority. An acute myocardial infarction occurs when there is a blockage in the coronary arteries. This client presents with renal clinical manifestations. The issue is urinary retention in the bladder due to benign prostate hyperplasia and not in the kidney. Urosepsis would likely be more prevalent than kidney failure.

NCJMM Step: Prioritize Hypothesis
Reference: Tyerman & Cobbett (2023), pp. 1121–1142, 1402–1403.

Answer 10.4

POTENTIAL NURSING INTERVENTIONS	INDICATED	NOT INDICATED
Complete a bladder scan	✔	○
Offer oral fluids to increase fluid intake	○	✔
Request an order to insert a Foley catheter	✔	○
Suggest client consume bananas	○	✔
Request an order to insert a venous access device	✔	○
Speak in a calm, reassuring voice to the client	✔	○

Rationale: Prior to requesting an order to insert a Foley catheter, it is important to know how much urine is being retained in the bladder. The assumption is that urinary retention is causing the abdominal pain, but knowing as much objective data as possible is necessary to rule out other abdominal conditions. Small oral fluid intake should be suggested to maintain hydration; however, when a client has urinary retention, monitoring fluid intake is imperative to understand fluid balance. Since the client has hyperkalemia, the intent is to drain the bladder and the serum potassium will correct itself; however, in the event the client suffers a life-threatening dysrhythmia, it is best to have venous access. Suggesting banana intake will only increase the serum potassium level and should be avoided. The client is agitated with the increase in pain. Speaking calmly and reassuringly to the client when in an acute episode will be better than a rushed cadence.

NCJMM Step: Generate Solutions
Reference: Tyerman & Cobbett (2023), pp. 1165–1173.

Answer 10.5

- ☐ Place the client in high-Fowler's position
- ☐ Provide water at the bedside to assist with insertion
- ✔ Ensure client education about not "tugging" on the catheter
- ✔ Maintain sterile technique
- ✔ Educate the client about maintaining perineal care at least twice per day
- ☐ Place the drainage system on the raised bed rail

Rationale: Clients need to be reminded that a balloon at the tip of the catheter holds 10 mL of sterile water, which will cause significant discomfort if it is pulled out of the urethra. Thus clients need to avoid unnecessary "tugging" of the catheter. The client needs to be careful when rising from the bed to ensure the drainage system follows him when not in the bed. Insertion of a Foley catheter is a sterile procedure. If the nurse contaminates the sterile field or sterile container, they should start over. This is imperative so as to not introduce any further bacteria into the bladder. Maintaining proper perineal cleanliness is also imperative so as to avoid introducing more bacteria into the bladder. If a man is uncircumcised, the foreskin must be pulled back and properly cleaned around the meatus. If a man is circumcised, proper hygiene is a must to eliminate bacteria. A client is placed supine with the head of the bed slightly raised during the insertion of a Foley catheter. High-Fowler's position will close off the urethra, making the insertion more difficult for the nurse and more uncomfortable for the client. Water is unnecessary to have at the bedside for the client. This is not a nasogastric insertion. The closed drainage system should be placed lower than the client's bladder to ensure proper drainage and to avoid urinary retention.

NCJMM Step: Take Action
Reference: Tyerman & Cobbett (2023), pp. 1165–1173.

Answer 10.6

ASSESSMENT FINDINGS	IMPROVED	NO CHANGE	WORSENED
T: 37.7°C (99.9°F)	✔	○	○
2 out of 10 pain on numerical rating scale	✔	○	○
Found wandering, unable to locate room	○	✔	○
S1, S2, and S3	○	✔	○
Pulse oximetry 92% on room air	○	✔	○
Urine output: 750 mL	✔	○	○
BP: 92/65	○	○	✔

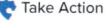

Rationale: The client could have developed an inflammatory response when they were admitted to the hospital. When the urine was drained, the client's ability to have a normal physiological inflammatory response eliminated any bacteria. The WBC level did not indicate an infection. Draining the urine improved the client's pain level. The client remains confused and wandering. This has not changed since admission as there have been periods of confusion mixed with periods of lucidness. The client is 92 years old, which could indicate some cognitive decline. The client continues to have an S3 heart sound. Further investigation is necessary to determine why the additional volume remains, even after the urine has been drained. The client will likely need an echocardiogram, as he may have developed an element of heart failure given his age and suffering the myocardial infarction with PCI. There was significant urine output after the catheter was inserted for urinary retention. At times, when there is a large volume depletion, there is a fluid shift, causing the client to experience a drop in blood pressure temporarily. This is a clinical manifestation that will need to be monitored.

NCJMM Step: Evaluate Outcomes
Reference: Tyerman & Cobbett (2023), pp. 1165–1173.

Medical-Surgical 11.0 (Musculoskeletal)

Answer 11.1

- ✔ Pupillary response
- ✔ Alertness
- ☐ Respirations
- ☐ Lung sounds
- ✔ Pulses
- ☐ Pulse oximetry
- ✔ Skin temperature

Rationale: Clients who return from a surgical procedure often will have received anaesthetic, either general or spinal, and analgesic delivered through intravenous access. It is important to monitor for neurological improvement and pupillary response. Lethargy and sluggish pupillary response could be an indication of anaesthetic medication or analgesic administered in the operating room or recovery room and these symptoms should improve as the pharmacological effect diminishes. The client's right dorsalis pedis pulse is weaker than the left pulse. This requires immediate follow-up to identify if there are any perfusion issues distal to the hip fracture. The skin temperature differences between the right and left leg also indicate a concern about perfusion. The respirations at 12 are slow but able to support the pulse oximetry level even on 2 L of oxygen administered through nasal prongs. Lung sounds are diminished, but there are no adventitious breath sounds to indicate something more serious that can occur when fluids are administered during surgical procedures. Pulse oximetry is stable with oxygen being administered through nasal prongs.

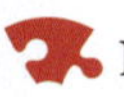

NCJMM Step: Recognize Cues
Reference: Tyerman & Cobbett (2023), pp. 1625–1628.

Answer 11.2

CLIENT FINDINGS	STROKE	HEMATOMA	VENOUS THROMBO-EMBOLISM
Weak dorsalis pedis pulses	✔	✔	✔
Level of consciousness	✔	○	○
Sluggish pupil response	✔	○	○
Skin temperature	✔	✔	✔
Bruit at the surgical site	○	✔	○
Moving extremities equally	○	✔	✔

Rationale: A client who is experiencing a stroke will exhibit neurological conditions with potential hemodynamic changes. These clients may experience weaker pulses and cool-to-touch skin as a result of blood flow being constricted in their peripheries to accommodate cerebral pressure changes. A client may even experience one side with blood flow and be warm to touch, while the opposite or contralateral of the body may be cool to touch. With strokes or any head injuries, level of consciousness (LOC) and pupillary response must be monitored. This client's LOC and sluggish pupillary changes may be a result of the anaesthetic and analgesic administered during the surgical procedure; however, if a client has suffered a stroke during the procedure, these two neurological assessment data will be important to consider. A client who is experiencing stroke symptoms could experience a carotid bruit, indicating turbulent blood flow. It is important to understand the location of the bruit. Clients who experience a stroke may have unequal movement of their extremities. A client who has developed a hematoma at the surgical site and in the femoral location may develop weaker pulses distal to the surgical site, indicating a lack of perfusion and blood flow to the leg. If this is severe enough and lasts for long enough, the extremity may require amputation. There will not be any neurological changes with a hematoma at the right hip surgical site. If a hematoma develops at the surgical site and there is a reduction in perfusion to the extremity, the skin may be cool to touch, but a bruit would also be auscultated at the site. With this client, no bruit was auscultated. With any surgery, venous thrombosis can occur as long as Virchow's triad is met, which is endothelial damage, venous stasis, and hypercoagulability of blood. The client will continue to move all extremities independently.

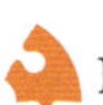

NCJMM Step: Analyze Skills
Reference: Tyerman & Cobbett (2023), pp. 692 (hematoma), 914–915 (venous thromboembolism), 1485–1510 (stroke).

Answer 11.3

The client is at highest risk of developing **venous thromboembolism**.

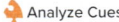

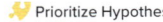

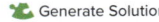

Rationale: Venous thromboembolism (VTE) can occur after lower extremity orthopedic surgery. The client's body sends platelets to the surgical site, which in turn travel down the extremity. Lying in the bed and lack of movement account for venous stasis. The surgery itself causes endothelial damage. A client who may be experiencing a VTE presents with sudden onset of intense, sharp, deep muscle pain that may increase with sharp dorsiflexion of foot. Objective assessment reveals increased warmth, swelling, redness, dependent cyanosis, and tenderness to palpation. If a client was rejecting a femoral prosthesis, this would accompany an inflammatory response with heat to the site and signs of infection with an increase in temperature. This client is afebrile; warmth is noted when touching the lower leg and foot, not the hip. Dry gangrene occurs as a result of degenerative changes accompanied by certain chronic diseases, such as atherosclerosis or diabetes, when the blood supply to the lower extremities is gradually reduced. Wet gangrene is the rapid elimination of blood flow seen in a severe burn or traumatic crushing injury. The presentation of this client is not similar to that of gangrene. Osteomyelitis is a severe infection of the bone, bone marrow, and surrounding soft tissue. There would be a febrile response, as well as night sweats, chills, restlessness, nausea, and malaise. Locally, there would be bone pain unrelieved by rest and that worsens with activity, swelling, tenderness, and warmth at the infection site. The client would also have restricted movement. This client is not expressing any of these clinical manifestations. Peripheral arterial disease occurs when there is an obstruction of collateral circulation and tends to be a chronic condition, not an acute presentation, as in this case.

NCJMM Step: Prioritize Hypothesis
References: Jarvis et al. (2024), pp. 553–565, 572; Tyerman & Cobbett (2023), pp. 219 (gangrene), 914–915 (venous thromboembolism), 1625–1628 (hip fracture), 1642–1643 (osteomyelitis).

Answer 11.4

- ☐ Elevate the right leg while in bed
- ✔ Use a pillow between the legs
- ☐ Apply a warm blanket to the affected area
- ✔ Notify health care provider
- ☐ Contact client's partner with status

Rationale: The client must be given proper care after orthopedic surgery. A pillow between the legs is recommended for at least 8 weeks after surgery when lying on their side or when supine. The nurse should keep the client's hips neutral and notify the surgeon if severe pain, deformity, or loss of function occurs. The affected surgical side should not be elevated when the client is in bed. This position is recommended when the client is sitting in a chair, but not in the middle of the night. A warm blanket should not be provided to the area with the VTE. This would only vasodilate the vessels, engorging the area with blood and increasing the obstruction and VTE. The client is not at risk for death. The client is be able to contact their partner on their own.

NCJMM Step: Generate Solutions
Reference: Tyerman & Cobbett (2023), pp. 1625–1628.

Answer 11.5

It would be a priority for the nurse to request a prescription for **unfractionated heparin IV**.

The nurse should prepare the client for the procedure **Doppler ultrasonography** to confirm diagnosis.

Rationale: Given the rapid progression of the client undergoing a surgical procedure to repair the hip fracture, there was not sufficient time for proper preoperative management for VTE prophylaxis. As a result, a clot has formed. Unfractionated heparin would be the best choice of anticoagulation therapy to prevent further clots from forming, given the quick onset of the mechanism of action. Low-molecular-weight heparin would be a second choice, but given the fresh surgical procedure, unfractionated heparin could be discontinued with a reversal of anticoagulation in a shorter time frame as compared to the other choices, such as the oral anticoagulant Rivaroxaban. Clopidogrel is an antiplatelet medication used more for coronary or cerebral conditions and is not a proper choice for VTE prophylaxis.

The client will be ordered to undergo a Doppler ultrasonography diagnostic procedure. This will indicate the location and extent of severity of the clot in the vein. The client would not be prepared for a spiral CT scan. This is prescribed for clients who are experiencing symptoms associated with pulmonary embolisms. A client will proceed to a coronary angiogram with confirmed myocardial infarction to identify the extent of coronary artery disease. An X-ray would not be an appropriate diagnostic procedure to identify blood clots in the venous system.

NCJMM Step: Take Action
Reference: Tyerman & Cobbett (2023), pp. 914–915 (venous thromboembolism), 1625–1628 (hip fracture).

Answer 11.6

Nurses' Notes

Day 2 Postoperative:
0800h: Client reports ambulating the hallways several times a day with the use of a walker and increased mobility each day. Right lower leg remains slightly edematous, foot similar in size to the left foot. Dorsalis pedis pulses strong and palpable on the left foot, weak but palpable on the right foot. Capillary refill less than 3 seconds on bilateral toes. Right leg remains cooler to touch as compared to the left. Bilateral lower extremity colour noted to be pink.

Rationale: Improvement indicates the frequency of ambulation. The client reports ambulating several times a day, which is an improvement in his hip repair. The edema in the left lower extremity has improved, with bilateral feet now the same in size. The location of the clot will take time to reduce in size. The dorsalis pedis pulse is not palpable and does not require the Doppler procedure to identify if it is present or absent. Bilateral colour has improved to pink, which indicates perfused.

NCJMM Step: Evaluate Outcomes
Reference: Tyerman & Cobbett (2023), pp. 914–915 (venous thromboembolism), 1625–1628 (hip fracture).

Medical-Surgical 12.0 (Immunity)

Answer 12.1

Progress Notes

April 20: Client presents to the clinic to request sexually transmitted infection (STI) testing. She reports flulike symptoms: fatigue, fever, muscle aches, headaches, dysuria, and purulent urethral discharge after having condomless intercourse with a male partner. Client is requesting STI panel be completed. Full panel including chlamydia, gonorrhea, HIV, herpes, genital warts completed with specimens taken for testing.

Rationale: The client is presenting with common STI symptoms that require follow-up. Although the symptoms of fatigue, fever, muscle aches, headaches, and dysuria could be related to the flu or a urinary tract infection, the fact that the client had condomless intercourse with her partner is a concern. Purulent drainage from the urethra requires further follow-up.

NCJMM Step: Recognize Cues
Reference: Tyerman & Cobbett (2023), pp. 1355–1371.

Answer 12.2

- ✔ Chlamydia
- ☐ Genital herpes simplex type 2
- ☐ Syphilis
- ✔ Human immunodeficiency virus (HIV)
- ✔ Gonorrhea
- ✔ Pregnancy

Rationale: When a client presents with STI-like symptoms, it is important to rule out other conditions, such as urinary tract infection, while also testing for STIs. Since the client reported engaging in condomless intercourse, a pregnancy test would be added to the STI panel to identify early health promotion for the fetus and provide supportive counselling. Clients who test positive for chlamydia often are asymptomatic, although some clinical manifestations associated with chlamydia include dysuria, urethral discharge, rectal discharge, and pain during defecation if anal intercourse occurred. Clinical manifestations associated with syphilis mimic other conditions. Clients present with a chancre, lymphadenopathy, genital ulcers, flulike symptoms, lesions, malaise, sore throat, rash, weight loss, and alopecia. There can also be latent clinical presentations, which include a positive test, lesions, aneurysms, aortic valve insufficiency, and neurosyphilis. Clinical manifestations associated with gonorrhea include dysuria, purulent urethral discharge, menstrual changes, and frequency of voiding. At the time of infection with HIV, clients often report flulike symptoms. The virus can lie dormant in the body until a test is required, as in this case, or the client presents with opportunistic infections. Anytime a client has condomless intercourse with a male partner, there is a possibility of pregnancy; therefore, a pregnancy test must be completed.

NCJMM Step: Analyze Cues
Reference: Tyerman & Cobbett (2023), pp. 1355–1371.

Answer 12.3

The client is at highest risk of developing **gonorrhea** and **human immunodeficiency virus**.

Rationale: It is not uncommon for clients to discover a positive HIV result at the time they are being tested for other STIs. The most common STIs associated with positive HIV results are gonorrhea and chlamydia, both of which can be treated. The client's presentations do not align with the other conditions.

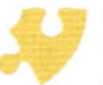
NCJMM Step: Prioritize Hypothesis
Reference: Tyerman & Cobbett (2023), pp. 279–306, 1355–1371.

Answer 12.4

- ✔ Assess for client suicide risk
- ☐ Report both gonorrhea and HIV to public health
- ☐ Contact client's partners
- ☐ Rebook client for follow-up appointment
- ✔ Reassure client about new antiretroviral medications to lower viral loads
- ✔ Leave client alone to process information

Rationale: With a new diagnosis of gonorrhea and HIV, the client is provided space and silence to absorb the information and to express any emotions or concerns. The client should be reassured that new antiretroviral medications are available and that people diagnosed with HIV can live long lives. The nurse should provide medical and emotional support resources for the client and evaluate if the client is a suicide risk and provide follow-up as needed. Maintaining client safety is most important. The nurse will report both gonorrhea and HIV to public health as these are both reportable STIs. Statistics are maintained to monitor for changes to population health and the need for health promotion and early interventions across each province and across Canada. It is not the nurses' responsibility to contact the client's partners but the client themselves. The client will be rebooked for a follow-up; however, immediately after delivering difficult news to the client, rebooking another appointment is inappropriate.

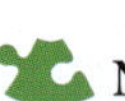
NCJMM Step: Generate Solutions
Reference: Tyerman & Cobbett (2023), p. 300.

Answer 12.5

- ✔ Initiate antiretroviral (ARV) medication regimen at the time of diagnosis
- ☐ Consult spiritual care
- ✔ Initiate cefixime and azithromycin
- ✔ Inform client of abstinence from all sexual activity until gonorrhea infection is cleared

Rationale: The client should begin AVR therapy at the time of diagnosis to significantly reduce viral loads. The client will need to be informed that Undetectable = Untransmissible.

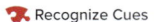

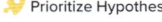

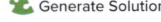

ARV therapy has been improved where viral loads remain low, and clients live a fairly normal life despite HIV diagnosis. HIV has become a chronic illness instead of a life-threatening illness. Clients can resume intimate relationships with clients. It is recommended to use condoms as part of prophylaxis; however, with viral loads low, HIV is untransmissible. Cefixime and azithromycin would be the correct antibiotics to prescribe for the gonorrhea infection. The client should be reminded to maintain strict adherence to either the ARV therapy or dual therapy for gonorrhea infection. Clients should abstain from all sexual activity until gonorrhea infection has been treated and not detected any longer. Gonorrhea is highly transmissible.

NCJMM Step: Take Action
Reference: Tyerman & Cobbett (2023), pp. 300, 1358.

Answer 12.6

CLIENT STATEMENTS	UNDER-STANDING	NO UNDER-STANDING
"I can still be intimate with a partner; I will need to use condoms and know my viral load."	✔	○
"I do not have to disclose my HIV status to any new partner."	○	✔
"I will be taking this ARV therapy for the rest of my life."	✔	○
"I can do this on my own."	○	✔
"I will contact all partners to recommend getting tested."	✔	○

Rationale: Clients can be informed that, despite HIV status, as long as they are taking ARV therapy and using condoms, the risk of transmission is very small, especially when viral load is undetectable by blood tests. Strict adherence to the medication regimen will keep the client as healthy as possible and for as long as possible. Clients take the ARV regimen for the rest of their lives. This is the only way to maintain a lower viral load, as ARV attacks the replication of the HIV at many intersections within the cell. The client is recommended to contact all her partners to inform them to get tested for HIV as well as gonorrhea and to inform all partners in the future of her positive status. It is a legal responsibility to disclose HIV status so that the consenting partner can make an informed decision to engage in sexual activity, or not. It is recommended that clients speak to other HIV-infected people who are willing to share with and assist clients with the new diagnosis. A community of support helps clients manage the new diagnosis.

NCJMM Step: Evaluate Outcomes
Reference: Tyerman & Cobbett (2023), pp. 300, 1358.

Medical-Surgical 13.0 (Multisystem)

Answer 13.1

- ✔ Vital signs
- ☐ Skin biopsy site
- ✔ Shortness of breath
- ☐ Radial pulses
- ☐ Bowel sounds
- ✔ Urine output
- ✔ Skin cool to touch

Rationale: This client is presenting with a compromised respiratory and cardiovascular system as evidenced by the lower blood pressure, higher heart rate, and increased respirations. The body is attempting to compensate for the acute inflammatory response with a high temperature, likely as a result of the skin biopsy. The decrease in or lack of urine output indicates the body is attempting to retain volume to compensate for the lower blood pressure. Given the age of the client, the compensatory mechanisms are creating a more stable presentation as compared to an older adult or pediatric client. The client data of cool-to-touch skin indicates vasoconstriction and another compensatory mechanism to maintain blood volume. The skin biopsy is important as that appears to be the source of entry for bacteria; however, the immediate concern is to maintain respiratory and hemodynamic status. Radial pulses are noted to be regular and strong, so no further follow-up is necessary at this time. Bowel sounds are present despite being hypoactive. Currently, there is blood flow to the area.

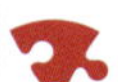
NCJMM Step: Recognize Cues
Reference: Tyerman & Cobbett (2023), pp. 751–771 (cardiovascular assessment), 1729–1751 (shock, sepsis).

Answer 13.2

The nurse should recognize that the client is potentially experiencing a **sympathetic nervous system response** as indicated by **low urine output** and **skin temperature.**

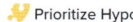

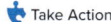

Rationale: The client is experiencing a high fever, lower blood pressure, higher heart rate, skin cool to touch, and reduced urine output. During the compensatory phase of shock, the body activates neural, hormonal, and biochemical compensatory mechanisms in an attempt to overcome the increasing consequences of anaerobic metabolism and to maintain homeostasis. A classic clinical sign of shock is hypotension, which activates the sympathetic nervous system (SNS). The SNS stimulates vasoconstriction and releases potent vasoconstrictors such as epinephrine and norepinephrine. Blood flow to the heart is maintained whereas blood flow to nonvital organs (such as the kidneys, gastrointestinal system, skin and lungs) is shunted or diverted, which accounts for the reduced urine output and the cool skin temperature. The body is diverting blood back to the heart to maintain cardiac output. The client is not in a hypervolemic state, and the nurse would not identify an S3 during assessment as left ventricular pressures are not increased but decreased. The client has normal heart sounds. The client presents with a fever and is hyperthermic, not hypothermic. The parasympathetic nervous system cannot be stimulated when the client is exhibiting more SNS clinical manifestations. One nervous system exhibits more clinical symptoms than the other even if there are still responses occurring from each system at the same time. The client is not experiencing a fever from the urinary tract infection, as the client is not presenting with urgency, frequency, and dysuria.

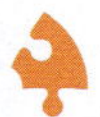
NCJMM Step: Analyze Cues
Reference: Tyerman & Cobbett (2023), pp. 1735–1736.

Answer 13.3

The client is at highest risk of developing **shock**.

Rationale: The client is no longer able to compensate for the infection and the body moves into the progressive stage of shock. The pulmonary system is the first to display signs of critical dysfunction. In response to decreased blood flow and the SNS stimulation, the pulmonary arterioles constrict, resulting in increased pulmonary artery pressure. As the pressure within the pulmonary vasculature increases, blood flow to the pulmonary capillaries decreases, and the ventilation–perfusion mismatch worsens. There is increased pulmonary permeability causing interstitial edema, bronchoconstriction, and a decrease in functional residual capacity. Clinical manifestations are tachypnea, crackles, and overall increased work of breathing. The cardiovascular system is profoundly affected. The cardiac output begins to fall, resulting in hypotension and decreased coronary, cerebral, and peripheral artery perfusion. This would explain the client's confusion, consistent decrease in blood pressure, and cyanosis around the lips and fingertips.

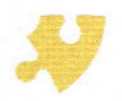
NCJMM Step: Prioritize Hypothesis
Reference: Tyerman & Cobbett (2023), p. 1738.

Answer 13.4

POTENTIAL NURSING INTERVENTIONS	INDICATED	NOT INDICATED
Plan for intubation	✔	○
Reposition client in Trendelenburg position	○	✔
Apply nasal prongs for oxygen administration	○	✔
Draw an arterial blood gas	✔	○
Obtain blood cultures	✔	○
Prepare client for a chest X-ray	✔	○
Request a nutritional consult for parenteral nutrition	○	✔

Rationale: The client is in respiratory distress and requires intubation. Applying oxygen via nasal prongs would be insufficient to meet the client's respiratory needs. Repositioning the client in Trendelenburg position would help with the blood pressure and increase the work of breathing. This choice of action would cause more harm to the client. At this stage, the client is confused and requires additional oxygenation, not repositioning. It is important to draw arterial blood cultures prior to initiation of antibiotics, which would offer a better chance of identifying the specific bacteria causing the infection. The client should have a chest X-ray to determine how severe the lungs have suffered. The client will not receive parenteral nutrition at this time and should be provided enteral feeds if intubated. This will help protect the stomach from erosion, which could lead to a gastrointestinal bleed.

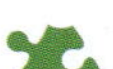
NCJMM Step: Generate Solutions
Reference: Tyerman & Cobbett (2023), pp. 1738–1740.

Answer 13.5

- ☐ Administer opiates for pain
- ✔ Initiate broad-spectrum antibiotics
- ☐ Insert intraosseous access to administer fluids
- ✔ Initiate 500 mL 0.9% sodium chloride IV bolus then 150 mL/hr continuous
- ✔ Insert a Foley catheter
- ✔ Contact general surgery for consult

Rationale: It is important to initiate broad-spectrum antibiotics to have some coverage for the client. Once the blood culture results are available, more specific antibiotic coverage can be ordered. The client requires a bolus at this time for hemodynamic instability. The client's blood pressure has continued to decrease, and a bolus would provide fluid resuscitation. Crystalloids are the initial fluid of choice for severe hypovolemia. Currently, normal saline is the most often used fluid in the initial resuscitation of shock. It is important to monitor for hyperchloremic metabolic acidosis to occur. Monitoring urine output will help assess how well the kidneys are perfusing. Urine output should be at 30 mL per hour or 05–1.0 mL/kg per hour if weight is known. A general surgical consult will be needed given the rapidly moving redness and left chest wall pain. Opiates would not be administered to the client, despite having a pain response. Once opiates would be given, a massive vasodilatory response would occur and the blood pressure would decrease considerably. It is safer to administer fluids first to have a hemodynamic response before administering opiates. Once the client is intubated, the respiratory system would be more supported as well. An intraosseous access device is not warranted for a client who likely still has peripheral access, until a central line can be inserted.

NCJMM Step: Take Action
Reference: Tyerman & Cobbett (2023), pp. 1738–1747.

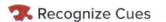

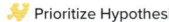

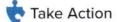

Answer 13.6

- ☐ The client cannot wiggle toes on command
- ✔ BP 100/75; P 78
- ☐ Diaphoresis
- ✔ Capillary refill greater than 3 seconds with no cyanosis noted
- ✔ Urine output documented at 50 mL/hr
- ☐ Right pupil 3 mm and left pupil 2 mm in size

Rationale: With fluid resuscitation and inotropic support, the client's blood pressure has improved enough to allow for renal perfusion. The cardiovascular system requires support, which will allow the body to fight the necrotizing fasciitis. No documentation of cyanosis indicates the client is finally adequately delivering oxygenated blood to the tissues, now that he is on ventilatory support. Urine output is measured above 30 mL per hour, which indicates the kidneys are perfusing minimally but still perfusing. If the client cannot follow commands, this may be due to the anaesthetic used during the surgical procedure and must be closely monitored. Diaphoresis may be a SNS response; however, acute myocardial infarctions can occur due to a reduced oxygen supply to the myocardium. Any changes in pupillary size must be monitored closely as this indicates changes in cerebral perfusion and increased pressure.

NCJMM Step: Evaluate Outcomes
Reference: Tyerman & Cobbett (2023), pp. 1738–1747.

Medical-Surgical 14.0 (Integumentary)

Answer 14.1

- ☐ Lung sounds
- ☐ Heart rate, respirations, and pulse oximetry
- ✔ Blood pressure and temperature
- ☐ Motor power
- ☐ Pulses
- ✔ Mucous membranes
- ☐ Weight
- ☐ Cough
- ✔ Wounds

Rationale: Initial assessment begins with airway, breathing, and circulation. The client presents as stable with assessment findings that need to be addressed. The primary assessment data that require immediate follow-up include the blood pressure and mucous membranes, which indicate dehydration, and the temperature, which indicates a febrile process and a potential infective/inflammatory process occurring, likely as a result of the bilateral wounds located in the antecubital fossa. The heart rate, respirations, and pulse oximetry are within stable parameters. The client's motor power is strong × 4 and the client is able to follow all commands, indicating normal neurological functioning. Although the client presents as undernourished and underweight, this would not be an immediate concern for the nurse.

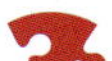
NCJMM Step: Recognize Cues
References: Jarvis et al. (2024), Chapter 13; Keatings & Adams (2024), pp. 10–23; Tyerman & Cobbett (2023), pp. 224, 486–490.

Answer 14.2

The nurse should recognize that the client is potentially experiencing **dehydration** and **infection**.

Rationale: The client's blood pressure, dry mucous membranes, and cracked lips indicate dehydration despite pulses being palpable. Urine output has not been reported but would be a consideration for further assessment data. Collecting fluid status would be another indictor to identify overall status and monitor if the status is deteriorating or improving. The client's temperature and wound description indicate an infection with poor perfusion as evidenced by the nonblanching erythema and yellow-green drainage. The client's lung fields when auscultated and the pulse oximetry are excellent, therefore removing the possibility of hypoxemia, pneumonia, and pulmonary embolus as potential answers. The client is not bleeding from other wounds and does not present with anemia-like symptoms, so anemia can be eliminated. The client's pulses are regular, and there is no associated shortness of breath indicating a potential dysrhythmia. The client answers questions appropriately, speech is clear, and the client has equal motor power, eliminating impaired cognition and the possibility of a stroke. The client presents as underweight, not overweight, removing obesity as a possible answer.

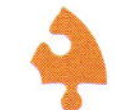
NCJMM Step: Analyze Cues
References: Jarvis et al. (2024), Chapter 13; Keatings & Adams (2024), pp. 10–23; Tyerman & Cobbett (2023), pp. 224, 486–490.

Answer 14.3

The client is at highest risk of developing **sepsis**.

Rationale: The client's condition has deteriorated over the past 2 days and has the potential to progress to sepsis. The client's initial presentation of chills and feeling unwell × 2 days, poor nutritional intake, hypotension, temperature, and poor perfusion at the wound beds indicate a more serious complication as a result. The client has not progressed to zero perfusion leading to gangrene in a wound; therefore, this would not occur at this time. Gangrene has the potential to develop if the wound remains untreated; however, given the wounds are a result of intravenous drug usage, the risk for sepsis remains higher than for gangrene. The client does not present with clinical manifestations associated with meningitis or neurological impairment since the client is able to obey commands, has motor power strong × 4, is alert and orientated to person, place, and time, and does not report any headache or stiffness in the neck. A client with melanoma would not present with a fever. The wound bed description does not align with impetigo, which has superficial pustules covered by a thick, honey-coloured crust.

NCJMM Step: Prioritize Hypothesis
References: Jarvis et al. (2024), Chapter 13; Keatings & Adams (2024), pp. 10–23; Tyerman & Cobbett (2023), pp. 224, 486–490.

Answer 14.4

POTENTIAL NURSING INTERVENTIONS	INDICATED	NOT INDICATED
Request an order to initiate intravenous fluids	✔	○
Prepare to draw blood cultures	✔	○
Administer an antipyretic then obtain a covering order from the health care provider when they assess the client	○	✔
Prepare to apply oxygen per nasal prongs	○	✔
Request to insert a peripheral venous access device	✔	○
Place the client in semi-Fowler's position	○	✔

Rationale: The client's blood pressure is decreasing, indicating early sepsis leading to vasodilation. Initiating a peripheral venous access device as well as initiating intravenous (IV) fluids, particularly an isotonic solution, would be an anticipated intervention. The client's temperature is increasing, which indicates an inflammatory process is occurring. The nurse needs to draw blood cultures before administering IV fluids and initiating antibiotic therapy to accurately identify the bacteria or virus. Administration of IV fluids leads to dilution of intravascular volume, and initiating a broad-spectrum antibiotic before drawing blood cultures may alter the laboratory results. Administering an antipyretic medication is not indicated. The client has not been seen by a health care provider yet. Anticipating interventions is different than performing an intervention. Note the difference in language as it says "administer." The client's pulse oximetry remains greater than 92% despite taking short, shallow breaths and an increase in respirations. The client is able to determine the position they want to be in for comfort. There is no need for the nurse to place the client in a specific position. Client comfort would be an important need to meet for this client.

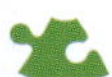
NCJMM Step: Generate Solutions
References: Keatings & Adams (2024), pp. 10–23; Tyerman & Cobbett (2023), pp. 500–501.

Answer 14.5

- ✔ Administer cefazolin 1 g IV q8h
- ☐ Initiate oxygen therapy at 2 L to 6 L to maintain pulse oximetry greater than 92%. Notify health care provider if respiratory status changes
- ✔ Elevate and apply heat to the wound beds
- ✔ Draw borders of erythema and inform health care provider if borders increase in size
- ☐ Insert an in-dwelling Foley catheter if urine output drops below 30 mL/hr
- ☐ Insert a peripheral venous access device in the left forearm
- ✔ Initiate 0.9% normal saline (sodium chloride at 125 mL/hr)
- ✔ Laboratory draws: complete blood count, electrolytes, and blood cultures (culture and sensitivity)
- ☐ Consult social work
- ☐ Consult addiction services

Rationale: The client requires intravenous access to administer fluids and broad-spectrum antibiotics such as cefazolin to improve hypotension. Labs should be drawn prior to initiating antibiotic therapy. Monitoring changes in the areas of cellulitis requires the nurse to draw the borders to identify if these areas increase or decrease in size. It is helpful to determine if treatment is effective or not. The client does not need oxygen therapy at the moment. The client does not require a Foley catheter as this may increase the client's susceptibility for a urinary tract infection and the nurse will want to encourage self-care. A peripheral venous access device is necessary; however, this order needs to be clarified as it is not good practice to insert a venous access device below the level of a wound. The venous access device is better inserted in the right antecubital to avoid the cellulitis that has developed on the right forearm and the increased size of the left antecubital cellulitis. Consulting social work and addiction services can be achieved when the client's acute presentation has improved.

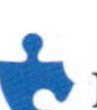
NCJMM Step: Take Action
References: Keatings & Adams (2024), pp. 10–23; Tyerman & Cobbett (2023), pp. 500–501.

Answer 14.6

ASSESSMENT FINDINGS	IMPROVED	NO CHANGE	DECLINED
Erythema less than original borders on right forearm	✔	○	○
BP 125/73	✔	○	○
Urine output 700 mL documented at 0730h	✔	○	○
RR 20	○	✔	○
Erythema extending beyond the left shoulder border and now documented at the collarbone	○	○	✔

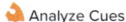

Rationale: Monitoring the client for improvement after treatment has been established is important. The client's right forearm cellulitis has improved whereas the left arm cellulitis is extending beyond the identified borders. The client's blood pressure has improved with the administration of intravenous fluids. Urine output from admission is approximately 117 mL per hour, indicating adequate perfusion of the kidneys. The client's respiratory status has not improved yet, but it can be monitored.

NCJMM Step: Evaluate Outcomes
References: Keatings & Adams (2024), pp. 10–23; Tyerman & Cobbett (2023), pp. 500–501.

Medical-Surgical 15.0 (Palliative Care)

Answer 15.1

Progress Notes	Nurses' Notes

0730h: Intended MAiD appointment is scheduled for tomorrow, for end-stage idiopathic pulmonary arterial hypertension. Client did not want to complete MAiD at home. Family to be arriving later in the day. Vital signs: T: 37.7°C (99.9°F); BP: 102/54; P: 105; RR: 26; with pulse oximetry of 92% on 6 L/min of oxygen via high-flow nasal prongs. Client presents as pleasant, cooperative, alert and oriented to person, place, and time. Gait steady, becomes ++ dizzy with sitting at the edge of the bed, requires two-person stand-by assist for ambulation and minimal changes to position (i.e., bed to chair). S1 and S2 heart sounds documented with no other adventitious heart sounds noted. Jugular venous distension noted at 7 cm. Apical heart rate regular, strong, and noted to be equal in rate to radial pulse. +1 peripheral edema noted to bilateral lower extremities. Client denies any pain with extremities. Reduced air entry noted throughout all lung fields. Client complains of ++ shortness of breath even with extended periods of talking. Client noted to have nonproductive wet cough. Client is voiding small amounts of clear amber urine. Client has reduced fluid and food intake over the past few days, states they are not feeling up to it. Hypoactive bowel sounds auscultated × 4 quadrants with abdomen firm and distended during palpation.

Rationale: The client's primary clinical priorities would be symptom identification and management related to respiratory status, as well as safety. The client has compromised gas exchange. Prior to admission, the client was on home oxygen therapy at 7 L per minute via nasal prongs. Now the client has progressed to high-flow prongs. Monitoring the progression of increased oxygen requirements is an indication of compromise. The client's respiratory rate is 26 breaths per minute, which is high and indicating increased work of breathing. It is important to monitor the heart rate as well, because there is typically a direct relationship between tachypnea and tachycardia. The client's change of status leads to dizziness, which could be a safety issue if the client attempts to ambulate without assistance. This indicates there is poor gas exchange because the heart cannot compensate quickly enough to increase oxygenated blood flow to the brain. The jugular venous distension noted at 7 cm indicates that the right side of heart is not pumping effectively, leading to backing up of blood. This decreases the amount of blood volume in the heart, leading to reduced systemic output. Reduced air entry correlates to poor gas exchange, oxygen requirements, and dizziness. Abdomen firm and distended is important to monitor for the client. Currently, the client has hypoactive bowel sounds, but a firm and distended abdomen would require monitoring and follow-up.

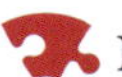
NCJMM Step: Recognize Cues
References: Astle & Duggleby (2024), pp. 117–118, 121, 434–440, 443; Cobbett (2025), pp. 445–457; Tyerman & Cobbett (2023), pp. 651–655.

Answer 15.2

- ✔ Cor pulmonale
- ☐ Bowel obstruction
- ☐ Deep vein thrombosis
- ✔ Pulmonary edema
- ☐ Atrial fibrillation

Rationale: The client's increased jugular venous distension (pressure) and impaired gas exchange indicate that the client is at risk for cor pulmonale and pulmonary edema. Cor pulmonale is caused by conditions that increase resistance in the pulmonary vasculature, such as chronic obstructive pulmonary disease (COPD), increasing the work of the right ventricle and causing a back-flow of blood. This complication contributes to less blood volume in the heart, which leaves less blood being ejected out of the left ventricle and ultimately less systemic oxygenated blood. Given the impaired gas exchange caused by the COPD and the increased jugular venous distension, there is less blood being delivered to the myocardium, causing an increased workload onto the heart, which pumps faster to increase the amount of oxygenated blood flow. With the high heart rate and impaired pump function of the heart, pulmonary edema is a potential finding. Currently, the client has hypoactive bowel sounds, which means gastric motility is reduced but remains intact. If the client loses bowel sounds in any of the quadrants, then a bowel obstruction or paralytic ileus may be a contributing factor. At present, this is not a complication to consider since bowel sounds remain in all four quadrants. The client is not exhibiting clinical manifestations associated with a deep vein thrombosis and could not develop this complication in the short time frame. Remember that the client is admitted to receive MAiD care. The client's heart rate is regular, not irregular as in the case of atrial fibrillation.

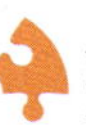
NCJMM Step: Analyze Cues
References: Astle & Duggleby (2024), pp. 117–118, 121, 434–440, 443; Cobbett (2025), pp. 445–457; Tyerman & Cobbett (2023), pp. 651–655.

Answer 15.3

The client is at highest risk of developing **acute myocardial infarction** as evidenced by **cardiovascular assessment.**

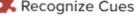

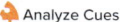

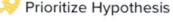

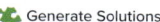

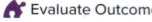

Rationale: The client's impaired gas exchange and increasing oxygen requirements have reduced the amount of oxygenated blood being delivered to the myocardium. The high respiratory rate, high heart rate, and low pulse oximetry level

that suction is patent is part of the daily safety checks. If suction is required during intubation or if the client vomits due to increased intrathoracic pressure, suction is prepared and ready. During a respiratory event, the client does not need blood cultures to identify the type of bacteria in the wound.

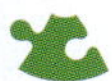
NCJMM Step: Generate Solutions
References: Astle & Duggleby (2024), pp. 725–811; Cobbett (2025), pp. 536–558; Tyerman & Cobbett (2023), 756–746.

Answer 16.5

- ✔ Initiate oxygen therapy with high-flow nasal prongs 0–8 L/min to maintain pulse oximetry greater than 92%
- ☐ Ambulate client as tolerated
- ☐ Give regular diet
- ✔ 0.9% normal saline (sodium chloride) 500 mL IV × 1 bolus then 150 mL/hr
- ✔ Administer bronchodilator
- ☐ Laboratory draws: complete blood count, electrolytes, lipid levels

Rationale: Ensuring airway management is vital to reducing the chances of intubation. Providing high-flow nasal prongs with oxygen delivery, followed by assessing the client's response, will provide evidence of bronchoconstriction. The client requires fluid resuscitation. With anaphylaxis, the systemic vasculature attempts to vasodilate while the airways bronchoconstrict. There is a decrease in blood pressure, an increase in heart rate, and increase in respiratory rate. Fluids will assist with increasing intravascular volume. A bronchodilator will dilate the airways, increasing the diameter of the airways with the intent to improve gas exchange. The client is not ambulating at the moment. Giving a regular diet is appropriate when the client can safely take food by mouth. Laboratory draws such as an ABG (arterial blood gas) are important; however, the ordered laboratory draws can be made after the client's respiratory status has improved and stabilized.

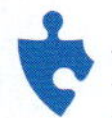
NCJMM Step: Take Action
References: Astle & Duggleby (2024), pp. 725–811; Cobbett (2025), pp. 536–558; Tyerman & Cobbett (2023), pp. 756–746.

Answer 16.6

CLIENT FINDINGS	IMPROVED	NOT CHANGED	DECLINED
Respirations 28	○	✔	○
T 37.9°C	✔	○	○
Short, shallow breaths	○	○	✔
Colour, pink	✔	○	○
No stridor noted	✔	○	○
Pulse oximetry 92%	✔	○	○

Rationale: The client suffered an anaphylaxis reaction to the Cloxacillin that was administered to them in error. Cloxacillin is a member of the penicillin family. After the code was called, the client continues to be tachypneic at 28 breaths per minute, indicating no change. The client is still catching their breath from the anaphylaxis. The client's temperature has improved significantly. The client presents as pink and perfused, whereas before the client was pale with cyanosis. Stridor is no longer present, which indicates respiratory distress has resolved. The addition of oxygen therapy improved the client's overall pulse oximetry.

NCJMM Step: Evaluate Outcomes
References: Astle & Duggleby (2024), pp. 725–811; Cobbett (2025), pp. 536–558; Tyerman & Cobbett (2023), pp. 756–746.

Medical-Surgical 17.0 (Respiratory)

Answer 17.1

- ☐ Orientation
- ☐ Motor power
- ☐ Pupillary response
- ☐ Pulses
- ✔ Pleuritic pain
- ✔ Lung sounds
- ✔ Breathing pattern
- ☐ Bowel sounds
- ☐ Urine output

Rationale: The client presents with a blunt traumatic chest wound from hitting the car's steering wheel with his chest. Respiratory symptoms that may compromise airway and breathing will impact circulation. Pleuritic chest pain may be a result of the impact and force of the injury. The absent breath sounds noted on the left lung will affect gas exchange since the remaining lung alveoli will be required to complete gas exchange. If the airway becomes compromised, the respiratory system will increase respirations, followed by an increased heart rate. The client's short and shallow respirations require immediate follow-up because the alveoli will not be inflated with this breathing pattern, reducing the ability of the alveoli to maintain appropriate gas exchange for the body. There are no concerns with orientation since the client presents as alert and oriented to person, place, and time. Pupillary response is brisk and pupils are equal in size. Pulses, radial and posterior dorsalis pedis, are palpable. Bowel sounds are present and auscultated in all four quadrants. The client has not expressed a need to void yet with the kidneys likely vasoconstricting as a sympathetic response.

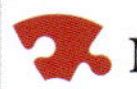
NCJMM Step: Recognize Cues
References: Astle & Duggleby (2024), pp. 996–1001; Cobbett (2025), pp. 774–794; Tyerman & Cobbett (2023), pp. 610–618.

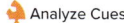

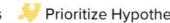

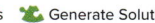

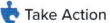

Answer 17.2

- ✔ Rib fractures
- ☐ Pulmonary embolus
- ☐ Deep vein thrombosis
- ✔ Pneumothorax
- ✔ Clavicle fracture
- ✔ Cardiac tamponade
- ☐ Bowel obstruction

Rationale: A client who presents with blunt-force trauma can present with rib fractures, develop a pneumothorax, have a clavicle fracture as a result of the seatbelt, and even a cardiac tamponade. Direct impact on the thorax area may present many respiratory and cardiovascular complications. Monitoring for clinical presentation of potential complications requires good assessment techniques and, at times, prevention of complications. This client cannot develop a pulmonary embolus just from blunt-force trauma to the heart unless there were pre-existing conditions not revealed. The client has not had enough time to develop a clot in the deep vein due to venous stasis. The client presents with active bowel sounds in all four quadrants, indicating that a bowel obstruction is not a complication.

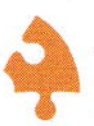

NCJMM Step: Analyze Cues
References: Astle & Duggleby (2024), pp. 996–1001; Cobbett (2025), pp. 774–794; Tyerman & Cobbett (2023), pp. 610–618.

Answer 17.3

The client is at highest risk of developing **pneumothorax.**

Rationale: The client presents with symptoms specific to a pneumothorax, such as asymmetrical breathing noted with bilateral inspiration and expiration, absent breath sounds noted over the entire left lung and tracheal deviation. There is increased intrathoracic pressure from the left side that is pushing the trachea to the unaffected side of the lungs, which is the right side. Pleurisy is inflammation of the pleura and does not present with these serious respiratory symptoms. There is an issue taking in air and expiring air, but there is no mention of crackles auscultated, which would represent fluid in the alveoli. The client may present with a fever; however, the cause of the client's respiratory symptoms is blunt-force trauma, not community-acquired or nosocomial-acquired pneumonia. A pleural effusion indicates fluid in the pleural space; however, again this does not present with tracheal deviation.

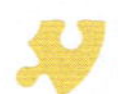

NCJMM Step: Prioritize Hypothesis
References: Astle & Duggleby (2024), pp. 996–1001; Cobbett (2025), pp. 774–794; Tyerman & Cobbett (2023), pp. 610–618.

Answer 17.4

POTENTIAL NURSING INTERVENTIONS	INDICATED	NOT INDICATED
Arrange a disposable water-seal chest drainage system with suction ready	✔	○
Prepare to administer intravenous fluids	✔	○
Reposition client in Fowler's position	✔	○
Prepare to insert a nasogastric tube	○	✔
Gather in-dwelling Foley catheter supplies	○	✔
Laboratory draw: type and cross-match	○	✔
Prepare to apply high-flow oxygen with a non-rebreather mask	✔	○

Rationale: Anticipating treatment plans is valuable to supporting the health care team and providing care for the client. Arranging a disposable water-seal chest drainage system and ensuring that suction is ready in anticipation of chest tube insertion is forward-thinking. Clients with a pneumothorax may present with a hemothorax too. Preparing for suction in anticipation of blood in the pleural space will assist with time management. The client has demonstrated increased intrathoracic pressure and requires immediate treatment with a chest tube. Airway management is important for this client. The client's blood pressure has decreased due to the increased intrathoracic and reduced filling time of the left ventricle, given where the pneumothorax is located. The nurse should reposition the client to have the head of the bed high so there is improvement in gas exchange and the abdominal muscles relax. High-Fowler's can be an uncomfortable position and should be reserved for circumstances where there is a need to increase alveoli expansion until a chest tube can be inserted. The client is oxygenated with high-flow oxygen via a nonrebreather mask until a chest tube can be inserted. At this point, the client requires a chest tube insertion to relieve the pressure in the chest. If the client continues to develop respiratory depression, then an intubation can occur at that time.

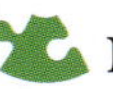

NCJMM Step: Generate Solutions
References: Astle & Duggleby (2024), pp. 996–1001; Cobbett (2025), pp. 774–794; Tyerman & Cobbett (2023), pp. 610–618.

Answer 17.5

- Initiate 0.9% normal saline (sodium chloride) 500 mL bolus then 125 mL/hr
- Chest X-ray
- Attach chest tube to high suction
- Oxygen 0–10 L per non-rebreather to achieve pulse oximetry greater than 92%

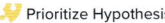

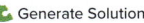

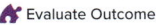

- Laboratory draws: complete blood count (CBC), electrolytes, arterial blood gas (ABG)
- Regular diet or diet as tolerated
- Monitor input and output

Rationale: The client's low blood pressure requires treatment to ensure hemodynamic stability. This will increase intravascular volume with a maintenance infusion. A chest X-ray is needed to ensure proper placement to drain fluid and air correctly. The pulse oximetry needs to be improved by increasing the oxygen flow in the mask until the alveoli are able to have proper gas exchange. The suction should be placed to low suction, not high suction, since high suction could cause complications. The laboratory draws are important to verify status; however, airway, breathing, and circulation remain priorities. The client can eat when their lung function has improved. A client could become nauseated with high-flow oxygen and a mask. Monitoring input and output is necessary to determine fluid status.

NCJMM Step: Take Action
References: Astle & Duggleby (2024), pp. 996–1001; Cobbett (2025), pp. 774–794; Tyerman & Cobbett (2023), pp. 610–618.

Answer 17.6

ASSESSMENT FINDINGS	IMPROVED	NO CHANGE	DECLINED
BP 101/70	✔	○	○
Pulse 102	✔	○	○
Respiratory rate 20	✔	○	○
4 out of 10 pain at insertion site	○	○	✔
Continuous bubbling in the water seal in the multichamber chest drainage system	○	○	✔
Chest tube drainage 130 mL for shift	○	✔	○

Rationale: Overall, the client's vital signs have improved since the chest tube has been inserted and the orders have been carried out. The client's lower blood pressure and heart rate indicate systemic stability and that the heart is not working as hard. The client's respiratory rate has improved and the client is not as tachypneic. There can be pain at the insertion site. Analgesics can be prescribed to assist with this discomfort. Continuous bubbling in the system may indicate a seal leak or a leak at the insertion site. Further investigation may be required to identify if there is indeed a leak or if it is the air from the pneumothorax. The nurse should document the bubbling and monitor whether it improves or declines. The chest tube drainage remains unchanged. Drainage is documented every shift and monitored for large amounts of pleural drainage, which can cause fluid shifts and affect hemodynamic stability.

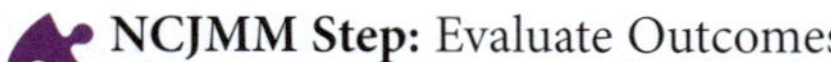

NCJMM Step: Evaluate Outcomes
References: Astle & Duggleby (2024), pp. 996–1001; Cobbett (2025), pp. 774–794; Tyerman & Cobbett (2023), pp. 610–618.

Medical-Surgical 18.0 (Respiratory)

Answer 18.1

- ✔ Skin colour characteristics
- ☐ Pleuritic pain
- ☐ Cognitive status
- ✔ Hemoptysis
- ☐ Temperature
- ✔ Blood pressure
- ✔ Respiratory retractions
- ☐ Lung sounds

Rationale: The client presents with poor perfusion as evidenced by their skin colour (grey), and hypotension with airway compromise (hemoptysis and respiratory retractions). The client is struggling to breathe, as evidenced by the indrawing and nasal flaring. This is an extension of abnormal to critical abnormal. Primary concerns revolve around the airway, breathing, and circulation first. Pleuritic pain is also abnormal; however, if extremities have lost perfusion, the hemodynamic instability extends beyond the thorax. Pleuritic pain indicates an obstruction of cardiac blood flow or inflammation of the pleura. The client's cognitive status remains intact since they are alert, oriented, and able to answer questions. Coarse crackles represent fluid in the alveoli, but the presence of hemoptysis indicates more than fluid in the alveoli, which is blood. The client's temperature is slightly elevated, indicating a systemic inflammatory response, but the priority is airway, breathing, and circulation.

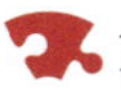

NCJMM Step: Recognize Cues
References: Astle & Duggleby (2024), pp. 1061, 1158; Cobbett (2025), pp. 938–949; Tyerman & Cobbett (2023), pp. 622–625.

Answer 18.2

- ✔ Sepsis
- ✔ Asymmetrical breathing
- ☐ Reduced gastric motility
- ☐ Migration of the central line into the carotid
- ✔ Perforation of the vein
- ☐ Dehydration

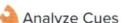

Rationale: There are risks associated with central-line insertion. The insertion site could become infected if employer policy is not followed correctly. The client is also at risk for sepsis, given the large abdominal surgery and placement of the colostomy. The client is at risk for asymmetrical breathing, which indicates a pneumothorax. The pleural space could be pierced during the time of insertion. Monitoring for the clinical manifestations of risks associated with line insertion is a key element of nursing practice for this client. During insertion, the central line will either be placed in the brachial vein, the internal jugular, or the subclavian on either the right or left side. This is not a tunnelled or port central line. A complication of line insertion in the subclavian site is that the tip of the central line can migrate toward the brain, but in the venous system, not the arterial system. When there is increased intrathoracic pressure as a result of a cough or heave, the tip of the line moves with the greatest flow during insertion. The carotid is an artery, not a vein. The line can perforate the vein, leading to a hematoma and additional bleeding for the client. This client is not at risk for dehydration given that Ringer's lactate has been infusing at 100 mL per hour.

NCJMM Step: Analyze Cues
References: Astle & Duggleby (2024), pp. 1061, 1158; Cobbett (2025), pp. 938–949; Tyerman & Cobbett (2023), pp. 622–625.

Answer 18.3

The client is at highest risk of developing **air embolus** based on the assessment data of **respiratory assessment**.

Rationale: The client presented with the classic triad of symptoms: dyspnea, chest pain, and hemoptysis, as well as coarse crackles, pleuritic chest pain, fever, and a sudden drop in blood pressure. Coarse crackles and a fever may indicate pneumonia; however, pleuritic chest pain is not associated with pneumonia. The client does not present with asymmetrical breathing, tracheal deviation, or absent breath sounds to suggest a pneumothorax. A pleural effusion may have transudative or exudative accumulation of fluid and cells. There is a dullness to percussion and absent or decreased breath sounds over the affected area. The primary assessment data indicate a respiratory complication. All other answers would be incorrect.

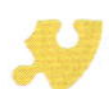
NCJMM Step: Prioritize Hypothesis
References: Astle & Duggleby (2024), pp. 1061, 1158; Cobbett (2025), pp. 938–949; Tyerman & Cobbett (2023), pp. 622–625, 589–594 (pneumonia), 610–612 (pneumothorax), 618–620 (pleural effusion), 1734 (sepsis).

Answer 18.4

POTENTIAL NURSING INTERVENTIONS	INDICATED	NOT INDICATED
Ensure all catheter connections are clamped	✔	○
Place the client in Trendelenburg position and turn on left side	✔	○
Provide supplemental oxygen	✔	○
Contact health care provider	✔	○
Prepare to administer narcotics for the pain	○	✔

Rationale: The nurse needs to ensure that all catheter connections are clamped in the event that air has entered the line. Placing the client in Trendelenburg position on their left side will float the air embolus to sit in the right atrium, allowing for additional supports to be in place. Providing supplemental oxygen to support airway and gas exchange is important for the client. The health care provider will need to be notified. Narcotics should not be administered for pleuritic pain; since the blood pressure is already low, the client's venous system will vasodilate and the blood pressure will decrease even further.

NCJMM Step: Generate Solutions
References: Astle & Duggleby (2024), pp. 1061, 1158; Cobbett (2025), pp. 938–949; Tyerman & Cobbett (2023), pp. 622–625.

Answer 18.5

Orders

- Piperacillin/Tazocin 2.25 g IV q8h
- Initiate anticoagulant therapy (IV heparin)
- Prepare the client for a spiral computed tomography (CT)
- Laboratory draws: PTT/INR, ABG
- Consult physiotherapy
- Oxygen therapy to maintain pulse oximetry greater than 92%

Rationale: Maintenance of gas exchange with supplemental oxygen and prevention of the formation of new clots with IV anticoagulant would be appropriate as immediate therapy. Antibiotic therapy is important, but not in the wake of an airway issue. The client has been ordered a spiral CT, which is a specific test to confirm whether a pulmonary or air embolus has occurred. Drawing PTT, INR, and ABG will ensure knowledge of how thin the blood is to prevent the formation of new clots, and a blood gas will determine acid–base balance. The client will be on bed rest; physiotherapy will assist with mobility.

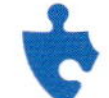
NCJMM Step: Take Action
References: Astle & Duggleby (2024), pp. 1061, 1158; Cobbett (2025), pp. 938–949; Tyerman & Cobbett (2023), pp. 622–625.

Answer 18.6

ASSESSMENT FINDINGS	IMPROVED	NO CHANGE	DECLINED
Pulse oximetry 94% on 3 L/min of oxygen via non-rebreather mask	○	○	✔
RR 22	✔	○	○
Client able to sit in semi-Fowler's position without chest pain	✔	○	○
BP 103/65	✔	○	○
T 37.8°C (100.4°F)	✔	○	○
Client has feeling of being unable to catch their breath	○	✔	○

Rationale: The client's health has declined since they required a non-rebreather mask instead of nasal prongs. Their respiratory rate has improved as a result of the mask, to the point they can now sit in semi-Fowler's position. Their blood pressure has improved to the point where there will be adequate hemodynamic status. Their temperature has improved, likely because of the antibiotic therapy. There has been no change in respiratory status as the client continues to recover from the embolus.

NCJMM Step: Evaluate Outcomes
References: Astle & Duggleby (2024), pp. 1061, 1158; Cobbett (2025), pp. 938–949; Tyerman & Cobbett (2023), pp. 622–625.

Medical-Surgical 19.0 (Integumentary)

Answer 19.1

Progress Notes

0730h: Client presents to the unit with failure to thrive. Previous comorbidities include cerebral palsy with bilateral contractures noted on wrists, elbows, and hips and a percutaneous endoscopic gastrostomy (PEG) tube in situ for nutrition. Vital signs: T: 38.4°C (101.1°F); BP: 91/67; P:76; RR: 14; with pulse oximetry of 92% on room air. On assessment, client presents as nonverbal but opens eyes to voice and tracks with eyes. Client is unable to follow commands but moves all extremities independently in the bed. Client moans with repositioning but does not express grimacing, guarding, tachycardia, or diaphoresis. Pupils equal in size, measuring at 3 mm and briskly reactive to light. Skin is cool to touch with dry mucous membranes, coating noted on tongue, and dry lips noted. Bilateral radial pulses strong with palpation and regular. Apical = radial pulse. Client takes short, shallow breaths with fine inspiratory crackles noted bilateral lower lungs with minimal cough reflex. Secretions pool at the back of the client's throat, requiring suction. Client positioned in semi-Fowler's position as they slide down the bed when the head of the bed is positioned too high. Foley catheter in situ because client incontinent of urine. Dark, concentrated urine noted in the Foley bag with 800 mL documented from 8-hour night shift. Client presents as cachectic with low body weight. Redness noted on bilateral shoulder blades, Loonie-sized area noted on coccyx with yellow slough, purulent drainage, and pink borders, and redness noted on bilateral heels as client rubs heels on the bed for self-soothing. Client to receive tube feeds as per dietitian's caloric requirements for basal metabolic rate through PEG tube, and all pill form medications to be crushed and administered as per institution policy. Skin around tube site has mild excoriation but is dry and intact. No open areas noted around PEG site. Bowel sounds hypoactive × 4 quadrants.

Rationale: This client presents with multiple pieces of information that require immediate follow-up because of the client's reduced mobility and high risk for infections. The client's higher temperature indicates that an infective process is occurring; the client is susceptible to skin, renal, and respiratory infections. The lower blood pressure requires further follow-up and monitoring. Given the client's smaller frame, a lower blood pressure and cardiac output can occur. Moaning is abnormal behaviour. The client may moan with stimulation as a neurological reflex, or this may be a result of pain. Nonverbal indicators do not point to pain as the cause of the moaning, but all potential indicators of pain should be further followed up. The skin presents as dehydrated as indicated by the dry mucous membranes, coating on the tongue, and dry lips. Another indicator of dehydration is the dark urine; however, there is adequate urinary output at 100 mL per hour overnight, which is within the expected range of at least 30 mL per hour. The client's skin breakdown as a result of the high risk of shearing forces due to the sliding down the head of the bed and the rubbing of heels on the bed is concerning.

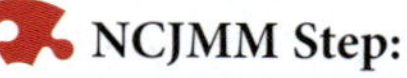

NCJMM Step: Recognize Cues
References: Astle & Duggleby (2024), pp. 619, 668, 906–926, 1164–1167, 1253, 1293–1306; Cobbett (2025), pp. 1088–1126; Tyerman & Cobbett (2023), pp. 142–146, 211–212, 230–235, 692, 835, 1103, 1178.

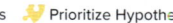

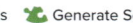

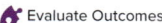

Answer 19.2

- ✔ Deep vein thrombosis
- ☐ Pneumothorax
- ☐ Pleural effusion
- ✔ Pneumonia
- ✔ Pressure injury
- ☐ Bowel obstruction

Rationale: The client's immobility and contractures can contribute to stasis of blood, endothelial damage, and an environment in which a blood clot could form. Ensuring adequate physiotherapy will help reduce the risk of a deep vein thrombosis forming. The client's clinical presentation of minimal cough indicates the risk for aspiration of secretions and the reduced air expansion, and immobility may also contribute to pneumonia occurring. Monitoring lung sounds will indicate if the fine crackles in the bases are from reduced lung expansion or if a more prominent infection is starting in this client. The lack of immobility, contractures, and cachectic frame contributes to an environment where a pressure injury is starting to develop. The client's bony prominences are red with a Loonie-sized open area already noted on the coccyx. The client does not present with asymmetrical lung expansion, tracheal deviation, or shortness of breath. The client's crackles are noted in the bilateral bases of the lung fields. Clinical manifestations of a client who presents with a pleural effusion include decreased or absent breath sounds, but no adventitious sounds noted.

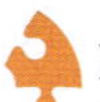

NCJMM Step: Analyze Cues
References: Astle & Duggleby (2024), pp. 619, 668, 906–926, 1164–1167, 1253, 1293–1306; Cobbett (2025), pp. 1088–1126; Jarvis et al. (2024), p. 497; Tyerman & Cobbett (2023), pp. 142–146, 211–212, 230–235, 692, 835, 1103, 1178.

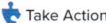

Answer 19.3

The nurse should first address the client's **skin integrity**.

Rationale: Because of the client's wiggling in bed and their incontinence, the wound has progressed from purulent drainage to bleeding. Attending to an open wound with the increased probability of being resoiled when the client has another bowel movement is a concern, especially with the client's increased temperature. The temperature is increasing because of the affected skin integrity and the likelihood of an infection. The vital signs are not to be addressed first since the client has just been stimulated, which increases cardiac output demands as well as respiratory requirements, just by turning. Monitoring the vital signs to identify whether the small change is a result of the increased movement or if there is a hemodynamic shift is important, but this is not a priority. The pulse remains strong and regular and does not need to be addressed. There has been improvement in the urine characteristics since it has changed from dark and concentrated to clear and amber in colour. The output remains appropriate since perfusion of the kidney requires at least 30 mL per hour of urine, and this client has 87 mL per hour (537 [total urine output] divided by 6 hours [time since the Foley bag was empty] equals 87). Nutrition remains a priority; however, the client's skin integrity remains the primary condition that needs addressing. Nutritional requirements need to be effective for proper wound healing. The client is already at a disadvantage due to their small frame and cachectic presentation. Movement initiated a cough response in the client clearing the airways by increasing lung expansion needed for increased body movement. This demonstrates that there are no infiltrates consistent with a pneumonia.

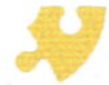

NCJMM Step: Prioritize Hypothesis
References: Astle & Duggleby (2024), pp. 619, 668, 906–926, 1164–1167, 1253, 1293–1306; Cobbett (2025), pp. 1088–1126; Tyerman & Cobbett (2023), pp. 142–146, 211–212, 230–235, 692, 835, 1103, 1178.

Answer 19.4

- ☐ Place the client in Trendelenburg position
- ✔ Reposition the client to stay off reddened areas
- ☐ Prepare to administer oral fluids
- ☐ Contact the family for update of status
- ✔ Provide reassurance to the client

Rationale: Repositioning the client to relieve pressure from the bony prominences is important. Using devices to reduce pressure and shearing forces is also important. Devices that should be used include foam wedges for back support when turning, pillows, pressure mattresses, foam dressings, lift sheets, wheelchair cushions, padded commode seats, and heel boots (foam, air). If the bed allows, there can be different bed positions or cardiac chairs, which will assist with proper wound healing and reduce shearing movement. Providing reassurance to the client is important. The client cannot be placed in Trendelenburg position because this may increase anxiety and create more shearing forces. The client has a PEG tube because of their inability to swallow and high risk for aspiration from oral secretions. Contacting the family about the change in wound status is not a nursing priority.

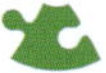

NCJMM Step: Generate Solutions
References: Astle & Duggleby (2024), pp. 619, 668, 906–926, 1164–1167, 1253, 1293–1306; Cobbett (2025), pp. 1088–1126; Tyerman & Cobbett (2023), pp. 142–146, 211–212, 230–235, 692, 835, 1103, 1178.

Answer 19.5

POTENTIAL NURSING INTERVENTIONS	INDICATED	NOT INDICATED
Administer laxatives	○	✔
Implement the Braden scale	✔	○
Place client in an adult incontinence product and secure sides	○	✔
Irrigate the wound	✔	○
Use friction-reducing sheets	✔	○
Hold the tube feeds to reduce risk of tube becoming loose again	○	✔
Incorporate a turning schedule	✔	○

Rationale: Maintaining skin integrity and creating optimal environments for healing are the priority nursing actions. These goals can be achieved by irrigating the wound to ensure the wound bed is clean, using friction-reducing sheets that will reduce the shearing forces when the client wiggles in the bed, incorporating a turning schedule to ensure the health care team keeps the client off the coccyx to allow for better blood flow to the area, and implementing the Braden scale, which is a tool used to predict pressure injury risk. Administering laxatives would only increase the number of bowel movements and contaminate the wound bed. Keeping the client off the wound and exposed to open to air will allow for enhanced tissue granulation by reducing and trapping moisture (which is often associated with incontinence products). The client requires adequate protein and caloric intake for proper wound healing. Holding the tube feeds would only increase the client's healing time.

NCJMM Step: Take Action
References: Astle & Duggleby (2024), pp. 619, 668, 906–926, 1164–1167, 1253, 1293–1306; Cobbett (2025), pp. 1088–1126; Tyerman & Cobbett (2023), pp. 142–146, 211–212, 230–235, 692, 835, 1103, 1178.

Answer 19.6

ASSESSMENT FINDINGS	IMPROVED	NO CHANGE	DECLINED
Wound identified as a stage 1 on Braden scale	✔	○	○
Bleeding of wound with fecal incontinence	○	✔	○
Caloric and protein needs identified by a dietitian	✔	○	○
T 37.6°C	✔	○	○
Client wiggles in bed	○	✔	○
Client tolerating sitting in chair with foam supports	✔	○	○

Rationale: The client's overall status has improved. The wound has reduced from a stage 2 pressure injury to a stage 1 pressure injury. The caloric and protein needs have been identified by a dietitian. Typically, 2 000 to 3 000 calories are required to assist with wound healing. The client's temperature has decreased with the implementation of measures to help avoid recontamination. The client is able to tolerate sitting in a chair with foam supports. There was no change in the bleeding of the wound during periods of fecal incontinence, and the client continues to wiggle, increasing the risk of other pressure injuries developing.

NCJMM Step: Evaluate Outcomes
References: Astle & Duggleby (2024), pp. 619, 668, 906–926, 1164–1167, 1253, 1293–1306; Cobbett (2025), pp. 1088–1126; Tyerman & Cobbett (2023), pp. 230–238.

Medical-Surgical 20.0 (Musculoskeletal)

Answer 20.1

- ☐ Pupillary response
- ☐ Alertness
- ☐ Lung sounds
- ✔ Characteristics of the pulses
- ☐ Pulse oximetry
- ✔ Skin temperature
- ☐ Urine output
- ✔ Pain

Rationale: The client experienced a motor vehicle accident with the primary injury being to the left tibia and ankle. Prior to any treatment, a neurovascular assessment is a priority and includes a peripheral vascular assessment (colour, temperature, capillary refill, pulses, and edema) and a peripheral neurological assessment (sensation, motor function, and pain). The client's pulse on the left dorsalis pedis is weaker than the right dorsalis pedis pulse and the skin is cooler to touch as well. Maintaining perfusion to the area is important, so monitoring for colour, sensation, warmth, and movement of the affected extremity will occur while the client is in the hospital. The capillary refill is promising. The client's pain level requires immediate attention; however, the pain is in response to the broken tibia and ankle. When a client has been involved in an accident and is hit from behind, a consideration is to monitor for a coup contrecoup head injury as well as a concussion. EMS indicated that the client did not lose consciousness and remained alert and oriented to person, place, and time. Monitoring for any changes in neurological status will be a priority of the nursing assessment. The client remains alert and appropriate with questions. Lung sounds indicate only fine inspiratory crackles but clear with cough; this indicates the fluid has remained stationary but has not affected respiratory status. The client does not present with a fever, but this will be monitored as well. The pulse oximetry is above normal, indicating appropriate air entry and gas exchange. The client's kidneys are perfusing, with 450 mL of urine measured.

NCJMM Step: Recognize Cues
References: Astle & Duggleby (2024), pp. 573–595; 599–602; Cobbett (2025), pp. 414–427; Tyerman & Cobbett (2023), pp. 1612–1614.

Answer 20.2

- ☐ Anxiety
- ✔ Infection
- ☐ Reduced perfusion to kidneys
- ☐ Heart failure
- ✔ Fat embolism
- ☐ Depression
- ✔ Nerve damage
- ✔ Compartment syndrome

Rationale: Clients who have suffered an open fracture are at risk of developing an infection as a result of a break in the skin. Common bacteria live on the skin and could enter the bloodstream, causing severe infections, such as osteomyelitis or even sepsis. Clients who fracture a longer bone are at risk for a fat embolism. Fat is released from the marrow of the injured bone and enters the systemic circulation; trauma may also stimulate the release of free fatty acids that form fat emboli. For clients who fracture a bone, it is important to monitor for nerve damage. As a result of the bone fracture, there are soft tissue injuries to the muscle. A normal physiological response to injury is swelling and increased neutrophils to the site. The swelling and increased pressure within a limited space lead to a condition called *compartment syndrome*. This compression of the space may lead to nerve compression as well as reduced blood flow below the level of the injury, reducing tissue viability. Compartment syndrome can occur from the fracture alone or after surgical intervention. Although a fracture can be painful, which may increase the client's anxiety, in the case of this client, anxiety is not a concern. The client is voiding; therefore, there are no data to indicate there is reduced perfusion of blood flow to the kidney. The client does not present with crackles during lung auscultation or increased jugular venous distension that may indicate heart failure. The client has an acute injury with no clinical manifestations of depression.

NCJMM Step: Analyze Cues
References: Astle & Duggleby (2024), pp. 573–595; 599–602; Cobbett (2025), pp. 414–427; Tyerman & Cobbett (2023), pp. 1622–1635.

Answer 20.3

The nurse should first address the client's **complaints of pain.**

Rationale: The client's complaints of pain would be a priority to address, to obtain pain control. The client's airway, breathing, and circulation are stable at present. Pain is the final element of the neurovascular assessment. Assessing location, quality, and intensity of the pain is important. Monitoring the effectiveness of pain management is vital to rule out complications such as compartment syndrome. Increasing pain that is unrelieved by medication therapy and is out of proportion to the extent of injury can be an indication of compartment syndrome. Clients should be instructed to report any changes in their neurovascular status. Monitoring for circulation would be the next priority for the client, given the changes in temperature and pulses between right leg and left leg. This client likely suffered a whiplash injury, which is common when being struck from behind in a motor vehicle accident. At present, the client's pupils remain the same size, and the client does not complain of a headache, just a tender neck. Neurological status remains stable at present, too. The client complains of nausea in the absence of emesis. If emesis were present, there might be pressure on the medulla oblongata, indicating a head injury and increased swelling in the brain. This would be more concerning and something to monitor. The client's leg and foot are secured for bone alignment; however, the client is still able to wiggle their toes. This indicates that the impulse from the brain to the leg/foot for movement remains intact and that no spinal cord damage has occurred. Finally, the client is able to maintain proper gas exchange and an adequate pulse oximetry reading.

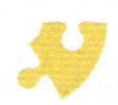
NCJMM Step: Prioritize Hypothesis
References: Astle & Duggleby (2024), pp. 573–595; 599–602; Cobbett (2025), pp. 414–427; Tyerman & Cobbett (2023), pp. 1612–1614.

Answer 20.4

POTENTIAL NURSING INTERVENTIONS	INDICATED	NOT INDICATED
Prepare to administer acetaminophen	○	✔
Place the affected bone in proper alignment	○	✔
Apply ice packs to the affected site of injury	✔	○
Maintain splinting of the affected fracture site	✔	○
Offer a warm blanket	○	✔
Prepare to administer opioid analgesic	✔	○
Mark location of pulses to facilitate repeat assessments	✔	○

Rationale: Ensuring that pain is adequately controlled either through pharmacological or nonpharmacological measures is a necessary nursing intervention. Understanding the effects and differences between an analgesic such as acetaminophen or an opioid will help determine which medication would be most appropriate when managing pain from a fracture. The acetaminophen would only be used for minor pain; an opioid would be more appropriate here given the severity of the injury. Learning the right medication to administer during a situation is good nursing practice and will ensure that the client receives excellent care while minimizing risk. Applying ice to the affected area may reduce swelling and reduce the chances of soft tissue complications such as compartment syndrome. Maintaining splinting of the fractured site is important to prevent further damage to surrounding tissues; however, it is out of the scope of practice for the nurse to place the affected bone in alignment. The nurse should not attempt to straighten or manipulate protruding bone ends. A warm blanket may increase blood flow to the area, increasing swelling to the area. Repeated neurovascular assessments will be important, and marking the location of pulses will assist if the swelling does occur or if another practitioner is trying to locate the pulses.

NCJMM Step: Generate Solutions
References: Astle & Duggleby (2024), pp. 573–595; 599–602; Cobbett (2025), pp. 414–427; Tyerman & Cobbett (2023), pp. 1612–1614.

Answer 20.5

Orders

1520h:
- Cefazolin 2.25 g PO q8h
- Administer tetanus toxoid intramuscularly × 1 dose
- 0.9% sodium chloride 100 mL/hr until able to tolerate fluids, then discontinue
- Elevate affected extremity
- Consult a dietitian to ensure adequate calcium and protein intake
- Hydromorphone 2 mg PO q6h prn
- Initiate full regular diet immediately
- Ambulate when ready

Rationale: With an open fracture, the risk of tetanus can be high. Administering a tetanus toxoid intramuscularly would be appropriate if there was no time to administer it prior to surgery. Only one dose is needed. Until the client has bowel sounds, maintenance fluids are necessary to provide volume and maintain blood pressure if administering pain medication. To reduce edema, the affected extremity is elevated on pillows. Nutrition is important for the reparative process of bones and tissues. Protein intake should be 1 g/kg body weight. Low protein levels interfere with tissue healing. Immobility and callus formation increase calcium needs. For adequate pain management, hydromorphone, NSAIDs (Tramacet or Ketorolac), and Percocet (acetaminophen with codeine) may be prescribed for pain management. Cefazolin is an appropriate antibiotic; however, the health care provider would need to be contacted to reassess the order. The dose, the route, and the time would need to be verified. The client cannot start on a full regular diet until the diet is advanced after bowel sounds are auscultated in all four quadrants; clear fluids progressing to a full diet is most appropriate. Initiating a full, regular diet too early may cause the client to aspirate or vomit. Opioid analgesics and anaesthetic may slow down the gastrointestinal tract. The introduction of food too early may lead to complications for the client. The client will be on bed rest; ambulation is not a priority.

NCJMM Step: Take Action
References: Abouli et al. (2023); Astle & Duggleby (2024), pp. 573–595; 599–602; Cobbett (2025), pp. 414–427; Tyerman & Cobbett (2023), pp. 1612–1614.

Answer 20.6

ASSESSMENT FINDINGS	IMPROVED	NO CHANGE	DECLINED
T 37.3°C	✔	○	○
Pain 10 out 10 on numerical pain scale	○	○	✔
Pulse oximetry 95% on room air	✔	○	○
Respiratory 16 breaths per minute	○	✔	○
Bowel sounds × 2 quadrants	✔	○	○
Complaints of numbness and tingling	○	○	✔

Rationale: The client's temperature has improved with the administration of cefazolin once the dose, route, and timing were corrected. The client's pain status has declined, and compartment syndrome may need to be considered. The client's overall respiratory status has improved as the client no longer requires oxygen therapy. The respiratory rate remains unchanged. Auscultation of bowel sounds indicates motility. The client is now complaining of tingling, leading to a possible compartment syndrome complication.

NCJMM Step: Evaluate Outcomes
References: Astle & Duggleby (2024), pp. 573–595; 599–602; Cobbett (2025), pp. 414–427; Tyerman & Cobbett (2023), pp. 1612–1614.

Medical-Surgical 21.0 (Respiratory)

Answer 21.1

- ☐ Alertness
- ☐ Pupillary response
- ✔ Vertigo
- ✔ Hemoptysis
- ☐ Vital signs
- ✔ Characteristics of the cough

Rationale: Cystic fibrosis is an obstructive lung disease in which there is obstruction of the airways with mucus. Cystic fibrosis can progress to a restrictive lung disease because of the fibrosis, lung destruction, and thoracic wall changes. The client presents with vertigo that may pose a safety issue if the client ambulates independently; blood-tinged sputum, when expectorating sputum is already difficult for a client with cystic fibrosis; and characteristics of the cough increasing over time and presenting with thick, purulent, and green sputum. Despite airway obstruction from the cystic fibrosis, the client is cooperative, and alert and oriented to person, place, and time. Bilateral pupillary response is comparable and brisk to light. The vital signs are stable at presentation despite a slight fever.

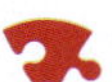
NCJMM Step: Recognize Cues
References: Astle & Duggleby (2024), pp. 955–976; Cobbett (2025), pp. 710–718; Tyerman & Cobbett (2023), pp. 671–676.

Answer 21.2

CLIENT FINDINGS	PNEUMONIA	ATELECTASIS	COR PULMONALE
Crackles with lung auscultation	✔	✔	○
Weight loss	○	○	✔
Pain with inspiration	✔	✔	✔
Febrile	✔	○	○
Shortness of breath	✔	✔	✔
Jugular venous distension	○	○	✔

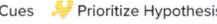

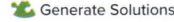

Rationale: When a client presents with increasing infections, it is important to consider whether the diagnosis is a result of an infective process or a complication of the natural disease progression of cystic fibrosis. A client who presents with clinical manifestations associated with pneumonia will have crackles in the lung fields and pain with inspiration due to inflammation of the airways. The client will present with a fever because the illness is related to a bacterial agent, and shortness of breath because alveoli and gas exchange are affected. For the client with atelectasis, which comprises collapsed airless alveoli, a complication is a pneumothorax, which is also associated with cystic fibrosis. Clients may present with crackles (only if the bronchus is patent, but none if the bronchus is obstructed), pain with inspiration as the lungs try to regroup all lung spaces to properly oxygenate blood to distribute systemically, and shortness of breath as a result. There are no cardiovascular complications, such as jugular venous distension, with pneumonia or atelectasis. Cor pulmonale is also a complication for clients living with cystic fibrosis, but it is a late complication. Over time, there will be weight loss due to increased respiratory rate and caloric expenditure with the demands of the lungs to oxygenate the blood despite fibrosis, shortness of breath due to the reduced blood flow from the right side of the heart into the lungs, and jugular venous distension due to impairment of the right ventricle. For a client living with cystic fibrosis, it is important to consider the conditions that may affect the client: pneumonia is an acute episode, atelectasis is associated with a pneumothorax, and cor pulmonale is a late-presentation chronic complication.

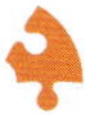
NCJMM Step: Analyze Cues
References: Astle & Duggleby (2024), pp. 955–976; Cobbett (2025), pp. 670–708 (airway management), 710–721 (chest physiotherapy); Jarvis et al. (2024), p. 494; Tyerman & Cobbett (2023), pp. 591–593 (pneumonia); 621 (atelectasis); 625–626 (cor pulmonale); 671–676 (cystic fibrosis).

Answer 21.3

The client is at highest risk of developing **sepsis** as evidenced by **respiratory assessment.**

Rationale: The client has had increasingly frequent infections over the course of the year. This clinical presentation has progressed to vertigo, even while driving, and now blood-tinged sputum. The primary concern for this client, who already presents with a fever, is that the condition may progress to sepsis because clients with cystic fibrosis are vulnerable to bacteria. The client does not present with any complications associated with failure to thrive; the client still has active bowel sounds and does not present with anorexia. The client does not have an obstruction for the same reason (since they continue to have active bowel sounds). Diabetes may occur in clients living with cystic fibrosis if the islets of Langerhans become fibrotic. Currently, this client does not present with clinical manifestations associated with this complication. The client is voiding and has not developed renal failure. The complication is determined as a result of the respiratory assessment. None of the other system presentation would be appropriate for determining the possibility of sepsis to develop.

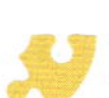
NCJMM Step: Prioritize Hypothesis
References: Astle & Duggleby (2024), pp. 955–976; Cobbett (2025), pp. 670–708 (airway management), 710–721 (chest physiotherapy); Tyerman & Cobbett (2023), pp. 955–976.

Answer 21.4

POTENTIAL NURSING INTERVENTIONS	INDICATED	NOT INDICATED
Plan to perform percussion, vibration, and postural drainage	✔	○
Encourage oral fluids	○	✔
Place client in reverse Trendelenburg position	○	✔
Ambulate client with physiotherapy	○	✔
Prepare client for a chest X-ray	✔	○
Place client on isolation	○	✔

Rationale: Clients with cystic fibrosis require consistent chest physiotherapy to assist with clearing secretions. Airway clearance is critical in reducing mucus and includes techniques such as chest physiotherapy (percussion, vibration), postural drainage, and positive expiratory pressure breathing. Even with adequate and frequent chest physiotherapy, when a client develops a respiratory infection with increased secretions, they may be at further risk for mucus plugs obstructing the airway. Proper positioning is dependent on the location for drainage and position. The client is placed in either an upright position, such as high Fowler's; upright in a chair; or in Trendelenburg position, whether side-lying, supine, or lying on the abdomen. With postural drainage, the principle of gravity is used to assist in bronchial clearance. Reverse Trendelenburg position is often used for vertigo and for clients with hemodynamic instability. The client is not alert enough for the nurse to encourage oral fluids. This would put the client's safety at risk by potentially leading to aspiration pneumonia. Ambulation and mobility would be encouraged for a client with cystic fibrosis; however, the client's alertness is limited at presentation and, therefore, the client may fall, leading to further musculoskeletal complications. The client would be sent for a chest X-ray to determine the severity of the respiratory infection. The client does not present with a condition that requires isolation, such as bacterial meningitis, tuberculosis, or COVID-19. The nurse needs to confirm isolation precautions with the facility's infection and prevention policy manual.

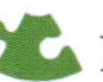
NCJMM Step: Generate Solutions
Reference: Astle & Duggleby (2024), pp. 955–976; Cobbett (2025), pp. 670–708, 710–718; Tyerman & Cobbett (2023), pp. 671–676.

Answer 21.5

- ✔ Initiate 0.9% sodium chloride (normal saline) 500 mL bolus × 1 then 125 mL/hr
- ✔ Oxygen 0–5 L per nasal prongs to maintain pulse oximetry greater than or equal to 92%
- ☐ Insert an in-dwelling urinary catheter
- ☐ Initiate a regular diet
- ✔ Laboratory tests: ABG, blood cultures
- ☐ Initiate metoprolol 25 mg PO twice a day

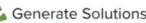

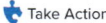

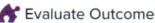

Rationale: Maintaining airway, breathing, and circulation for this client is the top priority. The client requires adequate oxygen support given that their pulse oximetry has decreased due to inadequate airway clearance. As a result of the inability to clear secretions along with having a respiratory infection, the client's blood pressure has decreased as well. To ensure adequate hydration, the client will need a bolus of fluid and then continuous hydration to increase intravascular volume. Identifying if there is a ventilation–perfusion mismatch will assist with treatment modalities. Drawing an arterial blood gas will provide this information. Finally, the client has a fever. Identifying which bacteria are causing the infection will assist with proper antibiotic therapy treatment modalities. The client may benefit from oral or intravenous therapy. The client does not require an in-dwelling catheter to assist with renal function. At present, the client requires treatment for airway management. Although nutrition is important for a client with cystic fibrosis, at the moment, initiating this treatment immediately is not warranted. An order of metoprolol would need to be clarified with the health care provider who prescribed this medication. Metoprolol is a beta blocker, a cardiac medication that reduces blood pressure and heart rate. This order may be an error; clarification is necessary prior to initiating this order. A more appropriate order would be an inhaled bronchodilator, especially if it is administered prior to chest physiotherapy. Clients living with cystic fibrosis are at risk for distal intestinal obstructive syndrome leading to constipation. A regular bowel protocol would be appropriate as well. Clients living with cystic fibrosis have difficulty digesting fats and proteins. Therefore, vitamin deficiencies are common and require pancreatic enzymes and supplementation.

NCJMM Step: Take Action
References: Astle & Duggleby (2024), pp. 955–976; Cobbett (2025), pp. 670–708, 710–718; Tyerman & Cobbett (2023), pp. 671–676.

Answer 21.6

ASSESSMENT FINDINGS	IMPROVED	NO CHANGE	DECLINED
Posterior lung sounds become clear with auscultation	✔	○	○
Expectorating green-tinged sputum only	✔	○	○
Absent bowel sounds	○	○	✔
Pulse oximetry level 96% on 3 L/min of oxygen therapy	✔	○	○
Respiratory rate 22	✔	○	○
Chest X-ray shows atelectasis to right lower lung	○	○	✔
Voiding clear, amber urine	○	✔	○

Rationale: Upon treatment, improved airway clearance is the expected result. Clear lung sounds indicate that there is adequate mucus clearance. Expectorating only green-tinged sputum without any blood is an improvement because this characteristic is typical for clients living with cystic fibrosis. Absent bowel sounds may indicate constipation or a bowel obstruction. The pulse oximetry has improved with oxygen therapy. Monitoring the status of gas exchange and oxygen requirements will indicate continued improvements. A chest X-ray demonstrating collapse of airways may require further lung recruitment therapy. This is a decline in the client's status. Finally, the client's kidneys remain constant and are perfusing well.

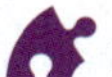
NCJMM Step: Evaluate Outcomes
References: Astle & Duggleby (2024), pp. 955–976; Cobbett (2025), pp. 670–708, 710–718; Tyerman & Cobbett (2023), pp. 671–676.

Medical-Surgical 22.0 (Cardiovascular)

Answer 22.1

- ☐ Motor power
- ☐ Stress
- ✔ Jugular venous distension
- ✔ Radial pulse characteristic
- ✔ Shortness of breath
- ☐ Bowel sounds
- ☐ Urine quality

Rationale: The client presents with an irregular pulse and shortness of breath as a result. At present, the client's hemodynamic status remains stable since their blood pressure is documented at 132/72. An irregular pulse has the potential to develop static blood in the atrium because the blood is not completely ejected into the ventricle; therefore, clots may form. This is called *loss of atrial kick*, which can be identified by the jugular venous distension. There is not enough atrial kick to expel all of the blood from the right atrium into the right ventricle and with the pressure of venous return, blood is backing up into the jugular venous system. The client's motor power is strong and independent. The client indicates they are experiencing stress, which can be tackled once the client's heart rate and breathing have improved. The client has active bowel sounds present in all four abdominal quadrants. The urine is clear and amber in colour.

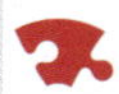
NCJMM Step: Recognize Cues
References: Astle & Duggleby (2024), p. 1006; Cobbett (2025), pp. 796–811, 710–718; Tyerman & Cobbett (2023), pp. 858–859.

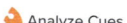

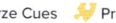

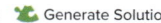

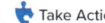

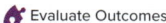

Answer 22.2

CLIENT FINDINGS	RIGHT-SIDED HEART FAILURE	ATRIAL FIBRILLATION	PERICARDITIS
Irregular pulse	○	✔	○
Jugular venous distension	✔	✔	○
"Racing heart"	○	✔	○
Shortness of breath	✔	✔	✔
Fatigue	✔	○	✔

Rationale: Right-sided heart failure causes a backward blood flow from the right ventricle to the right atrium and into the venous circulation. There is venous congestion leading to peripheral edema, hepatomegaly, splenomegaly, vascular congestion of the gastrointestinal tract, and jugular venous distension. The primary cause of right-sided heart failure is left-sided heart failure; shortness of breath may be a clinical manifestation. Fatigue is a sign of chronic heart failure. Clients who present with atrial fibrillation have irregular heart rates and may present with jugular venous distension due to the backward flow of blood from the right atrium into the venous circulation. If the heart rate is fast enough, clients may present with the sensation of a racing heart, and they present with shortness of breath as there is a decrease in cardiac output due to loss of atrial kick, rapid ventricular response, or both. Pericarditis is an inflammation of the pericardial sac. Clients with this condition present with severe chest pain that is sharp and pleuritic in nature and relieved by sitting upright, dyspnea, and a friction rub.

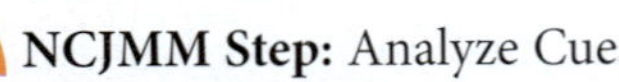
NCJMM Step: Analyze Cues
References: Astle & Duggleby (2024), p. 1006; Cobbett (2025), pp. 796–811, 710–718; Tyerman & Cobbett (2023), pp. 832 (right-sided heart failure); 858–859 (atrial fibrillation); 877–879 (pericarditis).

Answer 22.3

The client is at highest risk of developing **atrial fibrillation**.

Rationale: The client presented with nonspecific complaints of fatigue, shortness of breath with minimal exertion, and palpitations. The shortness of breath with minimal exertion and palpitations indicate that there is a cardiac and respiratory connection to the condition. The irregular pulse, feeling of a "racing heart," and increased jugular venous distension point toward atrial fibrillation as the primary condition. The vital signs include a fast heart rate (greater than 100 beats per minute), which indicates a tachycardia rhythm. Further assessment data are required to determine the type of rhythm the client is experiencing. During the assessment, there is a finding of an irregular pulse. Out of the potential conditions listed, the only irregular pulse is atrial fibrillation, which contributes to the initial presentation the client experienced. The client could not be experiencing bradycardia (heart rate less than 60 beats per minute). The client does not present with ventricular tachycardia because the client is able to speak in sentences, has not lost consciousness, and maintains a blood pressure. The client does not present with heart block.

NCJMM Step: Prioritize Hypothesis
References: Astle & Duggleby (2024), p. 1006; Cobbett (2025), pp. 796–811, 710–718; Tyerman & Cobbett (2023), pp. 858–859.

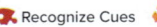

Answer 22.4

POTENTIAL NURSING INTERVENTIONS	INDICATED	NOT INDICATED
Prepare the consent form for the health care provider	✔	○
Allow the health care provider to answer all the questions	○	✔
Ensure suction is connected and working	✔	○
Collect oral pharyngeal airway and bag-valve mask device	✔	○
Allow the client to eat a regular diet	○	✔
Review policy and procedure	✔	○

Rationale: A transesophageal echocardiogram (TEE) is a diagnostic procedure used to rule out the presence of blood clots in the atrium prior to a cardioversion. If blood clots exist and a cardioversion occurs, the client may develop a stroke as a result of a clot being distributed to the brain. Consent needs to be obtained for this procedure. The health care provider administering the TEE will conduct the consenting process since the cardioversion will occur immediately after the TEE and once the cardiologist deems the cardioversion can proceed safely. The nurse can answer questions as well about the procedure and can be an advocate for the procedure, as well as for the client. Suction must be checked and verified that it is working. A client may drool or vomit once the camera is inserted into the mouth, and once sedation is given, the client is at risk for aspiration. Sedation is provided prior to the test being completed. An oral airway and bag-valve-mask device ensures the airway is protected during the procedure. A respiratory therapist assists with the procedure. A cardioversion should be completed only in a critical care environment where there is available support. The client must be nothing by mouth (NPO) prior to the cardioversion, to reduce the risk of aspiration pneumonia. Prior to a procedure, the nurse needs to review the policy and procedure document to ensure all steps are taken correctly.

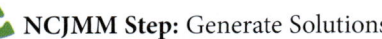

NCJMM Step: Generate Solutions
References: Astle & Duggleby (2024), p. 1006; Cobbett (2025), pp. 796–811, 710–718; Tyerman & Cobbett (2023), pp. 858–859.

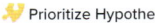

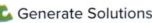

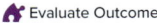

Answer 22.5

- ✔ Insert a peripheral venous access device
- ✔ 0.9% normal saline (sodium chloride) IV to keep vein open
- ✔ Ensure medications are available for conscious sedation (propofol and midazolam)
- ☐ Monitor input and output
- ☐ Complete a chest X-ray post-procedure

Rationale: A peripheral venous access device must be inserted into the client prior to the procedure being completed. Direct intravenous access will ensure that the medications are delivered safely. If the client becomes hypotensive during the procedure, fluids can be administered quickly. It is important to initiate intravenous fluids prior to the procedure and to keep the vein open until fluids are needed to administer medications or to give a bolus for a low blood pressure or for maintenance. During conscious sedation procedures such as a TEE followed by a cardioversion, it is important to utilize anaesthetic agents such as propofol (as an example only) and sedative agents such as midazolam (as an example only). The client should not be awake during the cardioversion. Monitoring fluid status is a nursing responsibility. A chest X-ray is not needed post-procedure unless an error is made.

NCJMM Step: Take Action
References: Astle & Duggleby (2024), p. 1006; Cobbett (2025), pp. 796–811, 710–718; Tyerman & Cobbett (2023), pp. 858–859.

Answer 22.6

ASSESSMENT FINDINGS	IMPROVED	NO CHANGE	DECLINED
Temperature	○	✔	○
Respiratory rate	○	○	✔
Heart rate	✔	○	○
Rhythm	✔	○	○
Pulse oximetry	○	○	✔

Rationale: Post-conscious sedation and after a procedure such as a TEE followed by a cardioversion, the nurse needs to place the client in the recovery position and monitor their vital signs and cognitive status. This client's temperature was unchanged. The respiratory rate declined as a result of the sedation because it was lower than previously. Monitoring whether the respiratory rate returns to a normal rate will ensure proper gas exchange. The client's heart rate and rhythm improved. Finally, the pulse oximetry declined in status only as the client was waking up; additional oxygen is needed until the client is more alert and the sedation effect has diminished.

NCJMM Step: Take Action
References: Astle & Duggleby (2024), p. 1006; Cobbett (2025), pp. 796–811, 710–718; Tyerman & Cobbett (2023), pp. 858–859.

Medical-Surgical 23.0 (Gastrointestinal)

Answer 23.1

- ☐ Pupillary size
- ☐ Cognitive status
- ☐ Heart sounds
- ☐ Lung sounds
- ✔ Frail-looking
- ✔ Nausea with emesis
- ✔ Diarrhea × 4 days ago
- ✔ Hygiene
- ✔ Urine characteristics
- ☐ No social supports

Rationale: The client presents with poor hygiene, is frail-looking, collapsed in the store, and has nausea, emesis, and diarrhea. The client's nutritional status requires further follow-up to ensure the client is meeting their own needs. Pupillary size is important to monitor given that the client collapsed on the floor, even though they think they did not hit their head. Older adults can develop complications from hitting their head and can display symptoms weeks after the event occurred. The pupils are equal in size and reactive to light. The client is alert and oriented to person, place, and time, so cognitively they are intact. The client does not demonstrate any abnormal heart sounds. There are clear lung sounds. The urine characteristics are dark and concentrated, with a strong odour. If this finding were solely on its own with a stable blood pressure, concentrated urine would be something to monitor; however, in this situation, the client also presents with cracking and flaking skin and dry and cracked lips, so there is more to the client's hydration status, even if the blood pressure remains intact. The fact that the client does not have any social supports is a concern. Human connection is necessary for good mental health and daily functioning. Isolation contributes to more serious conditions physically and mentally.

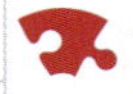

NCJMM Step: Recognize Cues
References: Astle & Duggleby (2024), pp. 416–424, 426–427; Cobbett (2025), pp. 885–891; Tyerman & Cobbett (2023), pp. 956–964.

Answer 23.2

The nurse should recognize that the client is potentially experiencing **malnutrition** and **dehydration.**

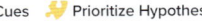

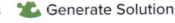

Rationale: The client presents with dysfunction of the gastrointestinal system, small stature, and a frail appearance for an older adult. *Frailty* is defined as the presence of three or more of the following: unplanned weight loss (>4.5 kg in the past year), weakness, poor endurance and energy, slowness, and low activity. Malnutrition is the result of inadequate intake of protein, or calories that could be organic or nonorganic, and requires further investigation, especially given that the client collapsed at the grocery store. The client's dehydration status is problematic as evidenced by the clinical presentation of dry skin, cracked lips, and dark, concentrated urine. There is not enough information to indicate if the client is at risk for dysrhythmias since there were no irregularities with palpating the pulses. The client does not have impaired gas exchange because their pulse oximetry levels are greater than 92%. Dark, concentrated urine does not indicate renal failure; further assessment data would be necessary to confirm that complication.

NCJMM Step: Analyze Cues
References: Astle & Duggleby (2024), pp. 416–424, 426–427; Cobbett (2025), pp. 880–881, 885–891; Tyerman & Cobbett (2023), pp. 380, 956–964.

Answer 23.3

The client is at highest risk of developing **seizures**.

Rationale: On review of the newest client data, such as results of blood work, the sodium levels are elevated. Hypernatremia can exacerbate with an increased risk of seizure activity. Given the low muscle wasting as a result of the malnutrition, the client is at an increased risk of having a seizure. The client's hemoglobin level is low, indicating anemia. Polycythemia vera is described as having too many red blood cells, not too few. The client's potassium level is on the upper level of normal and would need to be monitored to rule out dysrhythmia activity. The client presents as afebrile with clear air entry; therefore, pneumonia would be eliminated as a cause. Malnutrition causes weakness and poor wound healing. These are both complications; however, the client is at highest risk for seizure activity, which could have greater effects on the client's hospital stay.

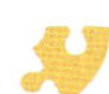

NCJMM Step: Prioritize Hypothesis
References: Astle & Duggleby (2024), pp. 416–424, 426–427; Cobbett (2025), pp. 880–881, 885–891; Tyerman & Cobbett (2023), pp. 349–351, 380, 956–964.

Answer 23.4

POTENTIAL NURSING INTERVENTIONS	INDICATED	NOT INDICATED
Determine frailty level through use of the Clinical Frailty Scale	✔	○
Maintain NPO status	○	✔
Request a consult for dietitian	✔	○
Identify whether the client is experiencing food insecurity	✔	○
Monitor for nausea	✔	○
Request a consult for social work	✔	○

Rationale: Determining the severity of the frailty the client is experiencing would be appropriate for rehabilitation and supportive care. The client does not need to remain NPO (nothing by mouth) and should be encouraged to order foods that are pleasurable and that appeal to the client's taste buds. There is no contraindication indicating that the client cannot swallow or has trouble digesting food. Complications of malnutrition include nausea and diarrhea, so monitoring for nausea and treating it, if necessary, would help the client take in oral food. Social work and a dietitian should be consulted for this client, given the poor nutritional state in which the client arrived at the unit and their lack of personal hygiene. Possibly, the client is experiencing challenges in their life that require additional support.

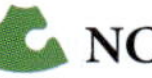

NCJMM Step: Generate Solutions
References: Astle & Duggleby (2024), pp. 416–424, 426–427, 429–431, 1111; Cobbett (2025), pp. 880–881, 885–891; Tyerman & Cobbett (2023), pp. 956–964.

Answer 23.5

- ✔ Record the client's height and weight.
- ☐ Complete a food diary for the client.
- ✔ Avoid interrupting the client during meals.
- ✔ Encourage friends to bring food and to visit during mealtimes.
- ☐ Plan tasks during mealtimes.
- ☐ Reduce between-meal nutrition supplements.

Rationale: Recording the client's height and weight at the start will provide baseline data. Monitoring for weight gain would be the priority. The nurse should avoid interrupting the client with unnecessary tasks during the meal. The client's environment should be conducive to eating: quiet, with the bedside table cleared of clutter, and with urinals, bedpans, and emesis basins placed out of sight. Encouraging friends and foods the client may like can encourage nutritional intake. Eating is a social experience that is often affected when clients are admitted to the hospital. The client should be encouraged to keep a food diary. The nurse should not take away autonomy of the client when they are tasked with managing their needs outside of the hospital. Enabling a person will not help their success upon discharge. The nurse should avoid planning tasks during mealtimes to avoid interruptions. Clients who are malnourished should be encouraged to eat food, not withhold nutrition.

NCJMM Step: Take Action
References: Astle & Duggleby (2024), pp. 416–424, 426–427; Cobbett (2025), pp. 880–881, 885–891; Tyerman & Cobbett (2023), pp. 956–964.

Answer 23.6

ASSESSMENT FINDINGS	IMPROVED	NO CHANGE	DECLINED
Client gains 1.5 kg	✔	○	○
Bowel movements become more solid	✔	○	○
Client able to choose nutritionally dense food on a budget	✔	○	○

ASSESSMENT FINDINGS	IMPROVED	NO CHANGE	DECLINED
Client develops a stage 2 wound on their left scapula	○	○	✔
Dizziness persists with standing	○	✔	○

Rationale: The nurse can help the client gain weight by paying particular attention to increasing their protein intake to help with tissue repair and improve wound healing. As the client eats more nutritionally dense food, the bowels will not excrete so much fluid, and the stool will bind together more. Helping the client choose and budget for dense foods will help the client retain some weight. Often, older adult skin is thin, and these clients are at risk for pressure injuries. The dizziness will persist until the client's body can regulate its volume better.

NCJMM Step: Evaluate Outcomes
References: Astle & Duggleby (2024), pp. 416–424, 426–427; Cobbett (2025), pp. 880–881, 885–891; Tyerman & Cobbett (2023), pp. 956–964.

Medical-Surgical 24.0 (Respiratory)

Answer 24.1

Progress Notes

1124h: Client was a direct admission to the unit accompanied by their partner for further gastrointestinal investigations. The client has had difficulty swallowing fluids and solids × months, but it has grown increasingly worse over the past 2 days. Vital signs: T: 37.6°C (99.6°F); BP: 102/58; P: 87; RR: 22; with pulse oximetry of 96% on room air. Client presents as pleasant and cooperative. Motor power strong × 4 extremities with client ambulating independently. Gait steady. Pupils equal in size and shape, measured at 3 mm, and respond briskly to light. Client denies pain. S1 and S2 heart sounds, apical heart rate regular and equals radial pulse. Bilateral radial pulses palpable, bilateral dorsalis pedis pulses palpable and strong. No edema noted. Capillary refill less than 3 seconds. Bilateral fine inspiratory crackles noted in right and left base lung fields when auscultated posteriorly. Client has a weak cough reflex; coughs when takes in too much fluid at one time. Respirations regular but tachypneic. No indrawing, nasal flaring, or use of accessory muscles noted. Abdomen flat with hyperactive bowel sounds auscultated in all four quadrants. BMI 17.1. Client states nausea on occasion with emesis if able to tolerate food and fluids. Takes sips to avoid emesis. Client states no pain with urination, no frequency or urgency. Urine concentrated when able to void.

Rationale: The admission documentation indicates that the client has had difficulty swallowing fluids for months and that this has become increasingly worse over the past 2 days. The concern is whether the client can protect their airway. The bilateral fine inspiratory crackles indicate fluid in the alveoli. There is no indication of an infection because there is no fever. Fluid should not be in the alveoli. The client has a weak cough reflex, indicating that if fluids were to travel from the intended esophagus to the trachea, the client would not be able to protect their airway as intended, which is evidenced by them coughing after fluids. The client presents as tachypneic but in no distress. Over time, the client has likely developed compensatory methods to maintain gas exchange. The client's BMI is 17.1, which is underweight. As a result of not being able to take in food and fluids, the client may present as malnourished. Finally, the urine is concentrated, indicating possible dehydration, even if the blood pressure does not reflect this yet.

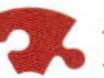
NCJMM Step: Recognize Cues
References: Astle & Duggleby (2024), pp. 757, 908, 930–934, 986, 1115–1120, 1141–1152; Cobbett (2025), pp. 908–936; Tyerman & Cobbett (2023), p. 590.

Answer 24.2

- ☐ Stroke
- ✔ Dehydration
- ☐ Deep vein thrombosis
- ☐ Bowel obstruction
- ✔ Pneumonia
- ✔ Failure to thrive

Rationale: The primary complications for which the client is at risk due to their dysphagia are dehydration and pneumonia (specifically, aspiration pneumonia). Silent aspiration is a condition that occurs when there is abnormal entry of secretions or substances into the lower airway. Once the immune response is overwhelmed with secretions, aspiration pneumonia develops. As a result of the client's inability to take fluids and their concentrated urine, the client is at risk for complications of dehydration and failure to thrive. Poor nutritional intake can reduce a person's immune response. The client has no peripheral edema to indicate that a clot has formed. The client's heart rate is regular, indicating no reason for a clot to have formed on the left side of the heart. The client does not present with any neurological symptoms like headache or confusion that would indicate the possibility of a stroke. The client presents with active bowel sounds in all four quadrants, which eliminates bowel obstruction as a complication.

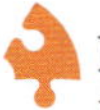
NCJMM Step: Analyze Cues
References: Astle & Duggleby (2024), pp. 757, 908, 930–934, 986, 1115–1120, 1141–1152; Cobbett (2025), pp. 908–936; Tyerman & Cobbett (2023), p. 590.

Answer 24.3

The client is at highest risk of developing **aspiration pneumonia**.

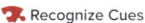

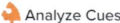

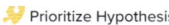

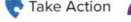

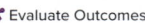

Rationale: The client's dysphagia is the direct cause of the aspiration pneumonia. The client's condition will deteriorate without correcting the issue and providing nutrition. The client does not indicate any classic symptoms of gastroesophageal reflux disease, such as abdominal discomfort after the client eats. The client's heart rate remains regular and in a normal range (60–100); therefore, there is no indication of any life-threatening dysrhythmias. The client does not present with type 1 or 2 diabetes mellitus. Diabetic ketoacidosis is primarily a complication of type 1 diabetes and can occur in clients with type 2 diabetes mellitus if ketones are produced. However, this client does not exhibit any clinical manifestations of diabetic ketoacidosis. The client is voiding without issue, and their blood pressure indicates there is still perfusion of the kidneys, ruling out renal failure. A client who does not eat sufficient nutrients will still produce hydrochloric acid and is at risk of developing a peptic ulcer, which can progress to a gastrointestinal bleed.

NCJMM Step: Prioritize Hypothesis
References: Astle & Duggleby (2024), pp. 757, 908, 930–934, 986, 1115–1120, 1141–1152; Cobbett (2025), pp. 908–936; Tyerman & Cobbett (2023), p. 590.

Answer 24.4

POTENTIAL NURSING INTERVENTIONS	INDICATED	NOT INDICATED
Keep client NPO (nothing by mouth)	✔	○
Encourage client to position self in the chair or semi-Fowler's position	✔	○
Plan to administer thickened fluids for hydration	○	✔
Prepare the client for a barium swallow	○	✔
Consult speech-language pathologist	✔	○
Ensure mouth swabs are close to the client	✔	○
Request an order to insert a peripheral venous access device	✔	○

Rationale: Until the cause of the dysphagia is determined, in order to minimize the highest risk (which is aspiration pneumonia), the client is kept NPO, nothing to eat or drink. Aspiration pneumonia could cause the client to remain in the hospital longer than expected. The nurse should maintain the client in an upright position to reduce the chances of secretions falling down the trachea. Until further diagnostic tests are completed, NPO status is maintained, which includes thickened fluids. A speech-language pathologist can conduct a swallowing assessment. A swallowing assessment can help identify clients at high risk for aspiration and the location of the swallowing problem and can determine which food consistencies are safest for the client to eat. The speech-language pathologist can also determine and provide swallowing exercises and proper head and neck positioning, as well as teach swallowing techniques. To rehydrate the mucous membranes, the client can use mouth swabs. Maintenance of oral care will also minimize the risk of infections pertaining to dysphagia. The nurse should request an order to insert a peripheral venous access device for fluid administration and in preparation for diagnostic procedures.

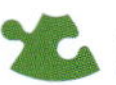
NCJMM Step: Generate Solutions
References: Astle & Duggleby (2024), pp. 757, 908, 930–934, 986, 1115–1120, 1141–1152; Cobbett (2025), pp. 908–936; Tyerman & Cobbett (2023), p. 963.

Answer 24.5

- ☐ Obtain chest X-ray
- ✔ Insert nasogastric tube and initiate tube feeds as per policy
- ☐ Obtain a swallowing assessment
- ☐ Consult physiotherapy
- ✔ Initiate 0.9% normal saline (sodium chloride) at 75 mL/hr
- ✔ Heparin subcutaneous as per weight

Rationale: The client requires nutrition and hydration. The goal of nutrition intervention in the management of dysphagia should be to minimize weight loss and maintain hydration. Until a swallowing assessment can be performed, inserting a nasogastric tube as per institution policy and initiating tube feeds based on the recommendations of the dietitian will ensure that there is some nutritional component being delivered to the client and that the stomach is coated with liquid, minimizing the risk of a peptic ulcer and, at worst, a gastrointestinal bleed. The client already has a peripheral venous access device, and hydration is important to provide intravascular volume and maintain perfusion of the kidneys. A chest X-ray is necessary if the client aspirates. Obtaining a swallowing assessment will be the best way to determine what the issue may be for the client. Physiotherapy will prevent the formation of blood clots by ensuring mobility. Heparin administered subcutaneously will prevent the formation of blood clots as well.

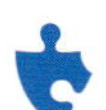
NCJMM Step: Take Action
References: Astle & Duggleby (2024), pp. 757, 908, 930–934, 986, 1115–1120, 1141–1152; Cobbett (2025), pp. 908–936; Tyerman & Cobbett (2023), pp. 963, 1046–1047.

Answer 24.6

CLIENT STATEMENTS	UNDER-STANDING	NO UNDER-STANDING
"I can still take sips of water."	○	✔
"I need to perform good mouth care as needed."	✔	○
"If the tube falls out, let someone know."	✔	○
"I am going to have the tube forever."	○	✔

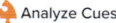

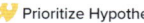

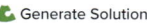

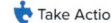

CLIENT STATEMENTS	UNDER-STANDING	NO UNDER-STANDING
"If I get the tube caught on something, let someone know."	✔	○
"I need to check the opening of my nose on both sides for irritation."	✔	○

Rationale: Even with the nasogastric tube, the client cannot take sips of water. The tube is for nutrition. The client must continue with good oral care, brush their teeth, rinse their mouth, and use petroleum jelly on their lips to prevent them from drying out. When a nasogastric tube is inserted, clients typically breathe through the mouth. If the tube falls out or gets caught, it is best to inform someone of the situation. If the client catches the tube and pulls it out of the correct position while infusing tube feeds, the client is at risk for aspiration pneumonia. The nurse should reassure the client that until all diagnostic tests are done, there is no reason to believe they will have the nasogastric tube forever. It is important to perform tests to determine the problem. The client and nursing staff must check the nares for irritation and skin breakdown. The skin of a nare is pliable and can cause necrosis if the tube placement is not correctly assessed.

NCJMM Step: Evaluate Outcomes
References: Astle & Duggleby (2024), pp. 757, 908, 930–934, 986, 1115–1120, 1141–1152; Cobbett (2025), pp. 908–936; Tyerman & Cobbett (2023), pp. 1046–1047.

Medical-Surgical 25.0 (Gastrointestinal)

Answer 25.1

- ☐ Pupillary response
- ☐ Blood pressure
- ☐ Cognitive orientation
- ☐ Dorsalis pedis pulses
- ☐ Lung sounds
- ✔ Hemoptysis
- ✔ Bowel sounds
- ✔ Abdomen firm and round
- ✔ Nausea
- ☐ Urine characteristics

Rationale: The client's symptoms requiring follow-up include gastrointestinal symptoms. Expectorating blood with clear air entry throughout indicates that the blood can only be originating from the esophagus or the stomach. The hyperactive bowel sounds accompanied by nausea indicate increased gastric motility. Despite no emesis at present, there is an increased risk that vomiting could happen. The firm and round abdomen indicates that there is gas buildup in the stomach, increasing pressure. These would be immediate findings to follow up on with this client. The client's bilateral pupillary response is brisk and the same size, which is a positive finding. The client's blood pressure is lower than normal; however, the client remains hemodynamically stable and does not require intervention. Bilateral dorsalis pedis pulses are documented as being weak, but they remain palpable; this is something to monitor for this client. Urine is dark and concentrated, indicating dehydration. Unless there are hemodynamic changes, monitoring urine output will be part of the nurses' assessment.

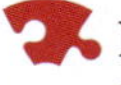
NCJMM Step: Recognize Cues
References: Astle & Duggleby (2024), pp. 1218–1221; Cobbett (2025), pp. 996–1022; Tyerman & Cobbett (2023), pp. 1016–1033.

Answer 25.2

CLIENT FINDINGS	BOWEL OBSTRUCTION	PULMONARY EMBOLUS	UPPER GASTROINTESTINAL BLEED
Nausea	✔	○	✔
Hemoptysis	○	✔	✔
Abdomen firm and round	✔	○	✔
Loss of appetite	✔	○	✔

Rationale: A client who is experiencing a bowel obstruction experiences nausea, a firm abdomen, and loss of appetite due to fluid, gas, and intestinal contents accumulating proximal to the intestinal obstruction. This causes distension. When an obstruction occurs in the small bowel, dehydration occurs quickly; there is a loss of bowel sounds, which indicates a loss of motility. However, this client continues to have active bowel sounds auscultated. When a client presents with hemoptysis, the nurse needs to consider conditions such as pulmonary embolus, pulmonary edema, or whether the bleeding is originating from the esophagus or stomach in the absence of adventitious breath sounds. With an upper gastrointestinal bleed, clients experience nausea and hemoptysis if there is frank bleeding in the esophagus, typically from a Mallory-Weiss tear, which is a weakened area in the esophageal wall. A firm and round abdomen may indicate bleeding in the stomach, which would lead to a loss of appetite.

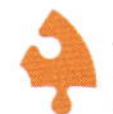
NCJMM Step: Analyze Cues
References: Astle & Duggleby (2024), pp. 1218–1221; Cobbett (2025), pp. 996–1022; Tyerman & Cobbett (2023), pp. 622–624 (pulmonary embolus), 1061–1062 (bowel obstruction).

Answer 25.3

- ☐ Gastroesophageal reflux disease
- ✔ Acute renal failure
- ☐ Pneumonia
- ☐ Pulmonary edema
- ✔ Acute myocardial infarction
- ✔ Hemorrhage

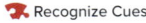

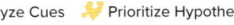

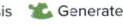

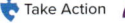

Rationale: The client is presenting with symptoms of an active acute upper gastrointestinal bleed. The potential conditions the client is at most risk of developing are acute renal failure from a major bleeding episode and loss of perfusion to the kidney, an acute myocardial infarction due to a loss of systemic blood flow and ultimately loss of flow to the myocardium, and a hemorrhage. The client is not at risk of developing gastroesophageal reflux disease because they already have a history of peptic ulcer disease, use of ibuprofen without taking pantoprazole, and a high-stress job. The client's lungs are clear, eliminating the possibility of developing pneumonia or pulmonary edema from the left ventricle not working properly in the absence of coronary artery disease.

NCJMM Step: Prioritize Hypothesis
References: Astle & Duggleby (2024), pp. 1218–1221; Cobbett (2025), pp. 996–1022; Tyerman & Cobbett (2023), pp. 1016–1033.

Answer 25.4

POTENTIAL NURSING INTERVENTIONS	INDICATED	NOT INDICATED
Insert another large-bore venous access device	✔	○
Packed red blood cells	✔	○
Clear fluids diet and advance to regular diet	○	✔
Insert a nasogastric tube and attach to low suction	✔	○
Chest X-ray	○	✔
Insert an in-dwelling Foley catheter	✔	○
Initiate Ringer's lactate	✔	○

Rationale: Establishing two large-bore peripheral venous access devices will assist with rapidly infusing blood and fluids into the client. The client's hemoglobin is 70 g/L (7 g/dL) and the client's blood pressure is low, which indicate hemodynamic instability requiring treatment. The preferred method would be to correct the circulation issues. The client will have a nasogastric tube inserted and attached to low suction to remove the gastric contents. The client is vomiting coffee-ground emesis, which is an indication of hemolyzed blood. There is a risk of aspiration. Removing the gastric contents will assist with improving the round, firm abdomen as well. Inserting an in-dwelling Foley catheter is a way to assess urine volume accurately. Feeding the client is not a priority right now because controlling the bleeding is more important. The client does not need a chest X-ray to verify whether the nasogastric tube is inserted correctly because gastric contents will be removed. Administration of an isotonic crystalloid solution will assist with the loss of volume.

NCJMM Step: Generate Solutions
References: Astle & Duggleby (2024), pp. 1218–1221; Cobbett (2025), pp. 996–1022; Tyerman & Cobbett (2023), pp. 1016–1062.

Answer 25.5

The nurse should insert a(n) **nasogastric tube** first.

It would be a priority for the nurse to request a prescription for **antiemetic**.

Rationale: The client already has one peripheral venous access device, which is infusing fluids. The priority would be to insert a nasogastric tube, decompress the abdomen, and drain the stomach of old blood. The tube will protect the client's airway by preventing a possible aspiration. This would be followed by insertion of the in-dwelling Foley catheter and then another peripheral venous access device. Later, the blood bank will be called to thaw the blood and arrange for a pick-up. Monitoring for fluid overload is important.

The nurse should request an order for an antiemetic to reduce the risk of vomiting blood and possible aspiration. A proton pump inhibitor is a medication used to reduce the amount of hydrochloric acid in the stomach and is appropriate for a client with peptic ulcer disease but who is not in the acute phase of an active gastrointestinal bleed. The medication chosen would be Sandostatin, also known as octreotide, which has a greater effect on reducing hydrochloric acid than a proton pump inhibitor. The client does not need an antipyretic; this would be acetaminophen, provided to clients who have a fever. This client does not have a fever.

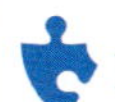
NCJMM Step: Take Action
References: Astle & Duggleby (2024), pp. 1218–1221; Cobbett (2025), pp. 996–1022; Sealock & Seneviratne (2025), pp. 649–651; Tyerman & Cobbett (2023), pp. 1016–1033.

Answer 25.6

ASSESSMENT FINDINGS	IMPROVED	NO CHANGE	DECLINED
BP 110/65	✔	○	○
Frank red blood with emesis	○	○	✔
Clear amber urine	✔	○	○
Dizziness	○	✔	○
Alert and communicative	✔	○	○

Rationale: The client's blood pressure has improved due to the packed cells and the fluid administration. The client continues to vomit, but this time frank red blood; this is likely a tear in the esophagus as a result of retching. The client's urine has improved from dark and concentrated to clear and amber. The client remains dizzy, likely as a result of the blood loss. The client is more awake and communicative instead of lethargic.

NCJMM Step: Evaluate Outcomes
References: Astle & Duggleby (2024), pp. 1218–1221; Cobbett (2025), pp. 996–1022; Tyerman & Cobbett (2023), pp. 1016–1062.

Medical-Surgical 26.0

Answer 26.1

- ✔ Pupillary response
- ✔ Speech
- ✔ Client orientation
- ☐ Vital signs
- ✔ Lethargy
- ☐ Radial pulses
- ☐ Lung sounds

Rationale: When the client returned from the visit with their friend, their pupils were pinpoint and sluggish to respond to light, which is a contrast from the previous assessment and is concerning. The pupils remained the same shape, but their reaction time was reduced. The client progressed from alert and orientated to person, place, and time with clear speech to being able to recognize self only and having slurred, disorganized speech. The client's lethargy is also concerning since the notes do not indicate that any medications were given to the client, yet the client's neurological status changed considerably. The vital signs were lower than the previously taken vital signs at shift change, but the client continues to maintain perfusion. The client presents with an adequate pulse oximetry level, which indicates appropriate gas exchange is occurring.

NCJMM Step: Recognize Cues
References: Jarvis et al. (2024), pp. 741–743; Keatings & Adams (2024), Chapter 7; Power-Kean et al. (2023), pp. 354–355.

Answer 26.2

CLIENT FINDINGS	STROKE	TRAUMATIC BRAIN INJURY	MEDICATION INGESTION (OPIOID)
Hypotension	○	✔	✔
Pinpoint pupils	○	○	✔
Altered level of consciousness	✔	✔	✔
Moves extremities independently	○	○	✔
Somnolence	○	✔	✔
Flushed face	○	✔	✔

Rationale: When a client has a stroke, there is an increase in blood pressure, not a decrease, due to the increased blood volume. Pupil size may be unilaterally different with different reactions to light from the right side compared to the left side, due to the occlusion. The client may present with altered level of consciousness depending on where the occlusion is located. Clients who are experiencing a stroke may develop hemiparesis as a result of the clot. Somnolence is not associated with a stroke. There is vasoconstriction as opposed to vasodilation when a stroke happens. When a client has a traumatic brain injury, the blood pressure becomes elevated before decreasing. Pupils are dilated, not pinpoint. There would be altered level of consciousness. The client should have no difficulty moving extremities independently. Somnolence, insomnia, and fatigue are clinical manifestations associated with head injuries. Concussions can cause a flushed face. If a client ingests an opioid or other substance, there will be vasodilation, a decrease in blood pressure, and a flushed face. There will be pinpoint pupils as a result of an opioid or heroin. The client may have an altered level of consciousness based on the response to the brain on the substance. The client would be able to move all four extremities independently, even if weak.

NCJMM Step: Analyze Cues
References: Keatings & Adams (2024), Chapter 7; Tyerman & Cobbett (2023), pp. 170, 1465–1472, 1490–1492.

Answer 26.3

The client is at highest risk of developing **respiratory distress**.

Rationale: There is nothing to indicate in the client's clinical presentation that they are experiencing a stroke or a traumatic brain injury such as a subdural hematoma. The client's somnolence, difficulty to rouse, and cluster breathing indicate the client has progressed to respiratory distress, and the client will not be able to protect their airway. Given the client's history, endocarditis is associated with intravenous drug misuse; however, the client does not present with a fever, pleuritic pain, flulike symptoms, or sore joints, which are common manifestations associated with endocarditis. When the pulses are palpable, they remain regular and unchanged. There is no indication that the client fell, and no bruising on their head, neck, or ears, ruling out a subdural hematoma. There are no clinical presentation associated with the renal system, therefore, eliminating renal failure.

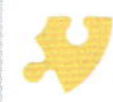
NCJMM Step: Prioritize Hypothesis
References: Keatings & Adams (2024), Chapter 7; Tyerman & Cobbett (2023), pp. 170, 1465–1472, 1490–1492.

Answer 26.4

POTENTIAL NURSING INTERVENTIONS	INDICATED	NOT INDICATED
Position the client in the recovery position supported by pillows	✔	○
Prepare to call a code blue	✔	○
Insert an in-dwelling Foley catheter	○	✔
Request an order to initiate oxygen therapy	✔	○

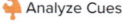

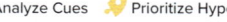

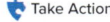

POTENTIAL NURSING INTERVENTIONS	INDICATED	NOT INDICATED
Ensure suction is working in the room with a Yankauer suction tip.	✔	○
Encourage oral fluid intake	○	✔
Prepare to administer naloxone	✔	○

Rationale: The client's pulse oximetry is low, and their respiratory rate is depressed, indicating the client likely ingested a narcotic or other substance. Placing the client in the recovery position will prevent aspiration. Given the low blood pressure and the low pulse oximetry, preparing to call a code blue may be warranted, given the client's breathing pattern. Inserting an in-dwelling Foley catheter is not a priority at the moment; airway, breathing, and circulation are the priorities. Oxygen therapy is warranted until the client is able to breathe independently. Ensuring suction is working in the room is a part of routine safety checks, and a Yankauer suction tip is appropriate if the client should present with emesis. This will assist in preventing aspiration. The nurse should not encourage oral intake, as the client cannot protect their airway. The nurse should be prepared to administer naloxone in the event the client ingested or injected an opioid. Be cautious of the rebound effect of any opioid after naloxone has been administered.

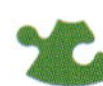
NCJMM Step: Generate Solutions
References: Keatings & Adams (2024), Chapter 7; Tyerman & Cobbett (2023), pp. 1760–1771.

Answer 26.5

- Oxygen 1–10 L/min nasal prongs or non-rebreather mask for pulse oximetry greater than 92%
- Insert a second peripheral venous access device
- Naloxone 0.4 mg IM and may be repeated q4min to a maximum of 10 mg
- 0.9% sodium chloride (normal saline) 500 mL IV bolus × 1, reconfirm for a second dose
- Chest X-ray
- Laboratory tests: toxicity screen, electrolytes, creatinine, BUN, arterial blood gas (ABG)
- Methadone 20 mg PO liquid solution
- Monitor input and output
- Regular diet
- Consult social work
- Consult addiction counsellor

Rationale: Initiating oxygen therapy to increase the pulse oximetry from 76% is a priority until the client is able to protect their airway. A second peripheral venous access device may be necessary to administer additional medication intravenously and fluids. Administration of naloxone is a priority to reverse the effects of the opioid ingestion/injection. At this time, it is unclear what the client may have taken as there is no indication of the specific drug. The nurse needs to exercise caution when administering naloxone, as the drug has a very short half-life. Once the half-life has been met and the naloxone excreted, the opioid will attempt to attach to the receptor, causing an additional overdose response. The nurse needs to stay with the client to monitor their symptom response. The client's blood pressure is low, so fluids may be necessary. A smooth muscle effect from the opioid has caused vasodilation initially; however, the body cannot respond accordingly, and the blood pressure decreases and fluids are required to increase intravascular volume. It will be imperative to identify the drug that was likely ingested or injected, as well as electrolytes, kidney function, and airway management to determine if the client may need to be intubated. All other orders are important; however, priority would be given to all orders to restore airway, breathing, and circulation priorities.

NCJMM Step: Take Action
References: Keatings & Adams (2024), Chapter 7; Tyerman & Cobbett (2023), pp. 178–181, 1760–1771.

Answer 26.6

ASSESSMENT FINDINGS	IMPROVED	NO CHANGE	DECLINED
Client awake and sitting upright	✔	○	○
Coarse crackles auscultated throughout bilateral anterior base lung fields	○	○	✔
Client on 4 L/min of continuous oxygen per nasal prongs for pulse oximetry of 97%	○	○	✔
Respiratory rate 18	✔	○	○
T 36.9°C (98.4°F)	○	✔	○

Rationale: The client has improved with orientation, ability to maintain airway, and posture. The client is able to sit upright and maintain a suitable pulse oximetry reading even if on 4 L per minute. The client did not require intubation, but this is a decline in status from their original baseline. The coarse crackles are a decline in status since data indicated fine inspiratory crackles. The client will need to be monitored for aspiration pneumonia and an increase in temperature. The respiratory rate has improved from 12 to 18 breaths per minute. The temperature remains unchanged.

NCJMM Step: Evaluate Outcomes
References: Keatings & Adams (2024), Chapter 7; Tyerman & Cobbett (2023), pp. 178–181, 1760–1771.

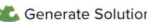

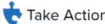

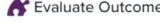

Medical-Surgical 27.0

Answer 27.1

BODY SYSTEM	PRIORITY FINDINGS
Neurological	○ Client orientation ✔ Dizziness ○ Motor power ✔ Tingling
Cardiovascular	○ Radial pulse characteristics ✔ Heart rate ○ Heart sounds ✔ Client perfusion
Respiratory	✔ Characteristics of the lung sounds ✔ Pulse oximetry ✔ Breathing patterns ✔ Tripod position
Gastrointestinal	○ Bowel sounds ○ Anorexia ✔ Characteristics of swallowing

Rationale:

Neurological: The client's dizziness may be an indication of vestibular complications, a sign of impaired perfusion to the brain from either a cardiovascular or respiratory issue. Tingling is related to an irritated nerve related to nerve tissue ischemia, constriction of the nerve or blood supply. Tingling is associated with afferent pathways, thinner c-fibres, and histamine. The client maintains orientation throughout despite a lower oxygen level. The client does not progress to being confused. The client's motor power remains strong × 4 extremities and they can move independently.

Cardiovascular: The client presents with tachycardia that remains regular. An increased heart rate reduces preload (or filling time of the ventricle). Without consistent accommodation, the heart rate cannot be maintained at a fast rate. The heart rate and blood pressure are inversely proportional, meaning as the blood pressure decreases, the heart rate increases to compensate for the lower cardiac output. The client's perfusion has minimized, indicating pale skin and pallor. In clients with darker skin and pallor, normal brown skin appears yellow-brown, and normal black skin appears ashen grey. The nurse needs to observe less pigmented areas such as the nailbeds, palms, or soles of the feet. The client presents with normal S1 and S2 heart sounds with no adventitious heart sounds of S3 or S4 noted.

Respiratory: The client's respiratory status remains a high priority requiring intervention. Coarse crackles in the right lower lobe have progressed to audible wheezing throughout all lung fields, indicating bronchoconstriction. The pulse oximetry has decreased from 94% to 82%, indicating a ventilation–perfusion mismatch. There is reduced gas exchange in the alveoli. The client is taking short, shallow breaths with retractions, indicating increased work or breathing. The tripod position is a positional change that increases the surface area of the alveoli to increase gas exchange.

Gastrointestinal: The client's inability to swallow is concerning and warrants further investigation. Either the client's esophagus is constricting or the trachea is constricting. The inability to swallow may increase the client's risk for airway compromise. If the client is drooling without swallowing, this is an indication of a closing airway.

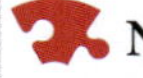
NCJMM Step: Recognize Cues
References: Keatings & Adams (2024), Chapter 7; Power-Kean et al. (2023), pp. 331, 670–673; Tyerman & Cobbett (2023), pp. 751–762, 899.

Answer 27.2

- ✔ Injury from falling
- ☐ Cerebral edema
- ✔ Shunting
- ✔ Hypoxemia
- ☐ Weight loss
- ☐ Mitral valve stenosis
- ☐ Coronary artery constriction

Rationale: Given the client's clinical presentation, the client would be at risk of falling due to the hypotension and impaired gas exchange. The client has already presented with dizziness when they had a higher blood pressure. Orthostatic hypotension would occur if the client were to walk long distances. The client is at risk of developing shunting and a ventilation–perfusion mismatch. Shunting is related to blocked ventilation (wheezing or bronchoconstriction) and collapsed alveoli (related to the coarse crackles upon admission). There is no impairment of the vascular circulation in the lungs, such as an embolus. The client is at risk for hypoxemia as a result of the low pulse oximetry and likely impaired gas exchange as evidenced by reduced perfusion (cyanosis, pale skin tone). The client does not present with any indication of a head injury resulting in cerebral edema. The client's few days of eating may account for loss of water; however weight loss is not a primary complication in this client. The client has no indication of mitral valve stenosis as evidenced through comorbidities or initial clinical presentation. The client does not present with cardiovascular-related complications such as coronary artery constriction (i.e., atherosclerosis). If the client developed chest pain, this would be as a result of impaired blood flow to the myocardium, not as a result of constriction of the coronary arteries.

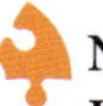
NCJMM Step: Analyze Cues
References: Keatings & Adams (2024), pp. 188–203; Power-Kean et al. (2023), pp. 331, 670–673; Tyerman & Cobbett (2023), pp. 751–762, 899.

Answer 27.3

The client is at highest risk of developing **anaphylaxis** and **respiratory distress** as evidenced by **respiratory assessment**.

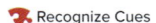

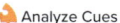

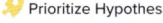

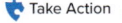

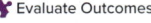

Rationale: The client has an allergy to penicillin and was given amoxicillin in error. This resulted in an allergic response that has the potential to develop into anaphylactic shock and respiratory distress. The respiratory assessment indicates increased work of breathing (retractions), impaired gas exchange (cyanosis and pale in colour, low pulse oximetry), and increased respiratory rate. The client is not at risk for dysrhythmias as there is no indication of an electrolyte imbalance and, currently, the client presents tachycardic but in a regular rhythm. The client is not at risk for a stroke as there is no indication of a clot being present or causative factor for a stroke. The client is not at risk for renal failure as the client continues to have a blood pressure, albeit low.

NCJMM Step: Prioritize Hypothesis
References: Keatings & Adams (2024), pp. 188–203; Power-Kean et al. (2023), pp. 331, 627, 670–673; Tyerman & Cobbett (2023), pp. 258–260, 264, 1734.

Answer 27.4

POTENTIAL NURSING INTERVENTIONS	INDICATED	NOT INDICATED
Request an order to administer a bronchodilator	✔	○
Prepare an emergency kit with epinephrine	✔	○
Encourage oral fluids	○	✔
Reposition client in high Fowler's position	○	✔
Request an order to administer oxygen	✔	○
Prepare to insert a peripheral venous access device	✔	○

Rationale: A bronchodilator will assist with the bronchoconstriction, enabling more oxygen to be delivered for gas exchange. Preparing epinephrine for an emergency kit is indicated especially if the client decompensates to anaphylactic shock. Epinephrine is a $beta_1$ and $beta_2$ agonist which also assists with bronchodilation at lower doses. The client may aspirate if oral fluids are encouraged, leading to greater respiratory risk for the client. The client should be encouraged to find a comfortable position of their choice. High-Fowler's position can be confining and uncomfortable. The client will be anxious, thus a calm, reassuring voice can provide holistic care for the client. The client's pulse oximetry is 82% on room air. Oxygen is warranted treatment. The client did not require a peripheral venous access device in the emergency department. Inserting a peripheral venous access device would ensure prompt administration of fluids to assist with the hypotension.

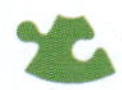
NCJMM Step: Generate Solutions
References: Keatings & Adams (2024), pp. 188–203; Tyerman & Cobbett (2023), pp. 264, 1743–1745.

Answer 27.5

- ☐ Initiate oxygen 1–10 L/min via nasal prongs or non-rebreather mask for pulse oximetry greater than 92%
- ☐ 0.9% normal saline (sodium chloride) 500 mL IV bolus × 1 then 100 mL/hr
- ☐ Insert an in-dwelling Foley catheter
- ☐ Laboratory draws: complete blood count, electrolytes, arterial blood gas (ABG), blood cultures
- ✔ Computed tomography (CT) chest
- ☐ Salbutamol sulphate 2.5 mg nebulizer q4h prn. Monitor heart rate
- ✔ Dimenhydrinate 25–50 mg PO/IV q4–6h prn

Rationale: It is important for the nurse to anticipate potential orders and to recognize orders that may need clarification or may be an error. The nurse is an advocate for client care and to ensure the delivery of safe care. The client will need to go for a chest X-ray to re-evaluate the pneumonia, which was the likely cause of the client seeking assistance; lung status post-exposure to penicillin; and the allergic response. A CT chest would be unnecessary as the client would have to lie flat for an extended period of time and it would be uncomfortable, whereas a chest X-ray is less invasive and can provide information needed to proceed with treatment. Dimenhydrinate is an incorrect medication name. The client has endured one medication error and does not need an additional error. The correct medication would be diphenhydramine, an antihistamine. All the other orders are appropriate.

NCJMM Step: Take Action
References: Keatings & Adams (2024), pp. 188–203; Sealock & Seneviratne (2025), p. 675 (dimenhydrinate); Tyerman & Cobbett (2023), pp. 264, 1743–1745.

Answer 27.6

CLIENT FINDINGS	IMPROVED	NOT CHANGED	WORSENED
Respirations 18	✔	○	○
T 38.9°C (102°F);	○	✔	○
Respiration rate to be regular	✔	○	○
Colour, pink, well perfused to mucous membranes and palms of hands	✔	○	○
No stridor noted	✔	○	○
Oxygen therapy 4 L/min	○	○	✔

Rationale: Due to a medication error, the client suffered an anaphylaxis reaction to the amoxicillin that was administered to them in error. Amoxicillin is a member of the penicillin family. After the code and based on the final nurses' note, the client's status improved with respirations, as they were breathing easily and at rest and at a reduced number of breaths; they were pink in colour whereas before, the client was pale with cyanosis; and stridor was no longer present, which indicates respiratory distress has resolved. There was no change in temperature as it had only changed by 0.2 degrees. Addition of oxygen therapy was the only client finding that indicated a worsening of clinical presentation.

NCJMM Step: Evaluate Outcomes
References: Keatings & Adams (2024), pp. 188–203; Tyerman & Cobbett (2023), pp. 264, 1743–1745.

Medical-Surgical 28.0 (Neurology)

Answer 28.1

- ☐ Pupillary response
- ✔ Shortness of breath
- ☐ Alertness
- ✔ Characteristics of pulses
- ☐ Lung sounds
- ✔ Headache
- ☐ Pulse oximetry
- ☐ Skin temperature
- ✔ Motor power
- ✔ Musculoskeletal weakness

Rationale: The client's shortness of breath is associated with the heart having to work harder with physical exertion—that is, long walks and climbing stairs. The irregular pulse and increased workload of the heart result in an inability to maintain appropriate systemic oxygenation, which is manifested by increasing the respiratory rate. An irregular heartbeat leads to the atriums and ventricles from fully expelling blood during systole either from the atrium to ventricle or right ventricle into the pulmonary system and left ventricle into the systemic circulation. All pulses remain palpable to touch, indicating appropriate perfusion. The client's persistent headache indicates a problem with the neurological circulation, as a result of either cerebrospinal fluid, edema, or vasoconstriction. The blurry vision associated with the headache is concerning. The client's right and left side motor power is abnormal as the left side indicates weakness and the right side indicates motor power as strong. Right and left side motor power should be equal, indicating equal corresponding responses from the right and left side of the brain. The musculoskeletal weakness reflects the brain not being able to send the same signals to the right and left side. There is either a dysfunction or abnormality within the brain structure, the neurological circulatory system, or the spinal system. The pupils remain the same size and shape and react to light equally on both sides. The client is alert and orientated, pleasant and cooperative. The lung sounds are clear anteriorly and posteriorly despite mild shortness of breath with increased activity. The pulse oximetry is documented at 97%, which indicates adequate gas exchange. The skin temperature is warm and dry to touch.

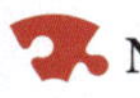

NCJMM Step: Recognize Cues
Reference: Tyerman & Cobbett (2023), pp. 1486–1492.

Answer 28.2

The nurse should recognize that the client potentially experienced a(an) **transient ischemic attack (TIA)** prior to admission as a result of untreated **atrial fibrillation**.

Rationale: The client's symptoms were brief and mostly resolved except for the motor power weakness on the right side as compared to the left side. A *transient ischemic attack (TIA)* is defined as any focal cerebral ischemic, even with symptoms lasting less than 24 hours typically; however, brain infarctions can be seen on magnetic resonance imaging (MRI) scans demonstrating lasting effects on the brain. TIAs are caused by microemboli or plaque temporarily blocking blood flow. They are a warning sign of progressive cerebrovascular disease. Stroke risk following TIA is greatest immediately after the event. Untreated atrial fibrillation is a modifiable risk factor associated with stroke. A clot can develop in the atriums and with a lack of atrial kick due to the fibrillation. If a clot forms on the left side of the heart and is ejected from the left ventricle, there is a risk of the clot travelling to the brain through the carotid artery delivering oxygenated blood to the brain. Plaque can also form in the carotid arteries as a result of atherosclerosis and break off, travelling to the brain and causing a disruption of blood flow. The client does not describe any risk factors associated with encephalopathic events, such as a recent infection, increased temperature, traumatic brain injury, or anoxic event. The client does not present with chest pain indicating an anginal event as a result of occlusion of the coronary arteries. The client's headache is a clinical manifestation of the transient ischemic event and did not cause the TIA.

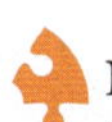

NCJMM Step: Analyze Cues
Reference: Tyerman & Cobbett (2023), pp. 1486–1492.

Answer 28.3

The client is at highest risk of developing a(an) **stroke**.

Rationale: Stroke risk following TIA is greatest immediately after the event. A TIA is a warning sign to seek further treatment and investigations. The client did not suffer a head injury based on the client presentation; therefore, a subdural hematoma is impossible. The question does not reflect subarachnoid or intracerebral hemorrhages that can occur with strokes. The client presents with clear air entry in the lungs and afebrile. The client does not have any respiratory concerns at presentation and assessment. There are no abnormal heart sounds indicating aortic stenosis or other clinical manifestations such as low cardiac output due to calcification from this progressive illnesses. The client presents with clear air entry and no evidence of jugular venous distension and peripheral edema, ruling out either left- or right-sided heart failure. The client does not present with chest pain indicative of an acute myocardial infarction.

NCJMM Step: Prioritize Hypothesis
Reference: Tyerman & Cobbett (2023), pp. 589–594 (pneumonia), 811–814 (acute myocardial infarction), 829–848 (heart failure), 887 (aortic stenosis), 1486–1492 (stroke).

Answer 28.4

- ☐ Insert a small-bore peripheral venous access device
- ☐ Nasogastric tube and attach to low suction
- ✔ Computed tomography (CT) scan of the brain
- ☐ Social work consult
- ☐ Speech-language pathology consult for swallowing assessment
- ✔ Antiplatelet medication
- ✔ Anticoagulation medication
- ☐ Culture and sensitivity (C&S) for pathogens
- ✔ Complete blood count (CBC), electrolytes, creatinine, BUN, lipid profile, fasting glucose, coagulation panel

Rationale: When a client is suspected of progression from a TIA to a stroke, a CT of the brain diagnostic test is done, which is quick and easy to complete. A result is obtained within 25 minutes and read within 45 minutes providing information about the size and location of the lesion. A CT scan of the brain will also indicate if the stroke is ischemic or hemorrhagic in nature. Administration of tissue plasminogen activator (tPA) would be irreversible and catastrophic if administered and the client had suffered a hemorrhagic stroke. There would be no way to stop the bleeding as there is no antidote for tPA. Proper anticoagulation and antiplatelet medication had not been prescribed yet as the client only just got to the neurology unit. Now that the TIA had progressed to a full stroke, antiplatelet and anticoagulation medication is warranted, especially since the cause was untreated atrial fibrillation. It is imperative to prevent the formation of further emboli extending the stroke, or the client will be at risk of experiencing another stroke. Knowing the foundational blood work before initiating treatment is important in order to verify the client's ability to clot (platelets), renal function, lipids to indicate atherosclerosis, and clotting factors. A large-bore peripheral venous access device is needed for a CT scan if contrast is provided, preferably an 18- or 20-gauge cannula. A small-bore cannula would be insufficient to administer fluids or contrast if that is warranted. The client does not require insertion of a nasogastric tube, nor is suction warranted for treatment at present. If the client cannot swallow, a swallowing assessment can be completed with a speech and language pathologist; however, acutely, the client will be placed on NPO to ensure adequate perfusion to the brain and minimize any swelling to the brain tissues. A social work consult is not warranted yet as the client has only just suffered a stroke. Follow-up will be important prior to discharge. The client does not have an infection; therefore, culture and sensitivity is not an appropriate order.

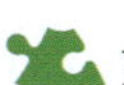
NCJMM Step: Generate Solutions
Reference: Tyerman & Cobbett (2023), pp. 1486–1492.

Answer 28.5

NURSING INTERVENTIONS	INDICATED	NOT INDICATED
Assess for presence of dysphagia	✔	○
Ensure left side of the body is supported by pillows	✔	○
Ask open-ended, multiple questions	○	✔
Place client on fluid restriction	○	✔
Monitor for Cushing's triad	✔	○
Assess client's ability to communicate, and choose best tool based on the client's ability	✔	○

Rationale: Clients who have experienced a stroke may be at risk of choking on fluids and food. Nutritional needs of all clients require prompt attention. Careful assessment of swallowing, chewing, gag reflex, and pocketing are important. Assessing for dysphagia promotes safe client care. After a stroke, clients may experience neglect syndrome, which results in decreased safety awareness. Anticipating any potential safety hazards will help protect the client from further injury as their sensory perception may be altered. Supporting the side of the body with the greatest deficits will assist with secretion drainage, ensure better gas exchange, and help with nutrition as well. Communicating with clients and meeting their needs are important. Questions should be kept simple with "yes" or "no" answers. This practice will help ensure that the client remains a part of the conversation. The client must be given time to respond to each question and not pushed to communicate. Assessing the client's ability to communicate is important if aphasia is present beyond simple questions. Communication tools are only valuable if the client has the dexterity to grasp a pen or marker. The nurse needs to assess the client's abilities before offering any communication tools. The client requires fluids for proper hydration and for cardiovascular function; fluids should not be restricted in this client. Given the client's reduced mobility, fluids will help reduce the risk of constipation and improve bowel function. After a stroke, the client is monitored for Cushing's triad (widened pulse pressure, bradycardia, and irregular respirations), which indicates increasing intracranial pressure. Post–ischemic stroke, a client may also develop bleeding in the brain.

NCJMM Step: Take Action
Reference: Tyerman & Cobbett (2023), pp. 1486–1492.

Answer 28.6

ASSESSMENT FINDINGS	IMPROVED	NO CHANGE	DECLINED
BP 130/76 mmHg	✔	○	○
Urinary incontinence requiring frequent toileting	○	○	✔
Lungs auscultated for fine inspiratory crackles that clear with cough	○	✔	○
Active bowel sounds × 4 quadrants	○	✔	○
Client presents as apathetic	○	○	✔

Rationale: The client's blood pressure has improved from the last documented pressure of 168/86 mmHg. The blood pressure must be high enough to maintain perfusion to the area but not too high to increase intracranial pressure and not too low, which limits oxygenation to the brain and tissues. The client's urinary incontinence is new and a result of the effects of the stroke. Frequent toileting may be a short-term intervention to retrain the bladder and enable the client to sense when their bladder is full. Nurses can assess a post-void residual using a bladder scanner. This will provide information as to how the bladder is emptying, reducing the possibility of a bladder infection. The lungs remain clear even after a cough. This is a positive sign, and unchanged, as the client is not aspirating, which could lead to pneumonia. Active bowel sounds remain unchanged from the last assessment, indicating the bowels are functioning normally. Assessment of the client's affect is important as clients who have had strokes often exhibit emotional responses that may or may not be appropriate. Some clients may appear apathetic, depressed, fearful, anxious, weepy, frustrated, or angry. Providing a supportive, calm environment for the client to feel and express emotions is important when atypical emotions are manifested.

NCJMM Step: Evaluate Outcomes
Reference: Tyerman & Cobbett (2023), pp. 1486–1492.

Medical-Surgical 29.0 (Endocrinology)

Answer 29.1

- ☐ Pupillary size
- ✔ Lethargy
- ☐ Motor power
- ✔ Lung sounds
- ☐ Dorsalis pedis pulses × 2
- ☐ Bowel sounds
- ✔ Nausea
- ✔ Speech pattern
- ☐ Pulse oximetry
- ☐ Anorexia

Rationale: The client's lethargy is concerning as the cause of the somnolence is unknown at the time of admission. The client's inability to remain awake even though they are being stimulated and their returning to sleep indicate the client is unable to maintain alertness, and cognitive factors will need to be investigated. The client's lung sounds of fine inspiratory crackles will need to be addressed and the fever monitored. Since the client has experienced vomiting for several days, there is a possibility the client could have aspirated stomach contents, though an inflammatory response had not begun at the time of admission. The client's nausea is concerning given the long duration of gastrointestinal illness, the lack of food, and the diabetes. Because of the client's compromised cognitive status, it is unknown at the time of admission if the client was still taking their Glucophage,. The client's speech pattern is concerning as there may be a neurological or endocrinological element that is causing the client's speech to fluctuate between clear and incoherent. The client's pupil size is equal in measurement and shape. The client's motor power is intact and strong × 4. The client's dorsalis pedis pulses are palpable and present. The client's bowel sounds are documented as hyperactive in all four quadrants. The pulse oximetry reading is documented to be above 92%, indicating adequate systemic oxygenation despite a low respiration rate. The client's lack of food is something to monitor; however, it is not an assessment finding that requires immediate attention.

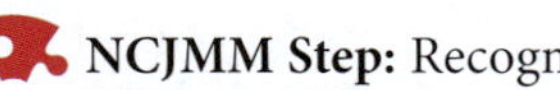
NCJMM Step: Recognize Cues
Reference: Jarvis et al. (2023), Chapter 19 (thorax and lungs), Chapter 20 (heart and neck vessels), Chapter 22 (abdomen), Chapter 25 (neurological system).

Answer 29.2

- ☐ Bowel obstruction
- ✔ Dehydration
- ☐ Heart failure
- ☐ Acute respiratory distress syndrome
- ✔ Hyperglycemia
- ✔ Hypoglycemia
- ✔ Ethanol (ETOH) intoxication

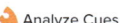

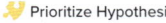

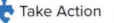

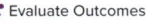

Rationale: Complications associated with 3 days of diarrhea and vomiting may be contributing to the client's dry mucous membranes and potential dehydration. At present, the blood pressure is intact and maintaining adequate cardiac output despite the cool skin temperature to touch. The nurse was unable to determine a blood glucometer reading with the portable machine indicating either too high of a blood sugar or too low of a blood sugar. Given that the client has been affected by the gastrointestinal illness for several days, the client may or may not have been taking their Glucophage. The client's speech pattern of being clear, followed by incoherent speech, could indicate an ETOH intoxication and this will need to be ruled out by further tests. The client presents with hyperactive bowel sounds in four quadrants and passing stool, eliminating the possibility of a bowel obstruction complication. The client does not present with additional heart sounds such as an S3 or previous cardiac conditions leading to complications of heart failure. The client's respiratory rate is low, not high, indicating acute respiratory distress syndrome. The client's respirations are regular and easy with no observation of indrawing or use of accessory muscles.

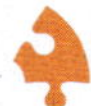

NCJMM Step: Analyze Cues
References: Goguen & Gilbert (2023); Power-Kean et al. (2023), pp. 458–459 (hyperglycemia); Tyerman & Cobbett (2023), pp. 594–595 (pneumonia), 1293–1296 (hyperglycemic emergencies), 1296–1297 (hypoglycemic emergencies).

Answer 29.3

The client is at highest risk of developing **dysrhythmias**, **hyperosmolar hyperglycemia state**, and **seizures.**

Rationale: The client's lab values indicate that the client is in a hyperosmolar hyperglycemia state as evidenced by the very high serum glucose level, which is associated with the type 2 diabetes mellitus diagnosis and the absence of ketones. If ketones were present, the client could be presenting with diabetic ketoacidosis; however, the absence of ketones eliminates this possibility. The client does not present as acidotic, which occurs with diabetic ketoacidosis due to the ketones, and the client's respiratory rate is low. A client who presents with diabetic ketoacidosis will attempt to compensate for the imbalance by increasing their respiratory rate to blow off (exhale) carbon dioxide, which is acidic. The client's hyponatremia predisposes the client to seizures, and the hypokalemia predisposes the client to dysrhythmias due to the sodium/potassium channel pump dysfunction resulting from the dehydration and the hyperactivity that occurs in the brain when there is too much or too little sodium in the blood. The client does not present with symptoms associated with stroke, hypoxemia, or renal failure, as evidenced by a normal creatinine level.

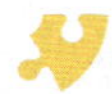

NCJMM Step: Prioritize Hypothesis
References: Power-Kean et al. (2023), pp. 120–122 (electrolyte imbalances), 458–459 (hyperglycemia), 465 (hyperosmolar hyperglycemic syndrome); Tyerman & Cobbett (2023), pp. 1293–1296 (hyperglycemic emergencies), 1296–1297 (hypoglycemic emergencies).

Answer 29.4

POTENTIAL NURSING INTREVENTIONS	INDICATED	NOT INDICATED
Monitoring intake and output	✔	○
Encourage independent mobilization	○	✔
Frequent vital signs with specific attention to blood pressure	✔	○
Prepare the client for cardiac monitoring	✔	○
Encourage oral fluid intake	○	✔
Allow the client to rest and recover with limited assessments	○	✔

Rationale: The client is at greatest risk of developing seizures, shock, coma, and death. Given the profound dehydration, the client is at risk for reduced renal perfusion leading to oliguria and even anuria. Adequate kidney perfusion is equal to 30 mL of urine production per hour or 0.5 to 1.0 mL/kg per hour if weight available. Monitoring adequate fluid resuscitation is important to minimize the risk for hypotension and hypovolemic shock. Monitoring the blood pressure frequently and, if possible, with an arterial line to accurately monitor the blood pressure will be imperative to monitor for decompensation and shock. The client is at risk for hypokalemia with the dehydration shift and initiation of intravenous insulin therapy. Cardiac monitoring is an important treatment preparation for identifying any life-threatening dysrhythmias or progression to acute myocardial infarction due to reduced systemic blood flow as a result of the profound dehydration. The client remains lethargic and rouses only with stimulation. Encouraging independent mobilization may predispose the client to falls and further injury. The client's level of consciousness and alertness may predispose the client to aspiration if the airway is not protected. The client requires frequent assessments to monitor the client's blood sugar, blood pressure, and level of consciousness. Limited assessments may cause the nurse to miss important assessment findings.

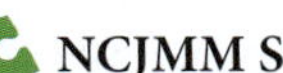

NCJMM Step: Generate Solutions
Reference: Tyerman & Cobbett (2023), pp. 1296–1297.

Answer 29.5

Orders

- 0.9% (sodium chloride) IV at 500 mL/hr × 4 hr then 250 mL × 4 hr
- Potassium chloride (KCL) 20 mmol/100 mL IV × 2 doses ASAP
- Humulin R IV as per protocol initiating at 0.1 unit/kg/hr once potassium level returns to greater than or equal to 3.3 mmol/L
- Place client on a cardiac monitor
- Insert arterial line for closer blood pressure monitoring
- Insert peripheral venous access device for additional fluid administration
- Transfer to ICU for observation and airway management
- Laboratory draws: complete blood count, electrolytes with serum glucose, creatinine, BUN, lipids, troponin q6h
- Point-of-care testing q30 min to 60 min prn
- Oxygen 2–6 L/min to maintain pulse oximetry greater than or equal to 92%

Rationale: The goal when treating clients with hyperosmolar hyperglycemia is to restore normal extracellular fluid volume and tissue perfusion, resolve ketoacidosis if present, correct electrolyte imbalances and hyperglycemia, and treat the cause. It is best for the client to be managed in a critical care area, such as an Intensive Care Unit or step-down setting for close observation. Initiating fluid hydration and restoring fluid balance is imperative to start the process of correcting glucose in the bloodstream through dilution and increasing urinary glucose loses. The preferred solution, as per Diabetes Canada, is through normal saline. The rapid rate of fluid administration with the hypertonic solution can lead to cerebral edema. Once the sodium level has returned to normal, IV solutions should be switched from 0.9% saline to 0.45% sodium chloride to replace ongoing fluid losses. The client will be monitored for cardiac dysrhythmias due to a hypokalemic state and the possibility of an acute myocardial infarction due to reduced blood flow to the myocardium. The client should also have an additional peripheral venous access device initiated for fluids and when dextrose 5% solution is started when insulin is initiated once serum potassium levels return to 3.3 mmol/L or greater. The potassium should be replaced; however, the order would need to be clarified before administering. Potassium chloride solutions can only be administered at 10 mmol/100 mL via a peripheral venous access device and 20 mmol/100 mL via a central line. The health care provider would need to determine if a central line is warranted and weigh the pros and cons of this invasive procedure. The potassium chloride can be administered at 10 mmol over 4 doses through a peripheral IV cannula. IV Humulin R will be initiated only when the serum potassium has reached a certain level. When insulin is initiated, the potassium moves into the cells, leading to further depletion of potassium levels and a higher probability of cardiac events. Careful monitoring of the potassium levels is necessary for treatment management. Transferring the client to the Intensive Care Unit will allow for proper and careful monitoring of the airway and glucose control. The health care provider will initiate the arterial line for close blood pressure monitoring. The client can have subsequent laboratory draws from the arterial line. The client does not need oxygen at the present time.

NCJMM Step: Take Action
References: Goguen & Gilbert (2023); Tyerman & Cobbett (2023), pp. 1296–1297.

Answer 29.6

ASSESSMENT FINDINGS	IMPROVED	NO CHANGE	DECLINED
Respiratory rate 26	○	○	✔
Creatinine 288 mcmol/L	○	○	✔
Urine output 35 mL/hr	✔	○	○
Heart rate 97	○	✔	○
T 38.4°C (101.1°F)	○	○	✔
Blood glucose 22 mmol/L	✔	○	○

Rationale: The client's respiratory rate has increased, which may be indicative of increased acidosis and a decline in status. An arterial blood gas should be drawn to determine if the increased respiratory rate is a compensatory mechanism or if there is another cause of the respiratory decline. A creatinine level increasing to 288 mcmol/L indicates the client has reduced kidney perfusion. Monitoring for acute renal failure after the prolonged dehydration would be important until the client's overall status improves. Urine output of 35 mL per hour is an improvement since the client had not voided at the time of admission. This indicates that the kidneys are attempting to increase perfusion, leading to oliguria instead of anuria. Careful monitoring of kidney function will be important during management of the client's condition. The client's heart rate remains unchanged. The temperature has increased, indicating there may be an underlying infection, which could be respiratory or renal in nature, given the dehydration due to the gastrointestinal virus. With fluid administration, a blood glucose of 22 mmol/L is an improvement from the admission level. The nurse will continue to monitor the potassium level, vital signs, cardiac rhythms, presence of shock, and further decompensation.

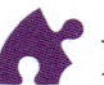

NCJMM Step: Evaluate Outcomes
Reference: Tyerman & Cobbett (2023), pp. 1296–1297.

Medical-Surgical 30.0 (Cardiovascular)

Answer 30.1

Nurses' Notes

1200h: The client was readmitted to the cardiac unit for further monitoring of chest pain. While shovelling their driveway, the client developed 8 out of 10 chest pain, as based on numerical pain scale, diaphoresis, and shortness of breath. Three years ago, the client had an acute myocardial infarction (MI) with angioplasty of the left anterior descending (LAD) coronary artery due to an 85% blockage. The ejection fraction of the left ventricle was documented to be 48% at the time of the acute MI. Client unable to remember subsequent results of their ejection fraction. The client has had no issues since the MI. Vital signs: T: 37.2°C (98.9°F); BP: 100/60; P: 105; RR: 18 at rest and 26 with speaking and ambulation; with pulse oximetry of 96% on room air. The client presents alert and oriented to person, place, and time. Obeys all commands. Motor power strong × 4 peripheral extremities. Client able to ambulate independently without any issue. Client pain free during assessment. The pain subsided en route to the hospital and has not returned since the shovelling. Jugular venous distension noted to be at 6 cm. S1 and S2 cardiac sounds auscultated with a noticeable S3. Bilateral radial pulses palpable and regular. Bilateral dorsalis pedis pulses palpable and regular. Capillary refill documented at less than 3 seconds. Skin warm and dry to touch. Dry mucous membranes noted. Coarse inspiratory crackles auscultated on anterior assessment with left lower lobe greater than right lower lobe. Client complains of shortness of breath at rest and states, "I feel like I cannot get enough oxygen when I am talking." Dry, nonproductive cough noted. Respiratory rate increases from 18 to 26 when client speaks. No diaphoresis, nausea, or emesis noted. Abdomen soft and flat with palpation, bowel sounds auscultated in all four quadrants. Urinal provided at the bedside in the event the client has to void. Client denies any issue with voiding prior to admission. Client states avoiding drinking excessively due to frequently needing to use the washroom. Denies any pain with voiding, only frequent, small amounts, and often at night. Venous access device inserted into left forearm infusing 0.9% normal saline infusing at 150 mL/hr.

Rationale: The client is presenting with respiratory compromise. The increase in respirations with exertion is concerning as that will also increase demand on the client's cardiac system. There is jugular venous distension measured at 6 cm, which indicates increased right atrial and ventricular pressures. A noticeable S3 relates to increased volume of the left ventricle, which correlates with the coarse inspiratory crackles noted in bilateral lung fields. The client notices the shortness of breath when speaking as well. There is a wet nonproductive cough that may begin to affect gas exchange at the alveoli step. When the nurse combines the information of a previous acute myocardial infarction with a stent placed in the left anterior descending coronary artery and a known ejection fraction of 48%, this leads to the strong likelihood of left ventricular compromise.

NCJMM Step: Recognize Cues
Reference: Tyerman & Cobbett (2023), pp. 811–823, 830–835.

Answer 30.2

- ✔ Oliguria
- ☐ Pneumonia
- ✔ Pulmonary edema
- ✔ Dysrhythmia
- ✔ Peripheral dependent edema
- ✔ Orthopnea
- ☐ Emesis
- ✔ Fatigue

Rationale: Oliguria is a consequence of low cardiac output, which leads to renal failure. Low cardiac output reduces perfusion in the kidney (prerenal failure) and leads to insufficiency or failure. Because of poor left ventricular function, the blood is unable to progress through the pulmonary vasculature. Clients with chronic heart failure can develop cardiomegaly or enlargement of the cardiac muscle. This condition requires greater electrical stimuli to contract the myocardial muscle. Clients are at risk of developing ventricular dysrhythmias such as ventricular tachycardia, ventricular fibrillation, and second-degree heart blocks. There is decreased venous return to the right side of the heart, which can lead to peripheral dependent edema and even ascites. Orthopnea is related to increased pressure in the pulmonary vasculature that increases when the client lies flat. A dry, nonproductive cough is one of the first clinical symptoms of heart failure. Due to decreased cardiac output, impaired perfusion, and decreased oxygenation to the tissue, fatigue is associated with heart failure. This client is not at risk of developing pneumonia as there are no bacteria in the alveoli. This client is not at risk of developing emesis. They may feel bloated or nauseated as a result of retention of fluid but not present with emesis.

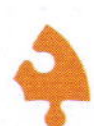
NCJMM Step: Recognize Cues
Reference: Tyerman & Cobbett (2023), pp. 830–835.

Answer 30.3

The client is at highest risk of developing **heart failure** as evidenced by the **respiratory assessment** and **cardiovascular assessment.**

Rationale: The client presents with volume overload due to the initial rate of the continuous intravenous fluid infusion. The client went into heart failure as a result of the increased volume leading to difficulty breathing as evidenced by the increased jugular venous distension, coarse crackles, worsening dry, nonproductive cough, and dyspnea. The client does not have anemia as there is adequate blood pressure and no indication of blood loss from a chronic condition. The client does not present with pulmonary hypertension as this would indicate reduced breath sounds and increased right-sided heart pressures, not crackles. The client does not have a pneumothorax as there is no sign of trauma or tracheal deviation, and shovelling snow would not lead to a pneumothorax with this client. The client is not dehydrated given a normal blood pressure.

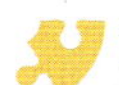
NCJMM Step: Prioritize Hypothesis
Reference: Tyerman & Cobbett (2023), pp. 830–835.

Answer 30.4

POTENTIAL NURSING INTERVENTIONS	INDICATED	NOT INDICATED
Request an order to administer a diuretic	✔	○
Request an order to administer a 500-mL bolus of an isotonic solution	○	✔
Request an order to draw electrolytes, BNP, creatinine, BUN	✔	○
Discontinue continuous intravenous fluid infusion	✔	○
Request an order to insert a Foley catheter	○	✔
Place the client on fluid restriction	✔	○

Rationale: Potential nursing interventions would include discontinuing the continuous intravenous fluid infusion, administering a diuretic (likely a loop diuretic for acute events and thiazide for chronic heart failure), drawing labs, and placing the client on fluid restriction (1.5 L per day). The plan would be to remove the workload of the heart in this situation for the client. A bolus of fluid would only cause a decline in the client's status, adding more volume to the clinical presentation. Electrolytes, brain natriuretic peptide (BNP), which is released with heart failure, and renal blood work are important to draw as a baseline. There is no indication the client requires a Foley catheter. A urinal would be the most appropriate drainage device.

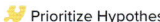

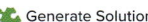

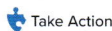

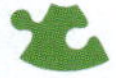
NCJMM Step: Generate Solutions
Reference: Tyerman & Cobbett (2023), pp. 830–835.

Answer 30.5

- ✔ Chest X-ray
- ☐ Arterial blood gas
- ☐ Continuous cardiac monitoring
- ☐ External pacemaker
- ✔ Echocardiogram

Rationale: Clients with heart failure would be ordered a chest X-ray to identify the amount of lung tissue affected by the additional volume in the circulatory system and an echocardiogram to identify if the ejection fraction of the left ventricle has been affected. An arterial blood gas would only be appropriate if the client required intubation or decompensated further even after pharmacological treatment (a loop diuretic such as furosemide). This client does not require continuous cardiac monitoring—only if the client's electrolytes demonstrate cardiomyopathy or hyperkalemia or hypokalemia. An external pacemaker is not appropriate since the client has a regular rhythm.

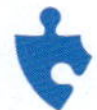
NCJMM Step: Take Action
Reference: Tyerman & Cobbett (2023), pp. 830–848.

Answer 30.6

ASSESSMENT FINDINGS	IMPROVED	NO CHANGE	DECLINED
BP 92/58 mmHg	○	○	✔
Urine output 200 mL	✔	○	○
ECG showing normal sinus rhythm	✔	○	○
Pulse oximetry measured at 92% on room air	○	✔	○
Respiratory rate 16	✔	○	○

Rationale: The client's blood pressure has decreased and declined. When there is diuresis, as evidenced by the urine output of 200 mL, which is an improvement, the blood pressure tends to drop slightly. This would need to be monitored. The electrocardiogram (ECG) shows normal sinus rhythm, which is an improvement from the tachycardia the client experienced previously. The increased heart rate indicated a sympathetic nervous system response and increased work of the heart. The client's pulse oximetry reading has not changed. The client's respiratory rate is an improvement, indicating that the diuretic has helped the client's respiratory status.

NCJMM Step: Evaluate Outcomes
Reference: Tyerman & Cobbett (2023), p. 830–848.

Medical-Surgical 31.0 (Neurology)

Answer 31.1

The top 4 findings include pupillary response, vertigo, nausea, and postauricular ecchymosis.

Rationale: Pupils are to react briskly to light. A sluggish response indicates that the client is taking either opioid medication or other street drugs; there is dysfunction of the cranial nerve and damage to the occipital area of the brain with the start of swelling in the brain. Vertigo indicates a dysfunction of the vestibular apparatus in the ear or in the vestibular nuclei in the brainstem. The gastrointestinal symptom of nausea could be accompanying the vertigo; however, nausea related to a neurological condition could indicate changes in status for a client and should be monitored. Postauricular ecchymosis is bruising noted behind the ears. This is also called a *battle sign* and indicative of a basal skull fracture. Otorrhea also accompanies a battle sign. Monitoring for bleeding in the brain is important nursing practice here. The pulses do not require immediate follow-up because bilateral radial and dorsalis pedis pulses are palpable but they should be monitored. The lung sounds are clear with auscultation and do not require immediate attention. The client has bowel sounds present.

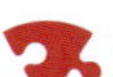
NCJMM Step: Recognize Cues
References: Jarvis et al. (2024), pp. 317–320, 708–716; Tyerman & Cobbett (2023), pp. 1465–1472.

Answer 31.2

- ☐ Blindness
- ✔ Changes in consciousness
- ☐ Pulmonary edema
- ✔ Increased cerebral pressure
- ☐ Deafness
- ☐ Hydrocephalus
- ✔ Bleeding

Rationale: With a neurological injury, any changes in levels of consciousness or pupillary responses indicate a change in status that requires further assessment. The client could become lethargic, obtunded, or even progress to a coma. Since the client hit their head on both the occipital and lateral sides, increased cerebral and cranial pressure could be a significant complication. The skull is a fixed object with limited available space for swelling and increased fluids to shift. Increased cerebral pressure is a normal inflammatory response to injury. The client is at risk of bleeding within the brain structure. There is no way to visualize the degree of lacerations or sheering forces that may have occurred by striking the head on a concrete surface. The client may have altered vision with a head injury but will not develop blindness. The client's lungs are clear and present without any respiratory issues or comorbidities; therefore, pulmonary edema will not occur. Given the location of the injury and the high likelihood of a basilar skull fracture, the client may experience tinnitus but not deafness. The client will not experience an overproduction of cerebrospinal fluid due to an obstruction. There will likely be more blood volume in the brain than cerebrospinal fluid.

NCJMM Step: Analyze Cues
References: Power-Kean et al. (2023), pp. 383–387; Tyerman & Cobbett (2023), pp. 1465–1472.

Answer 31.3

The client is at highest risk of developing **intracranial pressure** as evidenced by the client's **level of consciousness** and **emesis**.

Rationale: The clinical signs of the postauricular ecchymosis on the right side indicate a basilar skull fracture, which coincides with the narrative of the client hitting their head on the occipital and lateral right sides. Since the client has been in the emergency department their clinical status has changed. The new findings indicate increased pressure within the brain from a basilar skull fracture. The change in status with decreased level of consciousness and now emesis indicates a change in intracranial pressure. Based on the reports from friends, it is difficult to assess if the client lost consciousness. The nausea and now vomiting indicate increased pressure on the medulla oblongata in the brain. Abrupt vomiting is concerning and requires monitoring. Any changes in level of consciousness indicate increased neurological injuries and are a hallmark sign of change in status for any client. The client progressed from alert and oriented with some memory issues to somnolent, lethargic, and slurred speech. The Glasgow Coma Scale worsened from 13 to 11. The client's increased blood pressure may represent a change in pressure within the brain, but the change in level of consciousness and now emesis are more indicative of increasing pressure within the brain. The other vital signs are not indicative of any changes in status. The client's risk for stroke is low as the pupils remain equal in size and still sluggish. Traumatic encephalopathy is a chronic condition due to repeated concussions. Although the client has a headache that has gotten worse and there is emesis and they hit their head, there are greater risks associated with the client's change in status than to a migraine. The client does not present with a fever indicative of meningitis.

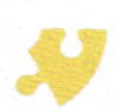

NCJMM Step: Prioritize Hypothesis
References: Power-Kean et al. (2023), pp. 383–387; Tyerman & Cobbett (2023), pp. 1465–1472.

Answer 31.4

POTENTIAL NURSING INTERVENTIONS	INDICATED	NOT INDICATED
Assess neurological vital signs every 8 hours	○	✔
Prepare to insert two large-bore peripheral venous access devices	✔	○
Position the head of the bed in the lowest position for comfort	○	✔
Keep the lights dimmed	✔	○
Regulate and keep number of visitors at a minimum	✔	○
Prepare bolus intravenous fluids	○	✔
Prevent shivering by keeping environment temperature comfortable	✔	○

Rationale: Managing a client with increased intracranial pressure requires careful monitoring and prompt attention to any changes as they could happen quickly. Assessment of neurological vitals would be more frequent than every 8 hours and may be every hour with the change in status, to minimize the risk of increasing intracranial pressure from the basal skull fracture. Monitoring for change in Glasgow Coma Scale, level of consciousness, and pupillary changes is important as these would be first signs of neurological changes. The client may require fluids AND diuretics to help reduce pressure within the brain tissue. Preparing to insert two large-bore peripheral venous access devices would be necessary for safety, especially with a client who is experiencing changes in status. The head of the bed should remain elevated to approximately 30 degrees and not be in a lowered position. Elevation will help reduce sagittal sinus pressure, promote venous drainage from the head, and decrease vascular congestion that can increase cerebral edema. Clients can benefit from a quiet, nonstimulating environment, which includes keeping the lights dimmed and reducing noise in the client's room by limiting the number of visitors. Bolus of intravenous fluids may be contraindicated as this would increase the volume in the brain. Adequate hydration is tempered with minimizing fluids to maintain intravascular volume and adequate cerebral perfusion. The room temperature should be kept warm and comfortable. A shivering client will increase their metabolic rate and experience increased cerebral pressure.

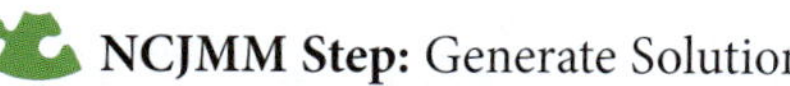

NCJMM Step: Generate Solutions
Reference: Tyerman & Cobbett (2023), pp. 1462–1465, 1470–1472.

Answer 31.5

Orders

- Initiate 3% normal saline (sodium chloride) at 0.5 mL/kg/hr
- Ondansetron 4–8 mg IV q12h prn
- Pantoprazole 40 mg IV od
- Head of the bed (HOB) to remain 30 degrees
- Insert an in-dwelling urethral catheter
- Computed tomography (CT) scan of the head to be completed without contrast
- Neuro vitals q1h × 4 hr and if stable q2h × 4 hr
- Draw arterial blood gas (ABG) now
- Laboratory draws: complete blood count, electrolytes, BUN, creatinine, liver function tests, INR, PTT
- Monitor intake and output.
- Blood glucose monitoring q4h
- Sequential compression devices to be applied while client is immobile

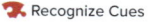

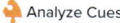

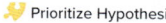

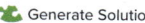

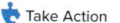

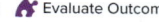

Rationale: Nonsurgical intervention includes the reduction of tissue volume related to cerebral tissue swelling and cerebral edema by using osmotic diuretics (if needed) and hypertonic solution. The 3% normal saline is a hypertonic solution that will reduce swelling and improve cerebral blood flow by drawing water out of the brain tissue. Infusions cannot be administered quickly as this can precipitate increased blood volume. Hypertonic solutions are a first-line treatment when compared with mannitol. Ondansetron will help reduce nausea and emesis. The retching would increase intracranial pressure. The client's status changed, and diuretics are not required at the moment. The head of the bed should remain at a 30-degree angle to assist with reducing venous pressure and with drainage. Finally, sequential compression devices would minimize the risk of a clot forming without administering an anticoagulant since the client suffered a head injury. Minimizing additional risk for bleeding in the brain would be taken. All other medications and tests would be necessary to minimize gastrointestinal bleeding until the client is able to tolerate food or a nasogastric tube. The in-dwelling catheter would prevent the client from moving too much and assist with obtaining accurate intake and output data. A CT head would be an appropriate diagnostic test to review the swelling in the brain if the client could tolerate the movement. All other laboratory draws and an ABG would provide information about oxygenation needs and foundational laboratory values.

NCJMM Step: Take Action
References: Sealock & Seneviratne (2025), pp. 651 (pantoprazole), 676 (ondansetron); Tyerman & Cobbett (2023), pp. 1462–1465, 1470–1472.

Answer 31.6

ASSESSMENT FINDINGS	IMPROVED	NO CHANGE	DECLINED
Pupils equal and briskly reactive to light at 2 mm	○	✔	○
Nausea only, no emesis	✔	○	○
Left lower leg increased edema and calf pain	○	○	✔
Negative 250 mL shift fluid balance	✔	○	○
RR 18	✔	○	○

Rationale: The client's pupils remain unchanged as per the previous assessment. No change in pupillary response and size remains positive as no further neurological complications have occurred. The client continues to be nauseated but has no further emesis, which is an improvement in the status. The left lower leg edema and calf pain could be indicative of a clot developing despite sequential compression devices (SCDs) being used. Without the use of an anticoagulant, which may increase bleeding, the SCDs may not be adequate enough to prevent clots from forming in the venous system. A negative shift in fluid balance indicates an improvement in reducing blood volume. If the client's overall status is improving and the kidneys are perfusing additional fluid, then there is a reduction in intracranial pressure. The client's respiratory rate has decreased as well, indicating improved respiratory effort.

NCJMM Step: Evaluate Outcomes
Reference: Tyerman & Cobbett (2023), pp. 1462–1465, 1470–1472.

Medical-Surgical 32.0 (Gastrointestinal)

Answer 32.1

Nurses' Notes | **Medications**

1752h: The client presents to the emergency department with sharp abdominal pain located in left lower quadrant, and right lower quadrant rated 6 out of 10 on a numerical pain scale along with extreme nausea and inability to keep any fluids down × 2 days. The client began semaglutide for weight loss × 3 weeks ago, taking the medication as prescribed, but reports having no bowel movement × 5 days with no flatus × 3 days. The client states the pain is nonradiating and intermittent throughout the night. Vital signs: T: 38.1°C (100.5°F); BP: 133/89; P: 114; RR: 18; with pulse oximetry of 99% on room air. Client presents as pleasant, cooperative, alert and orientated to person, place, and time. Gait steady, denies any dizziness. Bilateral pupils equal in size and shape measured at 3 mm and briskly reactive to light. Motor power strong × 4. S1 and S2 heart sounds, apical heart rate regular and equals radial pulse. Bilateral radial pulses and bilateral dorsalis pedis pulses palpable and regular. Skin warm to touch with mild diaphoresis noted due to abdominal pain. Client noted to be taking small, shallow breaths. Colour remains appropriate with no cyanosis noted. Capillary refill less than 3 seconds. No complaints of shortness of breath from the client. Hypoactive bowel sounds identified in bilateral upper quadrants and absent bowel sounds identified in bilateral lower abdominal quadrants with persistent eructation. Abdomen rounded and firm to touch. Tympany noted × 4 quadrants of the abdomen with mild percussion. Complaints of increased pain at 8 out of 10 with percussion. Client states feeling bloated and full despite reduced nutritional intake. Client denies difficulty voiding, no pain, but due to reduced fluid intake, voiding approximately 3 × per day for small amounts.

Rationale: The client is presenting with reduced fluid and nutritional intake and concerning gastrointestinal symptoms. The client reports no bowel movement × 5 days and loss of flatus with persistent eructation. This symptom presentation indicates the client has reduced mobility in the small and large intestine associated with increased gas in the abdominal cavity evidenced by the tympany. The abdomen is distended and uncomfortable for the client, resulting in small, shallow breaths, despite the client not reporting shortness of breath. The client is also experiencing increasing pain with mild percussion. The client complains of feeling bloated and full despite reduced nutritional intake, and hypoactive bowel sounds indicate the intestinal tract is filled with gas, delayed gastric emptying, and constipation.

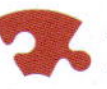

NCJMM Step: Recognize Cues
Reference: Tyerman & Cobbett (2023), pp. 1040–1043.

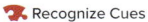

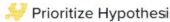

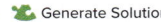

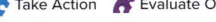

Answer 32.2

- ✔ Dehydration
- ☐ Irregular heart rate
- ☐ Reduced perfusion to the brain
- ✔ Anal fissures
- ✔ Hemorrhoids
- ☐ *Clostridium difficile*

Rationale: Complications the client may present with include dehydration, anal fissures, and hemorrhoids. At the moment, the client presents with an appropriate blood pressure and urine output, ensuring there is adequate cardiac output at the time of the assessment. Monitoring mucous membranes, urine output, fluid balance, vital signs, and electrolyte lab values throughout the hospital stay will assist with determining if the client develops dehydration. A client who has not had a bowel movement over several days may develop hard, constipated stool leading to anal fissures and hemorrhoids as the stool moves down the colon and can tear the anal mucosa when the client is having a bowel movement. The client presents with a regular heart rate. An irregular heart rate would be related to electrolyte imbalance or a previous cardiac issue. The client presents with increased weight gain as the only comorbidity. The primary issue is gastrointestinal, not neurological. Limited perfusion to the brain would not be associated with no bowel movement. The client is not at risk of developing infection with *Clostridium difficile*.

NCJMM Step: Analyze Cues
Reference: Tyerman & Cobbett (2023), pp. 1040–1043.

Answer 32.3

The client is at highest risk of developing **bowel obstruction** as evidenced by **absent bowel sounds**.

Rationale: The client's status has progressed from constipation only to a full bowel obstruction. Initially there were bowel sounds in the upper quadrants; now the abdominal pain has increased, with increased eructation, no flatus, increased blood pressure, and firm and round abdomen. The client continues to void, which indicates oliguria, not anuria with no indication of renal failure. There were no changes in the cardiovascular assessment, indicating a regular heartbeat, ruling out a dysrhythmia. A client who attempts to have a bowel movement may stimulate the Valsalva nerve, leading to bradycardia and even cardiac arrest. This client does not exhibit these concerns. The client has a poor appetite due to reduced nutritional intake; however, the cause is likely the semaglutide for weight loss since the symptoms began within the window of when adverse events, such as gastroparesis, can occur with these clients. The client is tachypneic due to the large abdomen, which is likely pushing up on their diaphragm, but the client is not hypoxemic since their pulse oximetry reading is greater than 92%. The client continues to have adequate gas exchange. Classic manifestations of a bowel obstruction include constipation, vomiting (may be foul-smelling and orange-brown in colour consistent with either fecal material or bacterial overgrowth), absent bowel signs, eructation, and no flatus.

NCJMM Step: Prioritize Hypothesis
Reference: Tyerman & Cobbett (2023), pp. 1040–1043.

Answer 32.4

POTENTIAL ORDERS	INDICATED	NOT INDICATED
Consult general surgery	✔	○
Insert a nasogastric tube and attach to low suction	✔	○
Transport the client to obtain a chest X-ray	○	✔
Laboratory tests: complete blood count, serum electrolytes, amylase, creatinine, and BUN	✔	○
Insert an in-dwelling Foley catheter	✔	○
Intravenous fluids: dextrose 5% and water preferred solution	○	✔

Rationale: Anticipating consulting of general surgery early in the progression of symptoms is a priority given the client's temperature increase. A client's temperature rise above 37.8°C (100.4°F) may indicate bowel strangulation or peritonitis leading to a bowel perforation or ischemic gut. A nasogastric tube will aid in the release of gastric gases and help relieve the nausea caused by stasis of stomach contents. Low suction of stomach contents will assist with prevention of further emesis and the possibility of aspiration. The client would be ordered a computed tomography (CT) abdomen and X-rays of the abdomen, not a chest X-ray. The client does not have anything concerning about their lungs at the present time. These laboratory tests would all be appropriate. An elevated white blood cell count may indicate an infective process is occurring related to bowel strangulation, peritonitis, perforation, or gut ischemia. Hemoglobin may indicate bleeding. Serum sodium, potassium, and chloride are decreased with bowel obstructions. An in-dwelling Foley catheter may be used for fluid monitoring as well as determining if intra-abdominal pressure is increasing or decreasing depending on the client's clinical manifestations. The client would be ordered normal saline 0.9% (sodium chloride) with potassium added to maintain fluid and electrolyte balance.

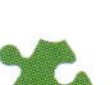
NCJMM Step: Generate Solutions
Reference: Tyerman & Cobbett (2023), pp. 1061–1063.

Answer 32.5

- ✔ Encourage deep breathing and coughing
- ☐ Administer oxycodone/acetaminophen for pain control
- ✔ Monitor for muscle guarding
- ✔ Insert two peripheral venous access devices
- ☐ Initiate bowel protocol

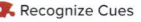

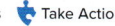

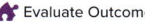

Rationale: Given the client's abdominal distension and tachypnea, ensuring deep breathing and coughing will help prevent nosocomial pneumonia. It is important to monitor for muscle guarding as this occurs with bowel strangulation and peritonitis. Inserting two peripheral venous access devices will assist with fluid management, replace electrolyte losses, and be available if packed red cells are required if the client starts to bleed. Although pain management is necessary for good client care, administration of an opioid such as oxycodone may further delay gastric emptying, resulting in further paralysis of the intestine. Administration of pain medication that does not slow down the intestine would be a better choice such, as a fentanyl patch if the pain is severe enough or nonsteroidal anti-inflammatory drugs (NSAIDs). The client does not need a bowel protocol to begin now but after their status has improved. Adequate bowel protocol, introduction of fibre into the diet, and proper hydration may be necessary topics for teaching. Overall goals are to relieve the obstruction and return bowel function to normal, reach minimal to no discomfort, have normal fluid and electrolyte status, and maintain adequate nutrition.

NCJMM Step: Take Action
Reference: Tyerman & Cobbett (2023), pp. 1061–1063.

Answer 32.6

ASSESSMENT FINDINGS	IMPROVED	NO CHANGE	DECLINED
Stoma brick red in colour postoperatively	○	○	✔
Urine output of 500 mL	✔	○	○
T: 37.7°C (99.8°F)	✔	○	○
Distended abdomen	○	✔	○
Fatigue	○	✔	○

Rationale: Postoperative care should focus on the stoma, protecting the skin and the stoma, selecting the pouch, providing client education on ostomy self-care, and assisting the client to adapt psychologically to a changed body. A new ileostomy is a decline in status that will improve the client's health overall. A brick red stoma with mild edema is an expected finding in the initial postoperative period. This indicates that the stoma is viable with a normal inflammatory process occurring. The client's urine output is an improvement. Orders would have been received at 2200h. This notation does not account for intake of fluid amount; however, over the nearly 7-hour period, the client would have voided approximately 71 mL per hour, indicating adequate perfusion to the kidneys. The temperature has improved considerably over the time of admission and intervention. Monitoring the temperature for a fever postoperatively will be a priority. The abdomen remains distended but is now soft. These are two different characteristics that describe the abdomen. The abdomen remains distended until the gas is relieved in the abdominal cavity. The fact that it is softer than in the previous assessment is an improvement. The client's fatigue is unchanged given all that they have endured in these past few days.

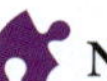
NCJMM Step: Evaluate Outcomes
References: Cobbett (2025), Chapter 45; Tyerman & Cobbett (2023), pp. 1061–106, 1070–1073.

Medical-Surgical 33.0 (Cardiovascular)

Answer 33.1

- ✔ Radial pulses
- ☐ Temperature
- ☐ Lung sounds
- ✔ Edema
- ☐ Bruising
- ☐ Mobility
- ☐ Dizziness
- ✔ Skin temperature
- ☐ Bowel sounds

Rationale: The client's clinical presentation is concerning because of reduced perfusion on the left arm. At this time, it is unclear if the fall is contributing to the reduced perfusion or if there is some other cause. The left radial pulse is weaker than the right radial pulse and the skin temperature on the left arm and forearm are also cooler to touch where the left upper arm is edematous, red, and warm to touch. The client does not present with a fever. Adventitious lung sounds noted on the left lower lobe when auscultated anteriorly with right lung field remain clear. Although this is an abnormal presentation, the fluid could be dependent given the length of time the client lay on their left side. At this point of presentation, the client has no fever, no cough, and no sputum to indicate anything further than fine inspiratory crackles. The bruising noted on the left shoulder and left hip are expected given the client's fall. The client complains of being sore only, but pain is manageable. The client is able to move independently with strong motor power and movement is not concerning. The client denies dizziness. Active bowel sounds are auscultated and do not require immediate attention.

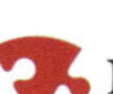
NCJMM Step: Recognize Cues
References: Jarvis et al. (2024), pp. 548–572; Tyerman & Cobbett (2023), pp. 751–794.

Answer 33.2

- ✔ Organ damage
- ✔ Limb ischemia
- ☐ Peripheral vascular disease
- ✔ Thrombosis
- ✔ Embolus
- ☐ Pleural effusions

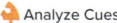

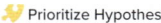

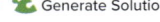

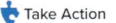

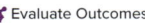

Rationale: Recognizing complications associated with poor perfusion in this client presentation is important. The client is at risk of developing organ damage, primarily kidney damage, given the length of time the client was on the ground and the potential dehydration (concentrated urine) despite perfused mucous membranes. Monitoring electrolytes, creatinine, and BUN serum levels and urine output will determine if kidney function is at risk. The client is at risk of developing limb ischemia given that the left arm and hand are cooler to touch and there is a difference in pulse pressure as compared to that in the other extremities. The client is at risk for a thrombosis, which is a clot in the vessel, given the amount of time the client was lying on the floor, their age, and the bruising around the shoulder and left hip. The client is also at risk of developing an embolus given the age of the client and the high likelihood of static blood flow due to the fall. Monitoring for pulmonary symptoms associated with an embolus will be important. Peripheral vascular disease is a chronic illness associated with reduced perfusion over time. This is an acute presentation, not a chronic presentation. The crackles auscultated are associated with settled fluid in the lungs, not fluid in the pleural cavity, therefore, limiting a complication of pleural effusions.

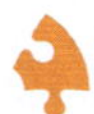
NCJMM Step: Analyze Cues
References: Jarvis et al. (2024), pp. 548–572; Tyerman & Cobbett (2023), pp. 751–794.

Answer 33.3

The client is at highest risk of developing **deep vein thrombosis**.

Rationale: The client is presenting with classic deep vein thrombosis (also known as a *venous thromboembolism*) of the left arm with clinical manifestations of Virchow's triad (hypercoagulability, venous stasis, and endothelial damage). The client presents after a fall leaving their left side of the body with clinical manifestations associated with reduced perfusion due to endothelial damage. They lay on the floor for an extended period of time, resulting in venous stasis, and they require platelets be delivered to the area in the event of bleeding increasing the potential for a clot to form. Symptoms that require immediate attention are the reduced pulses and difference in skin temperature on the left arm and hand and body soreness on the left side of the body. The client does not have any indication of a respiratory infection (afebrile) or signs of respiratory distress. The client presents with a regular rhythm and urine output. There is no indication of dysrhythmias or shortness of breath. The client's pulse oximetry is adequate at 97%, eliminating the possibility of hypoxemia. The client has active bowel sounds in all four quadrants, ruling out a bowel obstruction.

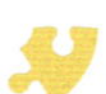
NCJMM Step: Prioritize Hypothesis
References: Jarvis et al. (2024), pp. 548–572; Tyerman & Cobbett (2023), pp. 898–928.

Answer 33.4

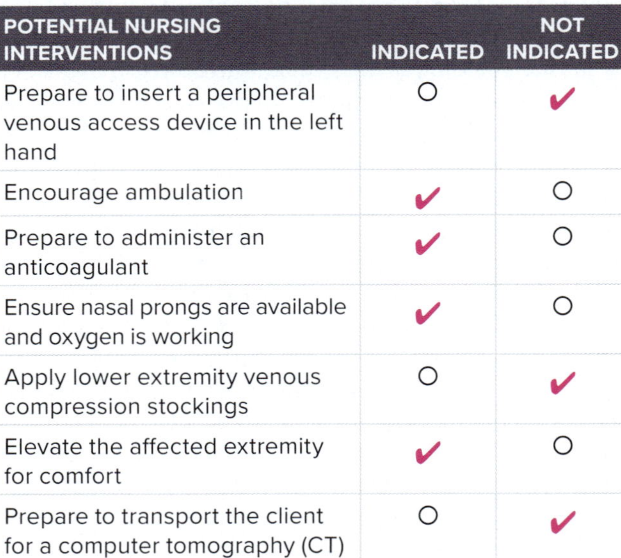

POTENTIAL NURSING INTERVENTIONS	INDICATED	NOT INDICATED
Prepare to insert a peripheral venous access device in the left hand	○	✔
Encourage ambulation	✔	○
Prepare to administer an anticoagulant	✔	○
Ensure nasal prongs are available and oxygen is working	✔	○
Apply lower extremity venous compression stockings	○	✔
Elevate the affected extremity for comfort	✔	○
Prepare to transport the client for a computer tomography (CT) chest	○	✔

Rationale: A peripheral venous access device will be necessary to administer fluids and may be required to administer anticoagulant by intravenous route. However, it is best to avoid using the arm that has the clot in the vasculature. Inserting a peripheral venous access device in the right arm is best practice, starting at the lowest point and moving up the arm. Encouraging ambulation, even moving from the bed to the chair and short distances to the washroom, will help prevent other clots from developing. An anticoagulant is also effective treatment in preventing other clots from forming. In the event the thrombus becomes an embolus, oxygen may be necessary if the embolus travels to the lung, obstructing pulmonary blood flow in the vasculature. Wearing venous compression stockings is a great idea; however, the clot has already formed in the arm due to the fall. A sequential compression device may be more comfortable for the client than wearing venous compression stockings. Pain management is a nursing priority. Elevating the affected extremity is a nonpharmacological intervention to begin managing the pain and improving blood flow. The client will not be transferred for a CT chest but could have a Doppler ultrasound of the left arm. If the client is suspected of developing a pulmonary embolus, then a spiral computed tomography (CT) could be used to assess the lungs.

NCJMM Step: Generate Solutions
Reference: Tyerman & Cobbett (2023), pp. 914–922.

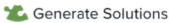

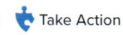

Answer 33.5

- Initiate heparin IV as per protocol with laboratory draw for INR and PTT 6 hr after starting therapy
- Venous Doppler ultrasound of the left upper arm
- Acetaminophen 500–1 000 mg PO q4–6h prn
- Laboratory tests: complete blood count, liver function tests, creatinine, BUN, and D-dimer
- Encourage oral fluids
- Regular diet
- Apply sequential compression devices to lower extremities while client is in bed

Rationale: Primary goals for care of a client with a clot is pain relief, anticoagulant therapy to prevent formation of other clots and reduce risk for a pulmonary embolus, and ambulation. There are several forms of anticoagulant therapy that could be ordered for a client and are dependent on the client presentation. This client experienced a trauma, a fall, and a clot forming due to venous stasis. Heparin via intravenous therapy is a good choice given the client's age and speed of the clinical presentation. Heparin has a short half-life and can be discontinued with quick effect. Other anticoagulants such as warfarin, dabigatran, apixaban, and rivaroxaban are oral and if bleeding is a risk, they have longer half-lives and could be an issue for an older adult. Heparin could also be administered as a low-molecular-weight heparin and administered subcutaneously. This route is prescribed for prophylaxis and low-risk deep vein thrombosis therapy. A venous Doppler ultrasound would confirm the location and size of the clot in the left arm. This would provide baseline assessment information and ability to monitor the reduction or increase in size of the clot. Pain management is necessary because of the venous congestion and inflammation of the tissues. Nonsteroidal anti-inflammatory drugs (NSAIDs), Aspirin, fish oil, supplements, garlic supplements, *Ginkgo biloba*, and certain antibiotics should be avoided as they can increase the risk of bleeding. All other orders would be important to assess baseline information for laboratory values and hydration since the client is able to take fluids and food by mouth. Use of sequential compression devices would help prevent clots from forming in the lower extremities and, given the age of the client, be necessary until heparin begins to take effect.

NCJMM Step: Take Action
Reference: Tyerman & Cobbett (2023), pp. 914–922.

Answer 33.6

CLIENT STATEMENTS	UNDER-STANDING	NO UNDER-STANDING
"I should avoid blowing my nose forcefully."	✔	○
"It is best to stay in bed and rest."	○	✔
"I need to stop drinking so much water."	○	✔
"I should watch not to bump into anything."	✔	○
"I will call for help if I notice any bleeding or bruising."	✔	○

Rationale: Providing client teaching when anticoagulant therapy has been prescribed is important nursing care. If the client is cognitively intact, the nurse will educate the client about the risk for bleeding and ways to reduce the risk for bleeding. The client should avoid blowing their nose forcefully and be careful with shaving or brushing their teeth. The client is encouraged to ambulate and should ambulate several times a day. This will help with prevention of additional clots, improve venous blood flow, and help with discomfort associated with a thromboembolism. If there are no contraindications for oral intake (i.e., heart failure and fluid restriction), a client should be encouraged to drink fluids, eat fruit, and, if necessary, take stool softeners to prevent constipation and hard stools that could tear the anal mucosa due to straining. Instructing the client to be careful and avoid further injury will minimize bleeding risk, especially for an older adult. Instructing the client to monitor for additional bleeding or bruising incorporates the client into their own care.

NCJMM Step: Evaluate Outcomes
Reference: Tyerman & Cobbett (2023), pp. 914–922.

Medical-Surgical 34.0 (Musculoskeletal)

Answer 34.1

- ✔ Pedal pulse characteristics
- ☐ Temperature
- ☐ Blood pressure
- ☐ Heart rate
- ☐ Lung sounds
- ✔ Peripheral edema
- ✔ Vertigo
- ✔ Skin temperature characteristics

Rationale: The client is presenting with symptoms associated with perfusion. Symptoms that require immediate attention involve the difference between right and left pedal pulses. The foot that is below the site of injury is displaying slower perfusion, putting the client at risk for further complications. Edema is a normal process for inflammation; however, the client's discrepancy between the right and left lower extremity and foot requires immediate attention. Increased swelling will compress the vasculature further, exacerbating reduced perfusion. The client's vertigo when the head of bed is raised indicates orthostatic hypotension, which could put the client at risk for injury. The difference in skin temperature for bilateral lower extremities is also another indication of reduced perfusion. The client does not have any infection; therefore, the temperature is not a concern, the heart rate and blood pressure are appropriate given the injury, and the lung fields are clear on auscultation.

NCJMM Step: Recognize Cues
References: Jarvis et al. (2024), pp. 548–572; Tyerman & Cobbett (2023), pp. 915–922.

Answer 34.2

✔ Headache
✔ Anxiety
✔ Impaired motor function
☐ Ventilation/perfusion mismatching
✔ Increased pain
☐ Increased preload
☐ Normal capillary refill

Rationale: The client's blood pressure is elevated due to the injury despite the client tolerating the pain well. Monitoring a cardiovascular response will be important for managing additional symptoms. The client may develop increased anxiety from reduced mobility and bed rest requests. Ensuring holistic stimulation to meet the client's needs will be important. Given the altered perfusion as already indicated by the clinical manifestations, the client may develop impaired motor function of the injured extremity. Assessing colour, sensation, warmth, and movement (CSWM) will provide data for improvement or decline in status. The client is also at risk for increased pain. Managing the pain threshold so the level remains manageable is important for client care. The client has clear air-entry throughout all lung fields and, at present, is not at risk for ventilation/perfusion mismatching, which could be associated with pneumonia. The client would experience a decrease in preload given the increased peripheral edema and reduced perfusion. This would in turn increase the workload of the heart. The client would likely experience a delayed capillary refill, greater than 3 seconds, further indicating reduced perfusion.

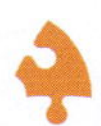

NCJMM Step: Analyze Cues
References: Jarvis et al. (2024), pp. 548–572; Tyerman & Cobbett (2023), pp. 915–922.

Answer 34.3

The client is at highest risk of developing **compartment syndrome**.

Rationale: The client's overall status has changed quickly, leading to a higher acute situation than initially presented in the morning assessment. The client's symptoms progressed to compartment syndrome as indicated by increased pain distal to the injury, increased pressure in the compartment, numbness and tingling, pallor, coolness of the skin distal to the injury, paralysis or loss of function of the extremity, and pulselessness or diminished or absent peripheral pulses. These six P's are the difference between compartment syndrome and the possibility of a deep vein thrombosis. The client presented with clinical manifestations of deep vein thrombosis with poor perfusion, weak pulse, and peripheral edema of the injured extremity and initially presented with two out of three qualities of Virchow's triad (venous stasis, endothelial damage, and, finally, hypercoagulability in the lab values taken at 0800h): a crushing leg injury (endothelial damage) that requires bed rest (venous stasis) and a high platelet value (hypercoagulability). Symptoms that require immediate attention are the loss of pulses on the right foot, increased peripheral edema on the right lower extremity, lab values demonstrating high platelet count, and the changes in skin temperature. The client does not have any infection; therefore, the temperature is not a concern. The sodium level is within normal parameters. The client is not at risk for contractures, an abnormal condition of the joint, characterized by flexion and fixation.

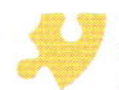

NCJMM Step: Prioritize Hypothesis
References: Jarvis et al. (2024), pp. 548–572; Tyerman & Cobbett (2023), pp. 350–351 (hyponatremia), 915–922 (deep vein thrombosis), 1622 (contractures), 1623–1624 (compartment syndrome).

Answer 34.4

POTENTIAL NURSING INTERVENTIONS	INDICATED	NOT INDICATED
Elevate the client's right lower leg higher than their heart level	○	✔
Request an order for analgesic	✔	○
Apply cold compresses to the injured area	○	✔
Request an order to add creatine kinase to the morning laboratory blood draw	✔	○
Measure the size of the right lower extremity	✔	○
Add a graduated cylinder to measure urine output	✔	○

Rationale: The nurse should not elevate the client's right lower leg as this may reduce venous pressure and decrease arterial perfusion. The extremity should not be elevated above the heart level. The client's pain level has increased since the morning assessment. The increased pain has increased their blood pressure and heart rate. Analgesic will reduce the cardiovascular workload of the heart and help reduce smooth muscle. The nurse should not apply cold compresses to the affected limb as this may lead to vasoconstriction and exacerbate compartment syndrome. The client is at risk of developing rhabdomyolysis. The nurse should monitor for evidence of muscle damage and urine output should be assessed. Elevated creatine kinase will indicate the destruction and breakdown of the muscle tissue. With rhabdomyolysis, myoglobin blocks the tubules in the kidney, leading to acute kidney injury. As a result, urine output is reduced and urine may be dark, reddish-brown in colour. A graduated cylinder will assist with monitoring the urine output overall status. Monitoring for clinical manifestations of hypocalcemia are also imperative if rhabdomyolysis is suspected. It is important to measure the size of the extremity and document the status. When there is increased swelling, it is difficult to determine if the client's condition is declining without accurate measurement around the widest area of the affected extremity. Assistance from other health care colleagues and an analgesic may be necessary to accomplish this task as it can be painful for the client.

NCJMM Step: Generate Solutions
References: Jarvis et al. (2024), pp. 548–572; Tyerman & Cobbett (2023), pp. 1623–1624 (compartment syndrome).

Answer 34.5

- ✔ Document the last time the client ate or drank anything
- ✔ Review all medications and inform the surgical team of all medications administered that shift
- ☐ Inform the client's family of impending surgery
- ☐ Ensure goals of care are discussed by the nurse with the client and documented in the chart
- ✔ Provide reassurance to the client to help reduce anxiety
- ✔ Place mark on the client's bilateral lower extremities indicating dorsalis pedis pulses and posterior tibial pulses
- ✔ Ensure the health care provider or orthopedic surgeon has obtained consent for the procedure

Rationale: The client refused lunch, which should be documented and the information provided to the surgical team. A client's risk for aspiration pneumonia increases if they eat or drink close to surgical times. The nurse should review all medications and ensure the surgical team is aware of any cardiac medications, anticoagulant medications, oral hypoglycemic agents, or antiplatelet medications. The client has no comorbidities and was not administered any medications. It is inappropriate for the nurse to notify the client's family and breach confidentiality, especially if the client can notify a family member themselves. The nurse can assist the health care provider with goals of care and obtaining consent. It is out of the scope of nursing practice to obtain goals of care designation independently without a physician or nurse practitioner present. Consent to the procedure must be obtained by the physician. Assessing and providing psychological support to the client is a part of holistic care. The swift response of the health care team may increase the client's anxiety. Marking all pulses is an important nursing action before any surgical procedure.

NCJMM Step: Take Action
References: Jarvis et al. (2024), pp. 548–572; Tyerman & Cobbett (2023), pp. 374–389 (preoperative nursing care), 1623–1624 (compartment syndrome).

Answer 34.6

ASSESSMENT FINDINGS	IMPROVED	NO CHANGE	DECLINED
RR 8	○	○	✔
Concentrated, urine output 35 mL/hr	✔	○	○

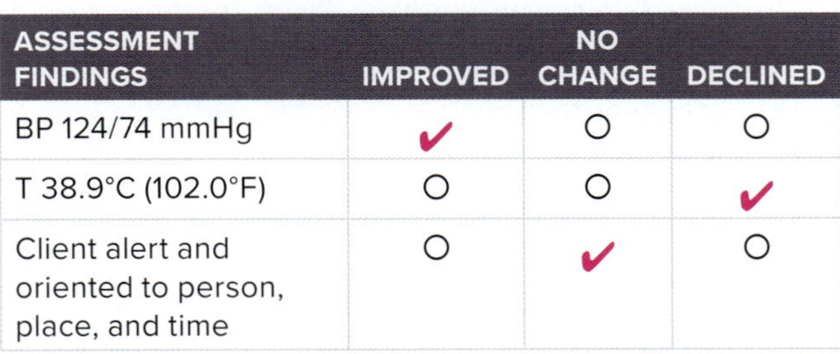

ASSESSMENT FINDINGS	IMPROVED	NO CHANGE	DECLINED
BP 124/74 mmHg	✔	○	○
T 38.9°C (102.0°F)	○	○	✔
Client alert and oriented to person, place, and time	○	✔	○

Rationale: When a client returns from a postanaesthetic recovery room, they may be lethargic and their breathing reduced. Monitoring their respirations and level of alertness is important to determine if the anaesthetic is being eliminated from their system. This client's creatinine level was elevated and given the potential for rhabdomyolysis, the client's fluid status is important to monitor. The client has concentrated urine output that meets the acceptable range of 30 mL per hour. Concentrated urine is better than dark, amber urine, which is indicative of rhabdomyolysis. The client's blood pressure has improved since preoperative. The client's temperature has increased, requiring antibiotics to prevent infection in the open wound.

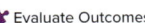

NCJMM Step: Evaluate Outcomes
Reference: Tyerman & Cobbett (2023), pp. 403–424 (postoperative nursing care), 1623–1624 (compartment syndrome).

Maternal/Birth Parent Health Unfolding Cases

Maternal/Birth Parent Health 1.0

Answer 1.1

TOP 3 FINDINGS
Fatigue
Output
Clear emesis

Rationale: Feeling nauseated during the first trimester is common for clients who are pregnant. This client is at risk for hemodynamic instability with dehydration, weakness, fatigue, low urine output (which indicates the client has positive 825 mL intake with negative 1 915 mL documented as output, putting the client in a negative 1 090 mL fluid balance), and dry mucous membranes. These clinical manifestations indicate that the number of times the client has emesis is becoming severe enough that it is putting the client at further risk for low volume. Currently, the blood pressure and heart rate can compensate, likely due to the client's age and health status before getting pregnant. Clear emesis is not an issue that requires follow-up; however, the number of times the client experiences emesis is an issue but was not one of the possible answers. This question is structured in a way that makes the student think beyond the initial presentation of multiple bouts of emesis to recognize potential hemodynamic instability.

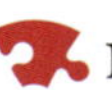
NCJMM Step: Recognize Cues
Reference: Keenan-Lindsay et al. (2022), pp. 278–280.

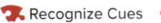

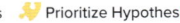

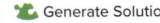

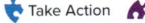

Answer 1.2

- ☐ Gastroenteritis
- ☐ Ectopic pregnancy
- ✔ Hypotension
- ☐ Appendicitis
- ✔ Fluid imbalance

Rationale: The client's hemodynamic status may be negatively affected, given the frequency of emesis that the client is experiencing. As a result, possible complications would lead to hypotension and fluid imbalance. The client is in a negative fluid balance, but given her age, she is able to compensate for the volume change. If the client develops hypotension, less blood may be delivered to the fetus. The client has lost more than 5% of prepregnancy body weight, indicating the fluid loss has been significant enough to bring the client to the hospital for further treatment. The client does not present with gastroenteritis symptoms as there is no fever, nausea, diarrhea, abdominal cramping, or distension. The client has already reached a 12-week gestation period for fetal development. An ectopic pregnancy is not a possible complication. The client does not present with abdominal pain; therefore, the client does not present with appendicitis.

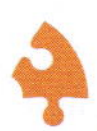

NCJMM Step: Analyze Cues
Reference: Keenan-Lindsay et al. (2022), pp. 278–280.

Answer 1.3

The client is at **highest** risk of developing **severe dehydration.**

Rationale: The client is hypotensive and has developed severe dehydration as a result of hyperemesis. The decreased normal sodium level indicates dehydration, as does the positive finding of ketones in the urine. Given that the client is not voiding, the potassium level is increasing and should be monitored for dysrhythmias. The client is not at risk for any neurological conditions such as SIADH, in which the client retains water or can develop cerebral edema, as this again is a condition in which the cells in the brain swell. The client is not at risk for acute renal failure, despite not voiding large amounts, as evidenced by the normal creatinine level. The white blood cell count is normal, and there are no presenting symptoms associated with pyelonephritis, such as lower back pain and previous urinary tract infection symptoms.

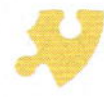

NCJMM Step: Prioritize Hypothesis
Reference: Keenan-Lindsay et al. (2022), pp. 278–280.

Answer 1.4

POTENTIAL NURSING INTERVENTIONS	INDICATED	NOT INDICATED
Place client in the side-lying position	✔	○
Anticipate blood draws	○	✔
Reassure client addressing fears	✔	○
Call a code blue	○	✔
Apply oxygen	○	✔

Rationale: Placing the client in a side-lying position is appropriate given her level of consciousness and potential risk for aspiration. As the morning lab work had already been drawn, a blood draw would not be warranted. The client may need reassurance because this is her first pregnancy, and she feels unwell due to the nausea and emesis. Although she is difficult to rouse, the client remains rousable and continues to present with a blood pressure and heart rate. She does not require a code blue to be called. The client also has adequate pulse oximetry, which was noted at 92%; therefore, she does not need oxygen applied.

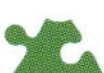

NCJMM Step: Generate Solutions
Reference: Keenan-Lindsay et al. (2022), pp. 278–280.

Answer 1.5

Orders

1030h:

- Insert an in-dwelling Foley catheter
- Draw an arterial blood gas
- Initiate oxygen therapy when pulse oximetry is less than 90%
- 0.9% sodium chloride (normal saline) 500 mL bolus × 1 then 125 mL/hr
- Insert peripheral intravenous catheter
- Monitor intake and output
- Begin to monitor with the Pregnancy-Unique Quantification of Emesis Scale
- Administer dimenhydrinate 50 mg IVPB q4h
- Administer acetaminophen 500–1 000 mg PO qid
- Consult dietitian

Rationale: The client requires quick fluid resuscitation and antiemetic therapy to assist with the consistent emesis. Normal saline would be the isotonic fluid of choice as the client is hyponatremic, and the bolus, followed by the rate, would be an appropriate therapy for this situation. The laboratory results, the hypotensive event, and lethargy indicate the client is severely dehydrated and requires fluids to increase the blood pressure and restore blood flow to the fetus. Dimenhydrinate is considered safe to administer during pregnancy and is readily available on postpartum units quickly, which is what the client needs.

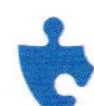

NCJMM Step: Generate Solutions
Reference: Keenan-Lindsay et al. (2022), pp. 278–280.

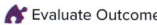

Answer 1.6

- ✔ Blood pressure
- ✔ Heart rate

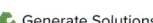

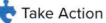

- ☐ Pulse oximetry
- ☐ Nausea with emesis
- ✔ Urine output

Rationale: The blood pressure, heart rate, and urine output indicate the client's status improvement. There is increased perfusion to the kidneys, improving the client's ability to produce urine after the intravenous fluid bolus and continuous intravenous fluids. Although the client has less nausea, she is still experiencing emesis, which could result in another episode of severe dehydration.

NCJMM Step: Evaluate Outcomes
Reference: Keenan-Lindsay et al. (2022), pp. 278–280.

Maternal/Birth Parent Health 2.0

Answer 2.1

TOP 4 FINDINGS
BP: 167/96; P: 85; pulse oximetry 94% on room air
Severe headache
Protein in urine
Spotting

Rationale: Two components to the diagnosis of pre-eclampsia are hypertension and new or worsening proteinuria. The client does not have any pre-existing conditions, so the hypertension is of new onset. Protein urea is defined as a concentration of 0.03 g/L or more in at least two random urine specimens at least 6 hours apart, with no evidence of infection. The nurse would follow up with a second urinalysis. The severe headache typically accompanies hypertensive events; however, the client is also at risk for seizures, blindness, and stroke. Bright red spotting or vaginal bleeding requires further follow-up to determine the care required. Clients with pre-eclampsia are at risk for placental abruption, so it is important to assess uterine tone and tenderness. The client's pupils are reactive to light, and the fundal height and fetal heart rate are appropriate for the gestation age.

NCJMM Step: Recognize Cues
Reference: Keenan-Lindsay et al. (2022), pp. 266–276.

Answer 2.2

- ✔ Thrombocytopenia
- ☐ Stroke
- ✔ Acute renal failure
- ☐ Confusion
- ✔ Blurred vision

Rationale: The client is at risk of developing organ dysfunction, including kidney or liver dysfunction. The client has reported small, pinpoint dots on her legs, which is likely thrombocytopenia. The client would be at risk for bleeding and potentially developing disseminated intravascular coagulation (DIC) or hemolysis. Given the high blood pressure, the client is at risk of developing neurological complications such as stroke, seizures, or blindness. The client is still voiding; therefore, she is not developing acute renal failure. There is nothing to indicate that confusion could occur, given that the client is 17 years old.

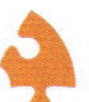

NCJMM Step: Analyze Cues
Reference: Keenan-Lindsay et al. (2022), pp. 266–276.

Answer 2.3

The client is at highest risk of developing **eclampsia** and **seizures.**

Rationale: Given the client's high blood pressure, the client is presenting with pre-eclampsia symptoms and is at highest risk of developing eclampsia, which is more severe, and seizures, as indicated by the low sodium levels. When sodium levels reach severe, neurological conditions can occur from the shift of fluid into the cell, causing cellular swelling. The question asks what the client is at highest risk for; therefore, fetal compromise is not an appropriate answer. It is too early in the gestational age to be concerned about postpartum hemorrhage. Given the client's presentation of spotting, placental abruption is a concern; however, there were no preceding symptoms, such as abdominal pain, uterine tenderness, and contractions. The white blood cell count is not elevated, which would indicate an infection, nor is there a febrile response.

NCJMM Step: Prioritize Hypothesis
References: Keenan-Lindsay et al. (2022), pp. 266–276, 292; Tyerman & Cobbett (2023), pp. 350–351.

Answer 2.4

POTENTIAL NURSING INTERVENTIONS	INDICATED	NOT INDICATED
Permit a highly stimulated environment	○	✔
Request an order to insert intravenous access (peripheral venous access device)	✔	○
Encourage mobility	○	✔
Monitor for HELLP syndrome	✔	○
Test suction equipment in the room	✔	○
Place bed in highest position	○	✔

Rationale: The client continues to be hypertensive; therefore, the nursing plan will include nursing actions to ensure the client remains safe. The client should have a quiet, nonstimulating, low-light environment. Loud, highly stimulating environments could increase the blood pressure. Reducing the number of visitors may be necessary at this time. Requesting an order to initiate peripheral intravenous access in anticipation of administering IV antihypertensive therapy is part of preparing for the potential medical plan. The client should be on restricted activity so as not to increase the blood pressure any further. Sequential compression devices or subcutaneous low-molecular-weight heparin would be recommended to prevent thromboembolism formation due to bed rest. The client is at high risk of developing HELLP syndrome or severe pre-eclampsia. HELLP stands for **h**emolysis, **e**levated **l**iver enzymes, and **l**ow **p**latelets. The nurse will need to monitor the client's hemoglobin to maintain pulse oximetry and adequate oxygen delivery to the fetus, monitor for liver toxicity and low platelet counts that could place the client at risk of bleeding, and monitor the coagulation profile to assess for disseminated intravascular coagulation (DIC). As routine safety checks, ensuring the suction works prior to a potential emergency is routine nursing practice. The client is at risk of developing seizures and may require suctioning at the time to prevent aspiration. The bed should be placed in the lowest position, not the highest position, which is also a safety precaution for a client who is at risk of developing seizures.

NCJMM Step: Generate Solutions
Reference: Keenan-Lindsay et al. (2022), pp. 266–276 (Box 14.5).

Answer 2.5

- ☐ Insert an in-dwelling urinary catheter
- ✔ Initiate magnesium sulphate IV loading dose 4 g, then initiate rate at 1 g/hr
- ☐ Apply oxygen 2–4 L/min per nasal prongs to maintain pulse oximetry greater than 90%
- ✔ Administer labetalol IV 2 mg/min
- ☐ Contact all family for family conference

Rationale: Two primary interventions for a client with pre-eclampsia are to prevent or control seizures and to control blood pressure. Magnesium sulphate must be administered through a loading dose and then a maintenance infusion. Labetalol can be administered with a bolus if necessary; however, the physician has ordered an infusion to maintain tighter blood pressure control. When administering magnesium sulphate, the client's blood pressure, pulse, and respiratory rate should be closely monitored. Oxygen saturation and electronic fetal monitoring activity are also warranted during the loading dose and throughout the administration of the magnesium sulphate. There is a risk of magnesium toxicity. Reduction in blood pressure reduces maternal morbidity and mortality rates associated with left ventricular failure and cerebral hemorrhage. A catheter is not warranted at this time as the client can move in the bed, and an in-dwelling catheter could risk causing a urinary tract infection. Oxygen therapy is used to maintain pulse oximetry above 90%; the client's oxygen saturation was measured at 92%. A family conference is not needed at this time.

NCJMM Step: Take Action
Reference: Keenan-Lindsay et al. (2022), pp. 266–276.

Answer 2.6

ASSESSMENT FINDINGS	IMPROVED	NO CHANGE	DECLINED
BP 145/77	✔	○	○
Oliguria	○	○	✔
Petechiae	○	✔	○
Loss of deep tendon reflexes	○	○	✔
Double vision	○	✔	○
RR 20	✔	○	○

Rationale: Monitoring for outcomes associated with blood pressure and potential seizure activity is a priority. A reduction in blood pressure and respiratory rate demonstrates improvement associated with the administration of labetalol. Reduced flow to the kidneys leading to oliguria and loss of deep tendon reflexes are signs of magnesium toxicity. Other signs of toxicity include loss of patellar reflexes, respiratory and muscular depression, oliguria, and decreased level of conscious. Adverse events associated with magnesium administration include lethargy, feeling of heat or warmth, headache, or nausea. Early signs of toxicity include vomiting, respiratory distress, hypotension, flushing, muscle weakness, decreased reflexes, and slurred speech. Since magnesium is excreted through the kidneys, reduced urine output exacerbates the toxic levels. Petechia and double vision are unchanged clinical manifestations since presentation in an emergency.

NCJMM Step: Evaluate Outcomes
Reference: Keenan-Lindsay et al. (2022), pp. 266–276.

Maternal/Birth Parent Health 3.0

Answer 3.1

- ☐ Disrespectful nursing staff
- ☐ No hormones for several months
- ☐ Expected pregnancy chest changes
- ✔ Started chest binding 2 weeks ago
- ✔ Right chest assessment data
- ✔ Vital signs
- ☐ Feelings of imposter syndrome
- ☐ Newborn weight

Rationale: Since the client has decided to bind his chest, the most concerning assessment data relate to his clinical presentation of chest tenderness, skin warm to touch, cracked nipples, and absent milk. The vital signs indicate the client presents with a fever. The client suffered disrespect at the hospital, which must be followed up with later, but it does not supersede the clinical presentation. The client will be provided information on how to file a formal complaint. The fact that the client stopped taking hormones and was able to conceive is positive. What would need to be considered is when to restart taking hormone therapy, which may address the feelings of imposter syndrome. The newborn weight is appropriate despite being lower. The child is gaining weight since birth and can be discharged from the hospital.

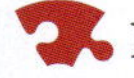

NCJMM Step: Recognize Cues
References: Keenan-Lindsay et al. (2022), pp. 657–660; MacDonald et al. (2016), p. 106; Wolfe-Roubatis, & Spatz (2015), pp. 32–38.

Answer 3.2

CLIENT FINDINGS	ENGORGEMENT	PLUGGED DUCT	INFECTION
Tender to touch	✔	✔	✔
Fever	○	○	✔
Sore nipples	✔	✔	✔
Swollen tissue of left chest	✔	○	✔

Rationale: With engorgement, chest fullness occurs around the third day postpartum and is a reassuring sign of healthy lactation. Parents can experience more intense fullness and sore nipples, and the chest may become enlarged, reddened, painful, shiny, and edematous. Frequent feedings would reduce engorgement. There will be no fever associated with engorgement. A plugged duct may cause an area of the chest to become swollen and tender. This area does not empty or soften with feeding or pumping. Clients may or may not experience sore nipples. The client would not experience a fever or generalized symptoms. Plugged milk ducts would increase the client's risk for infections. The client with an infection (candidiasis or mastitis) would experience swollen chest tissue, fever, and sore nipples.

NCJMM Step: Analyze Cues
Reference: Keenan-Lindsay et al. (2022), pp. 657–660.

Answer 3.3

The client is at highest risk of developing **mastitis.**

Rationale: The client is experiencing mastitis due to the chest binding, which resulted in plugged ducts. The fever indicates a source of infection and is unilateral compared to both chests being affected. The client is also experiencing chills and aches indicative of an infective process. As a result, there is a decreased milk supply in the right chest; however, the client has continued to chest feed using the left chest and should be applauded, given the difficult situation and stigma he experienced at the hospital. The nurse should ensure the client knows that the discriminatory comments will be addressed and provide information on how to file a formal complaint. The infant is feeding without issue; therefore, there is no issue with bonding or rejection of the birth parent.

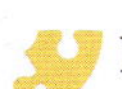

NCJMM Step: Prioritize Cues
Reference: Keenan-Lindsay et al. (2022), pp. 657–666.

Answer 3.4

POTENTIAL NURSING INTERVENTIONS	INDICATED	NOT INDICATED
Discuss potential causes of the mastitis	✔	○
Confirm chest is best for newborn feeding	○	✔
Collaborate with client about the best time to begin wearing chest binders	✔	○
Discuss alternate sources of newborn nutrition	✔	○

Rationale: The nurse should discuss with the client the best time to begin wearing chest binders. The chest binders likely contributed to the mastitis despite the mammary glands of the left chest still being able to produce milk. Discussing the needs of the client is important to help address body dysmorphia and additional negative emotions, such as the potential shame of feeling like an imposter. Chest feeding may not always be best, as the mental health of the client is important to address. Attending to the client's needs and their mental health will provide a nurturing environment for the newborn and parent. Returning to wearing chest binders is important for the client. Alternate sources of nutrition could be discussed with the client and his partner.

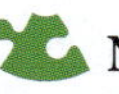

NCJMM Step: Generate Solutions
Reference: Keenan-Lindsay et al. (2022), pp. 657–660; MacDonald et al. (2016), p. 106; Wolfe-Roubatis & Spatz (2015), pp. 32–38.

Answer 3.5

- ☐ Suggest the client purchase lanolin ointment
- ☐ Draw complete blood count, electrolytes
- ✔ Assess latch of the newborn to left chest
- ☐ Encourage the use of cold compresses for milk production
- ✔ Request an order for antibiotic treatment

Rationale: The client has reported wanting to continue to chest feed; therefore, assessing if the newborn is latching correctly is important. A warm compress, not cold, could be applied to assist with milk expression. A cold compress could be used to reduce swelling. The more the newborn chest feeds, the more the mastitis will improve. If the client cannot feed the newborn off the right chest, he could use a pump to extract the milk and continue to feed off the left chest and supplement as needed. It is suggested that the newborn start feeding on the affected side, then move to the unaffected side until milk let-down, and then switch again. Antibiotic treatment would be appropriate, as would analgesics, and antipyretics may be required to help the client feel better. Lanolin ointment is used for sore nipples. Nurses must assess the client's allergies before applying lanolin ointment as it is made from sheep's wool.

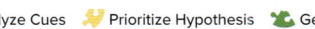

NCJMM Step: Take Action
References: Keenan-Lindsay et al. (2022), pp. 657–660; MacDonald, et al. (2016), p. 106; Wolfe-Roubatis & Spatz (2015), pp. 32–38.

Answer 3.6

STATEMENTS BY THE CLIENT THAT DEMONSTRATE UNDERSTANDING
"It is important to maintain hydration."
"I can use chest binders but gradually increase the time."
"Monitor for yeast to develop if the nipple does not heal."
"We can supplement with formula."

Rationale: The client needs to maintain adequate fluid intake and monitor for potential yeast to occur as sore, cracked nipples allow an entry point for yeast to develop. Supplementation of newborn nutrition may be necessary to support the child's healthy growth and development until the mastitis has cleared. Other client teaching to provide is monitoring stress and fatigue, identifying parental illness or ill family members, monitoring for chest trauma, and avoiding poor parental nutrition, all of which are factors for mastitis to occur. The use of chest binders will help the client with body dysmorphia and be closer aligned with the mental image he has of himself and how he wants to present himself to the world. Pregnancy creates a visual body adjustment despite the desire to chest feed. Addressing the client's mental health is also important. There will be some discomfort with chest feeding until the duct has been cleared, so if the client wants to continue chest feeding, discomfort is temporary. Nipple pain is not normal; however, nipples do require time to adjust to newborn feeding. If the client does not have an allergy to wool, lanolin cream can be suggested, or milk can be used on the nipple before feeding.

NCJMM Step: Evaluate Outcomes
Reference: Keenan-Lindsay et al. (2022), pp. 657–660; MacDonald et al. (2016), p. 106; Wolfe-Roubatis & Spatz (2015), pp. 32–38.

Maternal/Birth Parent Health 4.0

Answer 4.1

TOP 4 FINDINGS
Vital signs
Characteristics of the fundus
Low urine output
Oxygen requirements

Rationale: Despite several units of blood and fluid, the client's blood pressure has increased slightly but remains low post-delivery. Changes in the blood pressure, respiratory rate, heart rate, and temperature will be the first signs of hemodynamic changes and will need to be monitored. The uterus is boggy and unable to expel clots, which means that the uterus is not contracting enough to clot. Fundal massage can be uncomfortable but necessary to assist with clotting. Uterine atony and excessive bleeding can occur and should be monitored. Despite a high volume of fluid intervention, the urine output is low and needs to be monitored and followed. The oxygen requirements are concerning as she should be able to maintain normal oxygenation. The age of the client and the minimal blood loss are concerning but not a top priority at the moment.

NCJMM Step: Recognize Cues
Reference: Keenan-Lindsay et al. (2022), pp. 498, 532–539.

Answer 4.2

- ☐ Pneumosepsis
- ☐ Heparin-induced thrombocytopenia
- ✔ Disseminated intravascular coagulation
- ☐ Acute respiratory distress syndrome
- ✔ Acute renal failure
- ✔ Postpartum hemorrhage

Rationale: The primary issue is maintaining normal hemodynamic status. The client had significant blood loss during the Caesarean surgical procedure, requiring fluid boluses and replacement. The client is at risk for a postpartum hemorrhage given that the uterine tone is significantly reduced and not clotting. Since this is a potential bleeding issue, the client is also at risk of developing disseminated intravascular coagulation, in which the client both clots and bleeds. With a urine output of only 100 mL, the client is at risk of developing acute renal failure as the kidneys would not be perfused with inadequate cardiac output and low blood pressure. The client is afebrile with regular and easy respirations, eliminating the possibility that pneumonia or acute respiratory distress syndrome may be a complication.

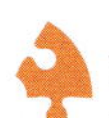
NCJMM Step: Analyze Cues
Reference: Keenan-Lindsay et al. (2022), pp. 498, 532–539.

Answer 4.3

The client is at highest risk of developing **hemorrhagic shock.**

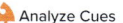

Rationale: The client's symptom presentation is consistent with hemorrhagic shock. The client's respirations are rapid and shallow, the pulse is rapid and weak, skin is cool and pale, urine output is zero, and there was a change in the client's level of consciousness. The clinical manifestations do not correlate with a venous thromboembolism, no shortness of breath such as in the case of a pulmonary embolism, no complaints of chest pain to indicate an acute myocardial infarction, and nothing to consider dysrhythmias as an issue.

NCJMM Step: Prioritize Hypothesis
Reference: Keenan-Lindsay et al. (2022), pp. 532–539.

Answer 4.4

POTENTIAL NURSING INTERVENTIONS	INDICATED	NOT INDICATED
Prepare to increase oxygen per nasal cannula	✔	○
Set up the rapid infuser	✔	○
Call a code blue	○	✔
Request an order to administer blood products	✔	○
Request an order to administer crystalloids	○	✔

Rationale: The pulse oximetry is low, requiring higher oxygen to be delivered. A rapid infuser can administer large amounts of fluid in a short amount of time. It requires two people to run the machine for client safety, as an air embolism could occur if no air detector is on the machine. The client requires prompt attention; however, a code blue is not warranted now. A health care provider should be notified first. If the client's status deteriorates and she becomes unresponsive and a pulse cannot be located, then a code blue should be called. Administration of blood products and crystalloids such as lactated Ringer's, normal saline, and colloids, such as albumin, packed red blood cells, and other blood products (platelets or fresh frozen plasma) may be ordered.

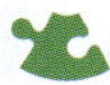

NCJMM Step: Generate Solutions
Reference: Keenan-Lindsay et al. (2022), pp. 537–539.

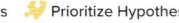

Answer 4.5

Orders

1645:
- Insert an in-dwelling urinary catheter
- Administer 0.9% sodium chloride (normal saline) 2 L bolus with rapid infuser
- Spiral computed tomography (CT) to be done in diagnostic imaging
- Insert another large-bore (at least 18 gauge) intravenous catheter
- Apply high-flow nasal prongs and titrate for a pulse oximetry of greater than 92%
- Administer 1 unit platelets
- Administer 2 units packed red blood cells now
- Laboratory tests: D-dimer, arterial blood gas (ABG)

Rationale: Additional fluids and packed red blood cells would need to be administered via the rapid infuser to increase intravascular volume. An additional large-bore peripheral intravenous access would need to be initiated to push more fluids into the client as fast as possible. The oxygen levels are low, so initiating high-flow oxygen through nasal prongs would be necessary at this time. Intubation would not be required as the client is not in respiratory distress. A urinary catheter would be needed. Monitoring hemodynamic status is important. The client does not require platelets at this time as the platelet level is 100 × 10^9/L. A D-dimer and arterial blood gas draw will be required, but it is not an immediate action.

NCJMM Step: Take Action
Reference: Keenan-Lindsay et al. (2022), pp. 537–539.

Answer 4.6

ASSESSMENT FINDINGS	IMPROVED	NO CHANGE	DECLINED
Skin cool to touch	○	✔	○
BP 90/64	✔	○	○
D-dimer result is positive	○	○	✔
Urine output 30 mL/hr	✔	○	○
Shortness of breath	○	○	✔

Rationale: The client's skin remains cool to touch as the body is maintaining vasoconstriction in the peripherals to increase blood flow to the heart, thereby increasing blood pressure. This is a physiological compensatory mechanism. After administration of the blood products and fluids, the blood pressure has increased, which is an improvement in the client's condition. A positive D-dimer indicates the client has developed a clot that has reached the lung. During administration with the rapid infuser, an air embolism could have entered the client's bloodstream. This client is at continued risk of developing disseminated intravascular coagulation and should be monitored carefully, given her recent Caesarean birth. An increase in urine output of at minimum 30 mL per hour indicates minimum renal output. There is some perfusion occurring at the kidney level now whereas there was none prior.

NCJMM Step: Evaluate Outcomes
Reference: Keenan-Lindsay et al. (2022), pp. 537–539.

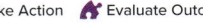

Maternal/Birth Parent Health 5.0

Answer 5.1

Progress Notes

May 12 at 0937h: Client was seen in the clinic for her 36-week appointment. Primary complaint is general malaise × 3 days, just a feeling of being unwell. The client's comorbidities include gestational diabetes mellitus and hypertension prior to pregnancy controlled through diet and exercise. The client presents as G2 T0 P0 A1 L0 with a previous miscarriage documented at 13 weeks. Client is accompanied to the clinic by their partner. Vital signs: T: 36.7°C (98.0°F); BP: 152/96; P: 97; RR: 22; with pulse oximetry of 97% on room air. Client presents with 8 out of 10 headache based on the numerical rating scale, without any relief from acetaminophen, complains of blurry vision, denies numbness or tingling in the hands or feet. Bilateral pupils equal in size and shape at 2 mm and react briskly to light. Motor power strong × 4 and gait steady with independent ambulation. Client indicates dizziness when rising too fast. Skin warm and dry to touch. Mild edema noted in the client's bilateral hands, with wedding rings on left hand noted to be tight. Finger remains warm to touch and capillary refill less than 3 seconds. Bilateral radial pulses bounding and palpable, with apical pulses equal to radial pulses. Bilateral dorsalis pedis pulses palpable and regular to touch. Client denies any chest pain but states able to "feel" heart beating in her head. Client thinks they are silly for even saying that. Upon auscultation, bilateral fine inspiratory crackles noted to anterior bases of lung fields. Client denies any cough and noted to be taking short, shallow breaths. Client states her breathing has become more difficult as the pregnancy has progressed. Client denies any pain with urination, denies changes in frequency. Urine sample collected in the office to complete a urine dipstick. Client indicates no change in appetite, eating healthy but × 2 days feeling nauseated. Fetal heart rate documented at 146 beats per minute. Client referred to the obstetrical unit for further investigation.

Rationale: A client who presents with a significantly high blood pressure (≥140/90 mm Hg), severe headache without any relief from acetaminophen, blurry vision, and swelling in the face or hands may be experiencing a cardiovascular event and requires immediate intervention for the safety of the client and their unborn child. There are different levels of hypertension with a pregnant person; the severity is to be assessed on the basis of clinical presentation. The levels of hypertension include nonsevere hypertension, severe hypertension, and pre-eclampsia. This client has risk factors for pre-eclampsia, such as age older than 40 years, presenting with gestational diabetes and pre-existing hypertension controlled with diet and exercise prior to this pregnancy, and a poor outcome (miscarriage) in a previous pregnancy. The client is feeling nauseated due to the vasospasms of the gastrointestinal tract.

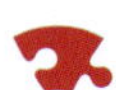 **NCJMM:** Recognize Cues
References: Keatings & Adams (2024), Chapter 9; Keenan-Lindsay et al. (2022); pp. 265–267.

Answer 5.2

- ✔ Blindness
- ☐ Impaired immunity
- ✔ Seizures
- ☐ Venous thrombosis
- ☐ Leukopenia
- ☐ Gastritis
- ☐ Viral stomach infection

Rationale: A pregnant client who presents with hypertension may be at significant risk for cortical blindness or retinal detachment due to the increased pressure on the optic nerve. If the client's blood pressure progresses from nonsevere hypertension (BP ≥140/90 mm Hg) to severe hypertension (BP ≥160/110 mm Hg), the client is at increased risk for seizures due to increased swelling in the brain and increased pressure within the cerebral vessels. The client may develop increased white blood cells, not reduced white blood cells. The client is not at risk of developing venous thrombosis unless there is an issue with both bleeding and clotting called *disseminated intravascular coagulation*. The nurse needs to confirm the hemoglobin, liver enzymes, and platelets blood levels. The client does not have anything wrong with their immune system. Often patients who present with high blood pressure will also present with nausea, vomiting, increased indigestion, and pain after eating, which can be mistaken for gastritis or a viral stomach infection. Early diagnosis of HELLP syndrome is critical because of the seriousness of the illness for the pregnant person and the fetus.

 **NCJMM:** Analyze Cues
References: Keatings & Adams (2024), Chapter 9; Keenan-Lindsay et al. (2022); pp. 265–267.

Answer 5.3

The client is at highest risk of developing **stroke** and **acute renal failure** with effects to the fetus that may include **oligohydramnios**.

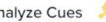

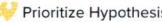

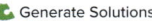

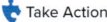

Rationale: The primary systems most affected by hypertension disorder in pregnancy include the neurological system (stroke or transient ischemic attacks), cardiovascular system (chest pain, myocardial ischemia or infarction), respiratory system (pulmonary edema, acute respiratory distress syndrome), and renal system (acute tubular necrosis, acute kidney injury, proteinuria, which indicates that the client has progressed to pre-eclampsia). Other conditions to be concerned about are bleeding disorders due to elevated liver enzymes, thrombocytopenia (low platelets), and disseminated intravascular coagulation. The client is not at a risk for anemia. If bleeding occurs, this would be a life-threatening condition for the client. The hypertension is a result of increased vascular resistance the heart is pumping against. There is nothing wrong with the conduction system of the heart. The client does not present with symptoms associated with an infection or manifestations associated with pneumonia. The client only presents with hypertension, and the exact duration of the symptom is unknown. As a result, oligohydramnios (too little amniotic fluid) occurs, which is an early indicator for neonatal morbidity. If the client has uncontrolled gestational diabetes, this may be more of a factor for the fetus's glycemia control than the hypertension. Placenta abruption may occur with clients with significant hypertension as opposed to placenta previa.

NCJMM: Prioritize Hypothesis
References: Keatings & Adams (2024), Chapter 9; Keenan-Lindsay et al. (2022); pp. 265–267.

Answer 5.4

POTENTIAL NURSING INTERVENTIONS	INDICATED	NOT INDICATED
Ensure the client is isolated from family	○	✔
Prepare to insert a nasogastric tube	○	✔
Create a nonstimulating and quiet environment	✔	○
Evaluate deep tendon reflexes at baseline assessment	✔	○
Instruct the client to remain on strict bed rest	○	✔
Limit fluid intake	○	✔
Ensure all safety equipment such as suction and oxygen are available	✔	○

Rationale: The client requires additional support from family and friends during this time. Minimizing the number of visitors will help maintain a quiet, nonstimulating environment with subdued lighting. Ensuring the client's environment is calming and soothing will help keep the blood pressure lower, minimizing risks to the client and fetus. Evaluating deep tendon reflexes at baseline assessment and throughout the hospitalization and pregnancy will be valuable information if the client is to be treated with magnesium to prevent or control seizure activity. Activity should be restricted; however, clients are not to remain solely on bed rest. There is no evidence to suggest that bed rest alone improves pregnancy outcomes. Reduced activity may be beneficial for decreasing blood pressure and promote fetal growth as well as improve amniotic fluid levels. The client is not experiencing a gastric illness but hypertension. A nasogastric tube is unnecessary. The client should be encouraged to take in oral fluids, a minimum of six to eight 250-mL glasses of water per day. Adequate fluid intake helps maintain optimum fluid volume and aids in renal perfusion and bowel function. If the client should have an emergency, oxygen, suction equipment should be readily available. An emergency medication tray should be easily accessible as well.

NCJMM: Generate Solutions
Reference: Tyerman & Cobbett (2023), pp. 270–273.

Answer 5.5

- ✔ Initiate magnesium infusion with a loading dose of 4 g followed by 1 g/hr IV
- ✔ Administer labetalol 100 mg PO to be taken twice a day
- ✔ Continuous external fetal monitoring
- ☐ Labs to draw q6h: complete blood count, electrolytes, creatinine, PT (INR), PTT, AST, ALT
- ☐ Ensure calcium gluconate is available
- ✔ Oxygen therapy 6 L/min (50% oxygen) for 1 hr then reassess
- ☐ Use a urine collection hat placed in the toilet
- ☐ Monitor input and output × 48 hr

Rationale: Prevention or control of seizure activity is an important goal and can be achieved by administration of magnesium sulfate per venous access device. Magnesium reduces decreased neuromuscular irritability by inhibiting the release of acetylcholine at the synapses. Administration of an antihypertensive medication is important treatment to reduce the client's blood pressure. Labetalol is the drug of choice, followed by nifedipine, methyldopa, acebutolol metoprolol, pindolol, propranolol, and hydralazine. Caution must be exercised to avoid decreasing the blood pressure to quickly, as this can impact uteroplacental perfusion and fetal status. Ensuring direct fetal monitoring is important to prevent perinatal mortality. Vaginal exams can also be used to evaluate the condition of the cervix. The client's pulse oximetry is less than 90%. Administration of at least 50% oxygen can be achieved through 6–10 L/min oxygen therapy. All the other orders are correct and appropriate, just not a priority.

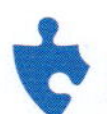
NCJMM: Take Action
Reference: Tyerman & Cobbett (2023), pp. 270–273.

Answer 5.6

ASSESSMENT FINDINGS	IMPROVED	NO CHANGE	DECLINED
Client noted to be indrawing and having difficulty speaking	○	○	✔
BP 135/85	✔	○	○
Urine clear and measured at 170 mL/hr	✔	○	○
Client presents with emesis ~50 mL of bile	○	○	✔
Bilateral pupils equal in size and shape at 3 mm and react briskly to light	○	✔	○

Rationale: Magnesium sulphate is a central nervous system depressant, so the nurse must monitor for signs of magnesium toxicity: lethargy, feeling of heat or warmth, headache, or nausea, vomiting, respiratory distress, hypotension, flushing, muscle weakness, decreased reflexes, and slurred speech.

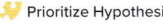

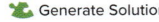

Diuresis should begin within 24 to 48 hours and not exceed 200 mL per hour, indicating a potential renal dysfunction. A decrease in blood pressure occurs with magnesium administration as there may be a drop in blood pressure at the start of treatment. The pupils remain unchanged. A sign of a potential stroke is a transient ischemic attack (TIA).

NCJMM: Evaluate Outcomes
Reference: Tyerman & Cobbett (2023), pp. 270–276.

Maternal/Birth Parent Health 6.0

Answer 6.1

- ☐ Newborn's Apgars
- ☐ Episiotomy site
- ✔ Pallor
- ☐ Pupillary response
- ✔ Palpitations
- ✔ Nasal flaring
- ✔ Skin temperature
- ✔ Uterine characteristics
- ✔ Cyanosis
- ✔ Lung sounds

Rationale: This client's airway, breathing, and circulation are most compromised and require immediate follow-up. The client's pallor as evidenced by pale conjunctiva and bilateral palms indicates reduced perfusion to the tissues. The client's ability to feel palpitations indicates the cardiovascular system is attempting to compensate with the respiratory system. The respiratory rate is elevated, as is the heart rate. The client's nasal flaring and cyanosis are indicative of difficulty breathing despite the client not recognizing the challenge. Fatigue from the delivery is likely the cause of the client not being able to recognize difficulty breathing. The client's cool skin to touch is another indication of reduced perfusion. A boggy fundus that does not stay firm even with massage is an early sign of a complication post-delivery. The newborn's Apgar scores are above 7 after the 1-minute and 5-minute marks, which is acceptable. The episiotomy site is sutured without any issue noted at the time of admission. The client's pupillary response is responsive and appropriate to light. The client presents with fine inspiratory crackles, which is concerning and may be contributing to the client's poor gas exchange.

NCJMM Step: Recognize Cues
Reference: Keenan-Lindsay et al. (2022), p. 481.

Answer 6.2

- ✔ Hypoxemia
- ☐ Anuria
- ☐ Respiratory acidosis
- ☐ Deep vein thrombosis
- ☐ Cerebral edema
- ☐ Anoxia
- ✔ Bleeding

Rationale: The two complications the client is at most risk of developing are hypoxemia and bleeding. The client is displaying difficulty with breathing and reduced gas exchange as evidenced by the cyanosis, cool skin to touch, and capillary refill at 3 seconds. The client is at risk for bleeding, specifically intrauterine bleeding with a boggy fundus. The client would be at risk for oliguria before anuria. The client has respirations of 24, which would lead to respiratory alkalosis, not respiratory acidosis. The client is blowing off CO_2, which is acidic, leaving the body to be alkalotic. The client does not present with deep vein thrombosis symptoms indicative of Virchow's triad (hypercoagulability, endothelial damage, and venous stasis). The client presents as orientated yet fatigued, therefore eliminating cerebral edema as a complication. Anoxia is described as the total absence of oxygen in the brain. The client does not have any indication of a brain injury leading to anoxia.

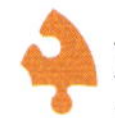

NCJMM Step: Analyze Cues
Reference: Keenan-Lindsay et al. (2022), p. 481.

Answer 6.3

The client is at highest risk of developing **amniotic fluid embolism.**

Rationale: An amniotic fluid embolism, also known as an *anaphylactoid syndrome of pregnancy*, is a rare complication; if this emergency occurs, there is an increased mortality rate for the client. A foreign substance was present in the amniotic fluid and introduced into the circulation of the labouring client, travelling to the lungs and presenting with symptoms similar to a pulmonary embolism. Risk factors for this type of emergency include advanced age, non-White individuals, placenta previa, pre-eclampsia, and forceps-assisted or Caesarean birth. Typical presentation can occur during labour, birth, or within 30 minutes after delivery. Clinical presentation includes respiratory distress, circulatory collapse, and hemorrhage. The client is experiencing an inflammatory response in association with delivery and the amniotic fluid embolism. The client presents with pulmonary edema as the crackles progressed from fine inspiratory crackles to coarse crackles. The client's respiratory status has decompensated.

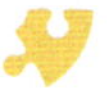

NCJMM Step: Prioritize Hypothesis
Reference: Keenan-Lindsay et al. (2022), p. 481.

Answer 6.4

POTENTIAL NURSING INTERVENTIONS	INDICATED	NOT INDICATED
Prepare to increase oxygen delivery or add a non-rebreather mask	✔	○
Place client in semi-Fowler's position	○	✔
Encourage rest for the client	○	✔
Request an order to administer blood products	✔	○

POTENTIAL NURSING INTERVENTIONS	INDICATED	NOT INDICATED
Provide emotional support to the client and partner	✔	○
Request an order to administer hypertonic intravenous solutions	○	✔

Rationale: The client's pulse oximetry reading indicates that the client requires additional oxygen support. The nurse should administer oxygen by a non-rebreather face mask at 10 L per minute or prepare to intubate the client. The client should be placed on her left side to allow for the amniotic fragment that is in the system to float to the right atrium, and in Trendelenburg position to increase cardiac output. If necessary, the client requires medical support through oxygen, fluids, blood products (packed cells and fresh frozen plasma), and critical respiratory support. The client and partner will require additional emotional support from the nursing staff. If the client develops an amniotic fluid embolism during labour or birth, additional support for the fetus will be necessary, too. The client requires an isotonic solution, not a hypertonic intravenous solution. The hypertonic solution will only increase the sodium level.

NCJMM Step: Generate Solutions
Reference: Keenan-Lindsay et al. (2022), p. 481.

Answer 6.5

Orders

1220:
- Insert an in-dwelling urinary catheter
- Administer 0.9% sodium chloride (normal saline) 500 mL bolus × 1
- Spiral computed tomography (CT) to be done in diagnostic imaging
- Insert another-large bore (at least 18 gauge) peripheral venous access device
- Apply non-rebreather mask at 10 L/min and titrate for a pulse oximetry of greater than 92%
- Contact the blood bank and administer 2 units packed red blood cells ASAP
- Laboratory tests: complete blood count, electrolytes, PTT, INR, type and cross-match, D-dimer, arterial blood gas

Rationale: The client requires fluids and packed red blood cells to increase systemic blood loss. Oxygen support is necessary to assist with gas exchange. The low hemoglobin level has low transport for oxygen through the bloodstream. Possible oxygen treatment with fluid support may improve the client's status. If not, the client will need to be intubated and monitored closely in a critical care area. Further lab testing will be required to monitor the client's serum levels, coagulation, oxygen levels, d-Dimer, and arterial blood gas. The nurse will insert an in-dwelling catheter and may take the client for a CT scan confirming an embolism is the cause of the client's symptoms. This is not immediate action to be taken. Another large-bore peripheral venous access device will be necessary to assist with fluid status but can be inserted when the blood is being thawed. Contacting the blood bank is the first action needed.

NCJMM Step: Take Action
Reference: Keenan-Lindsay et al. (2022), p. 481.

Answer 6.6

ASSESSMENT FINDINGS	IMPROVED	NO CHANGE	DECLINED
RR 16	✔	○	○
Urine output of 75 mL/hr	✔	○	○
Pedal pulses found with Doppler	○	○	✔
Ashen colour	○	✔	○
BP 97/54 mmHg	✔	○	○
Fundus firms up with massage	✔	○	○

Rationale: The actions of the medical staff have improved the client's status. The respiratory rate has decreased to a more appropriate level for the client. The client's kidneys have begun to perfuse, resulting in the production of urine. The pedal pulses were palpable but weak; however, now that pulses can only be found with Doppler, this could indicate a change in perfusion status or the client has received fluid hydration and developed pedal edema, making it difficult to palpate pulses. The client remains pale in colour and ashen, which can be observed regardless of skin tone. The blood pressure has improved with the packed cells and fluid hydration. The fundus has regained tone and is able to contract, which is an improvement.

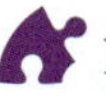
NCJMM Step: Evaluate Outcomes
Reference: Keenan-Lindsay et al. (2022), p. 481.

Pediatric Unfolding Cases

Pediatrics 1.0

Answer 1.1

- ☐ Apgars
- ☐ Birth weight
- ✔ Cyanosis
- ☐ Soft fontanel
- ✔ Systolic murmur
- ☐ Heart rhythm
- ✔ Respiratory rate
- ✔ Nasal flaring

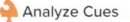

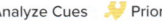

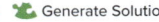

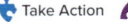

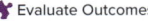

Rationale: Cyanosis, respiratory rate, and nasal flaring indicate signs of respiratory distress in the newborn. It is important to note the newborn was not in distress prior to nursing and it happened only at that time. If the client only developed cyanosis, acrocyanosis, and bluish discoloration of the hands and feet, these would be normal findings for the first 7 to 10 days; however, with the cyanosis there are respiratory symptoms. The indication of a systolic murmur is abnormal for a newborn and requires further investigation. The child may have an undiagnosed cardiac condition. Apgars are to be recorded as greater than 7; this newborn's Apgar scores at 1 and 5 minutes are appropriate. The birth weight of 3 750 g is between 2 500 and 4 000 g, which is considered a normal variation. Newborn fontanels are to be soft and flat, allowing for compression of the skull through the vaginal cavity, and flat indicates appropriate fluid status. It is concerning for the newborn to develop swollen or sunken fontanels as there could be an issue with fluid status. The heart rhythm is regular and strong, indicating this is a normal presentation.

NCJMM Step: Recognize Cues
Reference: Keenan-Lindsay et al. (2022), pp. 562 (signs of respiratory distress), 586 (newborn physical assessment), 593 (birth weight).

Answer 1.2

The client is at highest risk of developing **low pulse oximetry level.**

Rationale: The clinical presentation points to respiratory distress for the client with an undiagnosed heart murmur that requires further investigation. A potential complication for this client would be a low pulse oximetry level. Pulse oximetry readings can screen for congenital heart defects and early intervention. The newborn is not at risk for any fluid imbalances as identified by the anterior fontanel documented as soft and flat. The axillary temperature is considered a normal variation, with 37.0°C (98.6°F) being average. Newborns experience a transient decrease in glucose levels during the first 1 to 2 hours after birth. They can mobilize free fatty acids and ketones to help maintain adequate glucose levels. There are no indications the newborn is at risk for bleeding in the scenario presentation, as the birth was uneventful. Newborns may be at risk for bleeding if vitamin K is not administered; however, that is not the priority of this situation. Newborns often experience hypoglycemia, not hyperglycemia, after birth. With respect to recognizing hypoglycemia, newborns who experience traumatic births such as asphyxiation (cord around the neck) or any neurological injury may experience hypoglycemia. The delivery in this scenario was uneventful, so the newborn would likely be mobilizing free fatty acids to accommodate the limited ability for feeding. Cyanosis is not a clinical manifestation associated with hyperglycemia.

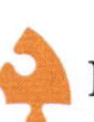
NCJMM Step: Analyze Cues
Reference: Keenan-Lindsay et al. (2022), pp. 595 (assessment of fontanels), 611–612 (hypoglycemia), 614 (screening for congenital heart defects), 593 (birth weight).

Answer 1.3

The client is at highest risk of developing **Tet spell** as evidenced by the client's **respiratory assessment.**

Rationale: A newborn who develops cyanosis when eating is most likely experiencing a Tet spell. Tet spells are associated with a cardiovascular condition called *tetralogy of Fallot*. This type of congenital heart disease has four defects: ventricular septal defect, pulmonic stenosis, overriding aorta, and right ventricular hypertrophy. Anoxic spells occur when the infant's oxygen requirements exceed the blood supply, usually during crying or after feeding. Tet spells or blue spells are acute episodes of cyanosis and hypoxia. In this scenario, the newborn had no signs of cyanosis at birth, with an uneventful delivery and normal Apgars; plus, during the initial assessment, the newborn did not appear to have any acute or mild cyanosis. Newborns and infants characteristically have a systolic murmur and respiratory distress as evidenced by the respiratory rate greater than 60 breaths per minute. The respiratory assessment provides further evidence of the Tet spell. Aspiration pneumonia can be common for infants to develop if they ingested meconium during delivery. There was no documentation to indicate this occurred, and the newborn is afebrile. The incidence of croup is not closely linked to clinical manifestations immediately after birth. There is no indication the client has bacterial endocarditis given the uneventful delivery. The vital signs point to afebrile and high respiratory rate, which is concerning for a possible respiratory or cardiovascular condition. The newborn's nutritional status highlighted the issue leading to a Tet spell; however, documentation supporting difficulty with feeding is an area of concern, but not something that caused the Tet spell. The parent-to-newborn connection is irrelevant as the new parent is trying to improve the connection through skin-to-skin contact.

NCJMM Step: Prioritize Hypothesis
Reference: Keenan-Lindsay et al. (2022), pp. 561–565 (newborn respiratory and cardiovascular assessment), 1129 (croup), 1140 (aspiration pneumonia), 1247–1248 (tetralogy of Fallot).

Answer 1.4

POTENTIAL NURSING INTERVENTIONS	INDICATED	NOT INDICATED
Prepare the client for a chest X-ray	✔	○
Encourage bottle feeding	○	✔
Give the family space to deal with new diagnosis	○	✔
Monitor pulse oximetry on the newborn	✔	○

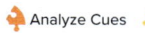

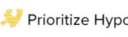

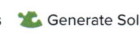

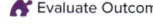

Rationale: Tetralogy of Fallot is the most common cyanotic defect with decreased pulmonary blood flow. To ensure proper assessment of cardiac function, the following tests could be ordered: X-rays, echocardiography, and cardiac catheterization. Completing chest X-rays and an echocardiogram would be noninvasive and quick as compared to a cardiac catheterization. Monitoring consistent pulse oximetry of the newborn will notify the health care team of possible impending life-threatening complications, such as pulmonary embolus, seizures, loss of consciousness, or sudden death following a Tet spell or anoxic spell. Caring for a child with congenital heart disease and their family requires support and resources, especially for a young new parent at 19 years old who did not share the news of the pregnancy with the biological grandparents. A better response would be to inquire what the new parent may need instead of leaving the new parent alone. The family will need help adjusting to the disorder and coping with the effects of the anomaly, as well as fostering growth and promoting family relationships. Maintaining adequate nutrition is important, as children with Tetralogy of Fallot may have poor weight gain, poor feeding habits, and fatigue during feeding. New parents may be hesitant during feeds to avoid Tet spells. The nurse should provide support as to what the new parent may need rather than encouraging bottle feeding at this time. The new parent has indicated they want to nurse the baby. If the newborn is not gaining weight and developing failure to thrive, then the discussion of supplementation may be necessary.

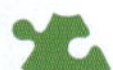
NCJMM Step: Generate Solutions
Reference: Keenan-Lindsay et al. (2022), pp. 1247–1248 (tetralogy of Fallot), 1277–1278 (care of the newborn with a cardiovascular condition).

Answer 1.5

- ☐ Prepare the newborn for surgery now
- ☐ Suggest meditation and yoga for coping
- ✔ Request a consult social work
- ☐ Contact the client's parents
- ✔ Provide client teaching about newborn heart failure

Rationale: The new parent will require additional support for themselves as well as their newborn. A social work consult will provide information to assist with housing, social support, and mental health support upon discharge. If the new parent withheld news of the pregnancy from the family, it is recommended to determine the needs of the new parent first and encourage them to seek additional supports from friends and other people in their lives. Clinical consequences of congenital heart defects include heart failure and hypoxemia. While in the hospital, the new parent will develop skills associated with recognizing symptoms associated with hypoxemia and to be monitored using pulse oximetry. The staff will assume responsibility to monitor for heart failure. Upon discharge, the new parent will need to recognize the signs and symptoms associated with right- and left-sided heart failure, given the large ventricular septal defect and the eventual increase in right ventricular size. New parents are taught how to assist in improving cardiac function, decrease cardiac demands, reduce respiratory distress, maintain nutritional status, promote fluid loss, and provide family support for newborns who may develop heart failure as a result of a congenital heart disease. Newborns less than 3 months and children older than 4 years of age have higher mortality rates with surgical interventions at this time. The newborn and parent will be supported until surgery is booked. The nurse should not assume the new parent is interested in meditation or yoga for coping strategies. A conversation is warranted to explore strategies to help with coping during this difficult and stressful time of becoming a new parent of a child with a congenital heart disease. The new parent has made it clear they did not involve their parents with the pregnancy. Providing emotional support to the new parent to determine what is best for them and their child allows for autonomous decision-making and minimizes bias for grandparent involvement.

NCJMM Step: Take Action
Reference: Keenan-Lindsay et al. (2022), pp. 526–526 (social support while parents transition to parenthood), 1159–1162 (family-centred care), 1277–1278 (care of the newborn with a cardiovascular condition).

Answer 1.6

CLIENT STATEMENTS	UNDER-STANDING	NO UNDER-STANDING
"I will need to notify the surgical team if the baby is not gaining weight."	○	✔
"If the baby turns blue, I need to put the baby against my chest with the knees up. I think you call it a knee–chest position."	✔	○
"Seizures do not run in my family so I do not think it would happen with the baby"	○	✔
"I have called my best friend who is going to stay with me and help with the baby."	✔	○
"If I see the baby is working hard to breath, I will call the nurse on call."	✔	○

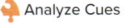

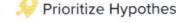

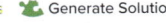

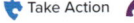

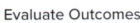

Rationale: The new parent will be instructed to consult the public health nurse, not the surgical team, to determine how best to manage failure to thrive. There are many public supports to help new parents. Failure to thrive is a concern for new parents with children who have a congenital heart defect such as tetralogy of Fallot. Parents will have to monitor nutritional intake, including hydration status. Putting the baby in a knee–chest position is suggested when treating hypercyanotic spells. The new parent can also use a calm, comforting approach, and administer 100% blow-by oxygen. In the hospital, there will be other supports in place, such as pharmacological intervention (morphine) and fluid replacement. Infants and children diagnosed with tetralogy of Fallot are at increased risk for pulmonary embolus, seizures, loss of consciousness, or sudden death following a Tet spell or anoxic spell. Information must be provided to new parents on how best to support children who seize. Increasing support for new parents with children diagnosed with congenital heart disease is important; it is good that the parent in this scenario will have new support when discharge arrives. Monitoring for clinical manifestations associated with heart failure is important for new parents when they are discharged home. Abdominal retractions and nasal flaring would indicate pulmonary congestion requiring prompt medical attention.

NCJMM Step: Evaluate Outcomes
Reference: Keenan-Lindsay et al. (2022), pp. 924–926 (failure to thrive), 1245–1255 (heart failure), 1255–1256 (management of hypoxemia), 1257–1262 (care of the newborn with congenital heart disease).

Pediatrics 2.0

Answer 2.1

Nurses' Notes	Vital Signs

1845h: Client arrived at ED accompanied by birth parents. Parents indicated client had low-grade fever all day and was lethargic. Parents felt client had a virus, administered children's acetaminophen (160 mg/5 mL × 1 dose) at 1200h, and encouraged fluid hydration by giving child almond milk and water; client vomits from cow's milk and has been drinking almond milk for 1 year. Client fell asleep on couch at approximately 1620h and parents found client with increased full-body stiffness, eyes open and deviating upwards, and unresponsive to voice or physical stimulation. Parents brought child to ED, who presents sitting on birth parent's lap resting head against upper chest. Client found to move all four extremities independently, able to follow commands and squeeze fingers moderately. Pupils equal in size at 2 mm and bilateral reaction to light. Heart rate regular and strong auscultated at the apical site. Skin warm and dry to touch. Lungs auscultated for bilateral clear air entry throughout anterior and posterior. Client has not eaten any food today, only drank almond milk and water. Bowel sounds remain hypoactive × 4. Parents estimate fluid intake at 700 mL of almond milk and 700 mL of water. Client has voided once today a small amount.

Rationale: The client presents with a viral infection and a low-grade fever. The most concerning assessment data relate to the birth parents finding the client with full-body stiffness, eyes open and deviating upward, and unresponsive to voice or physical stimulation. These symptoms indicate a possible neurological cause. Cardiovascular and respiratory assessments are unremarkable. The client not eating any food prior to the ED is concerning, as is the lack of urine, despite having drunk approximately 1.5 L, leading to possible dehydration.

NCJMM Step: Recognize Cues
Reference: Keenan-Lindsay et al. (2022), pp. 933–955, 1336–1376, 1530.

Answer 2.2

- ✔ Fluid imbalance
- ✔ Leukocytosis
- ✔ Confusion
- ☐ Dysrhythmias
- ☐ Bowel obstruction

Rationale: The client is at risk for a fluid imbalance given the possibility of dehydration. The client has consumed 1.4 L of fluid but has only voided once. The blood pressure remains normal but the heart rate is slightly elevated. This could be a result of the higher temperature and a normal physiological response. The client has a low-grade fever, which could account for a higher white blood cell (WBC) count in contrast to low or normal WBC levels. If the WBC count is elevated, then the presumed virus is likely a bacterial infection. Given the neurological presentation, the client could develop confusion depending on the cause of the clinical manifestations. For any client with neurological presentation, monitoring for confusion, changes in pupils, and changes in level of consciousness are key considerations. The client has not eaten all day prior to the ED visit, which is not unusual for a child who is feeling unwell; this does not mean there is a bowel obstruction. The client has hypoactive bowel sounds documented. Dysrhythmias are a potential concern for a client who is not voiding; however, for typically healthy individuals without previous cardiac issues, dysrhythmias would be less common. Laboratory values would determine if that was a potential complication for this client.

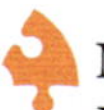

NCJMM Step: Analyze Cues
Reference: Keenan-Lindsay et al. (2022), pp. 933–955, 1336–1376, 1530.

Answer 2.3

The client is at highest risk of developing **seizure disorder** as evidenced by **sodium level**.

Rationale: The child is at risk of having a seizure disorder as evidenced by the low sodium levels. In the initial presentation at home, the client presented with seizure-like activity. The client presented with tonic clinical manifestations such as eyes rolling upward, stiffening in general with arms flexed and legs, head, and neck extended, apnea, and increased salivation, followed by some confusion, then a period of sleep, then return to full consciousness. Hyponatremia and hypernatremia can cause neurological presentation. Sodium depletion usually causes hypo-osmolality with the movement of water into cells. The most life-threatening consequence is cerebral edema and increased intracranial pressure. Neurological changes include lethargy, confusion, apprehension, seizures, and coma. The cause of the hyponatremia was a dilutional element of the blood as a result of the almond milk and water. Almond milk is mostly made up of water and in conjunction with water causes the serum sodium levels to be dilutional. Almond milk is typically used as a substitute for milk products. There is no evidence of maltreatment as presented in the narrative. Bacterial meningitis could be a consideration; however, the WBC results indicate no bacteria at play. The client does not present with clinical manifestations associated with hydrocephalus, such as pupils described as a setting sun, having a large cranium, or high-pitched crying. The lab results are normal except for sodium. The potassium levels are high and should be monitored.

NCJMM Step: Prioritize Hypothesis
References: Keenan-Lindsay et al. (2022), pp. 933–955, 1336–1376, 1521–1529, 1530; Power-Kean et al. (2023), pp. 120–121.

Answer 2.4

POTENTIAL ORDERS	INDICATED	NOT INDICATED
Computed tomography (CT) head	○	✔
Hypertonic intravenous fluids	✔	○
Chest X-ray	○	✔
Pulse oximetry	✔	○
Packed red blood cells	○	✔
Anticonvulsant medication	○	✔

Rationale: Hypertonic intravenous fluids would be chosen initially to increase the serum sodium levels. Once the sodium levels are corrected, the risk of a nonfebrile seizure would be reduced. Isotonic intravenous fluids must be administered at a rate consistent with the client's weight. Hypertonic solutions must be administered slowly to prevent cerebral edema. The only other order that would be appropriate for the client is to monitor pulse oximetry. If the client should have another seizure, monitoring for hypoxemia would be necessary. A CT head would not be warranted unless other clinical manifestations became more apparent to consider a test. The client would not have a chest X-ray as the lung sounds were clear. The hemoglobin level was normal, so initiating a blood transfusion would be unnecessary. Anticonvulsant medication would not be warranted at this time as the cause can be corrected. The medication would be ordered to help with symptom control if another seizure occurs, but the client would not require anticonvulsant medication.

NCJMM Step: Generate Solutions
Reference: Keenan-Lindsay et al. (2022), pp. 933–955, 1336–1376, 1521–1530.

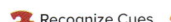

Answer 2.5

- ✔ Initiate 3% normal saline at a rate of 3 mL/kg
- ☐ Social work consult
- ☐ Encourage oral intake of food
- ✔ Document general observation of seizure
- ✔ Remove harmful objects around the client
- ☐ Restrain child

Rationale: The client will have hypertonic or isotonic intravenous solutions initiated to correct the hyponatremia. Once the electrolyte imbalance is corrected the client will make a full recovery. It is the nurses' responsibility to document any seizure activity, which would include describing the event, time of onset and how long it lasts, any changes in behaviour, movement, cardiovascular status, and hypoxemia. It is imperative to remove any objects around the client that could cause harm. There are seizure pads that can be applied on the bed rails to prevent injury to the client. The bed is placed at the lowest setting. If the birth parents are holding the child, the client is placed in the lowest and safest position. Social work can be consulted to provide support to the family; however, their services are not needed immediately. Encouraging oral intake can occur when the client is feeling better. The nurse should not restrain a client who is actively seizing.

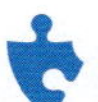

NCJMM Step: Take Action
Reference: Keenan-Lindsay et al. (2022), pp. 933–955, 1336–1376, 1521–1530.

Answer 2.6

ASSESSMENT FINDINGS	IMPROVED	NO CHANGE	DECLINED
New blood draw with sodium at 137 mmol/L	✔	○	○
Emesis	○	○	✔
Client sitting upright reading a book	✔	○	○
No further seizure activity	✔	○	○

Rationale: When the sodium level increases, the risk of seizure activity decreases. Emesis indicates potential pressure on the brain, which could be a decline in status and something to monitor in the client. If the client participates in play and social activities, then the status would be considered improved. The goal is no further seizure activity.

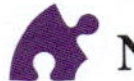

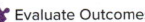

NCJMM Step: Evaluate Outcomes
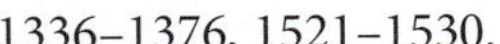
Reference: Keenan-Lindsay et al. (2022), pp. 933–955, 1336–1376, 1521–1530.

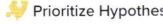

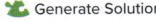

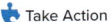

Pediatrics 3.0

Answer 3.1

- ✔ Mucous membranes
- ☐ Urine output
- ✔ Lung sounds
- ☐ Vital signs
- ✔ Dressing
- ☐ Nausea
- ✔ Pain
- ✔ Skin temperature

Rationale: Dry mucous membranes indicate dehydration despite adequate blood pressure with adequate cardiac output. This is a sign to consider in monitoring fluid status. The lung sounds are concerning specifically to the left side with no breath sounds noted on the left side of the lung anteriorly and posteriorly. Pain is a consideration despite the client indicating the value at 4. Any pain is not an expected finding despite a back stab wound. The dressing, and specifically the drainage on the dressing, is concerning as there could be a risk for bleeding. There is unknown information about the amount of blood lost at the site of the incident. The lower extremity skin temperature is concerning as this indicates vasoconstriction and possible hemodynamic involvement. The urine output is not concerning at this time as the hemodynamic status and gas exchange would be most concerning. The vital signs at this time are stable despite tachycardia. The client is compensating at the moment but is not experiencing hypotension or a fever. The pulse oximetry of 90% is something to monitor but does not require immediate follow-up. The client has nausea, but no emesis is documented. This is not an immediate life-threatening concern.

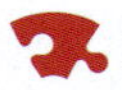
NCJMM Step: Recognize Cues
Reference: Power Kean et al. (2023), p. 501.

Answer 3.2

The nurse should recognize that the client is potentially experiencing complications of **bleeding** and **impaired gas exchange.**

Rationale: The dressing is saturated with sanguineous drainage, indicating there is a bleeding issue along with impaired gas exchange as addressed by the saturation level, decreased breath sounds on the left lower lobe anteriorly and posteriorly, and shallow breaths with increased depth with minimal movement. Impaired gas exchange with dehydration indicates the client could be at risk of developing hypovolemia or anemia. The client has not received any fluid hydration to allow for kidney perfusion. The client's gait was documented as steady without complaints of dizziness with a change in position. Petechiae has not been indicated on the assessment as this is a relatively new stab wound. There is no infection as the temperature is within normal range.

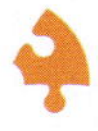
NCJMM Step: Analyze Cues
Reference: Power Kean et al. (2023), p. 501.

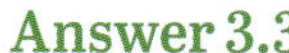

Answer 3.3

The client is at highest risk of developing **acute anemia.**

Rationale: The client is bleeding considerably from the stab wound. The most potential condition of concern is acute anemia. The client has clear air entry; therefore, pneumonia is not a consideration, and the client is afebrile. The client is a relatively healthy 16-year-old with no previous comorbidities indicating a concern for deep vein thrombosis. The client has not voided, but jumping to acute renal failure with a recent admission and no laboratory data to back that hypothesis up is not appropriate at this time. The client indicates no concerns for dysrhythmias despite no renal output since admission. There is no indication of thrombocytopenia such as petechiae, bruising, or any other hematological condition.

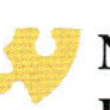
NCJMM Step: Prioritize Hypothesis
Reference: Power-Kean et al. (2023), p. 501.

Answer 3.4

POTENTIAL NURSING INTERVENTIONS	INDICATED	NOT INDICATED
Request an order to initiate oxygen therapy	✔	○
Prepare to insert an in-dwelling urinary catheter	○	✔
Encourage oral fluid intake	○	✔
Request an order to insert a second peripheral intravenous catheter	✔	○
Prepare the rapid fluid infuser	○	✔
Inform the client they will be receiving albumin, a blood product	○	✔

Rationale: The nurse should apply oxygen therapy as the client's oxygen saturation level has decreased from 90% to 84%. This client presents with acute anemia due to blood loss from a stab wound. With the loss of blood, the client has decreased oxygen-carrying capacity resulting in low oxygen levels. If there is no intervention, the client could become hypoxemic, resulting in organ damage. The client is attempting to compensate for the increase in heart rate. The other intervention, based on the possibilities, is to insert another peripheral intravenous catheter to provide additional intravenous fluids and potential blood products given the laboratory value. A urinary catheter is not indicated at this time as the client is able to void independently. Oral fluid intake will not be enough to compensate for the hemodynamic shifts for this client and necessary interventions. The client's presentation warrants caution and concern; however, rapid infusion is not needed yet.

NCJMM Step: Generate Solutions
References: Power-Kean et al. (2023), p. 501; Tyerman & Cobbett (2023), pp. 710–711.

Answer 3.5

- ☐ Monitor intake and output
- ✔ 0.9% sodium chloride (normal saline) 500 mL IV bolus × 1 then reassess BP
- ✔ Transfuse 1 unit of packed red blood cells (PRBC) ASAP
- ☐ Chest X-ray
- ✔ Oxygen therapy 0–6 L to maintain peripheral oximetry greater than 92%
- ☐ Administer hydromorphone 10 mg IV for pain every 1–4 hr

Rationale: The client's hemodynamic status has been deteriorating consistently over 4 hours. The client requires IV fluids, such as crystalloid solutions such as normal saline or Ringer's lactate, and whole blood products transfused as the client's hemoglobin is documented at 77 g/L. The client also requires additional oxygen support due to the low hemoglobin and decreased oxygen-carrying capacity. It will be important to monitor intake and output; however, stabilizing the client is the most important action at this time. A chest X-ray will be necessary to identify the severity of the injury, but the client's hemodynamic status has changed, and their breathing and circulation are compromised. Administering a narcotic is warranted; however, the order's dose is too high and could cause serious injury to the client, leading to respiratory depression. This order would need to be clarified by the nurse.

NCJMM Step: Take Action
References: Power-Kean et al. (2023), p. 501; Tyerman & Cobbett (2023), pp. 710–711.

Answer 3.6

ASSESSMENT FINDINGS	IMPROVED	NO CHANGE	DECLINED
Pulse oximetry reading 93%	✔	○	○
Dressing changes required every 1 hour	○	○	✔
Pale mucous membranes	○	✔	○
Dorsalis pedis pulses palpable	✔	○	○
BP 102/75	✔	○	○

Rationale: After fluid resuscitation and whole blood administration, improvements in hemodynamic status are the goal of treatment. Improved oxygenation is noted with a higher pulse oximetry reading, likely due to fluid and blood administration and oxygen support. There is an improved blood pressure as well. What remains concerning is the amount of bleeding and required dressing changes for the stab wound. Platelets may need to be administered if the bleeding persists and to monitor the hemoglobin levels. There is no change in the mucous membranes as they remain pale.

NCJMM Step: Evaluate Outcomes
References: Power-Kean et al. (2023), p. 501; Tyerman & Cobbett (2023), pp. 710–711.

Pediatrics 4.0

Answer 4.1

- ✔ Temperature
- ✔ Photophobia
- ✔ Stiff neck
- ✔ Listlessness
- ☐ Bowel sounds
- ☐ Lack of appetite
- ✔ Emesis
- ☐ Urine output

Rationale: Key signs of an inflammatory condition of the brain, specifically bacterial meningitis, are fever, severe headache, nausea, vomiting, and nuchal rigidity (resistance to flexion of the neck—called a *Brudzinski sign*). Additional signs are photophobia and a decreased level of consciousness. The clinical manifestations above indicate a possible inflammatory condition of the brain requiring further investigation. The client presents with active bowel signs in all four quadrants. Nausea and vomiting are also indications of increased pressure on the brain. Lack of appetite is not a finding that requires immediate follow-up. The client has not voided yet, but the blood pressure and heart rate are stable at present.

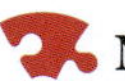

NCJMM Step: Recognize Cues
References: Keenan-Lindsay et al. (2022), pp. 1358–1361; Tyerman & Cobbett (2023), pp. 1478–1480.

Answer 4.2

CLIENT FINDINGS	MIGRAINE	GASTROENTERITIS	BACTERIAL MENINGITIS
Fever	○	✔	✔
Lethargy	○	○	✔
Neck stiffness	○	○	✔
Headache	○	○	✔
Nausea	○	✔	✔
Emesis	○	✔	✔

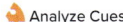

Rationale: A client experiencing a migraine exhibits the following clinical manifestations: nausea, vomiting, edema, irritability, sweating, photophobia, phonophobia, and prodrome of sensory, motor, or psychic phenomena. A tension-type headache presents with palpable neck and shoulder muscle tension, stiff neck, and tenderness. A client presenting with gastroenteritis, which is inflammation of the mucosa of the stomach and small intestine, will have clinical manifestations of nausea, vomiting, diarrhea, abdominal cramping, abdominal distension, fever, increased white blood cell counts, and blood or mucus in the stool. Clinical manifestations associated with bacterial meningitis include fever, severe headache, nausea, vomiting, and nuchal rigidity (resistance to flexion of the neck, called a *Brudzinski sign*). Additional signs are photophobia and decreased level of consciousness.

NCJMM Step: Analyze Cues
References: Keenan-Lindsay et al. (2022), pp. 1358–1361; Tyerman & Cobbett (2023), pp. 1050 (gastroenteritis); 1478–1480 (bacterial meningitis), 1511–1512 (migraine).

Answer 4.3

The client is at highest risk of developing **increased intracranial pressure** and **seizures.**

Rationale: As a result of the increased swelling of the meningeal tissues and obstruction of normal flow of the cerebrospinal fluid from the ventricles, increased intracranial pressure is a serious complication of bacterial meningitis. Most clients with the infection will develop increased intracranial pressure, altering the client's level of consciousness. The infective process of the illness causes inflammation, exudation, white blood cell accumulation, and varying degrees of tissue damage. The brain becomes hyperemic and edematous, and the entire surface of the brain is covered with a layer of purulent exudate that varies with the type of bacterial organism. As infection extends to the ventricles, thick pus, fibrin, or adhesions may occlude the narrow passages and obstruct the flow of cerebrospinal fluid. Seizures are often the first sign of a cerebral infection due to the hyperactivity of neurons firing as a result of the brain becoming increasingly edematous. Anticipating these primary complications will prevent further injury to the client. The client is also at risk for blindness, hearing loss, hemiparesis, aphasia, hemianopia, cerebral abscesses, subdural empyema, subdural effusions, bradycardia, coma, and even death. There is no increase in ectopy of the conduction in the myocardium because this is a neurological condition. The ventricles of the heart do not increase in size, leading to cardiomyopathy. The client is not at risk of gaining weight as a result of the condition.

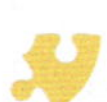
NCJMM Step: Prioritize Hypothesis
References: Keenan-Lindsay et al. (2022), pp. 1358–1361; Tyerman & Cobbett (2023), pp. 1478–1480.

Answer 4.4

POTENTIAL NURSING INTERVENTIONS	INDICATED	NOT INDICATED
Reposition the client in high-Fowler's position	○	✔
Prepare client for a lumbar puncture	✔	○
Place the client on contact isolation	○	✔
Ensure suction is working properly	✔	○
Provide reassurance to the parents	✔	○

Rationale: The client is exhibiting classic Cushing triad clinical manifestations, which is a sign of increasing intracranial pressure (widened pulse pressure, bradycardia, and irregular respiratory pattern). The client is also exhibiting changes in consciousness, requiring prompt attention for treatment and diagnosis. Projectile vomiting reflects pressure on the medulla oblongata, indicating that there is increasing intracranial pressure. The client is repositioned in the recovery position, not high-Fowler's, to prevent possible aspiration given that they are projectile vomiting. The client will need a lumbar puncture to analyze the cerebrospinal fluid. The client will need to be placed on droplet isolation, not contact isolation. Bacterial meningitis is spread through respiratory and throat secretions of the carrier. Ensuring suction is working is a good safety practice each time the nurse walks into the room. The parents will be scared; providing reassurance to them while their child is ill is part of holistic nursing care.

NCJMM Step: Generate Solutions
References: Cobbett (2025), pp. 275e.15–275e.22; Keenan-Lindsay et al. (2022), pp. 1358–1361; Tyerman & Cobbett (2023), pp. 1478–1480.

Answer 4.5

Orders

2200h:
- Acetaminophen for temperature greater than 38.5°C (101.3°F)
- Strict monitoring of input and output
- Initiate broad-spectrum cephalosporin (Ceftriaxone)
- Phenytoin to be administered per peripheral venous access device
- Initiate oxygen therapy at 2 L/min to 6 L/min to achieve pulse oximetry greater than 92%
- Laboratory tests: blood cultures, electrolytes, glucose, complete blood count, coagulation profile
- Computed tomography (CT) head
- Keep the head of the bed elevated to 45-degree angle
- Minimize stimulation in the room, lights dimmed

Rationale: Helping to reduce the temperature will help reduce the swelling in the brain. This reduction will help prevent further complications caused by increased intracranial pressure with the potential of death. A fever increases the frequency of seizures; therefore, the primary goal is to reduce seizure activity and to reduce the fever. High fevers increase metabolic rate and cause insensible fluid loss. The client needs to be monitored for seizure activity. Initiating antibiotics even before blood cultures and cerebrospinal fluid analysis are completed gets treatment started early. The Canadian Paediatric Society recommends Ceftriaxone as the antibiotic of choice. Monitoring for fluid status is important. High fevers contribute to an increase in metabolic rate and insensible fluid loss. Oxygen therapy is initiated to improve gas exchange for the client. Clients need to be monitored for dehydration and to ensure adequate fluid intake. Blood cultures and blood work provide a foundation for treatment. CT head will help in determining how edematous the brain is from the infection. Maintaining a low-stimulation environment (with reduced lights, music, and number of visitors) will decrease the body's response and thus help avoid the swelling.

NCJMM Step: Take Action
References: Astle & Duggleby (2024), pp. 678–680; Cobbett (2025), pp. 275e.15–275e.22; Keenan-Lindsay et al. (2022), pp. 1358–1361; La Saux (2020); Tyerman & Cobbett (2023), pp. 1455–1462, 1478–1480.

Answer 4.6

ASSESSMENT FINDINGS	IMPROVED	NO CHANGE	DECLINED
Client requests a popsicle	✔	○	○
T 39.7°C (101.6°F)		✔	○
Respirations become regular with good lung expansion	✔	○	○
Hemiparesis	○	○	✔
Nauseated with emesis	○	✔	○

Rationale: If the client is alert enough to ask for a popsicle, that is an improvement over their previous lethargic and listless response. The antibiotics, along with the other treatment measures, may be helping to reduce some of the swelling. It may take time for the fever to resolve. Fever management is a priority in treatment for the client. The respirations have improved, possibly on account of the antibiotic therapy or the addition of oxygen for the client. Hemiparesis may occur but usually resolves over time; if it does not resolve, further investigations, such as a cerebral abscess, subdural empyema, subdural effusion, or persistent meningitis, may still be present. Nausea with emesis indicates that there is still pressure on the medulla oblongata. There has been some improvement in swelling in the brain, but there are still residual effects of the infection.

NCJMM Step: Evaluate Outcomes
References: Cobbett (2025), pp. 275e.15–275e.22; Keenan-Lindsay et al. (2022), pp. 1358–1361; Tyerman & Cobbett (2023), pp. 1455–1462, 1478–1480.

Pediatrics 5.0

Answer 5.1

- ☐ Temperature
- ✔ Abnormal heart sounds
- ✔ Bilateral upper extremities warm, bilateral lower extremities cool
- ✔ Cyanotic lips
- ☐ Discontinuation of chest feeding
- ✔ Characteristics of the cry
- ☐ Weight

Rationale: The client's presenting symptoms of an S3 associated with inspiratory crackles indicate the client has reduced left ventricular systolic function. The bilateral warm upper extremities and bilateral cool lower extremities associated with the two differing blood pressures are also indicative of a possible congenital heart defect, such as coarctation of the aorta. The cyanotic lips are consistent with impaired gas exchange. At this point in the presentation, the infant's airway, breathing, and circulation are all compromised. Finally, the characteristics of the cry, described as shrill and piercing, may indicate increased intracranial pressure, which warrants further investigation. The temperature presents within normal limits. The birth parent attempted to alter the infant's feeding habits, changing from chest feeding to formula feeding, hoping to increase the infant's weight. The weight loss is concerning and will need to be monitored, but it does not warrant immediate action.

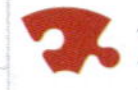

NCJMM Step: Recognize Cues
References: Jarvis et al. (2024), pp. 502–543; Keenan-Lindsay et al. (2022), pp. 1240–1245; Power-Kean et al. (2023), pp. 637–652.

Answer 5.2

- ✔ Impaired renal perfusion
- ☐ Peripheral edema
- ✔ Increased intracranial pressure
- ☐ Delayed gastric emptying
- ✔ Impaired gas exchange
- ☐ Respiratory infection
- ✔ Reduced cardiac output

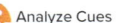

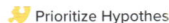

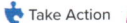

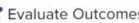

Rationale: The client presents with a concerning neurological presentation, including bulging fontanels, high-pitched cry, distended scalp veins, and poor feeding, which together indicate increased intracranial pressure in an infant. The petechiae on the lower extremities suggest thrombocytopenia and may require further investigation. The client presents with increased volume due to left ventricular dysfunction leading to an S3 and crackles in the lungs when auscultated. The client has warm upper extremities, cool lower extremities, and different blood pressures in upper and lower extremities as evidenced by extremity hypertension with readings 20 mm Hg higher than those of the lower extremity. The client has been losing weight, is unable to feed, and has tachypnea with pallor, which may be related to a cardiac condition. Low cardiac output will lead to reduced renal perfusion due to left ventricle dysfunction. The development of cyanosis and crackles is indicative of impaired gas exchange but is not a respiratory failure. The client does not present with peripheral edema, which is related to more chronic symptoms. Despite poor feeding, the client continues to have bowel movements, but this is unrelated to delayed gastric emptying. The client does not present with symptoms associated with a respiratory infection given that the client remains afebrile.

NCJMM Step: Analyze Cues
References: Jarvis et al. (2024), pp. 502–543; Keenan-Lindsay et al. (2022), pp. 693–694 (intracranial hemorrhage); 1240–1245 (congenital heart defects); 1337–1343 (intracranial pressure); Power-Kean et al. (2023), pp. 637–652.

Answer 5.3

The client is at highest risk of developing a **stroke** as a result of **coarctation of the aorta.**

Rationale: The client is at greatest risk for a stroke. Immediate attention is required for this client. The high-pitched cry associated with petechia and the classic presentation of coarctation of the aorta may increase the vascular resistance in the brain. Higher blood pressure on the upper extremities contributes to increased vascular resistance, especially with reduced cardiac output due to the narrowing of the aorta. The client is not at risk of developing anemia or low hemoglobin levels, given the clinical presentation. Dysrhythmias have the potential to occur, but the highest risk remains a stroke, as evidenced by coarctation of the aorta, given the blood pressure of the infant. Hypoxemia is already occurring, given the cyanosis and low pulse oximetry reading. The client could develop renal failure as a result of low cardiac output; however, the addition of intravenous fluids should prevent renal failure and increase perfusion to the kidneys.

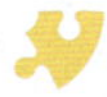
NCJMM Step: Prioritize Hypothesis
References: Jarvis et al. (2024), pp. 502–543; Keenan-Lindsay et al. (2022), pp. 693–694 (intracranial hemorrhage); 1240–1245 (congenital heart defects); 1337–1343 (intracranial pressure); Power-Kean et al. (2023), pp. 637–652.

Answer 5.4

POTENTIAL INTERVENTIONS	INDICATED	NOT INDICATED
Doll's head manoeuvre	○	✔
Computed tomography (CT) of the head	✔	○
Cardiac electrocardiography (ECG)	○	✔
Magnetic resonance imaging (MRI)	✔	○
Chest X-ray	✔	○
Cardiac echocardiogram	✔	○

Rationale: The client presents with two conditions: coarctation of the aorta that requires intervention and symptoms associated with increased intracranial pressure. The CT head and MRI will provide information about the inflammation in the brain and the cardiac echocardiogram will show the level of narrowing in the aorta. A treatment plan can be made with more diagnostic information. Understanding what tests will be needed for the client helps the nurse anticipate what the next steps will be for the client and the family. The client may need a chest X-ray to determine the severity of the fluid within the alveoli. The crackles would be associated with left ventricular dysfunction. A doll's head manoeuvre is associated with a client who is thought to have neurological death. This diagnostic test proves a dysfunction of the brainstem or oculomotor nerve. Cardiac electrocardiography will only provide information about the function of the electrical system of the heart, which creates a picture of the rhythm.

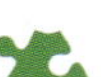
NCJMM Step: Generate Solutions
References: Jarvis et al. (2024), pp. 502–543; Keenan-Lindsay et al. (2022), pp. 693–694 (intracranial hemorrhage); 1240–1245 (congenital heart defects); 1337–1343 (intracranial pressure); Power-Kean et al. (2023), pp. 637–652.

Answer 5.5

- Ensure the client's hospital bed is prepared for the parent
- Check that all safety equipment is working, such as suction and oxygen flow meter
- Obtain baseline vital signs upon return to the unit
- Outline any bleeding on the dressing with a pen and document finding
- Monitor for pain by observing for rigidity or thrashing, crying, lowered brows

Rationale: Nursing action upon the client's return to the unit will be to monitor for airway, breathing, and circulation. Safety is of the utmost importance, so ensuring all safety equipment is in working condition for the client is a nursing priority. Obtaining baseline vital signs ensures foundational knowledge on which to base decisions if needed. Monitoring for improvements or a decline in temperature, heart rate, respiratory rate, and pulse oximetry is associated with good nursing care. Outlining the bleeding on a dressing ensures the nurse has knowledge that bleeding may occur after a surgical procedure, and monitoring the borders of the shadowing informs the nurse if the bleeding is improving or worsening. Good postoperative practice includes reinforcing dressings but not removing dressings, and monitoring for signs of bleeding on the bed or areas below the surgical site. Monitoring for pain is known as a fifth vital sign. Ensuring the client has proper pain management postoperatively enables the cardiovascular and respiratory systems to recover. The client's bed should be made, not the parents' bed. Although family support is important, prioritizing that the crib is ready for the client to increase comfort level is a therapeutic priority.

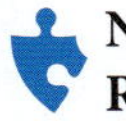
NCJMM Step: Take Action
Reference: Keenan-Lindsay et al. (2022), pp. 813–839, 1074–1084 (postoperative care).

Answer 5.6

BODY SYSTEM	NEW ASSESSMENT FINDINGS
Neurological	✔ Sunken fontanel ○ Moves all four extremities independently ✔ Requires q2h pain medication ✔ T 38.9°C (102.0°F)
Cardiovascular	✔ Capillary refill greater than 4 seconds ✔ Heart rate 170 ○ S1 and S2 heart sounds only ✔ Client extremities cool to touch × 4
Respiratory	○ Fine inspiratory crackles ○ Pulse oximetry measured at 97% on 3 L/min by mask ✔ Respiratory rate 68 ○ No cyanosis noted
Gastrointestinal	✔ 3% weight loss since last known weight ✔ Decreased tear production ○ Desire to take formula from bottle

Rationale: Monitoring client outcomes in the post-operative period is important for quality care. Upon review of this information system by system, the client is dehydrated as evidenced by the sunken fontanels, rapid heart rate of 170 (normal for 0–3 months is 100–160), tachypnea of 68 breaths per minute, weight loss of 3% (weight loss 3–5% for an infant is considered mild dehydration), and decreased tear production. The client is also demonstrating reduced perfusion as evidenced by capillary refill greater than 4 seconds and cool-to-touch extremities. The client has developed a fever postoperatively, which will need to be monitored in the event of an infection. The client's neurological status remains intact as they can move all four extremities. The heart failure has improved as evidenced by only auscultating S1 and S2 heart sounds, pulse oximetry maintaining on 3 L per minute of oxygen per mask, and no cyanosis noted. Fine inspiratory crackles remain unchanged from the previous assessment but have not progressed to coarse crackles. The client also wants to take formula from a bottle, which will help with hydration and nutrition, but only after bowel sounds have returned. Introducing fluids too early after surgery can lead to emesis and aspiration.

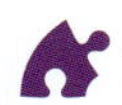
NCJMM Step: Evaluate Outcomes
Reference: Keenan-Lindsay et al. (2022), pp. 1074–1084 (postoperative care), 1179–1181 (dehydration).

Pediatrics 6.0

Answer 6.1

☐ Pupillary response
☐ Alertness
✔ Pain with swallowing
☐ Lung sound characteristics
☐ Pulses
☐ Pulse oximetry
✔ Respiratory breathing pattern characteristics

Rationale: The client presents with a sore throat, difficulty swallowing, and shallow breaths. They were not expanding their lung fields despite being clear with auscultation as no adventitious breath sounds were noted, except for quiet air entry. The fever is concerning as it relates to the sore throat; this would indicate the cause being more bacterial in nature, not viral. Monitoring the airway in a young child is a priority in this presentation. The client's bilateral pupils briskly respond to light. There is no notation of difference in size or shape. The client is alert and can answer questions, even stating they are tired. The lung sounds only present with quiet air entry but no adventitious sounds, such as crackles or wheezing. The pulses are weak but palpable. Pulse is not a priority to monitor, especially since the child has a blood pressure and heart rate. All initial vital signs are within normal range.

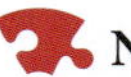
NCJMM Step: Recognize Cues
References: Keenan-Lindsay et al. (2022), pp. 1130–1131, 1530 (normal vital signs); Power-Kean et al. (2023), p. 703.

Answer 6.2

CLIENT FINDINGS	PNEUMONIA	ACUTE EPI-GLOTTITIS	RESPIRATORY SYNCYTIAL VIRUS
Fever	✔	✔	✔
Shallow breaths	✔	○	○
Sore throat	○	✔	○
Restlessness	✔	✔	✔
Lack of cough	○	✔	○
Clear air entry	○	✔	○

Rationale: A client who presents with clinical manifestations associated with pneumonia may have a preceding viral illness followed by fever with chills and rigors, shortness of breath, and increasingly productive cough. Auscultation indicates abnormalities such as crackles or decreased breath sounds. The client may also present with malaise, emesis, abdominal pain, and chest pain. A client who presents with an abrupt onset can rapidly progress to having severe respiratory distress. A child, typically between the ages of 2 and 7 years, who suddenly develops a fever can present with a sore throat and pain on swallowing. Other symptoms may include irritability, extreme restlessness, anxiety, apprehension, and fear. Initially, the client may present with slow, quiet breathing to enable better gas exchange. If the airway begins to be obstructed, the client may develop suprasternal and substernal retractions as well as stridor. The throat will present red and inflamed with a large, red, and edematous epiglottis. Clients who present with a respiratory syncytial virus (RSV) are usually under 2 years of age. Typically, there is an upper respiratory infection after an incubation of about 5 to 8 days. Clinical manifestations include rhinorrhea, low-grade fever, and otitis media and conjunctivitis may also be present. In time, a cough develops leading to a lower respiratory infection. Infants may also experience lethargy, poor feeding, or irritability when the upper airway is affected. Lower airway involvement leads to adventitious breath sounds such as wheezing, retractions, crackles, dyspnea, tachypnea, and diminished breath sounds.

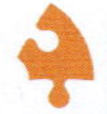

NCJMM Step: Analyze Cues
References: Keenan-Lindsay et al. (2022), pp. 1130–1131 (acute epiglottitis), 1133–1134 (RSV), 1134–1136 (pneumonia); Power-Kean et al. (2023), pp. 703 (acute epiglottis), 706 (bronchiolitis), 708 (pneumonia).

Answer 6.3

The client is at highest risk of developing **respiratory distress** as evidenced by **drooling** and **leaning over the bedside table.**

Rationale: The client is presenting with respiratory distress. Nasal flaring and use of suprasternal and substernal accessory muscles indicate respiratory distress. The classic tripod position (leaning over the bedside table) and drooling indicate that the client's airway is compromised, and if there is no immediate intervention, the client will go into cardiac arrest, requiring a code blue. Monitoring the deterioration of the airway is important to anticipate the most serious complication, respiratory failure. Epistaxis is a nosebleed. Atrophic glossitis is a big, beefy red tongue and is associated with pernicious anemia, folic acid deficiency, or iron deficiency anemia. The client did not ingest any object to consider a foreign body aspiration. If severe enough, this can also lead to respiratory distress or failure. The client does not exhibit any tracheal deviation or present with a cause for air becoming trapped in the pleural space. Candidiasis is a yeast infection often called *thrush*. The client did not present with white, cheesy, curd-like patches on the tongue or mouth. Clinical manifestations of pallor and the blood pressure indicate a hemodynamic shift for the client, which is another pattern of deterioration. The lung sounds are clear, and the pulses remain weak but palpable. This presentation does not indicate respiratory failure. Nasal flaring is associated with respiratory distress and should be monitored in the event the client's condition continues to deteriorate further to a severe critical abnormal scenario.

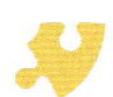

NCJMM Step: Prioritize Hypothesis
References: Keenan-Lindsay et al. (2022), pp. 1130–1131 (acute epiglottitis); Power-Kean et al. (2023), p. 703 (acute epiglottis).

Answer 6.4

POTENTIAL NURSING INTERVENTIONS	INDICATED	NOT INDICATED
Place the client in Trendelenburg position	○	✔
Ensure the difficult airway cart is present	✔	○
Encourage oral fluid intake	○	✔
Ensure suction is working correctly	✔	○
Prepare to insert a peripheral venous access device	✔	○
Ensure the client has a regular diet ordered	○	✔

Rationale: The client's airway, breathing, and circulation are of the highest priority for potential nursing interventions. The client is already presenting with clinical manifestations of airway inflammation as evidenced by drooling, tripod positioning, and difficulty swallowing. Ensuring the difficult airway cart is present is a safety consideration for the client, as a delay in intubation will delay appropriate treatment if the client's condition continues to deteriorate. Ensuring that the suction is working will be necessary if the client has any emesis, and suction will help during intubation, if necessary. Preparing to insert a peripheral venous access device will be a priority to initiate intravenous fluids and administer IV antibiotics. Placing the client in Trendelenburg position will assist with cardiac output but may exacerbate respiratory difficulty, increase airway edema, affect peak inspiratory pressures, and decrease lung volume. Offering oral fluids and food will only increase the client's risk for aspiration pneumonia.

NCJMM Step: Generate Solutions
References: Keenan-Lindsay et al. (2022), pp. 1130–1131 (acute epiglottitis); Power-Kean et al. (2023), p. 703 (acute epiglottis).

Answer 6.5

- ✔ Initiate humidified oxygen therapy at 2–6 L/min to maintain pulse oximetry greater than 95%
- ✔ Ceftriaxone 25 mg/kg IV q12h
- ✔ 0.9% normal saline (sodium chloride) 50 mL/hr
- ✔ Transfer to pediatric intensive care unit for close monitoring
- ☐ Monitor intake and output
- ☐ Vital signs q4h and prn

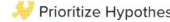

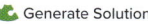

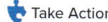

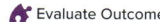

Rationale: Treatment for acute epiglottitis is airway protection, antibiotics, IV fluids, and reassurance. It is better to try humidified oxygen to see if the client's breathing improves. With no improvement, then nasotracheal intubation or tracheostomy would be considered. This treatment is best managed in an area that can easily and quickly accommodate critical care procedures such as a transfer to the pediatric intensive care unit. Bacterial epiglottis is best treated with antibiotic therapy and discontinued when the epiglottis is nearly normal in size, followed by oral administration for 7 to 10 days. Since the client cannot swallow, IV fluids are necessary to increase intravascular volume as evidenced by a lower blood pressure and to provide hydration to the client and perfusion to the kidneys. While these three main treatment plans are being initiated, the client needs to be transferred to a critical care area and an environment and staff who can handle changes in health status. Monitoring intake and output and vital signs are both important orders, but not priorities.

NCJMM Step: Take Action
References: Baxter (2020); Keenan-Lindsay et al. (2022), pp. 1130–1131 (acute epiglottitis).

Answer 6.6

- ✔ T 37.9°C (100.2°F)
- ✔ Client watching a movie on their parent's lap and laughing
- ✔ Able to eat a popsicle without complaining of sore throat
- ☐ Client has voided 250 mL in 8 hr since IV fluids initiated
- ✔ Respiratory rate 16 breaths per minute on 4 L of continuous oxygen via nasal prongs

Rationale: This client has responded well to the airway protection and antibiotics. The client's temperature has reduced, they are more alert and willing to engage in activities with their parents, they are able to eat a popsicle without difficulty, indicating a reduction in airway inflammation. Their respiratory rate has improved despite being on oxygen therapy via nasal prongs. The client does not present in respiratory distress any longer. They may be more dehydrated than initially thought, indicating small urine output.

NCJMM Step: Evaluate Outcomes
Reference: Keenan-Lindsay et al. (2022), pp. 1130–1131 (acute epiglottitis).

Mental Health Cases

Mental Health 1.0

Answer 1.1

Admission Notes

2138h: Police department called to scene and found the client wandering streets, barefoot, disheveled, poor hygiene, with no identification. Emergency medical service (EMS) were contacted to assess client. Client stated to EMS, "I need help. I can't sleep or eat; I can't seem to take care of my kids and I'm all they have." The client added more information: "I lost my job as a cook in a local restaurant 6 months ago because of the COVID-19 pandemic and cannot find another job. It's been really hard paying for food, not to mention the rent. I am going to be evicted. Where are my kids and I going to go? I feel so hopeless; what kind of a parent can't care for their children?" Client reports anxiety, type 2 diabetes mellitus as comorbidities treated by diet and exercise. Overall, client appears to be in good health. Client is appropriate, alert and orientated to person, place, and time, moves all extremities independently, no weakness noted. Chest remains clear upon air entry, client denies any chest pain, S1, S2 auscultated with no additional abnormal heart sounds noted. Client reports losing weight, approximately 2 kilograms in the last week due to loss of appetite. Denies any suicidal ideation, "I could never do that to my children." Bilateral bottom of feet assessed and noted to have four toonie-sized excoriated open areas with dried blood. No drainage noted.

Rationale: Identifying risk factors for depression is the priority for this client. Recognizing a stressful life event such as a job loss and income for 6 months may have detrimental effects on the family, nutrition, and stress levels. The loss of weight and inability to eat or sleep are risk factors associated with major depression episodes. The most common psychiatric presentations include depression and anxiety. These are cues indicating that there may be a bigger issue occurring with the client. These statements are important, so outpatient services may be consulted. They could address eviction and loss of income through social programs. The client requires further assessment to monitor for suicidal ideation despite none being present at the time of admission.

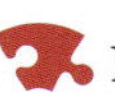
NCJMM Step: Recognize Cues
Reference: Pollard & Jakubec (2023), pp. 220–247.

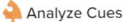

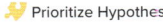

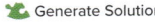

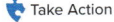

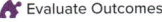

Answer 1.2

CLIENT FINDINGS OR STATEMENTS	ANXIETY	DEPRESSION	BIPOLAR DISORDER (MANIA)
"I can't eat or sleep."	○	✔	✔
Client found wandering and disheveled	✔	✔	✔
"I feel helpless."	○	✔	○
Possibility of eviction	✔	✔	✔
Denies suicidal ideation	○	✔	✔

Rationale: When a client arrives at the emergency department, the nurse must identify what similarities and differences present for conditions such as anxiety, depression, and bipolar disorder (mania). The nurse will need to consider all possibilities. When a client has been diagnosed with anxiety, there are three levels. Mild anxiety is exhibited by slight discomfort, restlessness, irritability, or mild tension-relieving behaviours such as nail biting, foot or finger tapping, fidgeting, and wringing of hands. A client can see, hear, and grasp information with the ability to problem solve. When a client exhibits moderate anxiety, only certain things in the environment are seen or heard unless pointed out. A client's ability to think is hampered, but learning and problem solving can still occur. A client may exhibit tension, pounding heart, increased pulse, and respiratory rate, as well as perspiration, gastric discomfort, headache, urinary urgency, voice tremors, and shaking. A client with severe anxiety may focus on one detail or many scattered details and be unable to notice their environment. There is difficulty with learning and problem solving. The client may exhibit behaviours to reduce anxiety, such as wringing hands, pacing, headache, nausea, dizziness, and increased insomnia. Trembling and a pounding heart rate are common. The client may hyperventilate and experience a sense of impending doom or dread. When a client presents with depression, they may exhibit symptoms of lethargy and fatigue; difficulty eating, sleeping, and eliminating; weight loss; neglect in grooming, dressing, and personal hygiene; and feelings of worthlessness, guilt, helplessness, hopelessness, and anger may be present, as well as feelings of suicidal ideation. When clients present with mania, there are sleep disruptions, leading clients to remain awake and forget to eat. They also may forget personal hygiene. When clients present in a manic state, they can forget to pay bills and may feel a sense of boundless energy, which can present as poor judgement and intrusive thoughts.

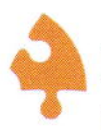
NCJMM Step: Analyze Cues
Reference: Pollard & Jakubec (2023), pp. 180–219, 220–247, 248–269.

Answer 1.3

The client is at highest risk of developing **major depressive disorder** as evidenced by the client's stated **feelings of hopelessness**.

Rationale: Acute depression is often characterized by a profound sense of hopelessness and worthlessness. It is the potential condition that the client is at highest risk of developing, and these characteristics can be triggers for serious safety risks. Insomnia and loss of appetite are known triggers for health issues and require medical attention, but these are not as likely to result in complications as quickly or as serious as those of acute depression. Extensive worry is a characteristic, and while worthy of the attention of mental health professionals, anxiety is not as likely to result in safety issues as is acute depression. Insomnia, loss of appetite and anxiety are likely treatable with outpatient services. Homelessness as a result of loss of employment is a serious issue, but not resolved by hospitalization. Neither suicidal ideations nor impaired health have yet to be established as diagnoses.

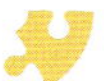
NCJMM Step: Prioritize Hypothesis
Reference: Pollard & Jakubec (2023), pp. 220–247.

Answer 1.4

- ✔ Client will be able to accurately describe rationale for prescribed antidepressant medication
- ✔ Client will collaborate on determining treatment goals
- ✔ Client will be able to accurately describe rationale for precautions that will be implemented for client safety
- ✔ Client will verbalize importance of attending unit-centred problem-solving group sessions
- ☐ Client with utilize extended periods of alone time for self-reflection
- ☐ Client will snack frequently on high-carbohydrate foods to supplement diet and manage weight loss

Rationale: The major goals of treatment are to help the client be as independent as possible, be free from self-harm, and achieve stability, remission, and recovery from major depression. Collaboration, medication, and therapy are the core interventions for achieving these goals and tend to help the client adhere to the plan of care. Some interventions should be tailored to the individual needs of the client. During hospitalization, clients often withdraw to their rooms and refuse to participate in unit activity. While depressed clients should be encouraged to set realistic goals to reconnect with their families and communities, the nurse needs to help the client balance the need for privacy with the need to return to normal social functioning. The same holds true of specific interventions related to dysfunctional sleep practices. If the client is experiencing difficulty sleeping, then interventions like deep breathing exercises may prove to be helpful. Nutrition is important, especially when a client is anorexic. A well-balanced diet of easily eaten foods provided in several small meals may be appropriate, but an emphasis on high-carbohydrate foods is not recommended, especially

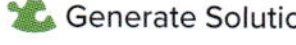

with the client's history of diabetes. Extended periods of isolation are not therapeutic and can even be dangerous, especially to a suicidal client.

NCJMM Step: Generate Solutions
Reference: Pollard & Jakubec (2023), pp. 220–247.

Answer 1.5

The nurse's first action should be to **assess client frequently for need to institute one-on-one observation.**

Rationale: Information about treatment will help ensure that the client will cooperate and adhere to the treatment. Escitalopram is a selective serotonin reuptake inhibitor (SSRI), not a monoamine oxidase inhibitor (MAOI), that can cause orthostatic hypotension resulting in dizziness. The rapid change in position, especially from lying or sitting to standing, often triggers the response. Various measures are implemented to help ensure the safety of a potentially suicidal client. Suicide precautions may vary somewhat from institution to institution but generally start with visual observation of the client at prescribed intervals but can progress to one-on-one continuous observation to observation that requires a staff member to always be within arm's reach of the client. The client is monitored for possible "cheeking" of medication to accumulate a sufficient quantity to be used in a suicide attempt. Even after the first episode of major depression, medication should be continued for at least 6 months to 1 year after the client achieves complete remission of symptoms.

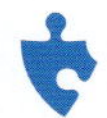

NCJMM Step: Take Action
Reference: Pollard & Jakubec (2023), pp. 220–247.

Answer 1.6

CLIENT STATEMENTS	UNDER-STANDING	NO UNDER-STANDING
"I need to keep my appointments with the clinic, so I won't get depressed again."	○	✔
"I'll call the clinic's hot line immediately if I start having suicidal thoughts."	✔	○
I'll need an electroencephalogram (EEG) done regularly."	○	✔
"The stress will go away as soon as I get a job."	○	✔

Rationale: The client verbalizes correct understanding of the need to notify a mental health professional if experiencing suicidal ideations, to receive the care needed to ensure continued personal safety. There may be a need for future hospitalization if depression symptoms become severe and include suicidal ideations. An EEG is not required to monitor a client prescribed an antidepressant medication since the medication is not known to affect brain activity. Depression is usually a result of a collection of ineffectively managed stressors. While being employed will lessen the client's stress level, it is not the only factor contributing to the diagnosis of depression.

NCJMM Step: Evaluate Outcomes
Reference: Pollard & Jakubec (2023), pp. 220–247.

Mental Health 2.0

Answer 2.1

TOP 4 FINDINGS
Unstable gait
Unable to follow commands
Hand tremors
Last known drink of alcohol 12 hours ago

Rationale: When a client is admitted to the unit with ETOH as a comorbidity, nurses will need to monitor for client safety, neurological compromise, hemodynamic compromise, and progression to alcohol withdrawal. The client presents as stable yet has alarming clinical manifestations. Nurses are to be aware of the need to monitor for alcohol withdrawal symptoms (identified in Table 18-2, Pollard et al. [2023], p. 359). The client presents with neurological symptoms that are concerning, such as unstable gait, inability to follow commands, hand tremors, and last known drink of alcohol 12 hours ago. Clinical manifestations consistent with client presentation of the time frame after last alcoholic drink for stages of alcohol withdrawal include minor withdrawal symptoms (insomnia, tremors, anxiety, gastrointestinal upset, headache, diaphoresis, palpitations, anorexia, nausea, tachycardia, hypertension, visual auditory or tactile hallucinations), withdrawal seizures, generalized tonic-clonic seizures, alcohol withdrawal delirium (delirium tremens), hallucinations (predominantly visual), disorientation, agitation, and diaphoresis. The nurse should assess the blood alcohol level, which should not remain high enough to consider the client intoxicated. The client presents with slurred speech and an unsteady gait, which is consistent with intoxication; the client also presents with effects of withdrawal that should be noted as significant. Symptoms will peak within 24 to 72 hours.

NCJMM Step: Recognize Cues
References: Pollard & Jakubec (2023), pp. 350–389; Tyerman & Cobbett (2023), pp. 164–188.

Answer 2.2

- ☐ Heart failure
- ☐ Pneumonia
- ✔ Seizures
- ✔ Delirium
- ✔ Respiratory depression
- ✔ Dysrhythmias
- ☐ Pulmonary embolus
- ☐ Diabetic ketoacidosis

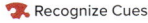

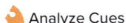

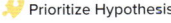

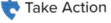

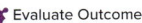

Rationale: Clients who exhibit symptoms associated with alcohol withdrawal require close monitoring. Complications associated with systemic compromises, such as seizures, delirium tremens, dysrhythmias (tachycardia), and even respiratory depression, may occur. Clients may have minor withdrawal symptoms (6–12 hours after last use), which include insomnia, tremors, anxiety, gastrointestinal upset, headache, diaphoresis, palpitations, anorexia, nausea, tachycardia, and hypertension. After 12 to 14 hours from last use, symptoms may include visual, auditory, or tactile hallucinations. After 24 to 48 hours from last use, the client may exhibit withdrawal seizures (generalized tonic-clonic seizures), and after 48 to 72 hours symptoms may include delirium tremens, hallucinations (predominantly visual) disorientation, agitation, and diaphoresis. Abrupt withdrawal of alcohol use may even predispose a client to a complete systemic response, leading to peripheral vascular collapse or cardiac failure.

NCJMM Step: Analyze Cues
References: Pollard & Jakubec (2023), pp. 350–389; Tyerman & Cobbett (2023), pp. 164–188.

Answer 2.3

The client is at highest risk of developing **grand mal seizures** as evidenced by the **sodium level.**

Rationale: This client is at increased risk for grand mal seizures. Symptoms of hypernatremia include convulsions. The alcohol withdrawal plus the high sodium result increases the client's risk of developing seizures. The client is not at an increased risk of developing a stroke or a deep vein thrombosis. The platelet levels are low; therefore, the components of Virchow's triad (venous stasis, hypercoagulability, and endothelial damage) are not present. The client does not present with a fever indicating an infection. The client's potassium level is elevated; however, this would result in cardiac instability leading to dysrhythmias specifically, premature ventricular contractions, ventricular tachycardia, and/or ventricular fibrillation. The white blood cell level is within normal range, also indicating no sign of an infection.

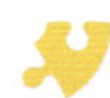
NCJMM Step: Prioritize Hypothesis
References: McDonald (2024), pp. 428–429 (hypernatremia); Pollard & Jakubec (2023), pp. 350–389; Tyerman & Cobbett (2023), pp. 342–372.

Answer 2.4

POTENTIAL NURSING INTERVENTIONS	INDICATED	NOT INDICATED
Prepare the client for Foley catheter insertion	○	✔
Reorient the client to the environment	✔	○
Prepare to administer an opioid	○	✔
Contact a family member to sit with the client	✔	○
Request an order to insert a peripheral IV	✔	○

Rationale: This client is progressing from anticipating a seizure to delirium tremens (DT). Features of alcohol withdrawal include perceptual disturbances such as visual or tactile hallucinations, requiring a nonjudgemental approach to decrease the client's anxiety and fear, contacting a family member or friend to sit with the client, and anticipating the need for peripheral IV access in the event an anticonvulsant may need to be administered. A Foley catheter does not need to be inserted. The nurse may offer a bedside commode (as the client remains unsteady with her gait, which increases her fall risk) or a bedpan if the client is unable to transfer. Only if both of these options cannot be carried out might a Foley catheter be necessary. It is important to recognize that insertion of a Foley catheter may increase the client's anxiety. An opioid is not the drug of choice for a client who has progressed to DT; a better choice is a benzodiazepine. The benzodiazepines lorazepam, diazepam, haloperidol, and chlordiazepoxide can be given either orally, sublingually, or intramuscularly to help manage these signs and symptoms. Nurses should recognize that in a client admitted with alcohol withdrawal, the progression to DT is serious and an acute episode requires constant management of care and monitoring for seizures, unconsciousness, hallucinations, and, above all, the safety of the client.

NCJMM Step: Generate Solutions
Reference: Pollard & Jakubec (2023), pp. 350–389.

Answer 2.5

- ✔ Administer lorazepam 1–2 mg SL × 1 dose now, then as per Clinical Institute Withdrawal Assessment for Alcohol–Revised (CIWA-AR) protocol
- ☐ Place client in bilateral wrist restraints
- ✔ Initiate 0.9% sodium chloride (normal saline) at 75 mL/hr
- ☐ Prepare for cardioversion
- ☐ Continue to monitor vital signs
- ☐ Client to remain NPO
- ☐ Administer Resonium calcium 15 g PO × 1
- ✔ Initiate CIWA-AR protocol

Rationale: This client is becoming more agitated with the swatting of her arm and calling out. Lorazepam is an appropriate benzodiazepine to use in clients with alcohol withdrawal. This may reduce agitation and inhibit the seizure threshold. The client should be placed on IV fluids as they will be NPO, and if a seizure occurs, peripheral IV access is required. From a safety perspective, the client should be placed on the CIWA protocol to maintain an appropriate level of sedation with hourly assessments for agitation and the need for medication. The CIWA protocol directs nurses toward monitoring hemodynamic, neurological, and respiratory status. Bilateral wrist restraints would only increase the client's agitation. Although the potassium is elevated, Resonium calcium powder is ordered when potassium levels are greater than 6 mmol/L. The client is at risk of developing cardiac arrest and should be monitored. The nurse will continue to monitor vital signs, but this is not a first priority.

The client will remain NPO except for medications to prevent aspiration pneumonia.

NCJMM Step: Take Action
References: Alberta Health Services (2018); Pollard & Jakubec (2023), pp. 350–389; Sanofi-Aventis Canada (2018); Sealock & Seneviratne (2025), pp. 278–279; Skidmore-Roth & Richardson (2024), pp. 815–817 (lorazepam).

Answer 2.6

ASSESSMENT FINDINGS	IMPROVED	NO CHANGE	DECLINED
RR 24	✔	○	○
BP 92/66	✔	○	○
Speech clear and appropriate	✔	○	○
Oxygen level at 3 L/min per nasal prongs	○	✔	○
Skin perfused	✔	○	○

Rationale: After an unwitnessed tonic-clonic seizure, the client's status has improved considerably since having delirium and high blood pressure. The client's hemodynamic status has improved, indicating the lorazepam was effective treatment. The client remains in a tenuous condition and continues to require close monitoring.

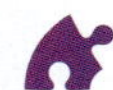
NCJMM Step: Evaluate Outcomes
Reference: Pollard & Jakubec (2023), pp. 350–389.

Mental Health 3.0

Answer 3.1

- ☐ Gastrointestinal presentation
- ✔ Client orientation
- ✔ Tremor
- ☐ "Pounding heart"
- ☐ Cardiovascular perfusion
- ☐ Mucous membranes
- ✔ Thirsty

Rationale: The client presents with nausea and vomiting along with a past medical history of bipolar illness and taking lithium. Lithium toxicity would be the most important diagnosis for this client. Dehydration leads to sodium depletion, where the kidneys will try to reabsorb sodium along with lithium, increasing the serum levels. Monitoring for signs and symptoms of lithium toxicity would be most important. Neurologically, scattered thoughts and tremors indicate early signs of lithium toxicity. This client would be hyponatremic, leading to the complaint of being thirsty. The client should be monitored for prolonged QT leading to dysrhythmias. Nausea and vomiting are contributing factors to the hospitalization and can be monitored but do not require immediate follow-up. The client may feel a "pounding heart" despite being bradycardic. The dry mucous membranes should indicate to the nurse that the client is dehydrated, as does the blood pressure, but these do not require immediate follow up. Bradycardia is due to dehydration and lithium toxicity.

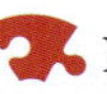
NCJMM Step: Recognize Cues
Reference: Pollard & Jakubec (2023), pp. 249–269.

Answer 3.2

The nurse should recognize that the client is potentially experiencing symptoms associated with **lithium toxicity.**

Rationale: Based on the symptoms, the client is experiencing lithium toxicity. There is no indication of facial droop, paralysis, or blood pressure referencing a stroke. The client reports no chest pain, so the condition cannot be myocardial infarction. The white blood cells are not elevated to indicate a urinary tract infection or sepsis inflammatory response syndrome, and the client's blood sugar is normal.

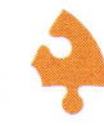
NCJMM Step: Analyze Cues
Reference: Pollard & Jakubec (2023), pp. 249–269.

Answer 3.3

The client is at highest risk of developing **convulsions** as evidenced by the client's **sodium level**.

Rationale: Based on the symptoms, the client is experiencing lithium toxicity and at greatest risk for convulsions. There are clinical manifestations indicating that the client is experiencing muscle weakness, pulmonary embolism, or cardiogenic shock. The client is hyponatremic, which means, because of the high sodium count, convulsions are potential with high levels of toxicity. The client is also at risk of developing dysrhythmias such as ventricular tachycardia due to high levels of displaced intracellular potassium. A right-hand tremor is not associated with lithium toxicity. The client will require cardiac monitoring. The respiratory rate does not indicate that the client will develop convulsions.

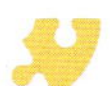
NCJMM Step: Prioritize Hypothesis
References: Chien et al. (2018), p. 13129; Pollard & Jakubec (2023), pp. 249–269; Sealock & Seneviratne (2025), pp. 279–280; Skidmore-Roth & Richardson (2024), pp. 807–809.

Answer 3.4

BODY SYSTEM	POTENTIAL NURSING INTERVENTIONS
Neurological	○ Sensory exam every 4 hours ✔ Monitor level of consciousness ✔ Seizure protocols
Cardiovascular	○ Vitals signs every 4 hours or more if needed ✔ Monitor cardiovascular rhythm for ventricular tachycardia ○ Insert arterial line
Renal	✔ Monitor output ○ Request 24-hour urine collection ✔ Urine test strip every morning

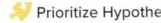

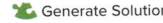

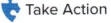

Rationale: This question asks the student to plan a phase of care for the client. The student must consider potential interventions based on their knowledge about the condition.

Neurological: The client is at risk for seizures based on lab values and may become more confused depending on the level of lithium in the blood. The nurse should be monitoring for any changes. A sensory test is only performed on clients with sensory deficits, as in the case of a spinal cord injury or after back surgery. This client would not require sensory testing.

Cardiovascular: The client is at risk for prolonged QT, requiring the nurse to monitor for ventricular tachycardia. The potassium level remains elevated, so even if the nurse was not aware of the prolonged QT, the elevated potassium should be reason enough to monitor for ventricular tachycardia. Completing vitals every hour could overwhelm the client. If their status changes, vital signs could be taken every 4 hours and increase in time as needed. An arterial line is unnecessary for this client and may exacerbate confusion.

Renal: The client is already dehydrated and hypotensive. Clients with lithium toxicity may develop polyuria due to the resistance to antidiuretic hormones, potentially leading to nephrogenic diabetes insipidus with chronic lithium toxicity. This would only increase the lithium concentration for the client. A urine test stick in the morning could be used to identify any glucose or protein in the urine. A 24-hour urine test would be a more appropriate assessment for renal concentration; 48 hours is too long.

NCJMM Step: Generate Hypothesis
References: Pollard & Jakubec (2023), pp. 249–269; Sealock & Seneviratne (2025), pp. 279–280; Skidmore-Roth & Richardson (2024), pp. 807–809.

Answer 3.5

- ✔ Initiate a large-bore peripheral intravenous catheter
- ✔ Administer 3% sodium chloride (normal saline) at 25 mL/hr
- ✔ Laboratory tests: CBC, electrolytes, lithium level, type and cross-match
- ☐ Prepare client for a computed tomography (CT) head
- ☐ Insert Foley catheter

Rationale: The client requires intravenous fluids as there is hemodynamic instability. In clients experiencing diabetes insipidus, fluids must be replaced slowly. Peripheral intravenous access must be started in the event more seizures occur. The client has oxygen applied with the appropriate pulse oximetry level. More laboratory levels will need to be drawn to identify if the client is even more hyponatremic due to diabetes insipidus. A CT head is not a priority, and neither is the Foley catheter. However, the Foley catheter would be valuable for monitoring urine output.

NCJMM Step: Take Action
References: Pollard & Jakubec (2023), pp. 249–269; Sealock & Seneviratne (2025), pp. 279–280; Skidmore-Roth & Richardson (2024), pp. 807–809.

Answer 3.6

ASSESSMENT FINDINGS	IMPROVED	NO CHANGE	DECLINED
Nausea	○	○	✔
Blood pressure	✔	○	○
Hemoglobin	○	○	✔
Oxygen level	✔	○	○
Skin perfused	○	✔	○

Rationale: Overall, the client's status has improved despite the return of nausea. The client responded to IV fluids to improve hemodynamic status. The client's lab values have improved as well.

NCJMM Step: Evaluate Outcomes
Reference: Pollard & Jakubec (2023), pp. 249–269.

Mental Health 4.0

Answer 4.1

Body System	Findings
Neurological	Client presents with flat affect. Found rearranging towels in the bathroom and placed within perfect distance on the counter. Denies hearing voices but adamant people were chasing him: "I know they will come for me. They will find me." States he does not shower. Client presents as disheveled as noted by his dirty clothes and uncombed hair. Client reports the shower in his apartment is broken. States he has thought about ending his life, has sent texts about this to his family and knows that when he decides to do it things will be better for everyone. He reports not feeling like doing anything, losing motivation.
Pulmonary	Bilateral fine inspiratory crackles auscultated posteriorly. Dry cough noted.
Cardiovascular	Client states he feels his heart is racing and can hear it pounding in his head. No edema noted. Pulses noted to be bilaterally strong in radials. Mucous membranes dry.
Gastrointestinal	Client presents with lower normal body weight. States he is not eating for fear "they will poison him." He has not told anyone but feels safe now.
Renal	Client has not voided since arrival at hospital. Smell of urine noted on clothes.

Rationale: Safety should always be the primary concern, and then airway, breathing, and circulation are priorities. In this situation, the client states he is not hearing voices, but the delusions of persecution are real to the client and should be verified. The client has had suicidal ideations, which is concerning and should be followed up with immediately. The rearranging of towels may seem insignificant; however, obsessive-compulsive disorder (OCD) is a common illness associated with schizophrenia. This observation is important to follow up with the physician to confirm schizophrenia. The client is conveying a suicide risk. Nurses must pick up on the presentation of clients when conducting a mental status exam. The statement of "racing heart" and of not having voided is important as there can be cardiovascular complications due to poor nutrition and dehydration. When clients are malnourished, there is a concern when medications are administered for toxicity, owing to dehydration and increased workload of the kidneys. Nurses must recognize mental health concerns in relation to the body during assessment.

NCJMM Step: Recognize Cues
Reference: Pollard & Jakubec (2023), pp. 270–303.

Answer 4.2

- ✔ Ventricular dysrhythmias
- ☐ Hypotension
- ☐ Pleural effusion
- ✔ Acute renal failure
- ☐ Hypertension

Rationale: The statement of "racing heart" and not having voided is important as there can be cardiovascular complications due to poor nutrition and dehydration. Although the client was admitted for a mental health assessment, the client is also at risk of developing ventricular dysrhythmias such as ventricular tachycardia and premature ventricular contractions, and not voiding means dehydration. This will cause the kidneys to reabsorb potassium, resulting in increased serum potassium levels, which will also contribute to ventricular dysrhythmias. The client has not eaten or drank anything because of the delusions. The lack of nutrition could further compromise the client's physical and mental health.

NCJMM Step: Analyze Cues
Reference: Pollard & Jakubec (2023), pp. 270–303.

Answer 4.3

The nurse should recognize that the client is potentially experiencing **psychosis** due to symptoms of **persecution.**

Rationale: The client is potentially experiencing psychosis due to symptoms expressed of persecution. Although the client is likely experiencing panic more than generalized anxiety disorder, these feelings cannot be dismissed. Panic is the most extreme level of anxiety and results in disturbed behaviour. Generalized anxiety disorder is characterized by persistent and exaggerated apprehension and tension. Clients experiencing mania express symptoms of euphoria and energy, engage in risky behaviour, and may even become psychotic and experience hallucinations, delusions, and dramatically disturbed thoughts and behaviour. The client in this situation has not experienced trauma, to the knowledge of health care staff. PTSD is an emotional response to a traumatic event or situation involving severe environmental stress. The client has indicated smoking cannabis, but in this instance, there is little evidence to support a problem with addiction. The cannabis likely contributed to the psychosis. A key point here would be that persecutory delusions are the only answer that aligns with the characteristic of schizophrenia. So, while the client may experience psychosis due to cannabis use (this would clear within a few days of abstinence), it would accentuate the underlying delusions.

Client findings: The client has indicated delusions of persecution. Suicidal ideation accompanies a diagnosis of schizophrenia and is a safety concern for clients experiencing a psychotic event. The client reports feeling isolated, as evidenced by being an out-of-province university student, living on his own, having a small social circle, and feeling like others see him differently (the client's self-perception is often a significant factor in feeling connected to others). Increased isolation is a risk factor to consider when assessing the client for safety.

The client reports anhedonia, not motivation for life. The client denies any hallucinations at the time of admission—auditory, visual, olfactory, gustatory, or tactile (see Table 15.2 in Pollard & Jakubec [2023], p. 278). A person may falsely deny hallucinations, requiring behavioural assessment to support or refute the person's report. Behaviours such as turning or tilting the head as if to listen to someone, suddenly stopping current activity as if interrupted, and moving the lips silently may indicate that the client is distracted by perceptual stimuli that are not evident to the nurse.

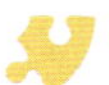

NCJMM Step: Prioritize Hypothesis
Reference: Pollard & Jakubec (2023), pp. 180–219, 249–270, 278.

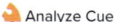

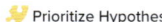

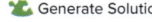

Answer 4.4

BODY SYSTEM	POTENTIAL NURSING INTERVENTIONS
Neurological	✔ Administer atypical antipsychotics, such as olanzapine ○ Encourage therapeutic group therapy ✔ Promote sleep–wake cycle
Cardiovascular	✔ Encourage oral intake of fluids ✔ Administer sodium polystyrene sulfonate powder (Resonium) (or Patiromer) ○ Monitor for atrial fibrillation
Gastrointestinal	✔ Encourage small meals and packaged foods such as crackers or peanut butter ○ Allow sugar drinks such as carbonated beverages ○ Encourage client to eat in his room

Rationale:
Neurological: The first and third options are correct to improve overall mental health and well-being. Atypical antipsychotics such as olanzapine will treat both positive and negative symptoms. Some atypical antipsychotics can be administered orally or intramuscularly. The route of administration depends on the clients' level of distress, safety concerns, and overall needs. Group therapy is not recommended for an individual with active psychosis. Therapeutic group activities are not recommended because increased stimulation may further agitate the client. Group therapy is excellent for promoting motivation, an environment for acceptable behaviours, opportunities to develop friendships, and increased social competence for clients who are nearing discharge. Maintenance of a regular sleep–wake cycle eliminates anxiety and stress that exacerbate psychosis associated with schizophrenia.

Cardiovascular: The lab values indicate the client is hyperkalemic and requires treatment. Resonium powder or kayexalate would be excellent choices since the client can take oral medications. The nurse needs to be careful to note that if clients are psychotic, they may refuse medication or cheek the medication. A thorough assessment would be necessary to document if the client has taken the medication. The client is dehydrated, so encouraging oral fluids will improve hemodynamic status and improve function of the renal system. Because of the client's age, he is adjusting to the dehydration, with no alterations in his blood pressure and heart rate. The client is at risk for ventricular dysrhythmias, not atrial dysrhythmias. The client is also at risk for toxicity related to medication if they are dehydrated, which would increase the antipsychotic medication in the body and could result in neuroleptic malignant syndrome.

Gastrointestinal: The client is nutritionally depleted because of his lower weight. Encouraging small meals and foods in packages will improve the client's energy and overall health. This may lead to increased participation in activities of daily living and willingness to engage with others. Food in packages may reduce delusions of persecution. Fluid intake is important, but not with sugary drinks. The client has already indicated anhedonia and may increase sedentary lifestyle and risk for obesity. Weight gain is also an adverse effect of many antipsychotics, which increases the risk for metabolic syndrome. The client can be encouraged to eat meals with others, which may enhance social skills.

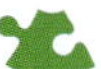
NCJMM Step: Generate Solutions
Reference: Pollard & Jakubec (2023), pp. 270–303.

Answer 4.5

- ✔ Request an order for sodium polystyrene sulfonate powder (Resonium) (or Patiromer)
- ✔ Administer antipsychotic medication, olanzapine
- ☐ Initiate 0.9% sodium chloride per peripheral intravenous catheter
- ☐ Prepare client to join group therapy activities
- ✔ Connect the client to continuous cardiac monitoring
- ☐ Insert a Foley urinary catheter.

Rationale: The highest priority would be to administer an antipsychotic medication followed by requesting an order for sodium polystyrene sulfonate powder (Resonium) (or Patiromer). While the client is actively psychotic, they are not able to make good decisions and present a high safety risk. In addition, when clients are psychotic, they may not want to take any medication. The immediate need is to reduce the psychosis so that the client is willing to participate in the larger treatment plan. In addition, several antipsychotics can be administered in intramuscular (IM) form if necessary. The nurse would monitor the client who is at risk for ventricular dysrhythmias.

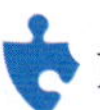
NCJMM Step: Take Action
Reference: Pollard & Jakubec (2023), pp. 270–303.

Answer 4.6

CLIENT STATEMENTS	UNDER-STANDING	NO UNDER-STANDING
"I need to keep my regular appointments with my psychiatrist."	✔	○
"I will have to withdraw from school to avoid stress."	○	✔
"It is ok if I miss a dose. I can take it when I remember."	○	✔
"If I do everything right, I can cure my illness."	○	✔
"Attending outpatient group therapy is important for me to feel connected to other people."	✔	○

Rationale: Clients living with schizophrenia require support, therapy, and pharmacological management to decrease the number and intensity of recurring psychotic episodes. It is common for individuals with schizophrenia to experience recurring psychotic episodes even if they take their medications. The goal is to decrease the number and severity of the episodes of psychosis. Interventions should promote self-care, independence, stress management, socialization, psychoeducation to provide understanding of and adaptation to their illness, milieu management, cognitive-behavioural interventions, cognitive enhancement, and medication administration. Nurses should also help clients maintain hope.

NCJMM Step: Evaluate Outcomes
Reference: Pollard & Jakubec (2023), pp. 270–303.

10 Answers and Rationales for Stand-Alone Case Studies

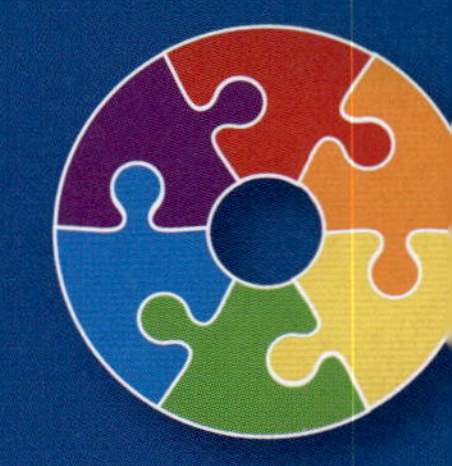

Medical-Surgical Bow-Tie Cases

Medical-Surgical 1.0

Answer

Action to Take	Condition Most Likely Experiencing	Parameter to Monitor
Provide a requisition to collect a urine specimen for urinalysis	Urinary tract infection	Temperature
Action to Take		**Parameter to Monitor**
Request an order for antibiotic therapy		Heart rate

Rationale:

Potential Condition: The client experienced a urinary tract infection (UTI), indicated by a fever, frequency, urgency, and burning sensation when initiating voiding. The client also has an overwhelming sense of generalized unwellness. The cause is likely due to lack of hygiene during intimate moments with a partner. The client is voiding, which eliminates renal failure and urinary retention. The client is not experiencing stress incontinence. The incontinence is associated with the frequency and urgency of the cystitis.

Actions to Take: The client requires further follow-up care to confirm a UTI beyond symptom presentation. The client should be provided with a laboratory requisition to confirm a UTI and started on antibiotic therapy as a fever has developed. If left untreated, there is a potential risk for the client to develop pyelonephritis or even sepsis. The client is voiding without difficulty; therefore, a urinary catheter or a bladder scan would not be necessary to determine how much urine the client may be retaining. Finally, there is evidence that the use of cranberry juice does little to treat an infection.

Parameters to Monitor: It is important to monitor for complications of the UTI, including pyelonephritis or sepsis. Monitoring the temperature and heart rate would be key indicators if the infection is progressing to beyond a UTI. The nurse should promote oral fluid intake; however, monitoring the balance is unnecessary. The client is voiding frequently, which would indicate the urine has minimal time to concentrate. The pulse oximetry would not require monitoring as the client does not present with any underlying respiratory conditions.

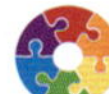

NCJMM Step: Recognize Cues, Analyze Cues, Prioritize Hypothesis, Generate Solutions, Take Action, and Evaluate Outcomes

References: Astle & Duggleby (2024), pp. 1162–1210; Tyerman & Cobbett (2023), pp. 1143–1146.

Medical-Surgical 2.0

Answer

Action to Take	Condition Most Likely Experiencing	Parameter to Monitor
Provide a urinal at the bedside	Postural hypotension	Blood pressure
Action to Take		**Parameter to Monitor**
Discuss with the health care provider the dosages and times of medications		Pain

Rationale:

Potential Condition: The client experienced postural hypotension given the clinical presentation of "the room was spinning" upon standing up, falling to the ground, and the documented changes in blood pressure. The client did not lose consciousness and denies bumping his head; however, older adults are prone to slow bleeding on the brain and should be monitored for a subdural hematoma after a fall. The client does not have any infection given a normal temperature throughout the day, despite incontinence. The client is not experiencing any dysrhythmias such as atrial fibrillation given the denial of palpitations and a normal and regular pulse.

Actions to Take: Preventing falls is a priority to reduce injury and length of stay in the hospital. Providing a urinal at the bedside will eliminate the need for the client to have to get up to use the washroom at night. Upon closer review of the medication list, the client is taking a diuretic at bedtime, and the antihypertensive medications (beta blocker or ACE inhibitor) may need to be adjusted accordingly to avoid postural hypotension from occurring in the future. The client does not require supplemental oxygen as the pulse oximetry was documented to be greater than 90%. The client does not have a source of infection, with a normal temperature documented throughout the day. The client is not in any distress; a code blue would not be needed as they were able to rise from the floor with help from the nurse.

Parameters to Monitor: Blood pressure would be a continuous parameter to monitor given the fall. The nurse has the options of take a lying, sitting, and standing blood pressure to aid in documentation and decision making. Even though the client denies pain at the time of the fall, it is important to monitor a pain response as there could be muscle or bone trauma requiring nonpharmacological and possibly pharmacological interventions. The client is not experiencing any infection; therefore, fever would not need to be monitored. The pulse oximetry was greater than 90% and there is no indication that the client was experiencing any respiratory distress. Urine output would be a factor to monitor during the day, but it is not a priority. If the medication list can be reconciled, the client may not feel the need to void in the middle of the night.

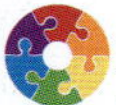

NCJMM Step: Recognize Cues, Analyze Cues, Prioritize Hypothesis, Generate Solutions, Take Action, and Evaluate Outcomes

References: Astle & Duggleby (2024), pp. 872–901; Tyerman & Cobbett (2023), pp. 789–790.

Medical-Surgical 3.0

Answer

Action to Take	Condition Most Likely Experiencing	Parameter to Monitor
Request an order to insert a peripheral venous access device	Dehydration	Heart rate
Action to Take		Parameter to Monitor
Request an order to administer intravenous fluids		Urine output

Rationale:

Potential Condition: The client presents with tachycardia, dry mucous membranes, and oliguric or reduced urine output over an 8-hour period (less than 30 mL per hour). Dehydration can present as a multisystem challenge, and in this case, the cardiovascular and renal systems were most affected. The client has reduced oral fluid intake as indicated by the need for a PEG tube and presented to the unit with the admitting diagnosis of diarrhea. The tube feeds are not currently meeting the demands of hydration or nutrition since the admitting diagnosis is failure to thrive and diarrhea. The client's blood pressure remains stable, which is likely due to the age of the client. Clients with PEG tubes can present with aspiration pneumonia if they are not placed in high-Fowler's position during tube feeds or medication administration. The fine crackles auscultated during lung assessment would be due to inability to cough and expand alveoli, reducing fine crackles. The client does not have aspiration pneumonia as there is no fever despite the respiratory rate being 24. Clients who are cachectic and frail tend to breathe faster to maintain cardiovascular stability. The client does not present with hypertension as the blood pressure is within a normal range. There are no clinical manifestations associated with diabetes.

Actions to Take: To improve hydration, a peripheral venous access device and intravenous fluids would help this client. Without prompt intervention, the client's hemodynamic status could be fatal as the client is not voiding and may precipitate hyperkalemia, leading to potential risk for cardiac arrest. Fluid resuscitation would be the most appropriate intervention at this time. The pulse oximetry at 90% does not require administration of oxygen. Positioning the client in semi-Fowler's would increase the risk for aspiration pneumonia. The client does not have aspiration pneumonia at present, and a chest X-ray is not required at this time.

Parameters to Monitor: Monitoring the heart rate and urine output would aid in determining whether the client's fluid status was improving. The heart rate would be within normal range (60–100 beats per minute) and urine output would exceed the minimum 30 mL per hour, indicating proper filtration of the kidneys. The client does not have an infection; therefore, monitoring temperature is not an appropriate parameter to monitor at this time. While mild excoriation of the PEG tube site was documented in the nurses' notes, improving cardiovascular and renal stability is of higher priority. The client does not indicate pain, even in a nonverbal manner.

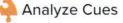

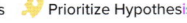

NCJMM Step: Recognize Cues, Analyze Cues, Prioritize Hypothesis, Generate Solutions, Take Action, and Evaluate Outcomes

References: Astle & Duggleby (2024), pp. 759 (Box 35.17), 1136–1156; Power-Kean et al. (2023), p. 120; Tyerman & Cobbett (2023), 211t–212t.

Medical-Surgical 4.0

Answer

Action to Take	Condition Most Likely Experiencing	Parameter to Monitor
Request an order for antibiotic therapy	Pneumonia	Temperature
Action to Take		Parameter to Monitor
Prepare the client for a chest X-ray		Respiratory status

Rationale:

Potential Condition: The client presents with respiratory changes indicating pneumonia as evidenced by the increase in temperature, changes in cough, increased oxygen requirements, and changes in lung sounds such as the crackles increasing throughout the lung fields. Postoperative pneumonias are one of the most common complications that can occur from reduced mobility and reduced lung expansion. Plus, this client received a general anaesthetic requiring intubation. The endotracheal tube provides a point of transmission where bacteria can enter the lungs. Nursing interventions are to encourage deep breathing and coughing, and analgesic can be provided. The client's blood pressure did not decrease indicating hypotension. The client is able to ambulate to the washroom with assistance, and pupils are equal and reactive to light without any changes to neurological status, thus reducing the likelihood of this presentation as a stroke. The client has denied chest pain throughout, indicating this is not an acute myocardial infarction.

Actions to Take: The client requires a chest X-ray for further assessment and will need antibiotic therapy specifically related to a pneumonia. Physiotherapy would be an appropriate intervention after treating the pneumonia. The oxygen level does not need to be increased as the client is maintaining pulse oximetry above 90%. The client does not require a CT head to rule out a stroke.

Parameters to Monitor: Monitoring the temperature and improvements in respiratory status would be the most appropriate parameters as this is the system most affected. All other systems require monitoring during normal postoperative recovery; however, respiratory status would be the highest priority in this clinical presentation. Monitoring the temperature helps determine early on if the infection is improving or status is decreasing.

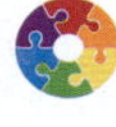

NCJMM Step: Recognize Cues, Analyze Cues, Prioritize Hypothesis, Generate Solutions, Take Action, and Evaluate Outcomes

References: Astle & Duggleby (2024), pp. 635–641, 1250–1254, 1365–1394; Tyerman & Cobbett (2023), pp. 590–595.

Medical-Surgical 5.0

Answer

Action to Take	Condition Most Likely Experiencing	Parameter to Monitor
Request an order for an antidysrhythmia medication	Atrial fibrillation	Respiratory rate
Action to Take		Parameter to Monitor
Prepare the client for an electrocardiogram		Heart rate

Rationale:

Potential Condition: The client presented with nonspecific complaints of fatigue, shortness of breath with minimal exertion, and palpitations. The shortness of breath with minimal exertion and palpitations indicate there is a cardiac and respiratory connection for the condition. The vital signs include a fast heart rate (greater than 100 beats per minute), which indicates a tachycardia rhythm. Further assessment data are required to determine the type of rhythm the client is experiencing. During the assessment, an irregular pulse is indicated. Out of the potential conditions, the only irregular pulse is atrial fibrillation, which contributes to the initial presentation the client experienced. The client could not be experiencing bradycardia (heart rate less than 60 beats per minute). The client does not present with pneumonia, which could present in a similar manner to the client's initial symptoms, but can be ruled out because there is no fever.

Actions to Take: Since the client is experiencing new-onset atrial fibrillation, administering an antidysrhythmic medication may alleviate the client's clinical manifestations. It would also be important to capture a 12-lead electrocardiogram (ECG) on this patient to determine if there are any other cardiac abnormalities. The client would not require a consultation with a dietitian as this is not a gastrointestinal concern. The client's pulse oximetry was documented at 92% on room air, which is satisfactory and greater than 92% saturation level. The client does not present with pneumonia and therefore does not require a chest X-ray.

Parameters to Monitor: Monitoring the client's heart rate and respiratory rate would help determine the effectiveness of the antidysrhythmic medication. If the heart rate remains elevated, another medication may need to be added. When the heart rate is high, there is a positive correlation that the respiratory rate would need to increase to compensate for the higher demand on the cardiorespiratory system. The urine output would not need to be monitored since the client voids independently and without issue. The pulse oximetry is within normal limits and does not need further monitoring. The client does not present with pneumonia and thus does not require monitoring of their temperature reflecting an infection.

NCJMM Step: Recognize Cues, Analyze Cues, Prioritize Hypothesis, Generate Solutions, Take Action, and Evaluate Outcomes

Reference: Astle & Duggleby (2024), pp. 641–650; Tyerman & Cobbett (2023), pp. 858–859.

Medical-Surgical 6.0

Answer

Action to Take	Condition Most Likely Experiencing	Parameter to Monitor
Request an order to administer a fluid bolus intravenously	Dehydration	Blood pressure

Action to Take		Parameter to Monitor
Request an order to draw electrolytes blood work (sodium and potassium)		Urine output

Rationale:

Potential Condition: The client presented with nonspecific complaints of weakness and confusion right after having the gastrointestinal illness. The client's daughter reports delirium as a result of the illness as well. Diarrhea and vomiting are key concerns related to dehydration in older adults. Clinical manifestations of dehydration in the case study are hypotension and tachycardia, oliguria and concentrated urine, dry mucous membranes, prolonged capillary refill time, and confusion. The client has a regular bilateral pulse when palpated, dismissing atrial fibrillation as the cause of the client's presentation. The client has clear lung sounds and no fever, eliminating pneumonia as the cause of the clinical manifestation. The confusion is due to the gastrointestinal illness, not dementia.

Actions to Take: The client's blood pressure is low, and the heart rate is elevated, indicating the need to replace fluids. A bolus of isotonic fluid will help initiate rehydration quicker than through oral intake. The client already has a peripheral venous access device inserted in the right antecubital fossa. It is important to monitor the client's electrolytes, paying particular attention to the sodium and potassium levels. When a client is dehydrated, the sodium levels may be low from prolonged vomiting. The client may also develop hypokalemia when the loss of fluid due to vomiting and a loss of sodium stimulates the secretion of aldosterone, leading to renal losses of potassium. With reduced perfusion to the kidneys, the client may also be at risk of developing hyperkalemia. Either way, blood for electrolyte lab values should be drawn. Administering a diuretic would only deplete the client's intravascular volume. The client does not need a psychiatry consult for the confusion as it is related to the dehydration. Older adults are more sensitive to fluid shifts. The client presents as weak and requires one-person standby assist but remains able to mobilize. It is better for an older adult to mobilize than have the intervention of a Foley catheter.

Parameters to Monitor: Monitoring the client's blood pressure and urine output will provide direct measurements of rehydration. Rehydration will correct the hemodynamic status and improve cardiac output, reducing workload of the heart. Monitoring the temperature and pulse oximetry is not necessary as the client does not have any signs of infection (clear lung fields, no shortness of breath) or a lower pulse oximetry level with clinical presentation. At this point, continuous monitoring of the heart rhythm is not necessary. An ECG may be ordered to have a baseline record; however, continuous monitoring is unnecessary.

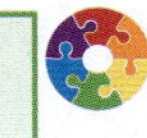

NCJMM Step: Recognize Cues, Analyze Cues, Prioritize Hypothesis, Generate Solutions, Take Action, and Evaluate Outcomes

References: Astle & Duggleby (2024), pp. 1028; Power-Kean et al. (2023), p. 120.

Medical-Surgical 7.0

Answer

Action to Take	Condition Most Likely Experiencing	Parameter to Monitor
Stop the transfusion immediately	Anaphylaxis	Respiratory rate
Action to Take		**Parameter to Monitor**
Prepare to administer epinephrine		Blood pressure

Rationale:

Potential Condition: Given the quick presentation of clinical manifestations, the client has developed anaphylaxis, a blood transfusion complication. The client presented with anxiety, difficulty catching their breath, scratchy throat, expiratory wheeze, and stridor, all of which indicate the airway may be constricting and thus reducing gas exchange. Anaphylaxis occurs when antibodies react to the donor blood product. This is an emergency situation where the priority is to maintain airway. The client does not have sepsis as the fever has not increased, nor has the client developed chills, vomiting, or diarrhea. The client's c-spine precautions have been removed after diagnostic tests ruled out a spinal cord injury, which means the client could not be developing spinal cord injury at 0330h. Although the client's blood pressure is hypotensive and the heart rate elevated, these would be consistent with hypovolemia. The quick acute response to the blood administration would be more closely aligned with a transfusion reaction as opposed to hypovolemia. There may be elements of hypovolemia given the blood on the sheets, but the respiratory distress is anaphylaxis, not hypovolemia.

Actions to Take: The first action a nurse must take is to stop the transfusion immediately. The nurse must follow the policy and procedure at the institution. The blood would not be flushed into the patient's peripheral venous access device if a reaction has occurred. The threat of respiratory compromise is already high. The blood would be disconnected from the peripheral access device and an infusion line of isotonic solution would be attached to maintain fluid hydration and a necessary line if other medications were needed. Given the client's clinical manifestations, it would be necessary to have epinephrine on hand. A code blue may be needed even after epinephrine was administered if there was no change in respiratory status. Sepsis could also be a transfusion complication; however, in this situation, the clinical manifestations present as anaphylaxis. Blood cultures would not be necessary. Airway, breathing, and circulation would need to be the priority. If pain medication were administered, there could be a further decrease in blood pressure. Maintaining airway is the priority. A chest X-ray is not a priority at the moment.

Parameters to Monitor: Monitoring the blood pressure and respiratory rate would be the priority to ensure the airway is maintained. Bowel sounds and capillary refill would be important after the acute incident of a transfusion reaction. Monitoring urine output is a measure of hemodynamic status and kidney function. This would be the priority after the airway has been secured.

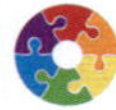

NCJMM Step: Recognize Cues, Analyze Cues, Prioritize Hypothesis, Generate Solutions, Take Action, and Evaluate Outcomes

References: Astle & Duggleby (2024), p. 1069; Power-Kean et al. (2023), pp. 210–211 (anaphylaxis), pp. 389–394 (spinal cord injuries), 627 (anaphylaxis), 627–630 (sepsis), 1045 (hypovolemia); Tyerman & Cobbett (2023), pp. 744 (TRALI), 1730–1731 (hypovolemic shock), 1734 (anaphylaxis), 1734–1735 (sepsis).

Medical-Surgical 8.0

Answer

Action to Take	Condition Most Likely Experiencing	Parameter to Monitor
Prepare to insert a Foley catheter	Benign prostate hyperplasia	Volume of urine in the bladder
Action to Take		**Parameter to Monitor**
Obtain a urine sample for culture and sensitivity		Intake and output

Rationale:

Potential Condition: The client is at greatest risk for benign prostate hyperplasia. The classic clinical manifestations include the need to void during the night, sense of urgency, trying to void then starting to void, and small stream. As people with prostates age, there is hyperplasia or thickening of the prostate gland. Over time, the prostate reduces the size of the urethra and causes urinary retention. The client does not present with a urinary tract infection as there is no pain with voiding, despite urgency, and the client does not have a fever. The client denies any discharge that could be indicative of a sexually transmitted infection. The client does not complain of any back pain and there is no sign of a fever, so the client is not presenting with kidney stones. A urinary tract infection and kidney stones are complications of benign prostate hyperplasia.

Actions to Take: The client is being admitted for further assessment of urinary retention. A catheter may be necessary to assist in completely draining the bladder. An in/out catheter may be necessary if the client presents with a high level of urine in the bladder. This can be uncomfortable, despite the issue presenting and the bladder growing in size. Over time, the bladder can lose tone and the ability to contract if extended due to volume for too long. It is important to rule out any bladder infections despite not presenting with any clinical manifestations associated with a urinary tract infraction. An antibiotic is not necessary at this point and requires further evidence to support the need for this treatment. It is important to maintain adequate fluid hydration. Intravenous fluids would be unnecessary at this point because the client is able to take fluids by mouth. A transurethral resection of the prostate (TURP) is a moderate surgical procedure used to reduce the size of the prostate. This would be a later intervention, not at the initial stages to determine what is making the client retain urine.

Parameters to Monitor: Monitoring the urine volume in the bladder and urine output would be the highest priority. Monitoring the urine volume in the bladder would be done as a minimally invasive procedure with a bladder scanner. An average amount of volume is derived from the bladder scanner. When the volume becomes elevated, an in/out catheter may be necessary to relieve the volume. Monitoring intake and output is important for determining the fluid status of the client. These should be relatively the same numbers, indicating a balance. If the client is retaining volume, there will be a positive fluid balance. If the client is voiding large amounts, there will be a negative fluid balance. It is not important at this time to monitor respiratory status or temperature as the client is not presenting with an infection. Capillary refill and identifying perfusion status are not priorities for this client.

NCJMM Step: Recognize Cues, Analyze Cues, Prioritize Hypothesis, Generate Solutions, Take Action, and Evaluate Outcomes

References: Astle & Duggleby (2024), pp. 1162–1209; Tyerman & Cobbett (2023), pp. 1402–1407.

Medical-Surgical 9.0

Answer

Action to Take	Condition Most Likely Experiencing	Parameter to Monitor
Change wafer of the two-piece ostomy system	Skin infection	Temperature
Action to Take		**Parameter to Monitor**
Clean the skin by the stoma with sterile normal saline		Wound discharge

Rationale:
Potential Condition: The client presents with a fever and skin breakdown with purulent discharge indicating a skin infection by the stoma. The client presents with fine inspiratory crackles that clear with a cough, but there are no other symptoms to indicate pneumonia. The client's breathing is not laboured. The client is voiding without issue as they deny pain, frequency, or urgency, which could indicate a urinary tract infection. The client is having a normal amount of bowel movements and does not present with emesis or nausea.

Actions to Take: It would be important to clean the skin under the wafer of the colostomy bag system with sterile normal saline and to replace the wafer. A cleansing enema is not necessary as the client reports regular bowel movements, and irrigating the stoma should be done with caution so as not to increase peristalsis, thus exposing the skin that is already broken down to more stool.

Parameters to Monitor: The client's temperature is monitored to determine if the infection is getting worse, and the wound discharge is important to check to keep the area clean. The client does not have a respiratory condition requiring the respiratory rate to be monitored. The client has bowel sounds indicating adequate peristalsis and intestinal motility. The client does not require monitoring of urine output as the client is not dehydrated.

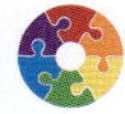
NCJMM Step: Recognize Cues, Analyze Cues, Prioritize Hypothesis, Generate Solutions, Take Action, and Evaluate Outcomes
References: Astle & Duggleby (2024), pp. 1210–1246; Tyerman & Cobbett (2023), pp. 1069–1070.

Medical-Surgical 10.0

Answer

Action to Take	Condition Most Likely Experiencing	Parameter to Monitor
Request a consult for wound specialists	Skin infection	Affect
Action to Take		**Parameter to Monitor**
Reposition client to reduce pressure on coccyx		Skin integrity

Rationale:
Potential Condition: The client presents with an infection as evidenced by the temperature, which is elevated for an older adult, due to a stage 3 coccyx wound from lack of mobility and proper nutritional intake. Pressure injuries occur on the skin covering bony prominences (scapulae, elbows, coccyx, and heels). The client's mental health status after their friend died led to poor nutrition, failure to thrive, periods of immobility with pressure on bony prominences, leading to skin breakdown and development of a wound. The LTC staff may have wanted to support the client in their sadness, but the lack of mobility and changes in position led to the development of a severe wound and longer healing time due to age. The client presented with a regular heart rate, which does not indicate a dysrhythmia. The client's refusal to eat does not equate to an eating disorder, which is a mental health condition. The client is not taking in enough nutrition to have consistent bowel movements. The client has clear air entry, only fine crackles throughout the lung fields, which would be due to the lack of mobility and increasing alveoli.

Actions to Take: It would be important to consult wound specialists to identify the proper treatment for the stage 3 wound. Given the client's poor nutritional status at the time of admission, wound healing and healing of the wound may take longer. Repositioning the client to stay off the area and to keep the area dry and intact would also help with healing. The client is able to eat but choosing not to, thus inserting a nasogastric tube is unnecessary. The client does not have difficulty swallowing. The client also does not need a venous access device or intravenous antibiotics at the present time. If the wound worsens, then more aggressive treatment options might be needed.

Parameters to Monitor: Monitoring the client's mood and affect as well as skin integrity will be beneficial to the wound healing. If the client increases ambulation and mobility, then less time will be spent placing pressure on the wound. It is not necessary to monitor the heart rate, bowel sounds (as the client does not present with constipation or a bowel obstruction), or range of motion.

NCJMM Step: Recognize Cues, Analyze Cues, Prioritize Hypothesis, Generate Solutions, Take Action, and Evaluate Outcomes
References: Astle & Duggleby (2024), pp. 1247–1289; Power-Kean et al. (2023), pp. 1024, 1028; Tyerman & Cobbett (2023), pp. 235–238, 511.

Medical-Surgical 11.0

Answer

Action to Take	Condition Most Likely Experiencing	Parameter to Monitor
Remove the client's wet clothing	Hypothermia	Temperature
Action to Take		**Parameter to Monitor**
Connect the client to a cardiac monitor		Dysrhythmias

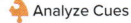

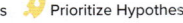

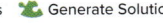

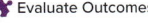

Rationale:

Potential Condition: The client narrative prior to admission to the ED indicates that the client was found in extremely cool temperatures leading to hypothermia. The client's temperature and bradycardia are also indicators of mild hypothermia, which is a temperature of less than 35.0°C. The client does not present with hypertension, hypotension, or hyperthermia as evidenced by the vital signs.

Actions to Take: To assist with the rewarming of the client, the first actions of the nurse are to remove any wet or frozen clothing, apply clean, dry clothing, and attach the client to a cardiac monitor. Obtaining a blood sugar may indicate the reason why the client did not respond to changing cool temperatures; however, the priority is to rewarm the client safely and within the parameters of institutional policy. The client does not present with hyperthermia (or a fever); therefore, administering an antipyretic (acetaminophen) to reduce the temperature is unnecessary. The client does not require additional respiratory or blood pressure support, nor has the client developed a life-threatening dysrhythmia as evidenced by the clinical manifestations.

Parameters to Monitor: It is important to monitor temperature and dysrhythmias for clients who present with hypothermia. Rewarming decisions for a client depend on the severity of the hypothermia. There should be gradual rewarming, typically 0.5–1°C per hour, but refer to your institutional policy. Rewarming a client too fast can lead to neurological complications such as increased intracranial pressure and reduced cerebral blood flow. The client's urine output would be monitored for dehydration and later parameters to consider. Rewarming the client is the priority here. Rewarming of a client with mild hypothermia may cause them to develop some mild hypotension; however, nothing life-threatening. When a client presents with severe hypothermia (<30°C), hypotension would be considered. The client denies any pain at present with no observed injury indicating that pain would be a priority parameter to monitor.

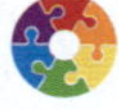

NCJMM Step: Recognize Cues, Analyze Cues, Prioritize Hypothesis, Generate Solutions, Take Action, and Evaluate Outcomes

References: Astle & Duggleby (2024), pp. 525–537; Cobbett (2025), p. 122; Tyerman & Cobbett (2023), pp. 1784–1785.

Medical-Surgical 12.0

Answer

Action to Take	Condition Most Likely Experiencing	Parameter to Monitor
Prepare to insert a peripheral venous access device	Hypertensive emergency	Blood pressure
Administer antihypertensive		Pupillary size and reaction

Rationale:

Potential Condition: The client presents with an extremely high blood pressure due to the use of cocaine, which is a stimulant. The client does not have any previous comorbidities to indicate that missed diagnosis of hypertension or missed medication would be the cause. An abruptly elevated blood pressure with a diastolic blood pressure above 120–130 mm Hg indicates a hypertensive crisis. A hypertensive crisis is further broken down into a hypertensive emergency (condition develops over hours to days, where the primary concern is end-organ damage) or a hypertensive urgency (condition develops over days to weeks and there is a severely elevated blood pressure but no clinical evidence of target organ damage). Another potential condition would be a stroke; however, the client's pupils are equal in size and shape and react accordingly to light, and the client is not experiencing any chest pain, which eliminates an acute myocardial infarction. An abrupt headache is a neurological condition in which a pulmonary embolus would present as a respiratory condition with shortness of breath and pleural chest pain due to a lodged clot in the pulmonary vascular system.

Actions to Take: A client with a hypertensive emergency will require hospitalization, continuous monitoring in a Critical Care Unit, and parenteral administration of antihypertensive medications to achieve a decrease in the mean arterial pressure. Lowering the blood pressure too quickly will result in less cerebral perfusion and may precipitate a stroke, or reduced perfusion to the myocardium may exacerbate an acute myocardial infarction. A peripheral venous access device would allow for the administration of intravenous fluids as well as administration of medications. In the event of a code situation, venous access has already been established. The client is not hypo- or hyperglycemic; therefore, taking a blood sugar would be inappropriate given the critical nature of the situation. While the client presents with coarse crackles, getting a chest X-ray would only prevent urgent treatment of the hypertensive crisis. The client has an open airway and currently a stable hemodynamic state.

Parameters to Monitor: Monitoring for signs of neurological dysfunction such as stroke, retinal damage, heart failure, pulmonary edema, and renal failure are important health assessments. Blood sugar monitoring is irrelevant at the moment. The client does not present with a fever or an infection that requires the monitoring of temperature. The client's gait is unsteady as a result of the high blood pressure.

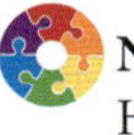

NCJMM Step: Recognize Cues, Analyze Cues, Prioritize Hypothesis, Generate Solutions, Take Action, and Evaluate Outcomes

References: Astle & Duggleby (2024), pp. 554–556, 644–649; Cobbett (2025), pp. 160–216, 551–552; Tyerman & Cobbett (2023), pp. 792–794.

Medical-Surgical 13.0

Answer

Action to Take	Condition Most Likely Experiencing	Parameter to Monitor
Prepare the client for a cardioversion	Atrial fibrillation	Clinical manifestations of a stroke
Action to Take		**Parameter to Monitor**
Obtain an electrocardiogram		Heart rate

Rationale:

Potential Condition: The client presented with nonspecific complaints of fatigue, shortness of breath with minimal exertion, and palpitations. The shortness of breath with minimal exertion and palpitations indicate there is a cardiac and respiratory connection for the condition. The vital signs include a fast heart rate (greater than 100 beats per minute), which indicates a tachycardia rhythm. Further assessment data are required to determine the type of rhythm the client is experiencing. During the assessment, there is a finding of an irregular pulse. Out of the potential conditions, the only irregular pulse is atrial fibrillation, which contributes to the initial presentation the client experienced. The client could not be experiencing bradycardia (heart rate less than 60 beats per minute). The client is able to speak in complete sentences and is alert and oriented to person, place, and time, indicating systemic and cerebral perfusion. Clients presenting in ventricular tachycardia present with complications associated with poor left ventricular function.

Actions to Take: Since the client is experiencing new-onset atrial fibrillation, preparing the client for a cardioversion would be one of the actions. Since the atrial fibrillation is new, the aim of treating the client's symptoms is to restore the heart's own intrinsic rhythm, resetting it to normal sinus rhythm. It would also be important to capture a 12-lead electrocardiogram (ECG) on this patient to determine if there are any other cardiac abnormalities and to confirm the client is indeed experiencing atrial fibrillation. The client would not require a consultation with a dietitian as there is no gastrointestinal concern. The client's pulse oximetry was documented at 92% on room air, which is satisfactory and greater than 90% saturation level. A chest X-ray is not required for this client.

Parameters to Monitor: Monitoring the client's heart rate and stroke symptoms would be the two most important parameters to monitor. If the heart rate remains elevated, additional treatment beyond cardioversion may be needed, with the likely addition of an antidysrhythmic medication. When the heart rate is high, there is a positive correlation with the respiratory rate, which needs to increase to compensate for the higher demand on the cardiorespiratory system. It would be important to monitor for clinical manifestations of a stroke. Untreated atrial fibrillation can create static blood flow in the chambers, increasing the likelihood of a blood clot to form. A complication of untreated atrial fibrillation can be pulmonary embolus if clots form in the right atrium, and a stroke if a pre-existing clot travels from the left atrium. The urine output would not need to be monitored since the client voids independently and without issue. The pulse oximetry is within normal limits and does not need further monitoring. The client presents with normal body temperature, which does not require additional monitoring.

NCJMM Step: Recognize Cues, Analyze Cues, Prioritize Hypothesis, Generate Solutions, Take Action, and Evaluate Outcomes

References: Astle & Duggleby (2024), pp. 536–567, 594–597, 955–976; Cobbett (2025), pp. 781–772; Tyerman & Cobbett (2023), pp. 858–860.

Medical-Surgical 14.0

Answer

Action to Take	Condition Most Likely Experiencing	Parameter to Monitor
Request an order to administer furosemide	Cardiomyopathy	Urine output
Action to Take		**Parameter to Monitor**
Request an order to initiate oxygen therapy		Continuous electrocardiogram (ECG) monitoring for dysrhythmias

Rationale:

Potential Condition: The client is experiencing symptoms associated with a cardiomyopathy. Although crackles are auscultated, reports of palpitations, irregular pulses noted, and shortness of breath, which align with atrial fibrillation. The client's symptoms of 3-cm JVD with +1 non-pitting edema is associated with increased right-sided pressures; however, the client's primary complaint is shortness of breath, reduced urine output, and related left-sided issues. The client denies any chest pain, and the heart sounds are also clear and not muffled, which would be consistent if the client presented with pericardial effusion. The client has low blood pressure associated with reduced cardiac output. Peripheral edema could be an indicator for chronic pericarditis; however, chronic pericarditis clinical presentation includes weight loss, edema, JVD, arial fibrillation, exercise intolerance, dyspnea on exertion, fatigue, and anorexia. The client has not had a change in weight and has only been hungry × 24 hours. Chronic pericarditis symptoms are not acute.

Actions to Take: The primary focus for this client should be airway, breathing, and circulation, thus administering a loop diuretic (furosemide) and applying oxygen therapy for a low pulse oximetry reading of 86% on room air are priorities. Preparing the client for a chest X-ray would be appropriate but not an immediate action. The appropriate blood test for this client would be a BNP. The client is already in volume overload due to the crackles; therefore, administering IV fluids would only put the client in further distress. There is no need to restrict the client's activity but to encourage movement as tolerated.

Parameters to Monitor: Urine output would need to be monitored, as well as dysrhythmias through ECG monitoring. When a client is in heart failure, furosemide would assist with pulmonary congestion and symptoms of heart failure, reduce peripheral edema, and improve oxygenation. Monitoring urine output would assist in identifying a fluid shift in the client. The client's left ventricle is not pumping adequately. These clients are prone to dysrhythmias, primarily atrial fibrillation, tachycardia, or bradycardia. The client does not have an infection so there is no need to monitor the temperature. Weight is appropriate for long-term monitoring parameters related to heart failure or if the diagnosis was chronic pericarditis. Monitoring for weight gain would be appropriate once the client's respiratory status has improved. The primary goal would be to reduce the volume overload by monitoring urine output and for any changes in the heart rhythm.

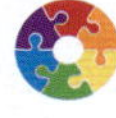

NCJMM Step: Recognize Cues, Analyze Cues, Prioritize Hypothesis, Generate Solutions, Take Action, and Evaluate Outcomes

References: Power-Kean et al. (2023), pp. 608–609; Sealock & Seneviratne (2025), p. 425; Tyerman & Cobbett (2023), pp. 891–895.

Medical-Surgical 15.0

Answer

Action to Take	Condition Most Likely Experiencing	Parameter to Monitor
Request antibiotic therapy	Cellulitis	Gangrene
Action to Take		Parameter to Monitor
Apply moist heat and elevate		Redness borders decreasing in size

Rationale:

Potential Condition: When administering an intradermal, subcutaneous injection or intramuscular injection, there is piercing of the skin. Cellulitis occurs when the skin was not prepped adequately with an alcohol swab to clean the skin. Cellulitis is described as a deep inflammation of subcutaneous tissue due to enzymes produced by bacteria. The client presented with typical clinical manifestations associated with cellulitis; the site of the injection was hot, tender, erythematous, and edematous with diffuse borders. The patient then developed chills, malaise, and fever. A cellulitis can be either a primary or secondary source of infection for the client. Usual causative agents are *Staphylococcus aureus* and streptococci because they live on the skin and are not harmful unless a person is immunocompromised or the agents are introduced into the tissues. Chicken pox presents as small, tight vesicles that first appear on the trunk and then spread to the face, arm, and legs. Vesicles erupt in succeeding crops over several days then become pustules and then crusts. Chicken pox is characterized by intense pruritus. Herpes zoster is also known as *shingles*. These present as small, grouped vesicles that emerge along the cutaneous sensory nerve, then pustules, then crusts. Shingles are caused by a reactivation of the dormant varicella virus or chicken pox. Psoriasis presents as a scaly, erythematous patch, with silvery scales on top. It is usually found on the scalp, outside of elbows and knees, low back, and anogenital area.

Actions to Take: Antibiotic therapy and application of moist heat with elevation are the primary actions to take to help minimize discomfort. Titre levels are drawn for chicken pox conditions. The client does not need a chest X-ray because they are presenting with a skin condition. There is no purulent drainage requiring a sample to be sent for culture and sensitivity.

Parameters to Monitor: If left untreated, cellulitis can progress to gangrene. The nurse needs to monitor for improvement and if the borders of redness minimize in size. This would indicate that the body's immune function is helping with the cellulitis. Pain level would be appropriate to monitor with herpes zoster (shingles) because this condition can be very uncomfortable, presenting with intense nerve pain. Blood pressure is irrelevant to monitor for skin conditions and this client is hemodynamically stable. The client does not present with an oozing wound; therefore, wound discharge would not need to be monitored.

NCJMM Step: Recognize Cues, Analyze Cues, Prioritize Hypotheses, Generate Solutions, Take Action, and Evaluate Outcomes

References: Astle & Duggleby (2024), pp. 732, 744, 773–783, 790; Cobbett (2025), pp. 617–643; Jarvis et al. (2024), pp. 270–272; Tyerman & Cobbett (2023), pp. 501–503.

Medical-Surgical 16.0

Answer

Action to Take	Condition Most Likely Experiencing	Parameter to Monitor
Prepare to initiate anticoagulant therapy (IV heparin)	Pulmonary embolus	aPTT and INR levels

Action to Take		Parameter to Monitor
Prepare to increase oxygen level		Pulse oximetry

Rationale:
Potential Condition: The client presents with clinical manifestations associated with a pulmonary embolus. The client was using only sequential compression devices in the ICU with limited mobility. The client's clinical presentation of a red left posterior calf with mild swelling indicates a deep vein thrombosis. Upon initial transfer, the tracheostomy site was dry and intact. The insertion was 6 days prior to the transfer, indicating the tissues would have healed by the time of the transfer. The client presented with frank red blood as opposed to dark streaks of blood in the mucus. The presence of frank red blood indicates irritation or, in this case, pulmonary edema of blood in the alveoli. Coarse crackles were documented after being suctioned. Crackles should improve with suctioning. The client does not present with pneumonia as that has resolved and the client does not have an infection as they are afebrile. The client does not have a pleural effusion as the frank red blood is from the airways, not the pleural space. The client has symmetrical air expansion, dismissing the possibility of a pneumothorax.

Actions to Take: The client needs an increase in oxygen therapy and anticoagulant therapy. The sequential compression devices were not enough to prevent a deep vein clot from forming, as evidenced by the swollen and red left posterior calf. Antibiotic therapy is not appropriate as the client does not have an infection. Increasing the suction pressure would only irritate the airway walls further and lead to increase in bleeding. The client will need to go for a spiral computed tomography (CT) scan, not a head CT. A spiral CT is specific for clients suspected of having a pulmonary embolus.

Parameters to Monitor: Monitoring the aPTT and INR would be appropriate as the client's clotting cascade has been affected. These are specific blood tests associated with bleeding disorders. It is important to monitor these laboratory parameters if there is a possibility of anticoagulant therapy being initiated. It is important to monitor the pulse oximetry levels; an increase in pulse oximetry indicates improved gas exchange. A decrease indicates a decline in status and further treatment may be needed. If the client exhibits renal failure and loses more blood, then urine output would be important to monitor. The client does not have a fever, thus temperature does not need to be monitored. The client has pain with inspiration, which is classified differently than chest pain. This is called *pleuritic pain* and is associated with pulmonary embolus.

NCJMM Step: Recognize Cues, Analyze Cues, Prioritize Hypothesis, Generate Solutions, Take Action, and Evaluate Outcomes
References: Cobbett (2025), pp. 723–760; Power-Kean et al. (2023), p. 692; Tyerman & Cobbett (2023), pp. 622–624.

Maternal/Birthing Parent Health Bow-Tie Cases

Maternal/Birthing Parent Health 1.0

Answer

Action to Take	Condition Most Likely Experiencing	Parameter to Monitor
Screen for other sexually transmitted infections	Syphilis	Educate client to practise abstinence until treatment is complete
Action to Take		**Parameter to Monitor**
Review nontreponemal and treponemal results		Jarisch-Herxheimer reactions

Rationale:
Potential Condition: Fever, sore throat, aches and pains, and loss of appetite all mimic the flu but are also the signs and symptoms of syphilis when there is a body rash present. A chancre sore on the genitals is typical in the first stage of syphilis but usually has healed by the time the patient has entered the second stage when a body rash can appear on the thorax, back, and/or hands. The client has denied any vaginal discharge, which excludes chlamydia and gonorrhea. The chancres point toward either syphilis or herpes. Given the timeline of symptom presentation, syphilis is the most logical answer. Chlamydia is caused by *Chlamydia trachomatis*, a gram-negative bacterium, and may present without any symptoms. Clinical manifestations may include urethritis, epididymitis, proctitis, cervicitis, hypertrophic ectopy, and dyspareunia. Herpes simplex virus presents when the virus enters through the mucous membranes or breaks in the skin during contact with an infected person. Primary presentation includes burning, itching, or tingling at the site of inoculation. Multiple small, vesicular, and sometimes painless lesions may appear on the inner thigh, penis, scrotum, and vulva and contain large quantities of infectious viral particles. The lesions may rupture. Clients who present with gonorrhea may be asymptomatic or have minor symptoms such as urethritis, dysuria, and profuse, purulent urethral discharge that develops 2 to 5 days after infection.

Actions to Take: The client should be screened for other sexually transmitted infections (STIs) and undergo serological testing; nontreponemal and treponemal would be taken from the lesions. Syphilis, chlamydia and gonorrhea are reportable STIs. Cultures are taken with gonorrhea, and diagnosis of chlamydia is done using nucleic acid amplification testing (NAAT). It is important to recognize which test is most appropriate for each condition.

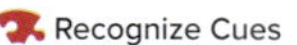 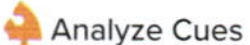 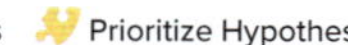 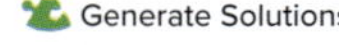
Recognize Cues Analyze Cues Prioritize Hypothesis Generate Solutions Take Action Evaluate Outcomes

Parameters to Monitor: The client should be educated to practise abstinence until treatment is complete about the occurrence of Jarisch-Herxheimer reactions with treatment. Clients require monthly follow-up and may need long-term serological testing even in the absence of symptoms. Abstinence is important until cure is demonstrated. Clients with gonorrhea and chlamydia may continue to have intercourse with the use of condoms. Triggers for stress are more related to an outbreak of herpes simplex virus. Clients need to be educated about the presence of Jarisch-Herxheimer reactions, which comprise an acute febrile reaction often accompanied by headache, myalgias, and arthralgias that develop within the first 24 hours of treatment. The reaction may be treated symptomatically with analgesics and antipyretics. If clients are pregnant and this reaction occurs in the second half of pregnancy, clients may be at risk for preterm labour and birth.

NCJMM Step: Recognize Cues, Analyze Cues, Prioritize Hypothesis, Generate Solutions, Take Action, and Evaluate Outcomes
Reference: Keenan-Lindsay et al. (2022), pp. 100–109.

Maternal/Birthing Parent Health 2.0

Answer

Action to Take	Condition Most Likely Experiencing	Parameter to Monitor
Prepare the client for dilation and curettage	Incomplete spontaneous abortion	Temperature
Action to Take		**Parameter to Monitor**
Prepare for laboratory draw of complete blood count, electrolytes, and coagulation		Signs associated with hemorrhage

Rationale:
Potential Condition: This client has experienced a late-pregnancy (12 to 20 weeks' gestation) incomplete spontaneous abortion or miscarriage. Incomplete miscarriages involve a heavy amount of bleeding with an open cervical os, seen with a speculum exam. Tissue may be present with the bleeding. Mild-to-severe uterine cramping may be present. Although uncommon, miscarriages can be septic, and they can include fever, abdominal tenderness, and vaginal bleeding, which may be slight to heavy and is usually malodorous. Placenta abruption involves the detachment of the placenta but typically occurs after 20 weeks of pregnancy. Placenta previa is when the placenta is implanted in the lower uterine segment so that it completely or partially covers the crevices or is close enough to the cervix to cause bleeding when the cervix dilates or the lower uterine segment effaces. The placental edge reaches or overlaps the internal cervical os between 18 and 24 weeks of gestation, requiring a follow-up examination. It is important to be aware of a client having a placenta previa prior to delivery. In this case, the client has not delivered and cannot have a postpartum hemorrhage.

Actions to Take: The nurse needs to prepare the client for a dilation and curettage (D&C) and prepare for laboratory drawing blood samples prior to the procedure. A client with an incomplete pregnancy loss can be given misoprostol orally or vaginally to induce labour and achieve vaginal delivery of the fetus. Mifepristone can be given safely concomitantly with misoprostol to facilitate cervical preparation and reduce procedure time. A D&C is required for this client. The cervix is dilated; if necessary, a curette is inserted to scrape the uterine walls and remove uterine contents. Pain relief is required post-procedure.

Parameters to Monitor: After D&C, the nurse must monitor for signs of an infection (temperature) and hemorrhage. An incomplete spontaneous abortion or miscarriage has the potential to develop into a septic process. After evacuation of the uterus, oxytocin is often given to prevent hemorrhage. For excessive bleeding, ergot products such as ergonovine or a prostaglandin derivative such as carboprost tromethamine (Hemabate) are given to contract the uterus. Analgesics such as ibuprofen may decrease discomfort from the cramping. Blood transfusions may be required for shock or anemia. If the client is Rh negative and not isoimmunized, they would be given Rh_o immune globulin within 48 hours of the pregnancy loss. Monitoring for hemorrhage is more important than extreme fluid shifts as there would be little effect on sodium and potassium cellular components. The client does not need to be intubated for the procedure; therefore, the chance of an ileus occurring is slim to none as a result of the D&C. Initiating support groups would be too early. The client and their partner need to be allowed to grieve. They should be offered the choice of spending time with the fetal remains. Support for grief and loss should be provided when appropriate for the client and their partner.

NCJMM Step: Recognize Cues, Analyze Cues, Prioritize Hypothesis, Generate Solutions, Take Action, and Evaluate Outcomes
References: Keenan-Lindsay et al. (2022), pp. 280–284, 288–293; Riggs et al. (2020).

Maternal/Birthing Parent Health 3.0

Answer

Action to Take	Condition Most Likely Experiencing	Parameter to Monitor
Prepare to administer an intravenous fluid bolus	Postpartum hemorrhage	Pulse oximetry

Action to Take		Parameter to Monitor
Initiate oxygen therapy		Blood pressure

Rationale:

Potential Condition: The client presents with symptoms associated with a postpartum hemorrhage. She had prolonged labour as documented, which is typically over 25 hours for a first-time parent and 20 hours for a parent who has previously delivered. This is her first child, and she presents with uterine atony (boggy fundus, golf ball–size clots, and bright red lochia). The client's hemodynamic status is unstable as her blood pressure has dropped significantly, and the uterus did not regain the appropriate tone. The client does not present with a fever or an infective process. The client denies any chest pain or difficulty breathing, excluding the possibility of a pulmonary embolus. The client is beyond the stages of dehydration given her unstable hemodynamic status and corresponding respiratory response.

Actions to Take: Management in treating a postpartum hemorrhage is to restore circulating blood volume and eliminate the cause of the hemorrhage. In this case, it is to improve uterine atony. The client already has two peripheral venous access devices. Administering an intravenous fluid bolus is a first priority to improve the client's blood pressure. Crystalloids such as lactated Ringer's, normal saline would be preferred initially until additional fluids could be administered. Colloids (albumin) blood or additional blood products (fresh frozen plasma or platelets) would also be a consideration to restore the client's circulating blood volume. Ensuring airway management is a top priority as well. Initiating oxygen therapy would assist with the client's gas exchange. The client does not present with an infection and would not require antibiotics of blood cultures. The client does not present with symptoms of a pulmonary embolus, such as pleuritic pain associated with rapid, shallow breaths, and shortness of breath; therefore, the client does not need a chest X-ray.

Parameters to Monitor: Monitoring the blood pressure for improvements in increasing circulating volume and pulse oximetry for improved gas exchange would be the priority. Monitoring urine output is a measure of hemodynamic status and kidney function. This would be the priority after the oxygenation has been established and the client's blood pressure has increased. Without circulating volume, the kidneys will not be perfused. The first sign of improved hemodynamic stability will be the blood pressure. The client's capillary refill was normal from the start, but if there is reduced perfusion if the client's status deteriorates, monitoring may be a consideration. The client's gait will improve after the client's blood volume is restored.

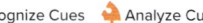

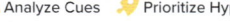

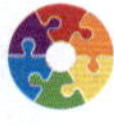
NCJMM Step: Recognize Cues, Analyze Cues, Prioritize Hypothesis, Generate Solutions, Take Action, and Evaluate Outcomes

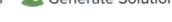

Reference: Keenan- Lindsay et al. (2022), pp. 532–539.

Pediatrics Bow-Tie Cases

Pediatrics 1.0

Answer

Action to Take	Condition Most Likely Experiencing	Parameter to Monitor
Administer humidified oxygen	Respiratory syncytial virus (RSV)	Pulse oximetry
Action to Take		**Parameter to Monitor**
Obtain nasal specimen sample for antigen detection		Number of wet diapers

Rationale:

Potential Condition: Clinical manifestations such as laboured respirations, abdominal retractions, nasal flaring, wet-sounding cough, and pallor indicate respiratory distress for the infant. Further respiratory clinical manifestations such as wheezing, diminished air entry, and being febrile indicate a virus or bacteria is the likely diagnosis. Asthma is chronic inflammatory condition of the airways typically caused by a trigger causing the airways to become narrow, leading to bronchoconstriction. Croup is an acute infectious process characterized by a bark-like cough, inspiratory stridor, and respiratory distress. Acute infections of the larynx are important to address in infants. The infant is too young to swallow anything in the middle of the night.

Actions to Take: Humidified oxygen via a mask or hood in concentrations to maintain adequate pulse oximetry at or above 92%. Humidified air will help break up nasal secretions that make feeding and breathing difficult. The nurse would also collect a nasal specimen sample to identify if there are any antigens present causing the RSV. No other conditions would require this confirmation of diagnosis. A peripheral venous access would only be inserted if the infant became dehydrated and required additional fluids. Fluid status is important to monitor throughout. A Foley catheter would be unnecessary for monitoring fluid status, and diuretics are not to be administered if adequate hydration is a concern.

Parameters to Monitor: Pulse oximetry is indicative of respiratory status. Continuous monitoring is a noninvasive way to monitor changes in oxygenation. Blood gas values may be drawn as well to guide therapy. Frequent feeds should be encouraged and breastfeeding supported. Supplemental oxygen can assist in these measures. In the hospital, wet diapers are weighed to determine hydration. There should be at least six to eight wet diapers within a 24-hour period, and the number of wet diapers should be monitored. A barking cough is a clinical manifestation of croup, which is not the potential condition. Bowel sounds are important to monitor with every client, but this is not a respiratory priority for this client.

The infant is only 5 weeks old so meeting developmental milestones is not necessary at this time.

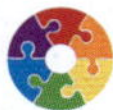

NCJMM Step: Recognize Cues, Analyze Cues, Prioritize Hypothesis, Generate Solutions, Take Action, and Evaluate Outcomes

Reference: Keenan-Lindsay et al. (2022), pp. 1129–1131 (croup), 1133–1134 (RSV), 1139–1140 (foreign body aspiration), 1143–1153 (asthma), 1153–1160 (cystic fibrosis).

Pediatrics 2.0

Answer

Action to Take	Condition Most Likely Experiencing	Parameter to Monitor
Prepare to insert a peripheral venous access device	Diabetic ketoacidosis	Glycated hemoglobin (hemoglobin A_1c)
Action to Take		**Parameter to Monitor**
Collect a blood specimen for glucose monitoring		Ketones in urine

Rationale:

Potential Condition: The client's clinical manifestations of weight loss, sweet fruity-smelling breath, excessive drinking, and frequent voiding are evidence of diabetic ketoacidosis, which is high blood sugar as a result of insulin deficiency or type 1 diabetes. Despite weight loss, the client is eating the same amounts and taking in fluids but not gaining any wait. The client is not experiencing a fever and does not complain of any burning with voiding; therefore, a urinary tract infection can be dismissed. The client does not have symptoms associated with a congenital heart defect.

Actions to Take: The client presents with dry mucous membranes and tenting of the skin indicating dehydration, likely as a result of frequent urination. It would be best to insert a peripheral venous access device in the event that intravenous fluids are ordered for hydration. It would be appropriate to collect a blood specimen to identify the glucose result. A urinalysis sample would be collected and antibiotics ordered if the client had clinical manifestations of a urinary tract infection. A cardiology consult is not necessary as the health problem is not a congenital heart defect.

Parameters to Monitor: It is important to monitor glycated hemoglobin to identify the client's average blood sugar levels for the past 3 months and to monitor for ketones in the urine. Blood glucose, glycated hemoglobin, and monitoring for ketones in the urine comprise nursing management for clients suspected of or diagnosed with diabetic ketoacidosis or type 1 diabetes mellitus. The client does not present with clinical manifestations associated with an infection; therefore, monitoring a temperature is not needed. The client does not present with failure to thrive as the client continues to eat despite losing weight. Loss of weight is a clinical manifestation for type 1 diabetes mellitus. Diet would not need to be monitored for this client. Diabetic snacks and patient and family education would be appropriate for this client and parent.

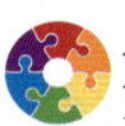

NCJMM Step: Recognize Cues, Analyze Cues, Prioritize Hypothesis, Generate Solutions, Take Action, and Evaluate Outcomes

References: Astle & Duggleby (2024), p. 1164; Keenan-Lindsay et al. (2022), Chapter 51, pp. 1395–1397.

Mental Health Bow-Tie Cases

Mental Health 1.0

Answer

Action to Take	Condition Most Likely Experiencing	Parameter to Monitor
Consult clinic nurse practitioner	Post-traumatic stress disorder (PTSD)	Use of drugs or alcohol for coping
Action to Take		**Parameter to Monitor**
Talk with the client of concern about coping strategies		Suicidal ideation

Rationale:

Potential Condition: The potential condition is PTSD. Major features of PTSD include recurrent, intrusive recollections of a disturbing event, dreams, and flashbacks, which are dissociative experiences in which the event is relived. There is also persistent avoidance associated with the trauma, causing the individual to avoid talking about the trauma or avoid activities, people, or places that rouse memories of the trauma, and persistent numbing as evidenced by the individual's feelings of emptiness inside or being disconnected from others. Persistent symptoms of increased arousal as evidenced by irritability, difficulty sleeping, difficulty concentrating, hypervigilance, or exaggerated startle response also occur. Difficulty with interpersonal, social, and occupational relationships nearly always accompanies PTSD, and trust is a common issue of concern. Clients may self-medicate.

Actions to Take: The nurse will want to consult a health care provider in the clinic to assist immediately with the father and his statements. The father should be praised for being brave, courageous, and vulnerable. The discussion of coping strategies begins with those regarding psychoeducation. Further coping strategies could include relaxation, mindfulness, and naming feelings. While normalizing emotions is important, what the father witnessed and is currently experiencing is not normal. He needs extra support. A crisis nurse is not warranted and may cause the client shame in this situation.

Parameters to Monitor: The father reports taking an SSRI. With this medication, suicidal ideation should be monitored. The father should also be monitored for unhealthy coping strategies such as drug and alcohol use, which can help alleviate feelings associated with forgetting the event. Treatments would include group psychotherapy and cognitive-behavioural therapy but parameters to monitor would be immediate and most at risk for, such as addiction and suicidal ideation.

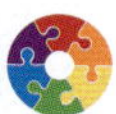

NCJMM Step: Recognize Cues, Analyze Cues, Prioritize Hypothesis, Generate Solutions, Take Action, and Evaluate Outcomes
References: Canadian Paediatric Society (2021); Pollard & Jakubec (2023), pp. 180–219; Skidmore-Roth & Richardson (2024), pp. 815–818 (lorazepam).

Mental Health 2.0

Answer

Action to Take	Condition Most Likely Experiencing	Parameter to Monitor
Assess risk for suicide	Borderline personality disorder	Effectiveness of mindfulness and relaxation techniques
Action to Take		**Parameter to Monitor**
Initiate therapeutic relationship with client		Depression

Rationale:
Potential Condition: The potential condition is borderline personality disorder (BPD). The major features of BPD include marked instability in emotion regulation, unstable interpersonal relationships, identity or self-image distortions, and unstable mood. People seek treatment for depression, anxiety, suicidal and self-harming behaviours, and other impulsive behaviours, including problematic substance use. Nurses are to minimize manipulative measures by clients with BPD. Staff should be aware of manipulative behaviour such as flattery, seductiveness, and instilling guilt. Physical violence toward intimate partners and nonintimate partners alike may occur.

Actions to Take: Two actions with this client will be to assess risk for suicide and initiate a therapeutic relationship with the client. Clients with BPD may engage in harmful self-soothing habits, such as cutting, promiscuous sexual behaviour, and numbing with substances. Such actions are common and may result in unintentional death. Chronic suicidal ideation is also a common feature of this disorder. Medications, therapy, or both can help individuals regulate emotions. Mindfulness, deep breathing, or relaxation techniques help the brain switch from the sympathetic nervous system to the parasympathetic nervous system. Specific medications include SSRIs, anticonvulsants, antipsychotics, and lithium to help dampen angry, impulsive labile behaviour.

Parameters to Monitor: With BPD there are high rates of comorbid illnesses, such as mood, anxiety, or substance use disorders, that may complicate the treatment and prognosis of BPD. Clients with BPD may also have other comorbidities, such as diabetes, high blood pressure, chronic back pain, fibromyalgia, and arthritis.

NCJMM Step: Recognize Cues, Analyze Cues, Prioritize Hypothesis, Generate Solutions, Take Action, and Evaluate Outcomes
Reference: Pollard & Jakubec (2023), pp. 390–412.

Mental Health 3.0

Answer

Action to Take	Condition Most Likely Experiencing	Parameter to Monitor
Request an order to administer potassium 10 mEq/50 mL D_5W via peripheral intravenous catheter	Anorexia nervosa	Seizure protocols
Action to Take		**Parameter to Monitor**
Establish therapeutic boundaries		Ventricular tachycardia

Rationale:
Potential Condition: Based on the low weight, frequent use of the gym, low blood pressure that is less than 90/60, hypokalemia, dehydration (sunken eyes, tenting, pallor of the eyes), constipation, lanugo, feeling chilled, and palpitations demonstrating previous cardiovascular concerns, the potential condition is anorexia nervosa. There are no clinical presentations of bulimia nervosa, binge eating, or eating disorder not otherwise specified (NOS).

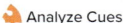

Actions to Take: The primary action is to administer potassium via IV as the potassium level is very low and places the client at risk for cardiac arrest due to a prolonged QT. The client is in renal failure given the lab values and is in starvation mode. The client requires hydration. The client does not require oxygenation given the stable vital signs and clear air entry. The client may require enteral nutrition, but not parenteral nutrition. Parenteral nutrition is used when electrolytes, carbohydrates, and lipids are administered through central venous access.

Parameters to Monitor: Electrolyte imbalances and complications of these imbalances are important to monitor for these clients. Because of the low sodium (Na) and potassium (K+) levels, the client is at risk for seizures (Na) and ventricular tachycardia (K+) and possible prolonged QT interval. Amenorrhea is a result of starvation. It is important but not the most important parameter to monitor. The client is anemic and may require blood administration if she becomes symptomatic. Polycythemia vera occurs when there are too many red blood cells.

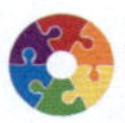

NCJMM Step: Recognize Cues, Analyze Cues, Prioritize Hypothesis, Generate Solutions, Take Action, and Evaluate Outcomes
Reference: Pollard & Jakubec (2023), pp. 304–323.

Mental Health 4.0

Answer

Action to Take	Condition Most Likely Experiencing	Parameter to Monitor
Complete a geriatric depression scale screening tool	Depression	Suicidal ideation
Action to Take		**Parameter to Monitor**
Prepare to consult psychiatry		Alcohol consumption

Rationale:
Potential Conditions: The client is experiencing symptoms of depression as indicated by lack of energy; withdrawal from family; recovery from an illness that has reduced her mobility and limited activities, leading to social isolation; being female (2:1 risk); having no family or close friends who live close by; and being a widow. Based on the wound assessment, the client's skin does not indicate cellulitis. Although the client experienced a traumatic event, there is no indication the client is re-experiencing the event. The client may present with avoidance. Client presents with alterations in cognition and mood, but in an acute phase, and does not demonstrate alterations in arousal and receptivity. Chronic osteomyelitis involves a bone infection that persists longer than 1 month. The client suffered the injury 2 weeks ago. The client is not exhibiting symptoms of anxiety; her vital signs are within normal parameters and the client presents calmly.

Actions to Take: The primary focus is on safety and confirming a possible diagnosis of depression. Assessment with a geriatric depression scale as well as consulting psychiatry would be the most important actions to take. Adding more pain medications could contribute to depression and withdrawal, leading to narcotic dependency. The client is managing well with 1 000 mg of acetaminophen twice a day. The client is not experiencing any signs of infection in the wound or with vital signs. The client remains afebrile. Consulting the client's daughter is not the role of the home care nurse. While encouraging social supports is appropriate to reduce isolation, the client is competent of being a participating member in her own care.

Parameters to Monitor: Monitoring for suicidal ideation and alcohol consumption contribute to the client's safety. The client has been home for only 2 days and has not participated in the care of her home. She has poor hygiene and is not cleaning up after herself. The realization of being alone, and recognizing early symptom presentation and suicidal ideation are important to document. The client has a bottle of liquor on the counter, so further monitoring of problematic alcohol use is important during this and subsequent visits. The client is not experiencing any infection; therefore, it is not necessary to monitor her temperature. The client's pain level is at a low level; monitoring for symptoms associated with mental health concerns is more important. The reduced use of mobility aids is an important concern but not a priority.

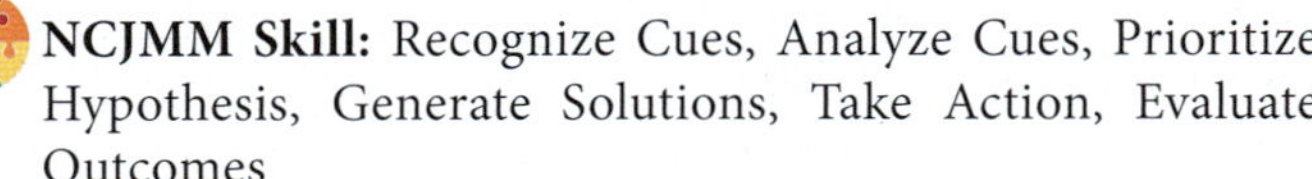

NCJMM Skill: Recognize Cues, Analyze Cues, Prioritize Hypothesis, Generate Solutions, Take Action, Evaluate Outcomes
References: Touhey & Jett (2020) pp. 343–367; Tyerman & Cobbett (2023), pp. 1642–1646.

Medical-Surgical Trend Cases

Medical-Surgical 1.0

Answer

POTENTIAL NURSING INTERVENTIONS	INDICATED	NOT INDICATED
Prepare client for chest X-ray	○	✔
Initiate isolation protocols	✔	○
Request a full-fibre diet from dietary	○	✔
Request an order to initiate intravenous fluids	✔	○
Apply barrier cream to coccyx	✔	○
Administer laxatives as per bowel protocol	○	✔
Request a cart with personal protective equipment such as gowns and gloves	✔	○

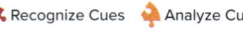

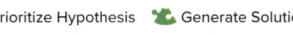

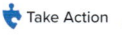

Rationale: The stool sample was positive for *Clostridium difficile (C-difficile)*, indicating that possible nursing interventions include isolation protocols, as *C-difficile* is very contagious and spread through contact isolation, requiring gowns and gloves when providing client care or upon entering the client's room. The client would require a single room. Based on the client presentation, the client is dehydrated. The low blood pressure and higher heart rate that is trending down require intravenous fluids as the client presents fatigued. The client's skin requires a barrier cream to prevent further breakdown, which would expose the client to increased risk for infection. The client presents with clear air entry, dismissing the need for a chest X-ray. A full-fibre diet and administration of laxatives for a bowel protocol would only exacerbate the diarrhea.

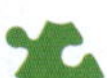

NCJMM Step: Generate Solutions
References: Astle & Duggleby (2024), pp. 676–724; Tyerman & Cobbett (2023), p. 1004.

Medical-Surgical 2.0

Answer

The client is at highest risk of developing **hypertension** as evidenced by the client's **cardiovascular assessment** and **vital signs.**

Rationale: The client presents with classic symptoms of hypertension: headache, double vision, palpitations (fluttering), feeling warm, and diaphoresis. These symptoms are related to the cardiovascular assessment as noted by the high blood pressure in the vital signs. The trend of the blood pressure remains elevated over several hours. The client does not present with hyperthermia or hypothermia, both of which are related to body temperature. There is not a reduced oxygen level in the blood as evidenced by the pulse oximetry levels. And the client reports no issues with emesis.

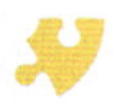

NCJMM Step: Prioritize Hypothesis
References: Astle & Duggleby (2024), pp. 522–571; Power-Kean et al. (2023), pp. 582–587; Tyerman & Cobbett (2023), pp. 773–795.

Medical-Surgical 3.0

Answer

POTENTIAL NURSING INTERVENTIONS	INDICATED	NOT INDICATED
Prepare to insert an 18-gauge peripheral venous access device	✔	○
Monitor urine output	✔	○
Prepare the client for an ultrasound	○	✔
Request an order for an analgesic	✔	○
Prepare to draw laboratory tests: electrolytes, creatine kinase, creatinine, BUN	✔	○
Administer sodium chloride per venous access device	○	✔
Elevate the forearm on pillows	✔	○

Rationale: The client's progression of symptoms indicates compartment syndrome, a condition in which swelling and increased pressure within a limited space reduce blood flow and nerve flow and compress tendons in the area. Key points to remember about compartment syndrome are as follows: it typically occurs with a fracture, crushing injury, fluid infusion, nephrotic syndrome, seizures, burns, casts that are too tight, and conditions that may affect microcirculation (diabetes, hypothyroidism, bleeding disorders, excessive anticoagulation, and malignancies). In the above case study, the nurse would anticipate inserting an 18-gauge peripheral access device in preparation for the surgical procedure fasciotomy, which is necessary if the intracompartmental pressures reach 30 mmHg. A large-bore peripheral venous access device is necessary, not a smaller gauge catheter. Clients with compartment syndrome are at risk of developing rhabdomyolysis, where myoglobin is released from damaged muscles leading to symptoms of acute renal failure; increased creatine kinase, creatinine, and BUN; and potential for increased potassium levels leading to cardiac dysrhythmias. The nurse should monitor for the 6 P's: pain, pressure, pallor, paralysis, pulselessness, and paresthesia. Ischemia can occur within 4 to 8 hours after the onset of compartment syndrome. Pulselessness and paralysis are late presentations of compartment syndrome. It is recommended that analgesic be administered in order to monitor if pain is relieved or persists, contributing to pain associated with a fracture (abnormal assessment) or a complication of the fracture (critical abnormal assessment). Elevating the affected extremity may help reduce the venous pressure and improve perfusion. The extremity should not be elevated above heart level. The client would not be prepared for an ultrasound test but may require direct measurement of the intracompartmental pressure using a manometer or an electronic transducer. Intravenous fluids would be necessary if the client is dehydrated or hemodynamically unstable. If an intravenous solution was necessary, maintaining intravascular volume would be the priority, as would minimizing extravascular leaking, which would only increase the compartment pressures.

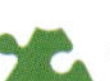

NCJMM Step: Generate Solutions
References: Power-Kean et al. (2023), p. 973; Tyerman & Cobbett (2023), pp.1623–1624.

Medical-Surgical 4.0

Answer

The nurse should recognize that the client is potentially experiencing **cellulitis.**

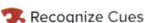

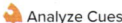

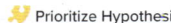

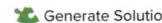

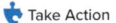

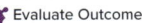

Rationale: When administering an intradermal, subcutaneous injection or intramuscular injection, there is a piercing of the skin. Cellulitis occurs when the skin was not prepped adequately with an alcohol swab to clean the skin. Cellulitis is described as a deep inflammation of subcutaneous tissue due to enzymes produced by bacteria. The client presented with typical clinical manifestations associated with cellulitis; the site of the injection was hot, tender, erythematous, and edematous with diffuse borders. The patient then developed chills, malaise, and fever. A cellulitis can be either a primary or secondary source of infection for the client. Usual causative agents are *Staphylococcus aureus* and streptococci as they live on the skin and are harmful unless the client is immunocompromised or these agents are introduced into the tissues.

NCJMM Step: Analyze Cues
References: Astle & Duggleby (2024), pp. 725–816; Power-Kean et al. (2023), p. 1035; Tyerman & Cobbett (2023), pp. 500–501.

Medical-Surgical 5.0

Answer

- ☐ Request an order to insert a Foley catheter
- ☐ Check the client's temperature every 1 hr
- ☐ Contact the client's clergy for last rites
- ✔ Initiate oxygen therapy at 2 L/min per nasal prongs
- ✔ Draw laboratory samples: complete blood count, electrolytes, troponin, blood cultures

Rationale: The client's oxygen level is decreasing, requiring therapy to increase the pulse oximetry levels, and blood work should be drawn for a client who is presenting with urosepsis. It is important to monitor the intake and output to determine if the patient is dehydrated and requires fluid resuscitation, which was the case at 1400h when a bolus was administered. The ongoing intravenous antibiotic therapy is used to treat the underlying infection. When the nurse monitors the intake and output, at the end of the shift there is a total. For example, the client has been receiving 09% normal saline at 125 mL/hr from 1000h until 1800h. This is 8 hours multiplied by 125 mL/hr, and the total fluid intake for that time period is 1 000 mL. The nurse must also add in the two antibiotic doses equalling 200 mL. The total fluid intake for the time the nurse was caring for this client was 1 200mL. The nurse must also monitor urine output. Good kidney perfusion is approximately 30 mL/hr or 0.5–1 mL/kg/hr if a weight is available. This client had a total of 650 mL output. To figure out the fluid balance for this shift, the nurse would subtract the output from the input (1 200 mL − 650 mL = 550 mL positive). This means the client had more fluid administered than the kidneys were able to perfuse. A client who presents with sepsis will require intravenous fluid resuscitation and antibiotic therapy support.

NCJMM Step: Take Action
Reference: Astle & Duggleby (2024), pp. 725–816, 1014–1072.

Medical-Surgical 6.0

Answer

- ✔ Gauze dressing secured on all four sides
- ☐ Dressing with dark red shadowing of blood
- ✔ Asymmetrical breathing
- ☐ Diaphoresis
- ✔ Indrawing and nasal flaring
- ✔ Tracheal deviation
- ☐ Temperature

Rationale: The client presents with a stab wound taped on all four sides, which is problematic for a client. Air remains trapped inside the pleural space, creating a tension pneumothorax. This client presented with clinical manifestations associated with increasing respiratory distress all related back to the gauze being taped on all four sides. Asymmetrical breathing is indicative of a lung collapse. Indrawing and nasal flaring represent respiratory distress and increased work of breathing, which is consistent with the decreasing pulse oximetry. Tracheal deviation is a late presentation of tension pneumothorax, which is a life-threatening situation. The dressing with dark red shadowing of blood not demonstrating an increase in bleeding does not require immediate follow-up. The diaphoresis is not associated with monitoring airway, breathing, or circulation. Increased work of breathing requires increased blood flow, leading to diaphoresis. The temperature is becoming elevated, indicating a possible sign of infection. This would be something to monitor; however, management of the airway is of highest priority.

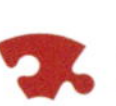
NCJMM Step: Recognize Cues
Reference: Tyerman & Cobbett, pp. 615–616.

Medical-Surgical 7.0

Answer

- ☐ Pupillary response to light
- ☐ Orientation to person, place, and time
- ✔ Oliguria
- ☐ Bowel sounds
- ✔ Interstitial peripheral venous access device

Rationale: This client presents with dehydration and requires fluid resuscitation. The interstitial peripheral venous access device, as described in the 1350h Nurses' Notes, will require replacement to maintain intravenous fluid hydration. The client presented with a low-level fall and denies hitting their head. At the time of presentation, the pupils remain equal in size and reactive to light. The pupils can be continued to be monitored if other clinical manifestations indicate a head injury or acute subdural/chronic subdural hematoma. The person answers questions appropriately and remains conscious. The bowel sounds are present and audible with auscultation. There is no sign of a bowel obstruction.

NCJMM Step: Recognize Cues
References: Astle & Duggleby (2024), pp. 1014–1072; Power-Kean et al. (2023), pp. 118–119; Tyerman & Cobbett (2023), p. 211.

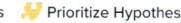

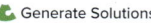

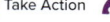

Medical-Surgical 8.0

Answer

The client is at highest risk of developing **pulmonary edema** as evidenced by the client's **respiratory assessment.**

Rationale: The client has presented to the cardiac unit for further monitoring of an acute myocardial infarction; however, acute respiratory tachypnea has developed as a result of the error in the infusion rate. The client previously had the rate infusing at 50 mL per hour, and an hour later, the nurse documented the infusion rate at 250 mL per hour. The additional increase in fluid hydration has caused the client to develop pulmonary edema or volume overload. The client had previous injury and angioplasty intervention to the left anterior descending coronary artery with an ejection fraction of left ventricular wall abnormality and mild heart failure. With the additional fluid, the client's left ventricle could not pump the extra volume effectively and blood pooled in the alveoli because of increased pressure, leading to pulmonary edema. This was evidenced by the respiratory assessment when there was a change from fine crackles to coarse crackles auscultated in the lung fields. The client also developed tachypnea and was found in the tripod position. Clients use the tripod position when they need to have lung expansion to improve oxygenation. The client does not present with an infection, which would eliminate pneumonia, pleuritis (inflammation of the pleura), and pericarditis (inflammation of the pericardium). The client's clinical presentation is more in alignment with volume overload and pulmonary edema, not a pleural effusion.

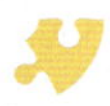

NCJMM Step: Prioritize Hypothesis
References: Astle & Duggleby (2024), pp. 725–816; Power-Kean et al. (2023), p. 678; Tyerman & Cobbett (2023), pp. 621–622, 832–834.

Medical-Surgical 9.0

Answer

The nurse should recognize that the client is potentially experiencing **hyperthermia** and **hypotension** as evidenced by the client's **temperature** and **blood pressure.**

Rationale: The narrative of the client indicates the client presenting with hyperthermia (heat exhaustion) as evidenced by the temperature greater than 39.7°C. There are neurological considerations when a client's temperature is greater than 40°C, with steps to take to prevent moving beyond 43°C. Hyperthermia can lead to increased intracranial pressure, seizure activity, and even coma. The client presents with confusion, fatigue, nausea, vomiting, tachypnea, hypotension (as a result of the dehydration), tachycardia, elevated body temperature, dilated pupils, pallor, and diaphoresis. Treatment begins by placing the client in a cool area and removing constrictive and wet clothing. The client is closely monitored for airway, breathing, and circulation complications, including cardiac dysrhythmias as a result of the extreme loss of fluid through diaphoresis. Fluid replacement is typically 0.9% sodium chloride solution via a peripheral venous access device until the client is able to take oral fluids as tolerated. An initial fluid bolus may be used to correct hypotension. Admission may be considered if the client's condition does not improve within 4 hours.

NCJMM Step: Analyze Cues
References: Cobbett (2025), Chapter 7; Tyerman & Cobbett (2023), pp. 1457, 1783–1785.

Medical-Surgical 10.0

Answer

- [ ] Provide the client with antibiotic samples to treat infection
- [x] Initiate social work support for the client
- [ ] Consult mental health resources
- [x] Instruct the client to go directly to the hospital for further assessment
- [x] Assess the client to see if she is experiencing any uterine cramping or preterm labour
- [ ] Provide education to the client about how to avoid reoccurrence of an infection

Rationale: The client is experiencing a urinary tract infection (cystitis) that has progressed to pyelonephritis based on the extension of symptoms noted at the Week 21 visit. The client requires further assessment beyond the clinic. The primary nursing actions in this clinical presentation would be to instruct the client to go directly to the hospital for further assessment, which would include additional lab work such as a complete blood count, electrolytes, and urine for culture and sensitivity. The outpatient low-risk clinic is not equipped to provide additional care to the client at this time given the complications of the pyelonephritis. The client should be assessed for preterm labour clinical manifestations, which would include determining if there have been cervical changes and any regular uterine contractions. Complications related to preterm birth contribute to high morbidity and mortality rates in newborns and infants. A final nursing action would be to initiate social work support for the client in the event the client is discharged home and does not receive further tertiary care support. If the client is unable to afford the antibiotics, then the client may need additional financial and nutritional supports. Providing antibiotic samples is not appropriate as the client's clinical manifestations have worsened and the client requires further assessment and possible treatment. The client does not present with any mental health concerns despite a difficult situation; the social work consult may be beneficial to the client. The client will require additional education about how to prevent further cystitis infections, but that is not the most immediate nursing action at this time.

NCJMM Step: Take Action
References: Astle & Duggleby (2024), pp. 1173–1180; Cobbett (2025), pp. 225–233; Keenan-Lindsay et al. (2022), pp. 295–296, 446.

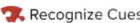

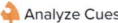

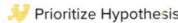

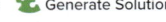

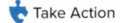

Medical-Surgical 11.0

Answer

- ✔ Pallor
- ☐ Alertness
- ☐ Bowel sounds
- ✔ Lung sounds
- ☐ Pulses
- ✔ Pulse oximetry
- ✔ Skin temperature
- ✔ Accessory muscles

Rationale: Airway, breathing, and circulation are the priorities for this client. The client presents with respiratory changes indicating pneumonia as evidenced by the increase in temperature, changes in cough, increased oxygen requirements, and changes in lung sounds such as the crackles increasing throughout the lung fields. The client also is cool to touch and has noticeable changes in dorsalis pedis pulses. Postoperative pneumonias are one of the most common complications that can occur from reduced mobility and reduced lung expansion. This client also received a general anaesthetic, requiring intubation. The endotracheal tube provides a point of transmission where bacteria can enter the lungs. The client remains alert and oriented to person, place, and time, indicating there has not been any cerebral compromise. There are bowel sounds in all four quadrants, indicating gastrointestinal motility has returned after the surgical procedure. Pulses remain palpable and present, even if the client is noted to have weak bilateral dorsalis pedis pulses.

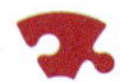
NCJMM Step: Recognize Cues

References: Astle & Duggleby (2024), pp. 955–976; Cobbett (2025), pp. 723–758; Tyerman & Cobbett (2024), pp. 589–594.

Medical-Surgical 12.0

Answer

ASSESSMENT FINDINGS	IMPROVED	NO CHANGE	DECLINED
Temperature 37.2°C (98.9°F)	✔	○	○
Concentrated urine	○	✔	○
Denies dysuria	✔	○	○
"Dribbling" incontinence noted	○	✔	○
Strong odour	○	✔	○
Blood pressure 92/62	○	○	✔

Rationale: The client is experiencing a urinary tract infection, based on the clinical presentation of pain with voiding (dysuria), urgency, and frequency. The client presents with a fever, which indicates that an infective process is occurring within the body. The client's confusion is common for both older adults and those with a urinary tract infection. With antibiotics, the client's fever has improved, and he has no pain with voiding, indicating the effect of the antibiotics. The client continues to have concentrated urine, which indicates hydration status. The client was likely avoiding drinking given the number of times he was needing to void. He was already having incontinence issues and stated he was embarrassed. The "dribbling" had not changed and may warrant further investigation for other issues, such as benign prostatic hyperplasia or inflammation in the urinary tract. The strong odour remains, which again could be a sign of dehydration. The client's blood pressure has not recovered yet and may be a further sign of dehydration, but it could also indicate a slower response to early sepsis where the body vasodilates. Monitoring the hemodynamic status of an older adult who is admitted with a urinary tract infection requires good nursing assessments in order to minimize the chance of the client becoming septic.

NCJMM Step: Evaluate Outcomes
References: Astle & Duggleby (2024), pp. 1165, 1171–1178, 1204–1206; Cobbett (2025), pp. 959–994; Tyerman & Cobbett (2023), pp. 1143–1148.

Medical-Surgical 13.0

Answer

The client is at highest risk of developing **sepsis.**

Rationale: The client presents with a fever and skin breakdown with purulent discharge, which indicates a skin infection by the stoma with the potential to become septic. The mixing of stool in a wound bed creates an environment for bacteria to enter the bloodstream. The client presents with fine inspiratory crackles that clear with a cough, but there are no other symptoms to suggest pneumonia. The client's breathing is not laboured. The client is voiding without issue since they deny pain, frequency, or urgency, any of which could indicate a urinary tract infection. The client is having a normal number of bowel movements and does not present with emesis or nausea.

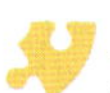
NCJMM Step: Prioritize Hypothesis
References: Astle & Duggleby (2024), pp. 1165–1169, 1232–1246, 1292–1295; Cobbett (2025), pp. 1024–1037.

Medical-Surgical 14.0

Answer

The client is at highest risk of developing **tension pneumothorax**.

Rationale: The client presents with a stab wound taped on all four sides, which is problematic for a client. Air remains trapped inside the pleural space creating a tension pneumothorax. This client presented with clinical manifestations associated with increasing respiratory distress, all related back to the gauze being taped on all four sides. Asymmetrical breathing is indicative of a lung collapse. Indrawing and nasal flaring represent respiratory distress and increased work of breathing, which is consistent with the decreasing pulse oximetry. Tracheal deviation is a late presentation of tension pneumothorax, which is a life-threatening situation. The client does not present with pneumonia despite presenting as febrile. There are absent breath sounds on the left lung and there is no indication of adventitious breath sounds. The client does not present with symptoms associated with a pulmonary embolus as there is no indication of an existing clot or a clinical history that would meet the parameters of Virchow's triad (hypercoagulability, venous stasis, and endothelial damage). The client would not have absent breath sounds if a pleural effusion was the complication developing. The client would present with clinical symptoms if the effusion was large. There is no indication of pulmonary edema as the client is 19 years old. Despite the injury, the left ventricle is able to maintain cardiac output to support a blood pressure, and there is no indication of volume overload in the alveoli as evidenced by auscultating crackles.

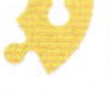

NCJMM Step: Prioritize Hypothesis
References: Power-Kean et al. (2023), pp. 674 (tension pneumothorax), 675 (pleural effusions), 678 (pulmonary edema), 689–691 (pneumonia), 692 (pulmonary embolus); Tyerman & Cobbett (2023), pp. 589–595 (pneumonia), 610–618 (tension pneumothorax), 618–620 (pleural effusion) 621–622 (pulmonary edema), 622–624 (pulmonary embolus).

Medical-Surgical 15.0

Answer

CLIENT FINDINGS	IMPROVED	NOT CHANGED	WORSENED
Respirations 18	✔	○	○
T 37.9°C (100.2°F)	○	✔	○
Respiration rate to be regular	✔	○	○
Colour pink	✔	○	○
No stridor noted	✔	○	○
Oxygen therapy 4 L/min	○	○	✔

Rationale: Because of a medication error, the client suffered an anaphylaxis reaction to the amoxicillin that was administered to them in error. Amoxicillin is a member of the penicillin family. After code blue was activated and based on the final nurses' notes, the client's status improved with respirations as the client was breathing easily and at rest and at a reduced number of breaths. They were pink in colour, whereas before, the client was pale with cyanosis. Stridor was no longer present, which indicates respiratory distress had resolved. There was no change in temperature as it had only changed by 0.2 degrees. Addition of oxygen therapy was the only client finding that indicated a worsening of clinical presentation.

NCJMM Step: Evaluate Outcomes
Reference: Astle & Duggleby (2024), pp. 725–816.

Medical-Surgical 16.0

Answer

The client is at highest risk of developing **phlebitis.**

Rationale: A complication of treatment from a peripheral venous access device is phlebitis. Typically, the solution is irritating the vein wall, or there is a chemical, mechanical, or bacterial cause. This client is not experiencing an infiltration of fluid as the redness is located above the site of the insertion and not at the site of insertion. Extravasation occurs when the solution is vesicant or irritating to the tissue if it leaks beyond the venous wall. Valves can obstruct insertion; however, this is not a complication when infusing normal saline solution. Clots can form in the catheter in situ in the vein; however, the peripheral venous access device continues to flush sluggishly, and the patterned assessment for phlebitis is to identify redness above the insertion site.

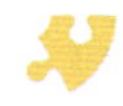

NCJMM Step: Prioritize Hypothesis
Reference: Cobbett (2025), pp. 814–859.

Maternal/Birthing Parent Health Trend Cases

Maternal/Birthing Parent Health 1.0

Answer

CLIENT STATEMENTS	UNDER-STANDING	NO UNDER-STANDING
"My grandpa has diabetes; I can use his medications."	○	✔
"I was trying to lose weight before getting pregnant and I want to continue walking."	✔	○
"I should test my blood sugar before driving."	○	✔
"I already eat healthy, so I do not have to make any dietary changes."	○	✔
"Controlling my blood sugar helps reduce complications for my baby."	✔	○

Rationale: All pregnant clients are screened for the presence of gestational diabetes mellitus at 24 to 28 weeks with a preferred "two-step" method (Fig 14.5, p. 277, in Keenan-Lindsay et al., 2022). This client's plasma glucose was above the threshold (11.1 mmol/L), indicating a diagnosis of gestational diabetes. This client has several risk factors, including age older than 35 years, high BMI of 30 indicating obesity, and a previous diagnosis of polycystic ovary syndrome. Other risk factors include being a member of a high-risk group (African, Arab, Asian, Latino, Indigenous, or South Asian); using corticosteroid medication; having pregestational diabetes or having gestational diabetes in a previous pregnancy; giving birth to a baby that weighs more than 4 kg; having a parent, brother, or sister with type 2 diabetes; or a previous diagnosis of acanthosis. Client education is provided and includes diet, exercise, monitoring of blood glucose levels, pharmacological therapy, and fetal surveillance. Clients are typically prescribed insulin therapy with testing done at fasting preprandial and postprandial times. Testing prior to driving is not necessary but is recommended for clients living with type 1 diabetes. This client cannot take her grandfather's medication as her treatment is individualized, just as is his treatment for his own illness. The client is encouraged to engage in moderate exercise programs as exercise may help lower blood glucose levels and reduce the need for insulin therapy. Dietary counselling is recommended, as needs may be different from those for individuals trying to lose weight, as in this client's case. Clients are recommended to have serial ultrasound assessments beginning at 28 weeks' gestation and repeated ever 3 to 4 weeks to monitor fetal growth and amniotic fluid levels. Once the patient reaches 36 weeks' gestation, fetal surveillance will occur weekly with nonstress testing.

NCJMM Step: Evaluate Outcomes
References: Berger et al. (2019); Keenan-Lindsay et al. (2022), pp. 276–278; McDonald (2024), pp. 248–253.

Maternal/Birthing Parent Health 2.0

Answer

The client is at highest risk of developing a **pulmonary embolus** as evidenced by the client's **laboured respirations.**

Rationale: Client presented to the ED with symptoms associated with a deep vein thrombosis meeting the factors associated with Virchow's triad: injury to the blood vessel endothelium (fall down the stairs), abnormalities of blood flow (pregnancy), and hypercoagulability of the blood (pregnancy). Pregnancy can compress the iliac veins and inferior vena cava by the uterus with increased venous pressure and reduced blood flow in the legs, except when the client is in a lateral position. Alterations in cardiovascular status contribute to edema, varicose veins, and hemorrhoids that can develop in the latter part of the term pregnancy and lead to increased risk for venous thromboembolism (VTE). Pregnancy is considered a hypercoagulable state in which clients are at a five- to sixfold increase risk for thromboembolic disease. When clients arrive at the emergency department, it is important to monitor the client as well as the fetus. Currently, the fetus status remains stable; however, this could change if the client's respiratory status and ability to oxygenate fetus and client change, too. The symptoms of shortness of breath and pain with inspiration, wheezing when lungs are auscultated, decrease in pulse oximetry, and increased respirations all indicate clinical manifestations of a pulmonary embolus. The client would experience atelectasis with pulmonary effusion, crackles with pulmonary edema, decrease in blood pressure with corresponding increase in heart rate with cardiac tamponade, and chest pain and diaphoresis with acute myocardial infarction. The client's respiratory assessment leads to the hypothesis that the client is at highest risk of developing a pulmonary embolus given the primary presentation. Pulses and increase in leg edema are associated with cardiovascular assessment and could indicate extension of a deep vein thrombosis. The changes in respiratory status indicate more of a respiratory involvement.

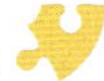
NCJMM Step: Prioritize Hypothesis
References: Jarvis et al. (2024), p. 499; Keenan-Lindsay et al. (2022), p. 183; Power-Kean et al. (2023), p. 533.

Maternal/Birthing Parent Health 3.0

Answer

POTENTIAL NURSING INTERVENTIONS	INDICATED	NOT INDICATED
Collect urine sample	✔	○
Draw arterial blood gas	○	✔
Recommend consultation with a dietitian	✔	○
Speak to the client's coach	○	✔
Suggest oral contraception	✔	○

Rationale: The client is experiencing amenorrhea due to her involvement in long distance running. The client does not have any menstruation due to lower body weight as evidenced by the drop in BMI. The nurse would have to consider other conditions that could cause amenorrhea, such as outflow tract obstruction, anterior pituitary disorders, polycystic ovary syndrome (documented acne), hypothyroidism or hyperthyroidism (ruled out as speech clear and appropriate), type 1 diabetes, medications such as phenytoin, substance use (opiates, marijuana, cocaine), eating disorders, strenuous exercise, emotional stress, or oral contraceptive use. The nurse would inquire further to rule out an eating disorder or type 1 diabetes by drawing blood work such as a complete blood count (CBC), urinalysis, thyroid-stimulating hormone (TSH) and prolactin levels, as well as fasting glucose. The client would need to have a urine sample to rule out a human chorionic gonadotropin (hCG) pregnancy test. The client would require follow-up appointments to monitor progression as the client is likely committed to performing at the national championships and could experience temporary amenorrhea. The nurse could provide counselling to assist with decision making. It is recommended that the client speak with a dietitian regarding healthy caloric nutrition to support overall health instead her of not eating. Information should be provided to the client about contraception use. Despite the absence of menstruation, the client could still become pregnant.

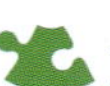
NCJMM Step: Generate Solutions
Reference: Keenan-Lindsay et al. (2022), pp. 92–93.

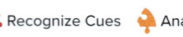

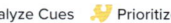

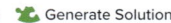

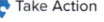

Pediatrics Trend Cases

Pediatric 1.0

Answer

POTENTIAL NURSING INTERVENTIONS	INDICATED	NOT INDICATED
Offer oral fluids to the client	○	✔
Request an order to insert a peripheral venous access device	✔	✔
Prepare to initiate oxygen therapy	✔	○
Initiate tube feeds to maintain regular schedule	○	✔
Prepare to take the client for a chest X-ray	✔	○
Place the client in high-Fowler's position	○	✔

Rationale: The client presents to the emergency department and eventually the pediatric inpatient unit with respiratory distress. The clinical manifestations appeared quickly within 24 hours with a fever, indicating that an infective process is occurring. Given the client's risk factors, such as dysphagia, tube feeds, and weak cough reflex, the client is at greatest risk for aspiration pneumonia from the PEG tube. Nursing interventions would be to maintain airway, provide oxygenation, and assist with procedures. The pulse oximetry level was noted to drop to 88% requiring oxygen therapy. The health care provider has been notified and orders would be imminent. The client will also need to have a chest X-ray to determine if they have aspiration pneumonia. A peripheral venous access device would be required for potential intravenous medications or additional fluid hydration until tube feeds can be restarted. The nurse would not offer oral fluids to a client with dysphagia and a weak cough reflex. This would only exacerbate the aspiration pneumonia or cause one if not happening at the time of admission. Starting tube feeds would be a contraindication given the client's presenting symptoms. It would be more prudent to place the client in semi-Fowler's than in high-Fowler's position. Semi-Fowler's position would offer the same benefits for enhanced gas exchange and make it easier to breathe and more comfortable for the client. Sitting at 60 to 90 degrees may increase the risk for development of a bed sore and be more uncomfortable for the client.

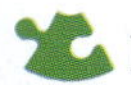

NCJMM Step: Generate Solutions
References: Astle & Duggleby (2024), pp. 1097–1161; Keenan-Lindsay et al. (2022), p. 1140.

Pediatric 2.0

Answer

- ✔ Initiate fluids through large-bore peripheral venous access device
- ✔ Call a code blue
- ☐ Provide ice chips to the client
- ✔ Draw an arterial blood gas
- ☐ Ask the client's parents to leave the room while the doctor completes the assessment
- ☐ Initiate antibiotic therapy
- ☐ Monitor urine output
- ☐ Draw CBC, electrolytes, and BUN

Rationale: This client is developing respiratory distress as evidenced by changing to tripod position, drooling, and edematous lips. The client's airway is occluding, and the child needs to be intubated immediately. During an emergency, the nurse needs to assess for airway compromise, respiratory distress, and circulatory dysfunction. This client requires fluids to prevent shock from developing. The primary emphasis during the emergent phase is the treatment of burn shock through giving fluids and management of pulmonary status. An ABG will help determine how compromised the client is at the time. Ice chips are not warranted now; airway, breathing, and circulation are the priority. The client's parents should stay and comfort the child, despite the busyness of the situation, not be asked to leave. It is important to maintain family-centred care. Antibiotics will be necessary to reduce infection; however, the child cannot breathe and requires immediate intervention. It is important to monitor urine output. For children weighting less than 30 kg, expect at least 1 to 2 mL/kg of urine output. For children weighing more than 30 kg, expect 30 to 50 mL/hr. Clients with burns lose fluid through the wound. Replacement and careful monitoring of electrolytes are important components of treatment, but not during an emergency. Children under 5 years of age account for 83% of all clients with scale burn injuries requiring hospital admission. Because of their thinner skin, children are more vulnerable to burns than adults. Significant burns can cause permanent scarring with contraction of the underlying tissues due to rapid growth and can lead to emotional scarring and physical disabilities.

NCJMM Step: Take Action
Reference: Keenan-Lindsay et al. (2022), pp. 870–871, 1430–1440.

Mental Health Trend Cases

Mental Health 1.0

Answer

The nurse should recognize that the client is potentially experiencing **thrombocytopenia** and **adverse event from medication** as evidenced by **small pinpoint, purple bruising** and **client proclaiming King of France status.**

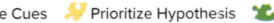

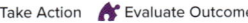

Rationale: Presenting symptoms of ADHD include impulsivity, hyperactivity, and inattention. Attention challenges and hyperactivity contribute to low tolerance of frustration, temper outbursts, labile moods, compromised school performance, peer rejection, and low self-esteem. Treatment includes behaviour management plans, individual and family counselling, play therapy for young children, cognitive-behavioural therapy, and pharmacological interventions for inattention and hyperactive-impulsive behaviours. Medications chosen are often psychostimulant medications, such as methylphenidate (Ritalin or Biphentin or Concerta), or a nonstimulant serotonin–norepinephrine reuptake inhibitor (SNRI), such as atomoxetine (Strattera). Nurses and educators should be aware of adverse effects of these medications. Clients taking methylphenidates should also be monitored for psychotic and manic symptoms as in this case study, suicide-related events, Raynaud's phenomenon, serotonin syndrome, and risk for priapism. The client is experiencing delusional thinking in proclaiming he is the King of France, and thrombocytopenia, as evidenced by the small pinpoint bruising noted on the legs.

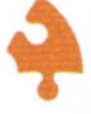

NCJMM Step: Analyze Cues
References: Canadian ADHD Resource Alliance (CADDRA) (2022); Pollard & Jakubec (2023), pp. 533–555; Skidmore-Roth & Richardson (2024), pp. 815–818.

Mental Health 2.0

Answer

- ☐ Leukopenia
- ☐ Sepsis
- ✔ Stroke
- ☐ Pulmonary embolism
- ✔ Increased intracranial pressure

Rationale: The client was found unconscious under traumatic circumstances. Bruising was noted all over the client's body with burn marks on her upper thigh. The trend indicated a head injury with likely increased intracranial pressure (ICP) as the client's level of consciousness progressed from awake and alert to unresponsive initially, then responding to painful stimuli only. Glasgow Coma Scale number was significantly decreased from the original documentation, as the client became unresponsive. At 1200h, client was exhibiting Cushing's triad, which is relevant to increased ICP: widened pulse pressure, bradycardia, irregular respirations. The change in pupils indicates neurological impairment. Stroke cannot be ruled out because of medications such as birth control pills. The client is likely going septic as well, given the high fever and clear lungs. It has not progressed to septic shock. Although it is concerning, the likely cause is neurological in nature and likely ICP. A CT head would be ordered next to rule out stroke and to identify the stroke or increased ICP. Clients experiencing domestic violence or trauma require nurses to recognize symptoms of medical conditions while caring for the client holistically. Psychotherapeutic modalities and other interventions can be determined in a plan of care. The client's age would need to be taken into consideration for the plan of care.

NCJMM Step: Analyze Cues
References: Pollard & Jakubec (2023), pp. 481–505; Power-Kean et al. (2023), pp. 367–369; Tyerman & Cobbett (2023), pp. 1453–1455.

Mental Health 3.0

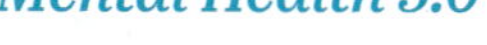

Answer

POTENTIAL NURSING INTERVENTIONS	INDICATED	NOT INDICATED
Draw blood cultures	✔	○
Request chest X-ray	○	✔
Nurse asks client, "Can you identify what happens before you feel you need to take a hot shower?"	✔	○
Monitor for septic shock	○	✔
Request an order to insert a peripheral venous access device	○	✔
Stay with the client	✔	○
Call security when the client attempts to take a shower again	○	✔
Group therapy will produce better results than cognitive-behavioural therapy	○	✔
Anticipate an order for lorazepam	○	✔

Rationale: The client is experiencing generalized anxiety disorder that would be classified as severe anxiety progressing to obsessive-compulsive disorder. In the narrative, the client is picking at their own skin, indicating a behaviour the client is using to attempt to reduce or relieve their anxiety. The showering has become a relief behaviour for this client as a way of coping, which effectively reduces her anxiety. It is important for medical and mental health care providers to realize the interrelationship between psychiatric and medical illnesses. The nurse on a medical unit will need to monitor for medical conditions such as sepsis-induced response syndrome (SIRS) in relation to the skin breakdown, as well as support the client's needs for mental health support. Blood cultures will need to be drawn as evidenced by the client's skin breakdown and the fever, which is indicative of SIRS, not septic shock. A chest X-ray is not needed as the client hyperventilates with the anxiety. The nurse asks the client to identify what is happening prior to the anxiety and the need for showering. This question is important in validating the client's feelings. A peripheral IV is not needed and may escalate the client's anxiety, as it will need to be wrapped before taking a shower. General mindfulness guidance is an important skill to teach this client. Contamination or washing excessively is a common obsession and compulsion. The nurse should remain with the client to promote trust and a safe environment, with minimal stimulation. A security guard or forced prevention of the behaviour may escalate the behaviour and anxiety, leading to a critical situation. The nurse should anticipate an order for fluoxetine (Prozac), citalopram (Celexa), or escitalopram (Cipralex), all of which are used for generalized anxiety disorders and obsessive-compulsive disorders.

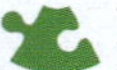

NCJMM Step: Generate Solutions
References: Pollard & Jakubec (2023), pp. 180–219; Power-Kean et al. (2023), pp. 1043–1046; Tyerman & Cobbett (2023), pp. 521–523, 525–526, 529–530.

Mental Health 4.0

Answer

The client is at highest risk of developing **anticipatory grief** as evidenced by **"how am I going to tell my family the news?"** and being **unable to speak** and **weeping.**

Rationale: Clients can experience grief in advance of loss, such as when a receiving a life-limiting diagnosis, known as *anticipatory grief.* Nurses need to recognize that people can experience symptoms of grief physically, cognitively, emotionally, socially, and spiritually and can intervene appropriately. Signs of anticipatory grief (Tyerman & Cobbett, 2023, Box 31.2) include periods of weeping, a feeling of unreality displayed as inability to speak, and the need to protect family. Complicated grief is unresolved grief where bereavement symptoms evolve into problematic substance use or chronic depression. Prolonged depression is the most common response to unresolved grief. Disenfranchised grief is when losses are not openly acknowledged, supported, or recognized as a loss, such as a suicide, loss of a pet, or the grief of someone who others thought could not grieve (i.e., a child or a person living with dementia). Prolonged grief disorder is characterized by severe and disabling, chronic grief, in light of multiple and global crises.

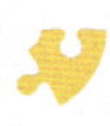

NCJMM Step: Prioritize Hypothesis
References: Pollard & Jakubec (2023), pp. 594–609; Tyerman & Cobbett (2023), pp. 203–204, 209.

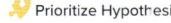

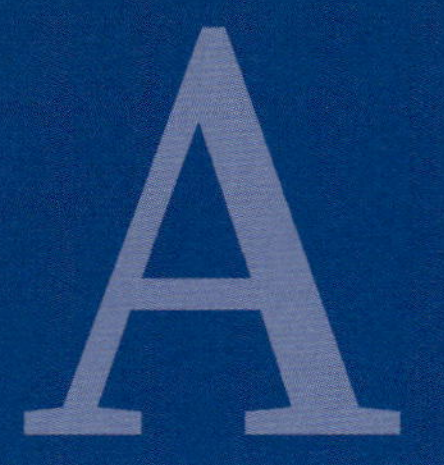

Normal vs. Abnormal vs. Critical Abnormal Condition Tables

Normal vs. Abnormal vs. Critical Abnormal

The concepts of normal → abnormal →, and critical abnormal are best presented visually to help students recognize patterns and learn how conditions can be grouped for ease of learning. The following information is presented in a head-to-toe format using conditions from Chapter 2 Tables 2.1 to 2.7. Use the following information to help study and recognize how conditions can improve for a client or lead to further physical deterioration. The list of conditions is not exhaustive, so you may wish to add additional information.

Each NGN unfolding or stand-alone case study will focus on a specific condition. When reviewing the client presentation in the narrative, minimize the clinical manifestations to a system that is the primary focus, then identify the potential complications or conditions that may develop. Once you have this information, identify possible solutions to treat the condition, including orders, nursing interventions, and laboratory and diagnostic tests, and then recognize how interventions have affected the client's outcome.

Chapters 7 (unfolding) and 8 (stand-alone) provide additional practise. Use the tables in Chapter 2 and these additional tables of conditions to identify strengths and gaps in learning.

Neurology

TRAUMATIC BRAIN INJURY

Normal	Abnormal		Critical Abnormal

Recognize normal neuro assessment:
LOC, pupil size and reactivity, motor power, pain, gait, GCS
	• Mild concussion
	• Moderate concussion
	• Severe concussion
	• Diffuse axonal injury
	• Hematomas
	  • Epidural
	  • Subdural
	  • Intracerebral
		• Postconcussion syndrome
		• Chronic traumatic encephalopathy
			• Seizures
			• Increased intracranial pressure

GCS, Glasgow Coma Scale; *LOC*, level of consciousness.

SPINAL CORD INJURY

Normal	Abnormal	Critical Abnormal
Recognize normal neuro assessment: LOC, pupil size and reactivity, motor power, pain, gait, GCS	Spinal cord injury	• Autonomic dysreflexia • Neurogenic shock

GCS, Glasgow Coma Scale; *LOC*, level of consciousness.

VASCULAR DYSFUNCTION IN THE BRAIN

Normal	Abnormal	Critical Abnormal
Recognize normal neuro assessment: LOC, pupil size and reactivity, motor power, pain, gait, GCS	Stroke • Ischemic • Hemorrhagic	• Further hemorrhaging • Increased intracranial pressure
	Cerebral aneurysm	• Ruptured aneurysm → bleeding • Increased intracranial pressure

GCS, Glasgow Coma Scale; *LOC*, level of consciousness.

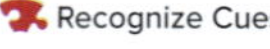
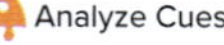
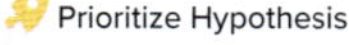
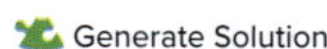
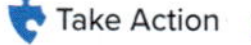
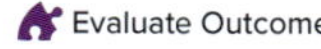

NEUROLOGICAL INFECTIONS

Normal	Abnormal	Critical Abnormal
Recognize normal neuro assessment: LOC, pupil size and reactivity, motor power, pain, gait, GCS	Bacterial meningitis	• Respiratory distress → ARDS • Increased intracranial pressure
	Encephalitis	• Respiratory distress → ARDS • Increased intracranial pressure

ARDS, Acute respiratory distress syndrome; *GCS*, Glasgow Coma Scale; *LOC*, level of consciousness.

SEIZURES

Normal		Abnormal	Critical Abnormal
Recognize normal neuro assessment: LOC, pupil size and reactivity, motor power, pain, gait, GCS	Seizures	Prolonged seizure activity	Status epilepticus
		Aspiration pneumonia	• Respiratory distress → ARDS • Inability to protect their airway • Sepsis

ARDS, Acute respiratory distress syndrome; *GCS*, Glasgow Coma Scale; *LOC*, level of consciousness.

DEMENTIA

Normal		Abnormal	Critical Abnormal
Recognize normal neuro assessment: LOC, pupil size and reactivity, motor power, pain, gait, GCS	Dementia	Dysphagia → aspiration pneumonia	• Respiratory distress → ARDS • Inability to protect their airway • Sepsis
		Dehydration→ hypovolemia	• AKI • Sepsis → shock (hypovolemic or septic)

		Risk of falls→ fractures	• Hematomas
			  • Epidural
			  • Subdural
			  • Intracerebral
			• Increased intracranial pressure

		Skin ulcerations	• Infections → cellulitis → sepsis → septic shock
		Urinary tract infection	• SIRS → urosepsis → septic shock

AKI, Acute kidney injury; *ARDS*, acute respiratory distress syndrome; *GCS*, Glasgow Coma Scale; *LOC*, level of consciousness; *SIRS*, systemic inflammatory response syndrome.

PARKINSON'S DISEASE

Normal		Abnormal	Critical Abnormal
Recognize normal neuro assessment: LOC, pupil size and reactivity, motor power, pain, gait, GCS	Parkinson's disease	Dementia	See above
		Seizures	See above
		Recurring infections • Respiratory • Urinary tract infections	• Respiratory distress → ARDS • Inability to protect their airway • Pneumonia • Sepsis → septic shock
		Visual changes	Blindness

ARDS, Acute respiratory distress syndrome; *GCS*, Glasgow Coma Scale; *LOC*, level of consciousness.

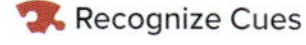 Recognize Cues 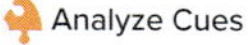 Analyze Cues 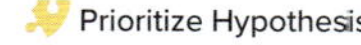 Prioritize Hypothesis 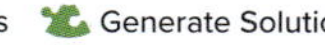 Generate Solutions 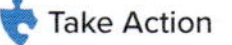 Take Action 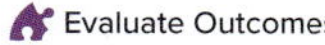 Evaluate Outcomes

MULTIPLE SCLEROSIS

Normal	Abnormal		Critical Abnormal

Recognize normal neuro assessment:
LOC, pupil size and reactivity, motor power, pain, gait, GCS
	Multiple sclerosis	Risk of falls→ fractures	• Hematomas
			  • Epidural
			  • Subdural
			  • Intracerebral
			• Increased intracranial pressure

		Recurring infections • Respiratory • Urinary tract infections	• Respiratory distress → ARDS • Inability to protect their airway • Pneumonia • Sepsis → septic shock

ARDS, Acute respiratory distress syndrome; *GCS*, Glasgow Coma Scale; *LOC*, level of consciousness.

GUILLAIN BARRÉ SYNDROME AND AMYOTROPHIC LATERALIZING SCLEROSIS

Normal	Abnormal		Critical Abnormal
Recognize normal neuro assessment: LOC, pupil size and reactivity, motor power, pain, gait, GCS	Guillain- Barre syndrome	Muscle weakness →	Respiratory distress → requiring intubation
	Amyotrophic lateralizing sclerosis (ALS)	Muscle weakness → dysmasesis (difficulty chewing)	Respiratory distress → requiring intubation • Aspiration pneumonia → respiratory distress → ARDS • Inability to protect their airway • Pneumonia • Sepsis → septic shock

ARDS, Acute respiratory distress syndrome; *GCS*, Glasgow Coma Scale; *LOC*, level of consciousness.

Cardiovascular

BLOOD PRESSURE—HYPERTENSION/HYPOTENSION

Normal	Abnormal	Critical Abnormal
≥95/60 mm Hg ≤135/85 mm Hg	Hypertension • Nonautomated BP ≥140/90 mm Hg • Automated ≥135/85 mm Hg • Diabetes ≥130/80 mm Hg • Hyperaldosteronism • Pheochromocytoma	Hypertensive crisis • Hypertensive emergency • Hypertensive urgency

	Hypotension (≤95/60 mm Hg)
	• Dehydration
	• Orthostatic hypotension
	• Acute myocardial infarction
	• Dysrhythmias that affect cardiac output
	• Bleeding
	• Intravascular fluid loss
	  • Second and third spacing
	• Insensible losses
		Shock
		• Hypovolemic shock
		• Cardiogenic shock
		• Distributive shock
		  • Septic shock
		  • Anaphylactic shock
		  • Neurogenic shock

DYSRHYTHMIAS

Normal	Abnormal	Critical Abnormal
Normal sinus rhythm 60–100 beats per minute	Sinus bradycardia <60 beats per minute	
	Sinus tachycardia >60 beats per minute	
	Atrial flutter Irregular atrial rate Normal ventricular rate	
	Atrial fibrillation Irregular atrial rate (quiver) Normal ventricular rate	
	Premature ventricular contractions Increased ventricular irritability	>10 may precipitate acute myocardial infarction or ventricular tachycardia (VTach)
		Ventricular fibrillation Irregular ventricular rate (quiver)
		Pulseless electrical activity
		Asystole

CORONARY ARTERY DISEASE

Normal	Abnormal		Critical Abnormal
Recognize normal CV assessment: BP, HR, pulses, S1, S2 skin temperature, diaphoresis, colour, capillary refill No chest discomfort or chest pain	Angina • Stable • Unstable • Prinzmetal or variant	Acute myocardial infarction • Inferior • Anterior • Lateral • Posterior Combination of any of the above	Cardiogenic shock

BP, Blood pressure; *CV*, cardiovascular; *HR*, heart rate.

HEART FAILURE

Normal	Abnormal		Critical Abnormal
Recognize normal CV assessment: BP, HR, pulses, S1, S2 skin temperature, diaphoresis, colour, capillary refill No clinical manifestations of heart failure	Left-sided heart failure	Pulmonary edema	Respiratory failure
		Reduced kidney perfusion	Acute renal failure
		Reduced LV function	Altered LOC Cardiogenic shock
	Right-sided heart failure	Cor pulmonale	Cardiogenic shock

BP, Blood pressure; *CV*, cardiovascular; *HR*, heart rate; *LOC*, level of consciousness; *LV*, left ventricular.

DISORDERS OF THE PERICARDIUM

Normal	Abnormal		Critical Abnormal
Recognize normal CV assessment: BP, HR, pulses, S1, S2 skin temperature, diaphoresis, colour, capillary refill	Pericarditis	Pericardial effusion	Cardiac tamponade

BP, Blood pressure; *CV*, cardiovascular; *HR*, heart rate.

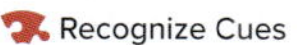 Recognize Cues 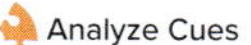 Analyze Cues 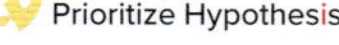 Prioritize Hypothesis 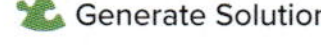 Generate Solutions 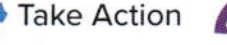 Take Action 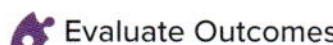 Evaluate Outcomes

INFECTIVE ENDOCARDITIS

Normal	Abnormal	Critical Abnormal
Recognize normal CV assessment: BP, HR, pulses, S1, S2 skin temperature, diaphoresis, colour, capillary refill	Endocarditis with known vegetations	Pulmonary embolus (if vegetation is present on the tricuspid or pulmonic valve and breaks loose travelling to the pulmonary vasculature)
		TIA or stroke (if vegetation is present on the mitral or aortic valve and breaks loose travelling to the brain)

BP, Blood pressure; *CV*, cardiovascular; *HR*, heart rate; *TIA*, transient ischemic attack.

VASCULAR CONDITIONS

Normal	Abnormal		Critical Abnormal
Recognize normal CV assessment: BP, HR, pulses, S1, S2 skin temperature, diaphoresis, colour, capillary refill	Deep vein thrombosis	Pulmonary embolus	Respiratory distress

BP, Blood pressure; *CV*, cardiovascular; *HR*, heart rate.

ARTERIAL CONDITIONS

Normal	Abnormal	Critical Abnormal
Recognize normal CV assessment: BP, HR, pulses, S1, S2 skin temperature, diaphoresis, colour, capillary refill	Abdominal aneurysm	Rupture → increased bleeding, reduced perfusion to the kidneys and lower extremities (limb ischemia), reduced LOC
	Spontaneous coronary artery disease (SCAD)	Acute myocardial infarction

BP, Blood pressure; *CV*, cardiovascular; *HR*, heart rate; *LOC*, level of consciousness.

Respiratory

RESPIRATORY INFECTIONS

Normal	Abnormal	Critical Abnormal
Recognize normal resp assessment: RR, pulse oximetry reading, colour (cyanosis), symmetrical or asymmetrical chest movements, use of accessory muscles, cough, LOC	Influenza	Respiratory distress → ARDS
	Pneumonia	

ARDS, Acute respiratory distress syndrome; *LOC*, level of consciousness; *RR*, respiratory rate.

DISORDERS OF THE PLEURAL WALL

Normal	Abnormal		Critical Abnormal
Recognize normal resp assessment: RR, pulse oximetry reading, colour (cyanosis), symmetrical or asymmetrical chest movements, use of accessory muscles, cough, LOC	Pleural effusion • Empyema • Blood	Pneumothorax • Spontaneous • Open • Tension Hemothorax Chylothorax	Respiratory distress

LOC, Level of consciousness; *RR*, respiratory rate.

LEFT- AND RIGHT-SIDED HEART FAILURE

Normal	Abnormal		Critical Abnormal
Recognize normal resp assessment: RR, pulse oximetry reading, colour (cyanosis), symmetrical or asymmetrical chest movements, use of accessory muscles, cough, LOC	Left-sided heart failure	Pulmonary edema	Hypoxemia → hypoventilation → Respiratory distress
	Right-sided heart failure	Systemic congestion	

LOC, Level of consciousness: *RR*, respiratory rate.

PULMONARY EMBOLUS

Normal	Abnormal	Critical Abnormal	
Recognize normal resp assessment: RR, pulse oximetry reading, colour (cyanosis), symmetrical or asymmetrical chest movements, use of accessory muscles, cough, LOC	Deep vein thrombosis	Pulmonary embolus	Respiratory distress

LOC, Level of consciousness; *RR*, respiratory rate.

PEDIATRIC INFECTIONS: EPIGLOTTITIS, RESPIRATORY SYNCYTIAL VIRUS (RSV)

Normal	Abnormal	Critical Abnormal	
Recognize normal resp assessment: RR, pulse oximetry reading, colour (cyanosis), symmetrical or asymmetrical chest movements, use of accessory muscles, cough, LOC	Epiglottitis	Airway obstruction	Respiratory distress
	Respiratory syncytial virus (RSV)	Retractions	

LOC, Level of consciousness; *RR*, respiratory rate.

ASTHMA

Normal	Abnormal		Critical Abnormal
Recognize normal resp assessment: RR, pulse oximetry reading, colour (cyanosis), symmetrical or asymmetrical chest movements, use of accessory muscles, cough, LOC	Allergic trigger	Asthma • Mild • Moderate • Severe	Respiratory distress

LOC, Level of consciousness; *RR*, respiratory rate.

CHRONIC OBSTRUCTIVE PULMONARY DISEASE

Normal	Abnormal	Critical Abnormal
Recognize normal resp assessment: RR, pulse oximetry reading, colour (cyanosis), symmetrical or asymmetrical chest movements, use of accessory muscles, cough, LOC	Chronic obstructive pulmonary disease • Emphysema • Chronic bronchitis	Respiratory distress → ARDS

ARDS, Acute respiratory distress syndrome; *LOC*, level of consciousness; *RR*, respiratory rate.

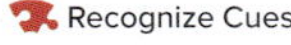 Recognize Cues 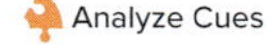 Analyze Cues 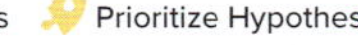 Prioritize Hypothesis 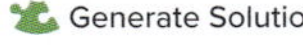 Generate Solutions 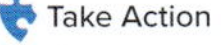 Take Action Evaluate Outcomes

CYSTIC FIBROSIS

Normal		Abnormal	Critical Abnormal
Recognize normal resp assessment: RR, pulse oximetry reading, colour (cyanosis), symmetrical or asymmetrical chest movements, use of accessory muscles, cough, LOC	Cystic fibrosis	Risk of infections	• Respiratory distress → ARDS • Inability to protect their airway • Pneumonia • Sepsis → septic shock
		Type 1 diabetes mellitus	Diabetic ketoacidosis
		Small bowel obstructions	Ischemic gut → SIRS → septic shock

ARDS, Acute respiratory distress syndrome; *LOC*, level of consciousness; *RR*, respiratory rate; *SIRS*, systemic inflammatory response syndrome.

PULMONARY ARTERY HYPERTENSION

Normal	Abnormal	Critical Abnormal
Recognize normal resp assessment: RR, pulse oximetry reading, colour (cyanosis), symmetrical or asymmetrical chest movements, use of accessory muscles, cough, LOC	Pulmonary artery hypertension	Cor pulmonale

LOC, Level of consciousness; *RR*, respiratory rate.

Renal

RENAL INFECTIONS

Normal	Abnormal		Critical Abnormal	
Recognize normal renal assessment: urine output (>30 mL/hr or 0.5–1.0 mL/kg/hr), 24-hour fluid balance, urine characteristics, absence of incontinence, frequency, absence of discharge	Cystitis	Pyelonephritis	Urosepsis	Septic shock

RENAL OBSTRUCTIONS

Normal	Abnormal	Critical Abnormal	
Recognize normal renal assessment: urine output (>30 mL/hr or 0.5–1.0 mL/kg/hr), 24-hour fluid balance, urine characteristics, absence of incontinence, frequency, absence of discharge	Kidney stones	Urosepsis	Septic shock
	Benign prostate hyperplasia		
	Neurogenic bladder		
	Overactive bladder		

ACUTE RENAL FAILURE

Normal	Abnormal	Critical Abnormal
Recognize normal renal assessment: urine output (>30 mL/hr or 0.5–1.0 mL/kg/hr), 24-hour fluid balance, urine characteristics, absence of incontinence, frequency, absence of discharge	Prerenal • Bleeding • Hypovolemia/dehydration • Heart failure Intrarenal • Inflammation • Toxins (antibiotics) • Infection (glomerulonephritis) Postrenal • Benign prostate hyperplasia • Tumours • Injury	Acute renal failure Acute kidney injury

RHABDOMYOLYSIS

Normal	Abnormal	Critical Abnormal
Recognize normal renal assessment: urine output (>30 mL/hr or 0.5–1.0 mL/kg/hr), 24-hour fluid balance, urine characteristics, absence of incontinence, frequency, absence of discharge	Immobility Infection Cocaine ingestion Statins Extreme muscle breakdown	Rhabdomyolysis

Gastroenterology

GASTROINTESTINAL BLEEDING (GIB)

Normal	Abnormal		Critical Abnormal	
Recognize normal gastrointestinal assessment: bowel sounds, abdominal symmetry, presence of nausea/vomiting, bowel habits, ease of swallowing, absence of pain, abdomen soft and flat, nutrition	Gastritis	Peptic ulcer disease	GIB	Hypovolemic shock

GASTROESOPHAGEAL REFLUX DISORDER (GERD)

Normal	Abnormal	Critical Abnormal	
Recognize normal gastrointestinal assessment: bowel sounds, abdominal symmetry, presence of nausea/vomiting, bowel habits, ease of swallowing, absence of pain, abdomen soft and flat, nutrition	GERD	Aspiration pneumonia	Septic shock

CELIAC DISEASE OR GLUTEN SENSITIVE ENTEROPATHY

Normal	Abnormal		Critical Abnormal
Recognize normal gastrointestinal assessment: bowel sounds, abdominal symmetry, presence of nausea/vomiting, bowel habits, ease of swallowing, absence of pain, abdomen soft and flat, nutrition	Celiac disease	Malnutrition	Celiac crisis

INFLAMMATORY BOWEL DISEASE

Normal	Abnormal		Critical Abnormal
Recognize normal gastrointestinal assessment: bowel sounds, abdominal symmetry, presence of nausea/vomiting, bowel habits, ease of swallowing, absence of pain, abdomen soft and flat	Ulcerative colitis		Severe inflammation → hemorrhagic erosions → abscesses → necrosis and ulcerations
			Toxic megacolon
	Crohn's disease	Dehydration	Hypovolemia Sepsis
		Weight loss	

SMALL AND LARGE BOWEL OBSTRUCTIONS

Normal	Abnormal		Critical Abnormal
Recognize normal gastrointestinal assessment: bowel sounds, abdominal symmetry, presence of nausea/vomiting, bowel habits, ease of swallowing, absence of pain, abdomen soft and flat	Paralytic ileus Adhesions Hernias Tumours Volvulus Strictures Intussusception	Infection	Ischemic gut → septic shock

LIVER DYSFUNCTION

Normal	Abnormal	Critical Abnormal	
Recognize normal gastrointestinal assessment: bowel sounds, abdominal symmetry, presence of nausea/vomiting, bowel habits, ease of swallowing, absence of pain, abdomen soft and flat, ability to clot	Cirrhosis of the liver Nonalcoholic steatohepatitis Nonalcoholic fatty liver disease	Hepatorenal syndrome	Acute renal failure
			Cognitive deficits/confusion

GALLBLADDER DYSFUNCTION

Normal	Abnormal	Critical Abnormal
Recognize normal gastrointestinal assessment: bowel sounds, abdominal symmetry, presence of nausea/vomiting, bowel habits, ease of swallowing, absence of pain, abdomen soft and flat, ability to clot	Cholelithiasis	Cholecystitis

PANCREATITIS

Normal	Abnormal		Critical Abnormal
Recognize normal gastrointestinal assessment: bowel sounds, abdominal symmetry, presence of nausea/vomiting, bowel habits, ease of swallowing, absence of pain, abdomen soft and flat, pancreatic enzyme production, glucose control	Pancreatitis	Severe pancreatitis	SIRS → septic shock → multi-system organ failure Respiratory distress → ARDS Acute kidney injury

ARDS, Acute respiratory distress syndrome; *SIRS*, systemic inflammatory response syndrome.

Endocrine

DIABETES

Normal	Abnormal	Critical Abnormal
Recognize normal endocrine assessment: absence of fatigue, weakness, weight, coping, stress levels, pancreatic enzyme production, glucose control	Type 1 diabetes mellitus	Diabetic ketoacidosis
	Type 2 diabetes mellitus	Hyperglycemia hyperosmolar state Diabetic ketoacidosis

METABOLIC DYSFUNCTION

Normal	Abnormal	Critical Abnormal
Recognize normal endocrine assessment: absence of fatigue, weakness, weight, coping, stress levels, pancreatic enzyme production, glucose control, energy, heat production, characteristics of skin, hair, nails	Hypothyroidism	Myxedema coma
	Hyperthyroidism • Graves disease • Goitre	Thyroid storm (thyrotoxicosis)

ALTERATIONS OF ADRENAL DYSFUNCTION

Normal	Abnormal	Critical Abnormal
Recognize normal endocrine assessment: absence of fatigue, weakness, weight, coping, stress levels, pancreatic enzyme production, glucose control, energy, heat production, characteristics of skin, hair, nails, absence of infections	Hypercortisolism • Addison's disease	Increased risk of infection
	Hypercortisolism • Cushing's syndrome	Addisonian crisis

ALTERATIONS OF ANTIDIURETIC HORMONE

Normal	Abnormal	Critical Abnormal	
Recognize normal endocrine assessment: absence of fatigue, weakness, weight, coping, stress levels, pancreatic enzyme production, glucose control, energy, heat production, characteristics of skin, hair, nails, presence of extreme fluid retention or excretion	Diabetes insipidus	Extreme fluid loss with hemodynamic instability	Hypovolemic shock
	Syndrome of inappropriate antidiuretic hormone (SIADH)	Severe hyponatremia Seizures Irreversible neurological damage	

Shock

HYPOVOLEMIC SHOCK

Normal	Abnormal		Critical Abnormal
Recognize normal CV assessment: BP, HR, pulses, S1, S2 skin temperature, diaphoresis, colour, capillary refill	Dehydration	• Severe dehydration • Bleeding (GIB, trauma, PPH, DIC) • Plasma (burns, insensible losses) • Second- or third- degree spacing	Hypovolemic shock

CV, Cardiovascular; *DIC*, disseminated intravascular coagulation; *GIB*, gastrointestinal bleed; *PPH*, postpartum hemorrhage.

CARDIOGENIC SHOCK

Normal	Abnormal		Critical Abnormal
Recognize normal CV assessment: BP, HR, pulses, S1, S2 skin temperature, diaphoresis, colour, cap refill	AMI	Left/Right ventricular heart failure	Cardiogenic shock
	Pericarditis	Pericardial effusion	Cardiac tamponade → cardiogenic shock
	Untreated AFib or DVT	Pulmonary embolus	Cardiogenic shock
	Ventricular dysrhythmia	Loss of ventricular pump	Cardiogenic shock

AFib, Atrial fibrillation; *AMI*, acute myocardial infarction; *BP*, blood pressure; *CV*, cardiovascular; *DVT*, deep vein thrombosis; *HR*, heart rate.

SEPTIC SHOCK

Normal	Abnormal		Critical Abnormal	
Recognize normal neurological, cardiovascular, respiratory, renal, and gastrointestinal assessment	UTI (Cystitis)	Pyelonephritis	Urosepsis	Septic shock
	Pneumonia	Respiratory distress → ARDS	Pneumosepsis	Septic shock
	Open wound on the skin	Cellulitis Burns Bacteria	Necrotizing fasciitis	Septic shock

ARDS, Acute respiratory distress syndrome; *UTI*, urinary tract infection.

ANAPHYLACTIC SHOCK

Normal	Abnormal		Critical Abnormal
Recognize normal neurological, cardiovascular, respiratory, renal, and gastrointestinal assessment	Allergic trigger	Respiratory distress	Anaphylaxis → anaphylactic shock

NEUROGENIC SHOCK

Normal	Abnormal		Critical Abnormal
Recognize normal neuro assessment: LOC, pupil size and reactivity, motor power, pain, gait, GCS	Spinal cord injury	Autonomic dysreflexia	Neurogenic shock

LOC, Level of consciousness; *GCS*, Glasgow Coma Scale

C Strategies for Faculty Using This Textbook

Introduction

Please use this textbook as a resource to guide individual teaching styles and enhance overall techniques in the classroom and clinical environments. The Nursing Clinical Judgement Measurement Model (NCJMM), clinical judgement, and higher cognitive referencing are familiar to each nursing educator, just by being a nurse. Each nursing educator has applied the necessary skills related to the cognitive domains as a practitioner; it is a manner of learning to include this cognitive processing as an educator now and make it accessible to students. Becoming familiar with the NCJMM and developing methods to adapt curricular content and frame for deeper cognitive engagement may take practice, just as it does for students.

Use this textbook to meet individual needs by providing examples in classroom or clinical environments, or assist in writing NGN case studies. Each NGN case study in this casebook is original and follows the same structure as the NCSBN. With practice, NGN case studies can be written to level students' learning needs based on their place in the curriculum. Please find strategies and tips for ways to incorporate NCJMM into lectures and clinical environments as well as strategies to assist in creating individual NGN case studies.

The following strategies may provide a reference for incorporating the NCJMM into current lectures and clinical environments.

Strategies for Teaching Content With the NCJMM as an Underpinning Theme

- Start with *understanding the six cognitive steps of the NCJMM* necessary for cognitive processing. Become familiar with developing a series of questions to help students achieve each step and recognize ways to improve student gaps to move to each step. This can be achieved more easily in the clinical environment as students work directly with clients and embody the NCJMM with each clinical experience.
- *Recognize personal strengths as an educator and identify gaps* in how to teach complex and complicated material. Be honest to narrow the gaps. For example, maternity and labour and delivery are specialized areas of nursing practice; however, teaching the presentation of a postpartum hemorrhage and the relevant nursing interventions is similar, yet different, to the presentation of a client who is hemorrhaging from a traumatic injury. It is a skill for the educator to recognize what makes these two presentations similar yet different. The ability to recognize the patterns by the educator and then articulate those patterns to students will demonstrate the cognitive steps of the NCJMM.
- *Become familiar with concepts and possible topics that may appear in NGN case studies* presented in tables found in Chapter 2. The information has been broken down into tangible material common to theory and clinical environments. These tables may help educators organize topics taught within nursing undergraduate programs and consider the presentation patterns of each condition when teaching the material. Educators new to teaching pathophysiology, assessment, pharmacology, and nursing interventions are encouraged to avoid overwhelming students with content. There also has to be a balance as educators are responsible for teaching complex conditions in a manner that is easy to grasp for the appropriate level of student. If students are overwhelmed while learning, remembering the patterns will become difficult. In the end, students will not be able to perform to the best of their ability. Experienced educators learn to recognize the patterns highlighted throughout the chapters and confer this information to student learners.
- *Develop pedagogical strategies to teach complex material.* Incorporating techniques while teaching nursing curricula content will stretch the educator's abilities. Developing creative methods to weave the NCJMM through lessons will enhance the student's ability to perform these cognitive steps when caring for clients. Adjusting the method for the student will enhance overall engagement with developing this skill. Be clear on the intended outcome of the chosen method. Learning does not have to be shiny to be effective, it just has to be meaningful for the student.

Strategies for Developing NGN Case Studies

- *Use personal clinical experiences as the central theme* of the NGN; however, ensure that all narrative elements are supported by evidence-informed and peer-reviewed information. All NGN case studies written for the casebook align with information from Elsevier textbooks. A deeper understanding of the NCJMM will be a foundation for effective writing of the NGN case studies. The References section provides a complete list of all Elsevier products and other references used throughout the casebook.
- *Plan out the story with a beginning, a middle, and an end.* Each NGN case study is a story with many moving parts to the whole picture. That is why the metaphor for this casebook is putting the pieces together. NGN case studies are structured narratives that reflect back to patterns

taught in classrooms and experienced in the clinical setting.

- *Each narrative presented in this textbook is written to set up student learning by dropping hints and cues within the story's basic structure.* NGN case study authors are recommended to have an excellent grasp of the material as this form of storytelling requires both general and expert knowledge. Each medical condition has a pattern to the clinical presentation, where students use their knowledge of pathophysiology, anatomy, and physiology to recognize key clinical presentation cues. This is foundational for any NGN case study. A narrative should have more than a few sentences to set up the story and be complete enough to allow for student progression. The outcome of any NGN case study is to solidify knowledge and make sound decisions based on the information presented. Too little information will not present a full picture of a client, and too much scattered information creates a chaotic narrative, leaving the student with a challenging experience in grasping the pattern. Remember, the answer cannot be given to the student, except in the case of a trend where that can be written in the introductory sentence, but not always. Teaching students how to arrive at a medical diagnosis based on the information provided will ensure that when working in clinical environments during the care of clients, students will be able to arrive at the same conclusions.
- *Each NGN case study is meant to reflect the clinical environment and a medical condition.* It should not be written to test a student's knowledge of theoretical concepts. Students who perform strong clinical judgement will be able to safely and competently care for clients. NGN case studies can have an element of a theoretical concept; however, the primary narrative should follow a clinical scenario. Testing for theoretical concepts can be achieved through summative and formative assessments or analytical papers.
- *Be kind when attempting this new skill.* It takes practice to develop and improve individual ability when writing NGN case studies, and it takes time. Learning how to implement the cognitive steps associated with NCJMM within the lecture and clinical environments AND attempting to write NGN case studies is a new skill.
- *Use the information in Chapters 5 and 6 to understand the structure of each NGN case study.* The narrative is written to accommodate the intended student outcome for each NGN case study. For example, when writing an unfolding case study, the story development and elements of the narrative should be planned before even writing the story with questions. The narrative provides the backbone for the question. The narrative associated with a bow-tie NGN case study has to have all the elements presented more concisely. In contrast, the trend NGN case study must have a developing narrative over time. Deciding on one element to develop for a trend is important as all elements should not be chosen. For example, if the purpose of the narrative for a trend is to ensure the student understands what to do when a client becomes symptomatic with hypotension, then do not add hyperkalemia to the story. Details of the study must be pertinent even if extraneous information is provided. Too many health abnormalities presented in a narrative only lead to student confusion, and the narrative has no direction.

Adjust each presented strategy tip to meet individual needs. These are only suggestions. Good luck with writing!

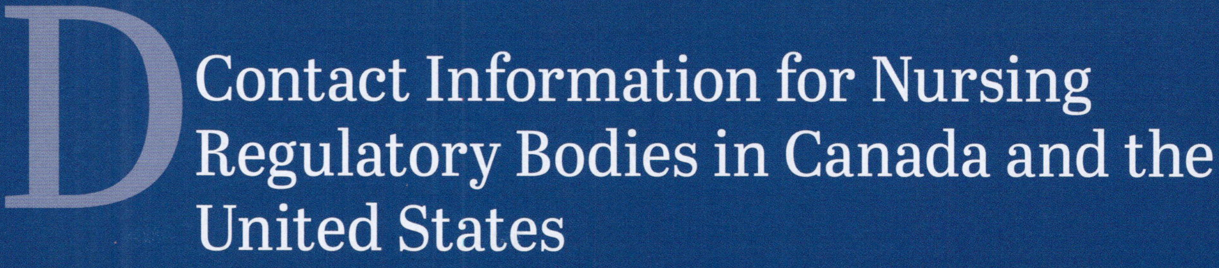

D Contact Information for Nursing Regulatory Bodies in Canada and the United States

Nursing Regulatory Bodies in Canada

BRITISH COLUMBIA
https://www.bccnm.ca
ALBERTA
https://www.nurses.ab.ca
SASKATCHEWAN
https://www.crns.ca
MANITOBA
https://www.crnm.mb.ca
ONTARIO
https://www.cno.org
QUEBEC*
https://www.oiiq.org
NEW BRUNSWICK
https://www.nanb.nb.ca
NOVA SCOTIA
https://www.nscn.ca
PRINCE EDWARD ISLAND
https://crnpei.ca
NEWFOUNDLAND AND LABRADOR
https://crnnl.ca
NORTHWEST TERRITORIES
https://cannn.ca
NUNAVUT
https://cannn.ca
YUKON
https://www.yrna.ca

Nursing Regulatory Bodies in the United States

ALABAMA
https://www.abn.alabama.gov/
ALASKA
https://www.commerce.alaska.gov/web/cbpl/ProfessionalLicensing/BoardofNursing.aspx
ARIZONA
https://www.azbn.gov
ARKANSAS
https://healthy.arkansas.gov/programs-services/topics/arkansas-board-of-nursing/
CALIFORNIA
https://www.rn.ca.gov

*Ordre des infirmières et infirmiers du Québec (OIIQ) has their own entry-to-practice examination. Other Canadian nursing regulatory body information is available if students want to work outside the province.

COLORADO
https://dpo.colorado.gov/Nursing
CONNECTICUT
https://portal.ct.gov/dph/public-health-hearing-office/board-of-examiners-for-nursing/board-of-examiners-for-nursing
DELAWARE
https://dpr.delaware.gov/boards/nursing
DISTRICT OF COLUMBIA
https://dchealth.dc.gov
FLORIDA
https://floridasnursing.gov
GEORGIA
https://sos.ga.gov/georgia-board-nursing
HAWAII
https://cca.hawaii.gov/pvl/boards/nursing
IDAHO
https://dopl.idaho.gov/bon/
ILLINOIS
https://idfpr.illinois.gov/profs/nursing.html
INDIANA
https://www.ncsbn.org/bon-member-details/Indiana
IOWA
https://dial.iowa.gov
KANSAS
https://ksbn.kansas.gov
KENTUCKY
https://kbn.ky.gov/Pages/index.aspx
LOUISIANA
https://www.lsbn.state.la.us
MAINE
https://www.maine.gov/boardofnursing/
MARYLAND
https://mbon.maryland.gov/Pages/default.aspx
MASSACHUSETTS
https://www.mass.gov/orgs/board-of-registration-in-nursing
MICHIGAN
https://www.michigan.gov/lara/bureau-list/bpl/health/hp-lic-health-prof/nursing
MINNESOTA
https://mn.gov/boards/nursing/
MISSISSIPPI
https://www.msbn.ms.gov
MISSOURI
https://www.pr.mo.gov/nursing.asp
MONTANA
https://boards.bsd.dli.mt.gov/nursing/
NEBRASKA
https://dhhs.ne.gov/licensure/Pages/Nurse-Licensing.aspx

NEVADA
https://nevadanursingboard.org
NEW HAMPSHIRE
https://www.oplc.nh.gov/new-hampshire-board-nursing
NEW JERSEY
https://www.njconsumeraffairs.gov/nur/Pages/default.aspx
NEW MEXICO
https://www.bon.nm.gov
NEW YORK
https://www.op.nysed.gov/registered-professional-nursing
NORTH CAROLINA
https://www.ncbon.com
NORTH DAKOTA
https://www.ndbon.org
OHIO
https://nursing.ohio.gov
OKLAHOMA
https://oklahoma.gov/nursing.html
OREGON
https://www.oregon.gov/osbn/Pages/index.aspx
PENNSYLVANIA
https://www.dos.pa.gov/ProfessionalLicensing/BoardsCommissions/Nursing
RHODE ISLAND
https://health.ri.gov/licenses/
SOUTH CAROLINA
https://llr.sc.gov/nurse/
SOUTH DAKOTA
https://www.sdbon.org
TENNESSEE
https://www.tn.gov/health/health-program-areas/health-professional-boards/nursing-board/nursing-board/about.html
TEXAS
https://www.bon.texas.gov
UTAH
https://dopl.utah.gov/nursing
VERMONT
https://sos.vermont.gov/nursing/
VIRGINIA
https://www.dhp.virginia.gov/Boards/Nursing/
WASHINGTON
https://nursing.wa.gov
WEST VIRGINIA
https://wvrnboard.wv.gov/Pages/default.aspx
WISCONSIN
https://dsps.wi.gov/pages/BoardsCouncils/Nursing/Default.aspx
WYOMING
https://wsbn.wyo.gov

References

Abouli, J. A., Curd, D. E., Mei, X. Y., et al. (2023). Attitudes and practices surrounding opioid prescriptions following open reduction internal fixation of distal radius and ankle fractures: A survey of the Canadian Orthopaedic Association Membership. *Advances in Orthopedics, 2023,* 9968219. https://doi.org/10.1155/2023/9968219

Alberta Health Services. (2018). *Provincial clinical knowledge topic: Alcohol intoxication withdrawal, adult, emergency department, V: 1.5.* https://extranet.ahsnet.ca/teams/policydocuments/1/klink/et-klink-ckv-alcohol-intoxication-withdrawal-adult.pdf

Almost, J. (2021). *Regulated nursing in Canada: The landscape in 2021.* Canadian Nurses Association. https://hl-prod-ca-oc-download.s3-ca-central-1.amazonaws.com/CNA/2f975e7e-4a40-45ca-863c-5ebf0a138d5e/UploadedImages/documents/Regulated-Nursing-in-Canada_e_Copy.pdf

Astle, B., & Duggleby, W. (2024). *Potter and Perry's Canadian fundamentals of nursing* (7th ed.). Elsevier Inc.

Baxter. (2020). *Ceftriaxone injection: Product monograph.* https://www.baxter.ca/sites/g/files/ebysai1431/files/2020-06/Ceftriaxone%20Injection%20USP_EN.pdf

Berger, H., Gagnon, R., & Sermer, M. (2019). Guideline no. 393—Diabetes in pregnancy. *Journal of Obstetrics and Gynaecology Canada, 393,* 1814–1825e. https://doi.org/10.1016/j.jogc.2019.03.008

Bradley, P., & Page Cutrara, K. L. (2022). *Elsevier's Canadian comprehensive review for the NCLEX-RN® examination* (3rd Canadian ed.). Elsevier.

Brown, P. C. Roediger III, H. L, & McDaniel, M. A. (2014). *Make it stick: The science of successful learning.* Harvard University Press.

Canadian ADHD Resource Alliance (CADDRA). (2022). *CADDRA guide to ADHD pharmacological treatments in Canada–February 2020.* https://www.caddra.ca/wp-content/uploads/Final-Laminate-Card-2019_9-1.pdf

Canadian Paediatric Society (CPS). (2021). *Schedule of well-child visits.* https://caringforkids.cps.ca/handouts/pregnancy-and-babies/schedule_of_well_child_visits#:~:text=Babies%20are%20usually%20checked%20by,Check%20for%20signs%20of%20jaundice

Canadian Paediatric Society (CPS). (2022). *Fever and temperature taking.* https://www.caringforkids.cps.ca/handouts/fever_and_temperature_taking

Chien, S. C., Liu, K. T., & Wu, Y. (2018). Lithium intoxication presenting as altered consciousness and arrhythmia with cardiogenic shock. *Medicine, 97*(45), e13129. https:/doi.org/10.1097/MD.0000000000013129

Cobbett, S. (2025). *Perry & Potter's Canadian clinical nursing skills and techniques* (2nd ed.). Elsevier Inc.

Eisenmann, N. (2020). An innovative clinical concept map to promote clinical judgment in nursing students. *Journal of Nursing Education, 60*(3), 143–150. https://doi.org/10.3928/01484834-20210222-04

Eli Lily Canada. (2019). *Mild, moderate, and severe hypoglycemia—What's the difference?* Diabetes Canada. https://www.diabetes.ca/managing-my-diabetes/stories/mild,-moderate-or-severe-hypoglycemia—-what-s-the-difference-

Goguen, J., & Gilbert, J. (2023). *Chapter 15: Hyperglycemic emergencies in adults.* Diabetes Canada. https://www.diabetes.ca/health-care-providers/clinical-practice-guidelines/chapter-15#panel-tab_FullText

Hall, L. E. (1955). *Quality of nursing care.* Manuscript of an address before a meeting of the Department of Baccalaureate and Higher Degree Programs of the New Jersey League for Nursing, February 7, 1955, at Seton Hall University, Newark, New Jersey. Montefiore Medical Center Archives, Bronx, New York.

Hartman, M. E., & Cheifetz, I. M. (2020). Pediatric emergencies and resuscitation. In R. M. Kliegman, J. W. St. Geme, N. Blum, et al. (Eds.), *Nelson textbook of pediatrics* (21st ed.). Elsevier.

Healthwise Staff. (2023). *Electrical cardioversion: What to expect at home. Your recovery.* myHealth.Alberta.ca. Network. https://myhealth.alberta.ca/Health/aftercareinformation/pages/conditions.aspx?hwid=zu2278

Heart and Stroke Foundation of Canada. (2023). *The DASH diet to lower high blood pressure.* https://www.heartandstroke.ca/healthy-living/healthy-eating/dash-diet?gclid=EAIaIQobChMIsJutg4vJgQMVeSytBh0KaQO5EAAYAiAAEgKeq_D_BwE&gclsrc=aw.ds

Jarvis, C., Eckhardt, A., Browne, A., et al. (2024). *Physical examination and health assessment* (4th ed.). Elsevier Inc.

Johnson, D. E. (1959). The nature and science of nursing. *Nursing Outlook, 7,* 291–294.

Keatings, M., & Adams, P. (2024). *Ethical & legal issues in Canadian nursing* (5th ed.). Elsevier Inc.

Keenan-Lindsay, L., Sams, C. A., O'Connor, C., et al. (2022). *Perry's maternal child nursing care in Canada* (3rd ed.). Elsevier Inc.

La Saux, N. (2020). *Position statement: Guidelines for the management of suspected and confirmed bacterial meningitis in Canadian children older than 2 months of age.* Canadian Paediatric Society. https://cps.ca/en/documents/position/management-of-bacterial-meningitis

MacDonald, T., Noel-Weiss, J., West, D., et al. (2016). Transmasculine individuals' experiences with lactation, chestfeeding, and gender identity: A qualitative study. *BMC Pregnancy and Childbirth, 16*(1), 106. https://doi.org/10.1186/s12884-016-0907-y

McDonald, S. A. (2024). *Pagana's Canadian manual of diagnostic and laboratory tests* (3rd ed.) Elsevier Inc.

National Council of State Boards of Nursing (NCSBN). (2018). Report of findings from the 2017 RN nursing knowledge survey. *NCSBN Research Brief,* 73. https://www.ncsbn.org/public-files/2017_RN_KSA_final.pdf

National Council of State Boards of Nursing (NCSBN). (2019a). Clinical judgement measurement model and action model. *Next Generation NCLEX News,* Spring, 2019. https://www.ncsbn.org/public-files/NGN_Spring19_ENG_29Aug2019.pdf

National Council of State Boards of Nursing (NCSBN). (2019b). *2019 NCLEX-RN® examination: Test plan for the National Council licensure examination for registered nurses.* https://www.ncsbn.org/publications/2019-nclexrn-test-plan

National Council of State Boards of Nurses (NCSBN). (2023). *Next Generation NCLEX: NCLEX-RN test plan.* https://www.ncsbn.org/publications/2023-nclex-rn-test-plan

Nibbelink, C. W., & Brewer, B. B. (2018). Decision-making in nursing practice: An integrative literature review. *Journal of Clinical Nursing, 27*(5–6), 917–928. https://doi.org/10.1111/jocn.14151

Orlando, I. L. (1961/1990). *The dynamic nurse-patient relationship: Function, process and principles.* National League for Nursing.

Petro-Yura, H., & Walsh, M. B. (1973). *The nursing process: Assessing, planning, implementing, evaluating.* Appleton & Lange.

Pi, Z., Zhang, Y., Zhou, W., et al. (2021). Learning by explaining to oneself and a peer enhances learners' theta and alpha oscillations while watching video lectures. *British Journal of Educational Technology, 52*(2), 659–679. https://doi.org/10.1111/bjet.13048

Pollard, C. L., & Jakubec, S. L. (2023). *Varcarolis's Canadian psychiatric mental health nursing: A clinical approach* (3rd ed.). Elsevier Inc.

Power-Kean, K., Zettel, S., & Toufic El-Hussein, M. (2023). *Huether and McCance's understanding pathophysiology* (2nd Canadian ed.). Elsevier Inc.

Prochaska, J. O., & DiClemente, C. C. (1984). *The transtheoretical approach: Crossing traditional boundaries of therapy.* Dow Jones Irwin.

Riggs, D. W., Pearce, R., Pfeffer, C. A., et al. (2020). Men, trans/masculine, and non-binary people's experiences of pregnancy loss: An international qualitative study. *BMC Pregnancy and Childbirth, 20*(1), 482. https://doi.org/10.1186/s12884-020-03166-6

Sanofi-Aventis Canada. (2018). *Resonium Calcium (calcium polystyrene sulfonate) prescribing information.* https://pdf.hres.ca/dpd_pm/00047479.PDF

Sealock, K., & Seneviratne, C. (2025). *Lilley's pharmacology for Canadian health care practice* (5th ed.). Elsevier Inc.

Skidmore-Roth, L., & Richardson, F. (2024). *Mosby's Canadian nursing drug reference* (2nd ed.). Elsevier Inc.

Tyerman, J., & Cobbett, W. (2023). *Lewis's medical-surgical nursing in Canada: Assessment and management of clinical problems* (5th ed.). Elsevier, Inc.

Wolfe-Roubatis, E., & Spatz, D. L. (2015). Transgender men and lactation: What nurses need to know. *MCN, the American Journal of Maternal Child Nursing*, *40*(1), 32–38. https://doi.org/10.1097/NMC.0000000000000097